CHOIC_ES

health and fitness

in

WELLNESS

health and

for

fitness

LIFE

THIRD EDITION

Sally A. Althoff
Portland State University

Milan Svoboda
Portland State University

Daniel Girdano

Gorsuch Scarisbrick, Publishers
Scottsdale, Arizona

Publisher:	Gay L. Pauley
Editor:	A. Colette Kelly
Consulting Editor:	Robert P. Pangrazi
Developmental Editor:	Katie E. Bradford
Production Manager:	Mary B. Cullen
Cover Design:	Kevin Kall
Typesetting:	Ashstreet Typecrafters

Gorsuch Scarisbrick, Publishers
8233 Via Paseo del Norte, Suite F-400
Scottsdale, AZ 85258

10 9 8 7 6 5 4 3 2 1

ISBN 0-89787-630-X

Copyright © 1988, 1992, 1996 by Gorsuch Scarisbrick, Publishers

Printed in the United States of America.

Library of Congress Cataloging-in-Publication Data

Althoff, Sally A.
    Choices in wellness for life / by Sally A. Althoff, Milan Svoboda,
Daniel A. Girdano. — 3rd ed.
        p.   cm.
    Includes bibliographical references and index.
    ISBN 0-89787-630-X (alk. paper)
    1. Health.   2. Physical fitness.   I. Svoboda, Milan.
II. Girdano, Daniel A.   III. Title.
RA776.A394   1996
613—dc20
                                                        95–49615
                                                        CIP

Contents

Preface

Being all that you can be is a dynamic, ever-changing process, and this process is directly affected by the personal choices you make every day. Indeed, these choices affect both the quality and quantity of your life. *Choices in Wellness for Life*, Third Edition, addresses this dynamic process and is written to serve as a helpful tool in your personal journey.

Your life has many dimensions—physical, emotional, social, intellectual, and spiritual—and research confirms that your choices in the areas of *fitness, nutrition, self-protection,* and *stress management* can enhance or detract from your ability to function in all of these dimensions. Of course, your choices in these areas can also alter the likelihood of your suffering from the major chronic diseases that affect so many people.

With the extensive and conflicting information available in the marketplace about fitness, nutrition, and stress, it is sometimes difficult to determine what information is correct and what is not. Which guidelines are reliable? Which guidelines are relevant to your life and goals? There are no easy answers to these questions. The best answer is simply to be as informed as you can, so that you can make informed choices and decisions. Our main objective in writing this book is to provide the basic information you need on the topics of fitness, nutrition, self-protection, and stress management regardless of your age and whether you are athletically inclined.

In presenting this information, we have assumed that, ideally, you would like to be fit, eat well, be able to protect yourself from harm, and not be over-burdened by stress. But we have tried also to acknowledge that your choices in these areas are personal and practical, affected by many aspects of your life. Thus, a central theme of this book is personal responsibility to explore and expand your potentials via the choices *you* make—choices bases on your schedule, your goals, your abilities, your budget, and so on.

To help you decide whether changes are in order in your current lifestyle, we have provided methods to assess your current fitness status, your nutritional habits, your risk of serious illness, your preparedness to protect yourself, and the level of stress in your life as these topics are discussed. Whenever possible, we have attempted to select tests that do not require specialized equipment. To help you develop as fully as you wish, we have described what we think are the best methods and techniques for building and maintaining positive health practices. Again, we have tried to make our recommendations as practical as possible, so that, if you prefer, you can do what you choose to do at home without investing large sums of money for special equipment or clothing.

Briefly, Chapter 1 of *Choices in Wellness for Life* introduces the concepts of quality living, health, and wellness, and their interdependent nature. Recognizing that it isn't always easy to act in accord with what you know, we have devoted Chapter 2 to examining the pathways and pitfalls involved in self-directed change. This chapter offers step-by-step methods for successfully undertaking change. Chapter 3 describes the primary biomarkers of the aging process, the major diseases, and their related risk factors that people in our culture typically encounter suggests behaviors that might lessen the impact. Most important, this chapter of these processes and promotes greater health and rigor throughout life.

Chapter 4 introduces the components of fitness, the general principles that underlie all forms of training, and common challenges encountered in exercise. Chapter 5 provides the rationale for and the methods to develop and maintain cardiorespiratory fitness. Chapter 6 offers procedures for developing and maintaining flexibility, strength, and muscle endurance. The focus of Chapter 7 is on weight control and the role of diet and of regular exercise in this process.

Chapter 8 discusses what is known and what is controversial about nutritional recommendations to maximize health and minimize disease. Chapter 9 provides instructions for analyzing your diet and building a healthy diet for yourself.

Chapter 10, much of which is new to this edition, examines the personal issues, attitudes, and choices involved in protecting yourself from STDs, drug abuse, and personal assault (a topic we believe is unique to our text).

Chapters 11 and 12 discuss daily stresses you may experience, their impact on your health, and techniques you may use to manage this problem. Chapter 12 allows you summarize all of your assessments and, if you choose, develop a personal behavior change strategy to follow. Finally, the appendices include a variety of tests and tables to aid in your evaluation. Appendix 9 provides the lab activities and instructions for assessments and planning activities described at the end of each chapter.

The content of this third edition has been updated to include new topics and concerns. We've updated our discussion of food labels, expanded our coverage of stress management, given you more information on STDs and AIDS, and have addressed the important topic of protecting yourself against violence. In short, we have made every effort to reflect today's issues and choices. As before, the information in this book will provide a basis for your choices; as before, the decisions will be yours.

Features new to this edition of *Choices:*
- Activities in the chapters to let you do quick "mini-assessments" as you read
- "FYI" boxes highlight information of special interest
- "Choices in Action" at the end of each chapter previews the end-of-book labs that accompany that chapter
- An in-depth, but optional, section of hands-on lab activities that allows you to determine you current level of wellness and then decide what course of action is best for you

ACKNOWLEDGMENTS

The authors wish to express gratitude to those who served as reviewers of this new edition of this book. In particular, we wish to thank William J. Pierce and his colleagues at Furman University for their suggestions regarding the content of this edition; Laurel Talabere of Capital University; Bernie Babcock of Treasure Valley Community College; and Stephen J. Virgilio at Adelphi University for helpful, constructive reviews.

The authors wish to make a special acknowledgment to Margaret Heyden of Portland State University for her important contribution to Chapter 10 regarding self-protection against assault, rape, and theft. Thanks also to James Ledridge, mathematician, and Gay Monteverde, Multnornah County AIDS Education Program, for providing, respectively, statistical and content advice regarding STDs.

We would like to thank Billie Anger for her thorough and extensive assistance in preparing the third edition manuscript. Thanks also to Kit Pratt and Lori Stumme for professional assistance. Thanks to the models for the book's photographs: Ally Britton, Gary R. Brodowicz, Rene Changsut, Steve Curtis, Dori Frame, Gordon Dunkeld, Nancy Gunther, Becky Hanscom, Angela Hewlett, Jennifer Himmelsbach, Eric Ludlow, Elise Whiting, Jane Mercer, and Belinda Zeidler.

Sally Althoff
Milan Svoboda
Dan Girdano

Introduction

CHOICES INFLUENCE QUALITY LIVING

Making informed choices and taking personal responsibility for your choices in the areas of fitness, nutrition, and stress management are themes that run throughout this book. These areas make up the *basic building blocks* of health. Almost everything you do involves making choices. If you are like most people, some of your choices are consciously thought out while others may not be. Sometimes a choice or a decision is made without adequate information, and as a result the choice may not be the best one possible. You can probably think of an example in your own past when, because of inadequate information, you made a choice that in hindsight did not prove to be the best choice. This book is written to provide you with basic, up-to-date information so that you will be better able to make informed decisions in the areas of fitness, nutrition, personal safety, and stress management.

Simply having access to this information will not automatically enable you to adopt behavior patterns different from those you have been following for some time, presuming changes seem warranted. Modifying behavior requires more than up-to-date information. Often less tangible factors are at play in determining whether or not you are able to change; your attitudes, goals, fears, and motivations are good examples. Because factors such as these can be so important in determining the success of an attempt at behavior change, suggestions for dealing with these issues are presented in this book.

GETTING THE MOST OUT OF THIS BOOK

Even though there are great similarities among people, individuals are unique biological organisms. This uniqueness demonstrates itself in the ways people are able to integrate fitness, nutrition, and stress management into their lives. For example, one person may have no difficulty to find the time or desire to exercise at all. Thus, to get the most out of this book it might be helpful to realize where you are in the behavior change process with respect to any particular issue. This process, as illustrated on the following page, consists of four basic steps: considering, attempting, achieving, maintaining. Accordingly, as you read the following chapters:

1. If some portion of the information is new to you, consider it with an open mind. Consider what it would mean to act on the information, to incorporate it regularly as a part of your lifestyle. Consider what you would be gaining and what you would be losing.

2. If you are already familiar with the information but have never attempted to apply it yourself, make an attempt. See what it feels like. Is it something you would find difficult to continue indefinitely? What changes could you make to help it be more to your liking?

3. If the information is something you have attempted to apply in the past but for one reason or another you have been unsuccessful, then spend some time analyzing what it is you need to change to be successful. What was it that caused you to discontinue the new behavior? What type of maintenance schedule would you be comfortable with?

When is the best time to make a change if one is needed? The answer, of course, depends on you and your circumstances. In general, the

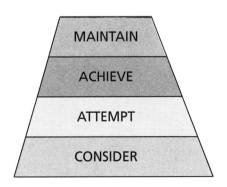

The process of changing behavior.

sooner you make a positive lifestyle change the better because such a change will enable you to operate at a higher quality of living for a greater length of time. Nevertheless, not everyone is willing or able to undertake self-directed change at a specific point in time. Certainly not everyone aspires to the same life goals or to the same health habits. For one person, eating in the most healthful way may be an appropriate goal under all circumstances. For another, it may create too much stress to be preoccupied with good nutrition at all times. Such a person may find it more in keeping with good mental health to be more spontaneous regarding nutrition decisions. All in all, you are the best guide as to whether and when a change is needed in your life. Only you can make that decision; no one can do it for you. Decision making and developing appropriate plans for implementing your goals are also discussed later in this book.

As you read this book you should not try to simultaneously make every one of the changes you might feel appropriate. To attempt to do so would be unrealistic, and it is unlikely that any changes you undertook would be maintained. Rather, it is recommended that you take small steps, one at a time. Small steps might be deciding to go for a 15-minute walk twice during the next week, switching to low fat milk from whole milk, or taking 5 minutes during the day to sit quietly and reduce the frenzy in your mind. By taking steps such as these you will slowly and realistically move yourself toward the end of the health continuum described as *optimal health*. We will discuss the health continuum in Chapter 1.

This book will provide you with the information, the methods, and the techniques you need to try one or more small steps toward becoming and being your very best. In fact, just by reading these pages and doing the suggested self assessments, you are taking the first step in the process of behavior change. You are CONSIDERING behavior changes. If your analysis reveals that *continuing* that behavior change process is what you really need to do, you'll be halfway there: you've started!

Quality Living

Your Personal Best

✔ What is your definition of quality living?

✔ What is the importance of health to quality living?

✔ How can you experience quality living even when you are seriously ill or when other aspects of your life are less than perfect?

✔ What does *lifestyle* have to do with quality of life?

What is "quality living"? According to the dictionary, the combination of these two terms means "excellent or superior existence." This definition presents a problem, however: After all, your concept of "excellent" or "superior" existence may be quite different from that of the person next to you. Think for a moment about the qualities of life that you believe would contribute to quality living. Would your family or friends come up with the same list? Probably not. With this in mind, quality living needs to be defined in such a way that everyone can relate to the concept and apply it to themselves.

Some common descriptors for quality living have emerged in psychological literature, particularly from the works of Abraham Maslow, Carl Rogers, and Fritz Perls. Maslow referred to quality living as *the process of self-actualization;* Rogers termed it *personal fulfillment;* and Perls called it a *condition of wholeness and happiness.* Essentially, the living condition each of those men described is *being all you can be.* Maslow referred basically to the process of quality living and the others referred to the feelings and emotions that quality living generates.

The process Maslow called **self-actualization** is that of becoming and being ever more of what you can be, ultimately expressing your full potential (an ideal, of course). In plain terms, this means making your best effort to develop yourself in all aspects of life and then using your talents and capabilities in creative and productive ways. Logically, this includes trying to be as healthy as possible, given that the more healthy you become, the more completely you will be able to fulfill your potential.

Quality Living = Health × Effort

Quality living, then, is the product of your health and your efforts. In this formula, **health** means how well you are able to function in each aspect of your life—physical, emotional, social, and so on. *Effort* actually refers to two things: (1) action —how much you are doing to improve or maintain your health; and (2) emotion—the feelings of fulfillment, wholeness, and happiness you derive from making the effort to develop yourself and be creative and productive.

Each of these factors influences the other to a certain extent, and each also has a direct impact of its own on quality living. How these factors interrelate and what levels of health and effort bring about quality living are the issues addressed in the rest of this chapter.

THE CRITERIA FOR QUALITY LIVING: THE HIERARCHY OF NEEDS

From his studies, Maslow found that, to be your most creative, productive self, certain basic needs—such as the need for food and shelter—must be satisfied, at least sufficiently to allow you to focus your attention and energies on your growth and development. This concept, with which you are probably familiar, has become known as Maslow's hierarchy of needs. As shown in Figure 1.1, it typically is presented in the form of a triangular stepladder to emphasize the dependency of the higher-level, more complex, needs on the fulfillment of the lower-level, more basic, needs. In order of the most basic to the most complex, these needs are:

1. Feelings of physical comfort in terms of hunger, sleep, bowel function, sex, and so on, and of energy and well-being in terms of overall health and physiological function.
2. Feelings of safety, security, and lack of danger or threat.
3. Feelings of belongingness and acceptance, of being one of a group or having a place; feelings of loving and being loved, of being worthy of love.

**FIGURE
1.1**   Maslow's hierarchy of needs.

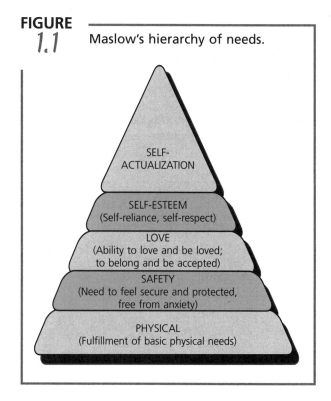

4. Feelings of self-reliance, self-respect, and self-esteem.
5. Feelings of self-actualization and fulfillment, of personal growth and development.

Clearly the foundation for achieving self-actualization is some basic degree of physical functioning. This is not surprising because life itself depends upon this. In terms of the hierarchy of needs, the more healthy and fit you are physically, the better able you will be to fulfill higher-level needs. Essential as it is, however, physical health by itself is not enough. As the hierarchy of needs indicates, self-actualization requires some degree of satisfactory or healthy functioning in *all* aspects of life, not just the physical. Thus, the emotional, social, mental, and spiritual aspects of your life also are important to self-actualization. As with physical functioning, the healthier you are in each of these areas, the greater is your potential for experiencing quality living.

HEALTH AND QUALITY LIVING: THE MEANS AND THE GOAL

Health is the term that describes your overall level of functioning at any particular point in time. As the word "time" indicates, health is a dynamic concept, fluctuating even from moment to moment. The range of fluctuation can be illustrated as extending on a continuum from optimal health to death. This continuum of health is shown in Figure 1.2. Optimal health represents the highest level of function possible. This is an ideal to strive for, but one that is probably never actually achieved. Death, of course, represents the complete loss of function.

Although the word "healthy" is often used to mean only the absence of physical illness or dysfunction, the continuum of health clearly shows that the absence of disease does not mean that you are even average in terms of overall functioning or health. Even if all disease were eliminated from the world, there would still be a continuum of health, and your position on that continuum would be a reflection of how functional you were in *all* dimensions of your life—the physical, emotional, social, mental, and spiritual.

To visualize this, imagine that the continuum representing health is not a two-dimensional line at all but, instead, a cylinder that may be sliced into a series of discs, as shown in Figure 1.3. Each disc may in turn be divided into five pie-shaped segments, each segment representing one of the basic dimensions of life.

Where you are on the continuum of health, then, is determined by the efforts you make to increase (develop) your level of functioning in each dimension, in combination with other factors such as genetics, illness, injury, medical expertise, the environment, and so on. The extent to which each of these factors influences your health is difficult to specify. It is possible for your level of effort to predominate over factors that might limit function. For example, you may have lost your legs as a result of an accident, but you do a marathon anyway, in the wheelchair division. You are blind, but you learn to ski. Conversely, it is also possible to exert your best effort and still have your health deteriorate due to an uncontrolled disease such as AIDS or advanced-stage cancer.

Time is also an issue in determining how much any one factor influences your health. A time lag may exist between effort and its impact on health. For example, exercising one day does not result in instant fitness, nor does resting one day from your usual exercise routine make you unfit. Breathing smoke-filled air for one evening or smoking one pack of cigarettes is highly unlikely to result in lung cancer. Over time, however, exercising does lead to increased fitness, and not exercising to loss of fitness. Likewise, being exposed to smoke-filled environments over time and smoking cigarettes greatly increase the risk of cancer. And certainly people who develop cancer or any other disease hope that the passage of time will have provided sufficient medical expertise to treat them.

Thus far, the examples used in this discussion of health have referred mainly to the *physical* dimension of life, because most people think of health in primarily physical terms. However, the formula really applies in each dimension of your life—the emotional, social, mental, and spiritual, as well as the physical.

To know what constitutes healthy functioning in each dimension of life is important. Knowing this can help you determine what factors may be influencing your health and what efforts you can make to move toward a higher level of overall health and, thus, toward a higher quality of living.

FACTORS AFFECTING HEALTHY FUNCTIONING

In their book *Health Through Discovery*, Dintiman and Greenberg offer the following definition of healthy function in terms of the five basic dimensions of life:

1. **Physical health:** The ability to carry out daily tasks with energy remaining for unforeseen circumstances; biological integrity.
2. **Emotional health:** The ability to control emotions and express them appropriately and comfortably.

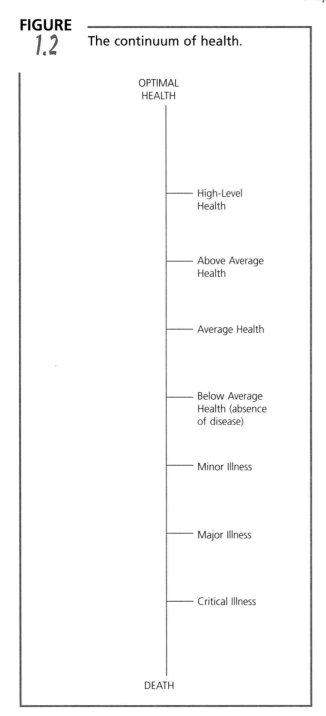

FIGURE 1.2 The continuum of health.

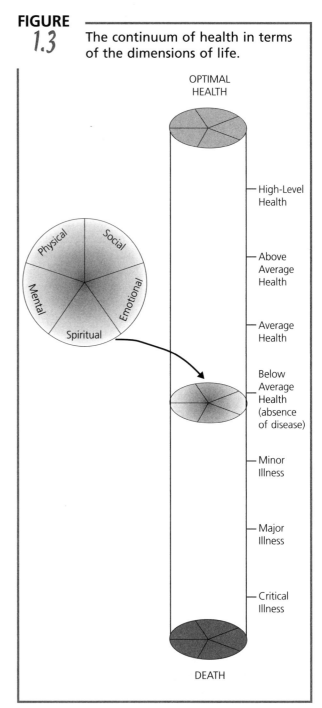

FIGURE 1.3 The continuum of health in terms of the dimensions of life.

3. **Social health:** The ability to interact well with people and the environment; having satisfying interpersonal relationships.
4. **Mental health:** The ability to learn, including intellectual capabilities.
5. **Spiritual health:** The belief in some unifying force such as nature, scientific laws, or a god-like entity.

As already indicated, how healthy you *really* are in each of these five dimensions of life depends on many factors. Some of these are directly within

your control and some are not. Although the factors are listed below in distinct categories, in reality these categories often overlap and influence one another.

As previously noted, lifestyle choices (your efforts) overlap many, if not most, of the factors to some degree. You can choose to lower your risk of disease by not smoking or by avoiding unsafe sex practices. You may be able to change your physical environment by moving from the city to the country, or improve your medical care by choosing another doctor. Although you cannot always prevent disease or accidental injury, you can choose how you will deal with these or any other factors should they become issues in your life.

1. *Lifestyle choices.* Many health experts rate lifestyle—the daily choices you make about how you will live your life—as the single most important factor influencing your overall health. Some examples of lifestyle choices that may affect your health are:

    a. To exercise or not; how much and how often to exercise

    b. What to eat

    c. How to handle stress and stressors

    d. To seek out or build a supportive environment

    e. To create or use opportunities to grow intellectually and spiritually

2. *Genetics.* Genetics determines your ultimate potential in each dimension of life. Manipulating your genetic endowment is not within your direct control, but lifestyle choices help you develop or utilize whatever potential you do have, be it extensive or limited. Some examples of genetic traits that may affect your health positively (+) or negatively (−) are:

    a. Hemophilia (−)

    b. Extra large lung capacity (+)

    c. Above average immune system function (+)

    d. Huntington's disease (−)

3. *Accident/injury.* Accidental injuries may limit your functional potential, and their impact is also subject to available medical expertise. Although you cannot always prevent or avoid accidents, the choices you make to protect yourself from these hazards to quality living can reduce the risk of their occurrence in your life. Some examples of injuries that may affect your health are:

    a. Broken arm

    b. Sprained ankle

4. *Disease/dysfunction.* As with genetics and accidents, you may not be able to avoid these health problems entirely, but your lifestyle choices can actually reduce your chances of disease. By eating well and exercising, for example, you may decrease your risks substantially. Even though a healthy lifestyle cannot assure that you will live free of disease, it can make you better prepared to deal with disease. The state of the art of medicine can also be a critical factor in determining the impact of disease on your life. Some examples of diseases/dysfunctions that may affect your health are:

    a. Physical: hepatitis, cancer, heart disease, diabetes, AIDS

    b. Emotional/mental: depression, schizophrenia, dyslexia

5. *Medical expertise.* As mentioned, the state of the art of medicine can be a critical factor in determining the impact of genetic abnormalities, injuries, and diseases. The knowledge level and skill of your personal physician and hospital/clinic staff are perhaps the most important of all because these people actually provide the care you receive. Although most of the issues in this area are not directly within your control, you can exert some influence by educating yourself and others and by taking direct action such as voting and working with organized groups on private and government programs for health. Some important examples of how medical issues may affect your health:

    a. State-of-the-art medical techniques may or may not be available to you.

    b. You may or may not be able to afford necessary treatment.

    c. Government allocations and budget considerations may make certain programs/treatments accessible or inaccessible.

    d. Sociocultural norms can limit access to help because of prejudices such as sexism, racism, and ageism.

    e. A medical solution/cure may simply not be possible or known at this time.

6. *Physical environment.* The physical environment in which you live and work most certainly can affect your health, primarily by increasing your risk of injury and disease. Today, environmental quality is controlled or not controlled largely by government and politics, business, and social policy, not necessarily in that order and not necessarily with human health as the main goal. Economics, politics, and nationalism often take precedence over health concerns. Nonetheless, you can take many actions every day to lessen your exposure to environmental hazards. Wearing seat belts when driving, avoiding smoke-filled rooms, refusing excessive exposure to X-rays, and not drinking and driving are but a few of these. Some examples of physical environment factors that may affect your health are:

    a. Overcrowding

    b. Air/water pollution

    c. Radiation

    d. Work hazards

7. *Psychosocial environment.* The people in your world and the quality of interaction you have with them constitute your psychosocial environment. Most immediately this consists of your family and

friends, but it also includes workmates and members of your community, state, region, and country. Today everyone is even a member of the world community. The beliefs, values, attitudes, knowledge, and actions of these people can have a significant impact on your opportunities to grow emotionally, mentally, and spiritually, as well as to be physically safe and well. Of course, you don't get to pick the family or the society into which you are born, but you can acknowledge for yourself an "unhealthy" situation and work to establish relationships with people whose values, attitudes, and actions encourage you to strive for full functioning in each dimension of your life. Some examples of psychosocial factors that may affect your health are:

a. Exposure to the beliefs, values, and attitudes in your circle of family and friends

b. Peer pressure to smoke, drink, "party" excessively, and so on

c. Being part of a family or group that is physically active and encourages you to be so

d. Social norms and political policies that may support racism, religious biases, and so on

In essence, as shown in Figure 1.4, health is a means to the goal of self-actualization, the quality living experience. In plain terms, your health is "what you've got to work with" at any point in time. As defined earlier, a healthy level of functioning in each aspect of life is basically synonymous with the capabilities Maslow identified in the hierarchy of needs as critical to becoming all you can be or moving toward self-actualization.

Of the numerous factors that can influence how healthy you are, your **lifestyle**—your everyday efforts to preserve and develop your capacities—is the single most important factor. As indicated earlier, your efforts not only enhance your functioning but also generate the feelings of a quality living experience: fulfillment, wholeness, and happiness. **Wellness** describes a health-promoting lifestyle.

QUALITY LIVING: A WELLNESS LIFESTYLE

Throughout the previous discussion of quality living and health, *effort* has emerged as a key to

quality living. It is critical to all the aspects of quality living—developing healthy functioning in each dimension of life, using your talents and capabilities in creative and productive ways, and experiencing feelings of fulfillment and happiness. Deliberate and consistent efforts to become more and more of what you can be in each dimension of life constitute a wellness lifestyle, the process of self-actualization, a quality living experience. The greater your efforts and the healthier you become, the more "actualized" you will be.

You may be wondering how a physical disability, temporary or permanent, or a decreased level of health affect your capacity to live a wellness lifestyle. It is important to remember that *wellness* refers to the efforts and the choices you make from moment to moment; it does not refer to your *functional status*. As long as you are striving to develop and expand your potential, you can experience a sense of personal fulfillment regardless of your actual level of health. Thus, if you find yourself at a low level of health because of inactivity, stress, or poor diet, by beginning to use and develop what capabilities you do have, you can experience increased quality in living as you work to become healthier. In the same way, you can experience quality in living even while struggling against disease or dysfunction. Until the problem condition obliterates the potential for function, you can express and develop the capacity you do have.

FIGURE 1.4 Health and self-actualization: The means and the goal.

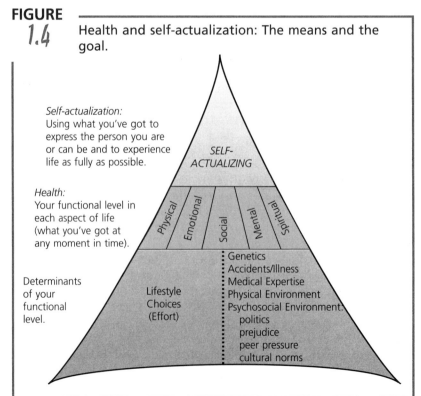

Self-actualization: Using what you've got to express the person you are or can be and to experience life as fully as possible.

Health: Your functional level in each aspect of life (what you've got at any moment in time).

Determinants of your functional level.

SELF-ACTUALIZING

Physical   Emotional   Social   Mental   Spiritual

Lifestyle Choices (Effort)

Genetics
Accidents/Illness
Medical Expertise
Physical Environment
Psychosocial Environment:
  politics
  prejudice
  peer pressure
  cultural norms

In essence, your level of health may not always reflect your level of effort at the moment, but the quality of your living experience will. Full expression of the person you can be may be the ultimate goal in the pursuit of quality living, but becoming what you can be at this moment provides the joy in daily living.

What does a wellness lifestyle really mean? By definition, a wellness lifestyle means striving to develop your abilities in each dimension of life. By doing this, you will be developing the capabilities specified by Maslow's hierarchy of needs (Figure 1.1) as being necessary for self-actualization. A wellness lifestyle, then, must include efforts to:

1. Achieve and maintain biological integrity. For example:
   a. becoming physically fit
   b. eating nutritious foods
   c. getting needed rest and relaxation
   d. protecting yourself from physical hazards and injurious agents/substances in the environment
2. Develop self-love and love for others. For example:
   a. acknowledging and expressing feelings and desires constructively
   b. creating a psychosocial environment supportive to your growth and development
   c. expressing affection and respect for others
3. Interact with other people successfully. For example:
   a. being interested in other people
   b. identifying other people with whom you enjoy talking and doing things
   c. establishing a sense of belonging with other people
4. Develop and apply intellectual capabilities and skills. For example:
   a. expanding your knowledge base
   b. applying your skills to become self-reliant and productive in society
5. Formulate a personal philosophy for living. For example:
   a. examining approaches to life proposed by science, philosophy, and religion
   b. identifying personal beliefs about life
   c. formulating answers for the basic questions "Why am I here?" and "What am about?"

Adopting a wellness lifestyle doesn't mean suddenly accomplishing all of these goals. It does mean making some effort to grow in each dimension of your life, beginning wherever you need to begin. Your efforts may not be equal in all dimensions. It is not unusual for someone to concentrate efforts in one or a few areas. A true wellness lifestyle, however, means giving at least some attention to each dimension of your life. The ultimate goal is to balance your efforts, striving to develop as much in one dimension as in another. The more balanced your efforts, the better you will be able to express, experience, and enjoy yourself. The *lifestyle circle* is a device that will help you determine how balanced your efforts are.

THE LIFESTYLE CIRCLE

The lifestyle circle is designed to allow you to determine whether you are living a wellness lifestyle and, if so, how balanced your efforts are. By estimating your level of effort in each dimension of life, using the scale of 1–10 provided on the circle, you can create a picture of your lifestyle. For example, if you rate your efforts in all dimensions relatively high—for instance, 7s, 8s, and 9s—your lifestyle circle will be filled out fairly completely and evenly. It will actually look like a large circle, as shown in Figure 1.5a. This "picture" shows a balance of efforts across dimensions. On the other hand, if you rate your efforts in one dimension as fairly high, but only average in three others and actually low in another, your lifestyle circle will appear lopsided, as shown in Figure 1.5b. This circle reflects effort in each dimension of life, but certainly not a balanced effort.

In essence, the more closely your lifestyle picture approximates a circle and the bigger the circle, the more completely you are becoming the person you can be, given your level of health at the moment. Likewise, the smaller or more lopsided your lifestyle picture, the less you will experience an overall sense of well-being.

FIGURE
1.5   Wellness lifestyle circles.

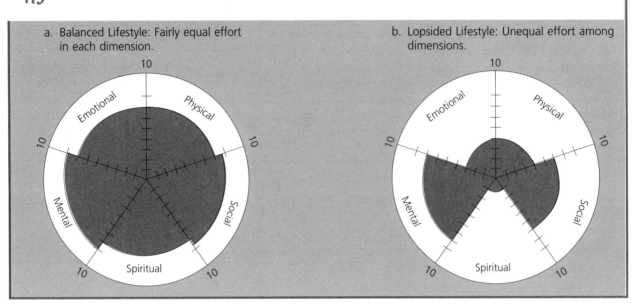

a. Balanced Lifestyle: Fairly equal effort in each dimension.

b. Lopsided Lifestyle: Unequal effort among dimensions.

SUMMARY

The concept of quality living presented in this chapter is based on the observations of Maslow, Rogers, and Perls that richness in living is experiencing the thrill of becoming and being all you can be. Becoming as healthy as you can be will provide the knowledge, the skill, the confidence, the fitness, and the energy for you to achieve whatever heights are possible for you. In the interim, the process of becoming—the practice and preparation, the hard work and effort it takes to develop your capacities—generates a feeling of quality living all its own. In essence, quality living is not just reaching a goal; it's also *reaching for the goal!*

REFERENCES

Ardell, D. 1985. *Fourteen Days to a Wellness Lifestyle.* Mill Valley, CA: Whatever Publisher.

Carlyon, W. 1984. "Disease Prevention/Health Promotion—Bridging the Gap to Wellness." *Health Values: Achieving High Level Wellness* 8 (May/June): 27–30.

Dintiman, G., and Greenberg, J. S. 1986. *Health Through Discovery*, 3d ed. New York: Random House.

Greenberg, J. 1985. "Health and Wellness: A Conceptual Differentiation." *Health Education* 16 (Oct./Nov.): 4–6.

Maslow, A. 1968. *Toward a Psychology of Being*, 2d ed. New York: Van Nostrand Reinhold.

Maslow, A. 1970. *Motivation and Personality*, 2d ed. New York: Harper and Row.

Perls, F. 1966. "Gestalt Therapy and Human Potentialities." Chapter 35 in *Explorations in Human Potentialities.* Herbert Otto, ed. Springfield, IL: Charles C. Thomas.

Rogers, C. 1968. *On Becoming a Person.* Boston: Houghton Mifflin.

CHOICES IN ACTION

Before going on to Chapter 2, take a moment to think about and assess your current efforts toward a wellness lifestyle. In Appendix 9, Labs 1 and 2 have been developed for this purpose. Lab 1, "Functional Status Worksheet," allows you to estimate your current level of functioning in each dimension of your life. While completing this worksheet, you may feel that you do not have all the information you need to be accurate—that's okay. The remainder of this book is devoted to helping you better assess your efforts; Lab 1 is intended as a "preassessment" for you.

In Lab 2, "Lifestyle Worksheet," you will have a chance to fill in your own lifestyle circle. Together, Labs 1 and 2 will help you see where you are now and perhaps give you a glimpse of where you want to head. Later, you will have an opportunity to compare these early assessments to those that you complete at the end of the course, in Chapter 12.

2

Making Choices About Wellness

✔ Willpower is not the key to changing behavior. Do you know what is?

✔ How can you motivate yourself to make changes in your life?

✔ What common pitfalls might you encounter when trying to change behavior, and how can you avoid these pitfalls?

✔ How healthy are you in each aspect of your life?

✔ What are your goals for each dimension of your life, and what must you do to reach them?

✔ What can you do *now* to get started?

In this chapter you will learn how you can change your behavior deliberately without relying on willpower and wishes, if you decide that doing so will enhance your quality of living. The basic actions involved in changing yourself in some way are *considering, trying, achieving,* and *maintaining*. These actions were illustrated in order of progression in the Introduction. The smaller size of each successive step represents proportionately the number of people who generally reach it. As indicated, many people consider changes in their lives but never quite get around to trying them. Of those who do try, many stop before they achieve their goal, and of those who do reach their goal, many do not maintain their new behavior in the long run.

Why do only some people advance from step to step in the behavior change process? Is it a matter of willpower? If so, what do you do if you don't have the necessary willpower? Without it, can you follow some procedure that guarantees success in changing your behavior? Is there some "best time" to try to make changes in your life? To help you take charge of your life and make the changes you wish to make, these questions are addressed in this chapter.

CHOOSING AND CHANGING OUR BEHAVIOR

Decide how you want to be
Do what you have to do

Epictetus, *Discourses*

Making Choices Versus Relying on Willpower

Amazingly, the simple ancient directive of Epictetus provides a succinct summary of what modern researchers have been learning about how people do make behavior changes. At this point you may be wondering, "How can something that sounds so easy be so hard?" Perhaps the reason is that we try to change ourselves without following Epictetus's basic steps; we don't *decide* first how we want to be. Many times we try to change ourselves according to someone else's beliefs and values without determining if we actually believe in and value that behavior ourselves. Most often we simply wish we were like this or that or hope that someday we will be, but we don't *decide* that we will be. We don't take action.

Furthermore, we usually don't analyze ourselves and our behavior sufficiently, if at all, to determine what we need to do to change. We may try to make total changes overnight when we are ready or able to take only one small step toward the change we want to make. Or we may try to make changes according to someone else's guidelines, which may not be right for us, or may not even be right at all. Witness the plethora of weight-loss diets offered to us in magazines and paperbacks, many of which result in short-term weight loss, malnourishment, and increased body fat!

We may understand Epictetus's directive, but this does not mean we know how to accomplish the steps he recommended. Many of us who try to change something about ourselves proceed in ways destined to fail, or perhaps manage to succeed without knowing how we did it. Thus, willpower or the lack of it has become the mystical explanation for success or failure. If you succeed, you are one of the lucky few with enough willpower. If you fail, you just don't have it. If you have ever made a New Year's resolution or similar type of self-promise to change something about yourself, you probably understand this challenge all too well.

The "PRE" Factors Versus Willpower

Fortunately, research has shown that willpower isn't the key to changing behavior after all. Specifically where health is concerned, three key categories of factors seem to determine our behavior: predisposing factors, reinforcing factors, and enabling factors (PRE).

1. **Predisposing factors** are thought to be the basis for motivation, or the predisposition to act one way versus another. These factors consist of our knowledge, beliefs, attitudes, and values, plus personal characteristics such as age, gender, race, socioeconomic status, and so on, which can influence the extent of our knowledge and what we believe and value. As used here, the term *belief* means a conviction that something is true or real. *Attitude* refers to a relatively constant feeling of positivity or negativity about something or someone. *Value* refers to something that we act to keep or gain.

2. **Reinforcing factors** refer to persons or events who/which support or encourage certain behaviors.

3. **Enabling factors** are our personal skills and resources—what we know how to do and the resources available to help us do what we want to do. These resources could include money, a swimming pool, a car, a clinic or hospital, a stop-smoking class, and so on.

The PRE factors and how they influence our behavior are illustrated in Figure 2.1. As the arrows in the figure indicate, we tend to choose behaviors that we know about, that we believe to be helpful in some way (or at least not immediately and drastically harmful), and that we enjoy or feel good about (arrow 1). Our choices, however, may be modified or limited by the absence or inadequacy of personal skills or "know how," the facilities and services necessary to carry out the behavior as we need to (arrow 2). The behaviors we eventually choose impact events and people in our lives in positive, negative, or neutral ways (arrow 3). They, in turn, influence our behavior. Behaviors associated with the desired outcome of events or found acceptable by other people, especially people we care about, will be positively reinforced. We will feel encouraged to repeat these behaviors. On the other hand, behaviors that others do not favor or that don't produce desired results or good feelings will be negatively reinforced or discouraged (arrows 4 and 5).

This model of how PRE factors influence behavior provides a way of analyzing why we have succeeded or failed at trying to change ourselves in the past. More important, it provides a way to plan successful behavior changes in the future. The prescribed plan involves developing a set of predisposing factors that moves us to behave in the desired way, a set of enabling skills and resources that allows us to perform the desired behavior successfully, and a sufficient number of supporters to reinforce our forward steps and encourage us to keep going forward. In essence, we have to create a new chain of events or PRE factors that lead to the desired behavior.

The Health Belief Model

Researchers in the area of health-related behavior change have found that we are most likely to succeed in changing our behavior when we believe the following to be true:

1. That our current behavior jeopardizes our health in some way.
2. That we could end up experiencing considerable pain, time lost from work, money problems, family problems, and so on because of our current behavior.

FIGURE

2.1   The "PRE" factors. The numbered lines indicate the direction of influence in usual order of occurrence.

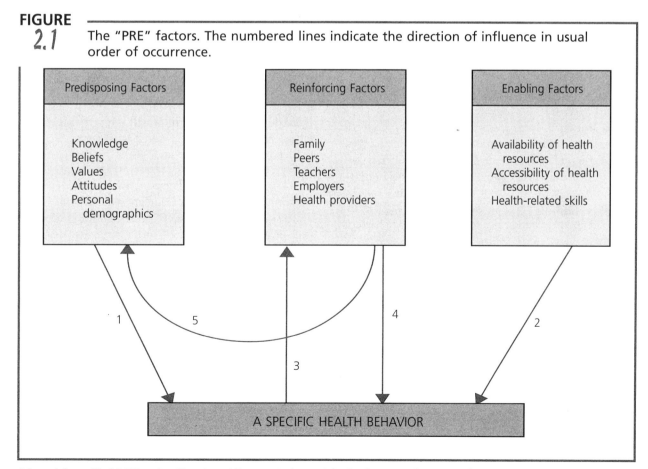

Adapted from *Health Education Planning: A Diagnostic Approach* by L. Green et al., © 1980 by Mayfield Publishing, Mountain View, CA.

3. That the benefits of a new way of behaving are ultimately achievable and worth the cost in terms of the time, effort, and money we might have to expend to change ourselves.

4. That we can, in fact, do this new behavior and that whatever we need to do it in the way of facilities, equipment, or assistance is within our grasp.

5. That once these beliefs are in place, a "cue to action" or precipitating force makes us feel the need to take action.

Officially known as the **health belief model,** these five conditions provide basic guidelines for constructing the chain of beliefs, attitudes, values, capabilities, and reinforcements that can link us with the way we want to be. Specifically, this model suggests that the pathway to change is made up of three segments or steps linked together:

1. Analyzing current and possible alternative behaviors

2. Deciding that a new way of behaving is desirable and worth working toward

3. Identifying and planning for the specific conditions, facilities, equipment, and assistance that seem most likely to promote success, *and* specifying a specific time for getting started

THE PATHWAY TO CHANGE

The three sequential segments or steps in the pathway to making behavior changes are presented below. For this discussion, the steps are: (a) analyze your current behavior; (b) decide how you want to be and begin an action plan; and (c) do what you have to do: Individualize your action plan. Suggestions are offered for accomplishing each step. In addition, common pitfalls or traps that lead away from successful change are identified for each step. Finally, ways to get back on track are discussed.

The first steps in the behavior change process are designed to work on predisposing factors: our knowledge, beliefs, attitudes, and feelings. We need to become aware of our actions, how we feel about our behavior, and the options open to us. Once we are aware of these factors, we can plan how to enable and reinforce ourselves to change.

Step 1: Analyze Current Behavior

The goal of the first step along the pathway to change is to determine the answer to two questions:

1. Is our current behavior jeopardizing our health, or our ability to work productively, to

support ourselves, and to build rewarding relationships?

2. Would another way of behaving produce results more in line with the quality of living we would like for ourselves?

To answer these questions with any degree of accuracy, we will need to gather some information about ourselves—what we actually do and how this affects our lives now and will affect us in the future if we continue our current behavior. We also need to learn what benefits we might gain if we choose a different way of behaving.

Because we are all busy with so many things each day, the only way to get an accurate picture of any given behavior we engage in is to keep a written record of it for at least one week, and perhaps even two or three weeks if our lives vary a lot from week to week. We need to record not only when the behavior occurs, but also where, with whom, the positive and negative outcomes, and our thoughts/feelings. A sample behavior record or diary focusing on stress is shown in Figure 2.2.

Not all of this information is necessary to determine if you are endangering your health and well-being. If you do decide to change your behavior, however, the additional information will help to identify the people, places, and times that tend to trigger or reinforce the behavior you are trying to change; the needs you will have to fulfill in other ways; and the self-talk (things you say to yourself about your behavior or your capabilities) that may impede or discourage your attempts to change. Knowledge of these things will allow you to individualize the behavior change process to fit your own particular circumstances—or, in the words of Epictetus, to "do what you have to do."

Another important aspect of the first step is personal assessment. Is your current behavior providing the degree of health and functional capabilities you want for yourself right now? You also will need to do some "personalized study" to determine the probable long-term impact of your behavior. Personalized study means more than just reading; it means projecting what you might be like ten, twenty, or thirty years from now, based on your personal assessments and what is currently known about the long-term benefits/consequences of various behaviors. This projection should show you whether you are headed up or down the quality living scale. The information and assessment tools and techniques needed to gather this data on a basic level are provided in the remaining chapters of this book.

If more information is needed to firmly substantiate or convince you of the impact of a specific behavior, talking with or reading about people who

FIGURE
2.2   A sample behavior diary page for stress.

When	What Happened	Where	With Whom	Outcomes N = negative P = positive	Thoughts/ Feelings
S L E E P					
5					
6					
7					
8					
9					
10					
11					
Noon	Top priority – Visit with mother Low priority – Stopped to get shoes at repair shop	On the way to Mother's	Alone	N: less time with mother – She felt bad	I felt bad and sad
1					
2					
3	Late for appointment because left mother's late	At office	With colleague	N: Not enough time to plan meeting	Embarrassed Annoyed
4					
5					
6					
7					
8					
9					

are enjoying the benefits or suffering the consequences of the behavior may help. The many clubs, self-help groups, and official organizations supporting or fighting almost any form of health behavior or condition will help you locate others who are like you or are like you want to be. You also can obtain more in-depth self-assessment data from a thorough physical exam, blood tests, an EKG, blood pressure screening, exercise stress test, and so on. These tests generally cost money and require trained personnel and time. If, however, the results of sophisticated tests and consultation with experts will impact your belief system more than self-assessments, the money and time will be well spent.

Pitfalls to change in Step 1. Minimizing the importance of any or all of the components of this first step may lead to some erroneous conclusions or assumptions about our behavior and ourselves. For example, it's easy to decide not to do the record-keeping, the personalized study exercises, or the assessments. We assume that we already know this information, or that we don't have the necessary time for such things. In reality, however, we all do much of the information-gathering required by Step 1 automatically, as we listen to news broadcasts and our friends and families and read magazines, newspapers, and books. What we usually don't do, however, is make a concerted effort to find out the nitty-gritty facts about recommended behaviors versus what we actually do. Consequently, we are generally aware of behaviors that are supposed to be harmful or helpful to our health, but we don't really know how our own behaviors compare to these and, therefore, what our own risks or benefits are. Rather, we simply assume that we are in fairly good shape, or eat a well-balanced diet, or handle stress well enough.

One reason we make these assumptions is that our bodies seem to be working all right, and spending time and effort and perhaps even money to check up on something that works is hard to justify in our busy lives. Ironically, most of us behave differently when it comes to our cars. We do take time to watch the gauges and look under the hood even when the car *is* working well. We do spend the money to refuel, change the oil and belts and so on, before the car sputters to a halt. We do these things to assure that the car will get us where we want to go when we want to go. That's the body's job, too, but our cars have some advantages when it comes to eliciting caring behavior from us: They come equipped with gauges and warning lights to tell us how they are running and if something needs our attention. They also come with maintenance schedules and repair manuals to tell us what we have to do to keep them operating in top form. If we ignore all of this "enabling" information, the car simply won't run, so we are "reinforced" quickly to take proper care of it.

The body, on the other hand, doesn't have gauges to indicate from moment to moment how much fat is accumulating on our blood vessel walls, if our fuel mixture is adequate, or how high our blood pressure or muscle tension is. It also doesn't come with a maintenance/repair manual. This manual is still being written, in fact, as we learn bit by bit why the body breaks down and how to prevent it or fix it. So, unless we make a special effort to assess the body's functioning level and obtain information about the best way to treat it, we may let it deteriorate unknowingly.

The body may give warning signals when it is starting to break down, but this is not always the case. Furthermore, because it is more durable and adaptable than our cars, the body can continue to run, although certainly not at full capacity, for a long time, even without proper care. In this way, the body reinforces lack of attention and sloppy maintenance. Unless we learn from others or through experience what higher-quality functioning (living) is like, we might sputter along ignorantly through life thinking our bodies are working just fine.

Our cars have one more advantage over our bodies: We know the value of our cars. They cost thousands of dollars. Most of us cannot afford to replace them very often, and we certainly don't want to be without a car, so we are predisposed or motivated to take good care of cars. It's hard to be similarly motivated to take good care of the body, though. We never paid anything for it; it came "free." Furthermore, because we've never been without it, it's hard to realize how valuable the body is even though we know all the money in the world couldn't buy a new one if we need it.

Only when the body breaks down do we get an inkling of its value. In fact, the body is our one vital vehicle in life, providing us with the potential to do what we want and to become what we can. Perhaps this is what Hugh Prather meant when, in his book *Notes on Love and Courage*, he wrote, "Learning to love [to value] yourself is the definition of change." Taking the time to learn about ourselves—what we are doing and how we can enhance our living experience—*is* an act of valuing. One thing is clear: We do spend time, effort, and money on the things we value.

Sometimes the time or money is not what makes us reluctant to assess our behavior but, rather, that we don't want to confirm our suspicions that we are behaving in harmful or at least unbeneficial ways. If we force ourselves to acknowledge this by recording our behavior, we might feel guilty or uncomfortable, or feel that we have to give up things we like doing or do things we won't like.

If comparing our actual behavior with what we think is right or best for us produces uncomfortable feelings, something *does* need to be changed—either our behavior or our opinion of it, or both. Such emotional discomfort indicates values or attitudes in conflict with each other. We can like or value doing something that we know could shorten our lives or at least reduce our vitality and vigor. Smoking, overusing salt, or having a regular diet of bacon and eggs or burgers and shakes are just a few examples. We know now that these behaviors are or can be harmful, but this wasn't always the case. Thus, though we now have new information and options to consider, we still may not be free to choose the healthiest way of behaving. We may find ourselves trapped in long-term habits or in behavior patterns that we find pleasurable or always have believed to be okay or perhaps even value as part of our family or ethnic heritage. In these cases, just knowing that another way of behaving would be more beneficial to our health might not be enough to overcome the influence of these beliefs and attitudes.

If the new information is strong enough, we might be moved to try the new behavior. Because any new behavior is initially awkward and uncomfortable, however, we have a tendency to return quickly to old habits. Our habits, whether good or bad, will feel more comfortable and natural than the new behavior. Until we can free ourselves from the reaffirming attitudes, beliefs, and values attached to our current behaviors, trying to change ourselves might be a losing battle. We may even conclude that we lack willpower or may decide we want to remain just as we are.

Although deciding we like ourselves as we are is certainly an acceptable possibility, we need to make sure we haven't made that choice simply because, even though we would like to be different, we don't want to give up the satisfaction or pleasure our current behavior brings. This distinction is important to make because what many of us fail to realize is that we don't (won't) give up something we like or habitually do unless another way of behaving becomes equally or more attractive. In his book *Toward a Psychology of Being*, renowned psychologist Abraham Maslow made the following observations about how we grow or change:

> We don't do it because it's good for us...or because someone told us to or because it makes us live longer.... Growth [change] takes place when the next step forward is more intrinsically satisfying than the previous gratification with which we have become familiar and even bored. . . .

To summarize, we don't have to worry about giving up something we like doing, because we probably won't. What we do have to be concerned about is finding a different behavior that provides as much or more satisfaction as the old behavior. Our chances of accomplishing this are best if we gather the information about our current behavior and about alternative ways of behaving as indicated in Step 1. We will then have personal guidelines for shaping the remaining steps in the behavior change process. These steps deal with learning and

coming to value behaviors that are more representative of how we would like to be and of the quality of life we desire.

Step 2: Decide How You Want to Be and Begin an Action Plan

After studying the probable consequences of our current behavior versus other ways of behaving, the second step begins with deciding how we *want* to be. This is not to be confused with the conclusion, "That's how I am." You may decide not to make changes, of course, but whatever your decision, you must be able to say, "I want to be like that." This step requires making a statement of desire: "I want to be a person who exercises regularly and is fit" or "I want to be a smoker."

Stating our desires doesn't presume that tomorrow or from now on we must be that way, or even that we want to go through the sometimes uncomfortable and awkward process of changing ourselves, if that's required. A statement of desires simply identifies what we would like to become and, thus, what we need to start becoming now. In essence, this is a decision that commits us to action—the action of becoming. Unless we complete this critical step, we probably won't be successful in changing ourselves because we won't do what we have to do.

To ensure that our decision about how we want to be evolves into a commitment to act, we will need to *build an action plan*. Otherwise our decision easily could become just another silent promise to ourselves that gets forgotten in the daily hubbub of our lives, overridden by old habits and thoughts. Therefore, the first concern in our action plan must be to keep our attention focused on the new way we want to be and the rewards and benefits we hope to gain. We can do this by developing and practicing new ways of thinking about ourselves that affirm and remind us of what we want to become. In his book *Increasing Human Effectiveness*, Bob Moawad calls this positive self-talk **constructive affirmation.** He emphasizes that we need to practice this technique two to three times a day for two to three weeks to begin displacing the attitudes and beliefs that have supported our old behavior. This might seem silly and unnecessary, but just as the body needs some time to get in shape, the mind needs time to move from thoughts such as "I don't have time to exercise" to "I take time to exercise."

If becoming a regular exerciser is your goal, "I take time to exercise" is an example of an affirmative statement. "I enjoy exercising 20 minutes a day, three to four times a week" is another example. FYI 1 offers guidelines for formulating constructive affirmations.

Guidelines for Affirmations

- Describe what you want to be rather than what you are or don't want to be.
- Use the personal reference "I."
- Use present tense, not future tense.
- Use "feeling" words such as "enjoy," "am proud of," and so on.
- State specifically what you are doing.
- Use realistic standards such as "regularly" or "consistently" versus "always" or "every day."
- Refer only to your own behavior without making comparisons to other people.

By reviewing the feelings and self-talk you recorded in your behavior diary for Step 1, you can see the attitudes and beliefs—the thinking patterns—that have sustained your old behavior. Using the guidelines in FYI 1, you can work on changing these thoughts by substituting constructive affirmations that will encourage you to choose behaviors to fit your goals. To complete Step 2 in a way that will keep you moving forward along the pathway to change, then, you will need to:

1. Clearly state your goal: how you want to be and why (the rewards and benefits you expect to gain).
2. Make a commitment to that goal by initiating an action plan.
3. Formulate constructive affirmations and practice them two to three times daily as the first component of your action plan.

One way to operationalize this process is to carry with you a 3" x 5" card with your goal and its rewards written on one side and three to four affirmations written on the other side. An example of this action plan reminder card is shown in Figure 2.3. While you are working on affirming how you want to be, you can begin to determine what you have to do to change yourself, Step 3 in the pathway to behavior change.

Pitfalls to change in Step 2. Deciding how we want to be but not taking any action usually means we haven't truly decided. Instead, we are *considering* how we might want to be. We are, in reality, still at Step 1. Many of us remain at this stage, never committing ourselves to action. Why? And how do we get out of this pit of inaction and back on the pathway to change?

We seem to get stalled at the considering stage of behavior change for two main reasons:

1. We don't really believe that our current behavior is jeopardizing our health or quality of living or that we could change ourselves even if we wanted to.
2. We can see that we need to change, but we are simply not motivated.

In both of these cases, collecting more data regarding the consequences of our current behavior and the benefits of changing might be the stimulus we need. Just doing more reading may not be potent enough, though. We may have to deliberately expose ourselves to those who currently are suffering the consequences of potentially damaging behavior or who have changed their behavior and currently are enjoying the benefits. We can find these people through organizations such as Alcoholics Anonymous, Overeaters Anonymous, the Cancer Society, and the Heart Association, as well as through teachers, counselors, and friends.

We also can do something to get ourselves motivated. According to Art Turock, who specializes in methods for generating motivation to exercise, **motivation** is "a function of what we choose to focus on." Thus, by focusing our thoughts on how we would like to be and the benefits that would be ours, we may be able to develop the motivation we've been waiting for. Probably the easiest way to do this is to formulate and use the constructive affirmations described earlier—whether we do or do not feel motivated. What we say to ourselves has a great deal to do with how we behave.

We may have to work on these issues for some time to get ourselves on the pathway to change. That's okay. No step in the pathway has a time limit. Each step does, however, require action. The key to changing ourselves is to keep acting. We will succeed only if we have tried.

Step 3: Do What You Have to Do—Individualize Your Action Plan

To determine what we have to do to change our behavior, we must deal with two key challenges. In

FIGURE

2.3   An action plan reminder card.

GOAL AND REWARDS/BENEFITS

*Goal: Decrease and prioritize the
number of things I do in a day.*

*Rewards: Enjoy what I do more.
Feel more relaxed.
Produce higher-quality work.
Have more time for people
and relationships.*

3" x 5" CARD

AFFIRMATIVE STATEMENTS

*I enjoy planning for people, as well as
things, in my day.*

I make time for myself regularly.

I budget time to do quality work.

FLIP SIDE

his analysis of how we grow, or make constructive changes in our lives, Maslow wrote, "The only way we can ever know what is right for us is that it feels better . . . than any alternative." He also pointed out, however, that we are "both actuality and potentiality" and that basically we don't (won't) move from safe, secure actuality (how we are now) toward potentiality unless the dangers are minimal and the attractions or rewards clearly evident.

To address these issues, we will have to try a new way of behaving for a long enough time to see if it really provides the benefits we want. In addition, we will have to do this in a way that minimizes the stress and discomfort that usually accompany change and maximizes our chances of being successful and feeling positive about what we are doing. The only way we can hope to meet these conditions is by carefully preparing and planning for the change we want to make.

When trying a new behavior, you can enhance your chances of success in several ways:

1. *Make sure you know how to work toward your goal step by step, safely and effectively.* Taking a class and reading books and articles written by legitimate experts are ways of doing this. If you injure yourself the first time you try to exercise or find yourself ravenous and depressed after not eating for three days, you most likely will not want or be able to continue your efforts to change.

2. *Identify a short-term goal—some action, no matter how small, that you know you can do to begin working toward your goal.* If becoming a nonsmoker is your goal but quitting completely isn't something you think you can do immediately, your goal should be reduced to something you *can* do, even if it's only cutting out one cigarette a day. Success breeds success *and* the confidence that we can change our behavior.

3. *Locate sources of, and arrange for, support and reinforcement.* Identify a support person or group. Any change you try to make, no matter how small, can be stressful. The discomfort can cause you to abandon your new efforts and return to old habits. Having someone to talk with when you feel distressed or discouraged can make the difference between continuing to try and abandoning the effort.

You should select a support person who appreciates the effort you are making and can provide the encouragement and reinforcement you need when you need it. Ideally, this person is someone who has lived through the experience you are attempting. If no personal acquaintance matches this description, self-help groups and behavior-change classes are excellent sources of help.

4. *Stipulate a reward that will be yours for* each day *you achieve your goal.* The reward must be something you can do or have *only* if you are successful. Examples of rewards are a sauna or luxurious bath, half an hour to read the paper or an interesting book, a television program, a favorite snack, and some "play time" with friends.

No matter how tough, determined, or capable you think you are in pursuing your goal, arranging for reinforcement of your efforts is important. Reinforcement is one of the major factors in shaping behavior, which is exactly what you are trying to do.

When you have completed these preparations, you can finalize the action plan you began in Step 2 by following the guidelines presented next.

▪ *Deciding what you will do and how you will do it is the key to "doing what you have to do."* Often the goal we are working toward means eliminating or reducing some behavior, such as smoking, drinking, eating cookies, or watching television. The key is to concentrate not on what we must stop doing but instead on what we will do in its place. Furthermore, if we decide to eat an apple rather than a cookie during our break, how will we manage if no apples are available or if everyone else is having luscious-looking brownies? We can bring an apple with us to solve the availability problem, take a walk instead of going to the snack room at break, or interest a friend in eating apples instead of brownies so we have some support.

Problems such as these can be resolved in a number of ways, but not all of them would be right for any one of us. Identify for yourself constructive behaviors that will be consistent with the long-term goal you are trying to reach. Keep in mind that each time we do not engage in our old behavior, we will be practicing a new way of being. Replacing one bad habit with another is unlikely to be anyone's goal.

We also have to determine how we will avoid or deal with the social and environmental cues or conditions that might trigger our old behavior instead of the new behavior we are trying to learn. The information you recorded in Step 1 about where and when and with whom your old behavior occurred should provide some guidance in meeting these challenges.

▪ *Deciding when to begin trying a new behavior sounds simple enough, but this decision may be one of the most difficult to make and adhere to.* "Tomorrow," "soon," or "next week, maybe" are the dates we prefer. The main reason for our hesitation is that changing is scary. It is uncertain. It is different. All of this can make us feel uncomfortable enough to decide not to decide when to begin.

We can do several things to minimize our concerns and get ourselves started. First, we can try visualizing our action plan. If we have carefully planned exactly what we will do, we should be able to "see ourselves" doing it. This mental rehearsal can help to alleviate our fears and boost our confidence. If we can't see ourselves behaving as we have planned, perhaps we need to revise our plan to better reflect what we can do.

Next we need to promise ourselves a review date, at which time we will evaluate how well we've done and how we feel, and alter our plans accordingly. In general, a week or two of trying our new behavior will be long enough for us to determine how we are doing. Knowing that we don't have to suffer interminably if our plan isn't working will let us feel more comfortable about trying it. If we have been able to do what we planned, and we feel confident and comfortable about it, we can expand our plan. If we have been only partly successful or don't yet feel comfortable with what we are doing, we can work with the same plan or revise it to better reflect what we can do.

Keeping a record of or charting our behavior and our feelings each day is probably the best way to ensure that we have the data we need to evaluate our progress and revise our plan. Record-keeping is also an effective motivation technique, so making the effort to do this might help us succeed.

▪ *We can help ourselves get started on the date we have set by utilizing a motivational device called a* **self-contract.** A sample self-contract is presented in Figure 2.4 and the self-contract form is provided as an activity at the end of this chapter. Essentially, this is a written promise to ourselves to try for a designated period the action plan we have developed. In a way, it is also a public declaration of our intent, because our helper or support person must read and sign the contract to confirm his or her participation.

Putting our intentions in writing, telling someone else we're going to do something, and asking someone to do something with us are all good ways to get ourselves going. Once we do get underway, asking our support person to help us with what we are trying or to check with us each day to see how we are doing also can be helpful in maintaining our momentum.

Self-contracting is a tool to help you get your plans out of your imagination and into action *now.* It works. You may not need this device to get you started (or to keep you going), but for many of us a tool like this will make the difference between studying the map and actually taking the trip!

Pitfalls to change in Step 3. Preparing and planning to change ourselves step by step is not something most of us want or expect to have to do. We want instant success without too much effort or too much discomfort. We ignore the reality that we may be trying to change behavior we have engaged in for ten to twenty years, which could mean, for example, that we have practiced not exercising between 3,560 and 7,300 times, eating in a certain way between 10,950 and 21,900 times, and smoking (one pack per day) between 73,000 and 146,000 times. We may be disappointed, then, when we expect to eliminate behaviors such as these from our lives in one fell swoop.

In essence, we try to do major surgery on our behavior without preparing for the operation by learning the steps involved in the procedure, whether we should expect discomfort and for how long, and what kind of help or support we will need to get us over the rough spots. We also don't plan how we are going to live without our old behavior, what we will do in its place, or how we will learn these new behaviors. Consequently, many of our behavioral surgeries get canceled or ultimately have to be repeated again and again because the procedure we followed produced only temporary improvement and our old behavior

FIGURE 2.4   Sample self-contract.

A CONTRACT WITH MYSELF

I, _Candy Daley_, hereby declare that I am ready and willing to commit myself to the following goals and activities. I realize that to achieve my long-term goals, I must be willing to work for small gains, I must seek support, and I must be prepared adequately. Therefore, for the next week I resolve to myself to do the following:

1. Long-term goal(s): _Eat more nutritious foods and less junk_

2. Specific goal: During the next week, I plan to: _Have a piece of fruit instead of a candy bar or chips for my afternoon snack when I'm at school on Monday, Tuesday, Wednesday, and Thursday._

3. I will ask my helper to assist me by: _Meeting me at snack time (before class) and bringing or buying something nutritious to eat with me._

4. I realize I can easily avoid fulfilling my action plan by: _Forgetting to take a piece of fruit to school. Buying a candy bar instead of some fruit at school "just for today."_

5. So I plan to avoid doing this by: _Putting a reminder on the refrigerator door and on the notebook I take to school. Meeting my "helper" for snack time someplace away from candy machines and counters._

6. My reward to myself when I fulfill the terms of my action plan each day will be: _Put 50¢ in kitty each day to use for a snack or movie on the weekend._

TODAY'S DATE: _2/22/96_   SIGNATURE: _Candy Daley_
REVIEW DATE: _3/1/96_   HELPER: _Karen Aboutu_

7. Action plan evaluation/revision
   a. After working on my action plan for one week, I found that: _Every day that my helper and I met as planned, I was successful and I saved money and felt pretty good about myself! However, on the day my helper was sick, I bought my usual candy bar. After I ate it, I was sorry I'd done that._

   b. To continue working toward my goal in small steps during the next week, I plan to:

   _✓_ Follow the same action plan because: _Even though I wasn't totally successful my first try, I do think I can do this. I want to try it one more week. If I don't succeed completely this week, I'll cut my goal back to three days per week instead of four so that I can feel fully successful._

   _____ Expand my action plan to include: _____

   _____ Cut back on my original plan for now because: _____

Adapted from *The American Way of Life Need Not Be Hazardous to Your Health* by James Farquhar. Copyright © 1978 by Stanford Alumni Association.

gradually grew back into place. So once again we fall off the pathway to change and into the pit of inaction, concluding that we lack willpower or are not motivated enough, or that we are what we are and can't change.

The truth is that the pathway to lasting change has to be traveled step by step because it requires learning and practicing, not just eliminating. What we must learn are the thoughts and feelings, skills and support systems that predispose, enable, and reinforce us to change—to become who we want to be. The way out of the "pit of inaction" is to learn what you have to do to change yourself and to start doing those things as best you can. Building an action plan and using self-contracts can help you succeed in accomplishing these goals.

The best time to change is always *now*. *Now* gives us the longest time to enjoy the quality of life being the person we want to be. If our current behavior is damaging to life itself, *now* also may give us a longer time to live. If, for some reason, *now* isn't right or possible for you, the next best time is always *as soon as you possibly can.*

SUMMARY

As Prather wrote:

> *Now is the time to take possession of my life, to start the impossible journey to the limits of my aspirations, for the first time to step toward my loveliest dream "If I had only known then what I know now"—but now I know enough to begin.*

The primary focus of this chapter has been a process for changing behavior based on personal analysis of current behavior patterns and taking into account the possible alternatives that might better reflect the person you would like to be. Factors known to influence behavior are discussed in terms of how they predispose, reinforce, and enable you to act one way versus another. Important among these factors are your attitudes, beliefs, and values; the people around you, especially those you care about; your personal skills; and access to needed resources.

The health belief model discussed earlier offers a guideline for developing the beliefs, attitudes, values, reinforcements, and capabilities that can lead to positive change in your life. This model suggests that the pathway to change consists of three basic steps. These steps and the specific actions involved in each are listed in FYI 2. Suggestions for accomplishing these steps, as well as the potential pitfalls that can lead away from successful change, are discussed in the chapter itself.

The Pathway to Change

1. Analyze current behavior:
   a. Keep a behavior diary for at least a week.
   b. Assess current physical and/or psychosocial status.
   c. Project probable long-term impact of current behavior.
   d. Obtain additional information if needed, by reading, talking with others, and making in-depth assessments.
2. Decide how you want to be and begin an action plan:
   a. Write a first-person statement of your goal or how you would like to be.
   b. Begin an action plan by formulating and practicing constructive affirmations.
3. Do what you have to do: Individualize your action plan:
   a. Learn how to progress toward your goal step by step and safely.
   b. Identify a short-term goal you know you can accomplish.
   c. Locate sources of support—person or group.
   d. Stipulate a reward for each day you achieve your goal.
   e. Finalize your action plan:
      - Decide exactly what you will do and when you will start doing it.
      - Visualize the situation, what you will do, and how you will handle obstacles.
      - Use the self-contract to get started.
      - Evaluate your progress and revise your plan accordingly within one to two weeks.

CHOICES IN ACTION

Take this opportunity to look at some behavior you do (or perhaps don't do, but think you should), just to see if a change is really needed. Perhaps you haven't noticed just how much you've changed from the way you'd like to be—or, perhaps your worry about a behavior is unwarranted. These assessments will give you the opportunity to take an honest, informed look at your behavior choices.

First, look back at your responses to Lab 1 and Lab 2. Do those items to which you responded "Don't know" or "Low" indicate areas where a change may be needed? Look again at your lifestyle circle—in which dimensions of life did you rate your level of effort as low?

Next, Lab 3, "A Biographical Sketch 2025+," gives you a chance to envision yourself in the future and thus may help you identify necessary changes in your current behavior. Lab 4, "Tracking and Analyzing Your Behavior," shows you how to monitor and analyze a particular habit or behavior you might want to change. If you do identify a behavior you would like to eliminate, modify, or add to your life, Lab 5, "The Pathway to Change," provides a process for implementing behavior change. Try it out. See how far down the pathway you can get.

REFERENCES

Becker, M. 1974. "The Health Belief Model and Personal Health Behavior." *Health Education Monographs* 2 (4): 409–419.

Braiker, H. 1989. "The Power of Self-Talk." *Psychology Today* 3 (December): 23–29.

Branden, N. 1994. *The Six Pillars of Self-Esteem.* New York: Bantam Books.

Farquhar, J. 1978. *The American Way of Life Need Not Be Hazardous to Your Health.* Reading, MA: Addison-Wesley Publishing.

Fiore, N. 1989. *The Now Habit: A Strategic Program for Overcoming Procrastination and Enjoying Guilt-free Play.* Los Angeles: Jeremy P. Tarcher.

Green, L. et al. 1980. *Health Education Planning: A Diagnostic Approach.* Mountain View, CA: Mayfield Publishing.

Maslow, A. 1968. *Toward a Psychology of Being,* 2d ed. New York: Van Nostrand Reinhold.

Moawad, B. *Increasing Human Effectiveness.* Tempe, AZ: Edge Learning Institute.

Pelletier, K. A. 1994. *Sound Mind, Sound Body.* New York: Simon & Schuster.

Prather, H. 1977. *Notes on Love and Courage.* New York: Doubleday.

Prochaska, J. O., Norcross, J. C., & Diciemente, C. C. 1994. *Changing for Good.* New York: William Morrow and Co.

Smith-Jones, S. 1991. *Choose to Live Peacefully.* Berkeley, CA: Celestial Arts.

Turock, A. 1984. *Getting Physical: Motivate Yourself to Stay Fit.* Seattle: Excel Fitness Publishing.

3

The Major Hazards to Quality Living

Aging and Chronic Disease

✓ Which two categories of disease account for almost seven of ten deaths?

✓ How susceptible are you to these diseases, and what factors can minimize your risk?

✓ How can you maintain vitality and vigor as you get older?

✓ Why do so many people develop disabling conditions such as diabetes, high blood pressure, and arthritis as they grow older?

✓ How can you tell if you are developing these problems, and what can you do about them?

The focus of this book is quality living. In the succeeding chapters, you will encounter much information and many choices that will help you achieve a quality living experience—that is, *doing the things that you want to do with your life*. To begin, however, we must be able to stay alive. We also have to have the functional capability to do the things we want to do. Clearly, aging and disease both present threats to these two necessities. Although most of this text is directed toward maximizing our capacities, we also must give some attention to preventing and avoiding or minimizing the processes of disease and aging, at least to the extent possible given current information.

THE ROLE OF CHOICE

In terms of disease, most deaths and disabling conditions in America today are attributed to cardiovascular disease and cancer. Many other health problems and diseases affect the quality of life for many people, but the prominence of these two diseases demands attention. We need to know which are most likely to be problems for us and what we can do to avoid them, or at least minimize their impact on our lives.

For example, if people would choose not to smoke, almost 160,000 deaths from cancer per year would be eliminated. This represents approximately one-third of all cancer deaths. Another striking example is the lower mortality rate from cardiovascular disease today compared to the early 1960s: 400,000 fewer deaths per year today. The lower rate represents a combination of people's choices and improved medical technology.

When asked, few people say they are looking forward to getting older. Of course, people do not want the alternative either—dying young. Although these statements may seem to be conflicting, they really aren't. We don't want to die young and capable nor do we want to become old and incapable. If we could continue to be capable as the years rolled by, though, we probably wouldn't care how old we were.

The good news is that we have, in effect, found the Fountain of Youth. Actually, it's not a fountain or a magic elixir. It's an active lifestyle with a young-at-heart attitude. It's a way of living that seems to provide a biological status twenty to thirty years younger than our chronological age. A person could be 50 years old but be functionally comparable to an average 25-year-old, or 80 years old but comparable functionally to the average 55-year-old. If you are in your 20s, having the functional capacity of a 55-year-old probably doesn't

seem that appealing, but a person can be impressive at just about any age. For example, about 42% of the runners who finished the 1989 New York Marathon (26 miles) were over 40 years of age. Of these runners, 56 were over age 70 and the oldest finisher was 91!

While being able to do the things you would like to do as you get older is certainly a desirable benefit, today it is becoming a necessity. To remain a viable society, the majority of people in it must be functionally capable. No society can survive with a large number of members who cannot contribute to its well-being. In the United States a growing proportion of citizens are becoming older, increasing the need to remain capable longer.

Average life expectancy, or how long we are likely to live given current rates of disease and accidents, has increased dramatically in this century. In the early 1900s average life expectancy was about 49 years of age, and 1% or less of that lifetime was spent in terminal illness. Today, life expectancy is 75.7 years, with a probable 10% or more of that time spent in terminal illness. Thus, life expectancy has increased 1½ times, but time spent in illness and disability has increased 10 times. With health care costs as they are, this additional time becomes a massive burden to families and society alike. The differential in time has been called the "failure of success." Technology has allowed us to be here longer but not necessarily to truly "live" that long. For society's sake, we also need to extend "active life expectancy," the average time people are able to be active and productive. "Active life" represents the additional time most people really want.

WHAT IS AGING?

Before proceeding, we need an operational definition for **aging.** The aging process refers to all changes that result from the passage of time. In reality, then, aging begins at the moment of conception and lasts until the moment of death. Because this span of time happens to be the same time period referred to as "living," aging is synonymous with living. For research purposes, however, the term has been restricted to post-maturation changes, those that occur during adulthood. The National Institute on Aging uses age 21 as that demarcation—to the shock of many who didn't know they were among the "geriatric set!"

Although positive changes do occur with aging, the basic biological change is one of gradual decline in all body systems, at an average rate of .75 percent to 1 percent per year beginning in the early to mid-20s. This is hard to believe, but the change is so gradual and the body has so much reserve capacity that declines usually don't become evident until the second half of life. This rate of decline is called "average" because research has literally been pouring in to demonstrate that those who choose not to be like the "average" sedentary person also are choosing not to age at the same rate. As we mentioned earlier, genetics does influence how we age and could counterbalance some of the efforts we might make to continue to be highly functional. On the other hand, our behaviors also can influence the impact of genetics.

WHAT IS OLD?

Some people identify a certain chronological age— 70 or 80 or 90—as "old," yet they see an 80-year-old marathoner and say she is so "young." We have learned by observation that people in their 70s, 80s, and 90s generally have lost speed, quickness, strength, and endurance. Because this is what aging involves, these people can be characterized as *old*. The 80-year-old marathoner, on the other hand, exhibits the strength and endurance normally associated with youth. Therefore, this person is thought of as "young."

The concept involved here is not chronological age. It is biological age. Whenever biological function is less than expected or desired, people say, "Well, I must be getting old!" In contrast, when older people demonstrate youthful biological function, we call them "young for their age." When people say "Wouldn't it be great to be young again," they are referring to biologic youth. Few people actually want to be a teenager again, with all those pimples and other problems. What they would like is to have a teenager's biological level of functioning to go along with an older person's intellect and emotional maturity.

THE FOUNTAIN OF YOUTH: HOW TO AGE WITHOUT BEING OLD

If you were to learn of a Fountain of Youth like the one Ponce de Leon searched for, from which you could drink to regain your biological youth, would you? How far would you go to get to that fountain? How much would you pay to drink from it? Your answers will suggest what you are going to do with the news that the Fountain of Youth is real. It's not exactly like the Fountain of Youth people have hoped for previously. It doesn't confer eternal youth or eternal life. What it does offer is the vim, vigor, and vitality to go along with the longevity we have attained and the youthful spirit we apparently carry in our hearts, even into the later years of life.

When he was an older man, Ralph Waldo Emerson said, "Within I do not have wrinkles and used heart, but unspent youth." Goethe is quoted as saying, "Say lively brisk old fellow, white hairs or not, you can still be a lover." Victor Hugo noted, "Winter is on my head but spring is in my heart." These men each wrote of feeling young at heart in an old body. And now we have discovered this Fountain of Youth, so the wisdom and maturity that come with age can be combined with a young spirit and a biological youthfulness.

How or where do you get this biological youthfulness? The answer is simple: from yourself. You build this Fountain of Youth. It's a do-it-yourself construction project. What you are really building, of course, is *you*—the most you can be at any successive age. The discussion that follows here about the Biomarkers of Aging provides a blueprint for building this fountain of youth. And you can customize the blueprint into a design that best fits you and your goals in life.

CHALLENGING THE BIOMARKERS OF AGING

A number of biological functions and features are widely recognized as biomarkers or reflectors of aging. The most prominent of these are muscle mass, strength, percent body fat, basal metabolic rate, aerobic capacity, blood cholesterol, blood pressure, glucose (blood sugar) tolerance, bone density, immune function, and intellectual capacity. In reading further, you will learn that the major building blocks for your personal fountain of youth are exercise and nutrition, combined with a youthful spirit. In this case, a youthful spirit means continuing enthusiasm for living, a mature but young heart. Very importantly, it will become clear that no matter how old you are now—20, 50, 80—you can begin to build your fountain of youth.

Muscle Mass, Strength, and Body Fat

Between ages 20 and 70, men and women both lose an average of about 30% of their total muscle cells. That's about 6–7 pounds of lean mass per decade. This leaves a person with an ever-increasing percent body fat. Strength also decreases by 30% to 50% in various muscle groups.

Studies now show that people who want to maintain, regain, or improve their strength, even into their 80s and 90s, can do so with exciting success. Researchers have reported that:

1. Men in their 60s and 70s who strength-trained developed muscles as strong and as large as those of 20-year-olds.

2. Older people (60–90 years) have achieved the same strength and muscle mass gains as younger people when both age groups trained at the same intensity (these gains averaged 175% in strength and 9% in muscle mass or size).

3. Even nursing home residents, with an average age of 87, who did strength training for their legs more than doubled their strength (113% increase), increased their walking speed by 12%, and increased their ability to climb stairs by 30%.

We are never too old to become stronger. It's more a matter of choosing to do strength exercises than a matter of being young or old.

Basal Metabolic Rate (BMR)*

Basal metabolic rate (BMR) is the rate at which the body spends calories for basic functions such as breathing and pumping blood. BMR declines about 2–3 percent per decade starting in the 20s. Basically, this means the body will need about 100 fewer calories each day with each passing decade, and that means the average person will have a more difficult time controlling weight. This is especially the case as "eat more and do less" rather than "do more and eat less" tends to describe the average aging American. For those who choose to maintain or improve their muscle mass, however, the problem of weight gain diminishes because muscle cells use more calories than fat cells and also because exercising uses more calories than being sedentary.

Maintaining or improving muscle mass also helps with another problem that seems to plague the average aging American: being able to eat enough calories to get enough vitamins and minerals without gaining a lot of weight. Eating fewer than 1500 calories a day (some say 1200) does not allow a person to get the daily recommended nutrients, let alone the quantities of antioxidants being discussed today (see Chapter 8 for a further discussion of antioxidants).

Muscle mass and exercise combine to allow more calories, and thus more vitamins and minerals, to be eaten without weight gain. Keeping weight (% body fat) from becoming excessive also means less risk for cardiovascular disease, cancer, and diabetes, as we will point out later in the chapter.

Aerobic Capacity

Aerobic capacity is the capability of the lungs, heart, and blood vessels to take in and deliver sufficient oxygen for muscles to use for sustained physical activity, whether to do work or to have fun. The aerobic capacity of the average sedentary person begins to decline in the 30s and may fall 40 to 60% by the 70s. Those who remain active decline only half as much or even less. In one study of men who exercised regularly between the ages of 50 and 70 versus men who did not exercise during this time, aerobic capacity declined 13% and 41%, respectively! Differences such as this between active and inactive individuals have been observed repeatedly. The active person can be half as old as an average person of the same age in terms of ability to do physical work or play.

Several benefits of exercise and good nutrition make this possible. As already stated, exercise can make muscles stronger. In this case, a stronger heart muscle can pump more blood and a stronger diaphragm and intercostal (between the ribs) muscles can bring in more air. Blood vessels that aren't narrowed and clogged up with fatty deposits can deliver the most blood to muscles. The sedentary lifestyle and typically high-fat diet of Americans promote fatty deposits on vessels, whereas an active lifestyle and a low-fat diet tend to decrease this problem. Specifically, exercise increases high-density lipoprotein (HDL) cholesterol (the "good" or protective cholesterol) in the blood. Exercise also helps to lower body fat, and lowering body fat tends to increase HDLs. In addition, a low-fat diet tends to decrease low-density lipoprotein (LDL) cholesterol (the "bad" or fatty-deposit-promoting cholesterol) in the blood. The higher HDL level and lower LDL level decrease the risk for cardiovascular disease, especially heart attack. More information on HDLs and LDLs is offered later in this chapter.

Blood Pressure

Exercise and diet also can combine to lower high blood pressure, which tends to increase with age. Increasing stiffness in the walls of arteries (arterial stiffness) has been considered a natural part of aging and contributes to higher blood pressure. Recent studies show that rigorous exercise may lessen arterial stiffness by as much as 30%. Also, most studies examining the impact of exercise on high blood pressure report an average decrease of 10 points in both systolic and diastolic pressures (the top and bottom numbers of the blood pressure reading).

*BMR is gradually being replaced by the term *resting energy expenditure* (REE), used later in this book.

Taking off weight also helps to lower blood pressure, and exercise and diet both are critical to weight loss. Further, a diet that is adequate in potassium and calcium and lower in salt also contributes to normal blood pressure levels. High blood pressure (hypertension) is discussed in more detail later in this chapter.

Glucose Tolerance

Glucose tolerance, the body's ability to process glucose, or blood sugar, is another function that has been thought to decline with age beginning in the mid-40s. The cells seem to lose their sensitivity to insulin, the hormone that facilitates movement of glucose from the blood into the cells. If this decline becomes severe enough, the condition is called adult onset diabetes, or Type II diabetes.

Now this decline is associated strongly with inactivity and overweight rather than age itself. Exercising and maintaining or improving muscle mass while minimizing increases in body fat seem to enhance cell sensitivity to insulin and minimize or prevent declines in this system.

Bone Density Loss

Yet another biomarker of aging that can be minimized by exercise and diet is loss of bone density. Men and women alike begin to lose bone density in their 30s at an average rate of 1% per year. The rate of loss for women is greater than for men and more than doubles after menopause. The serious problem of osteoporosis develops if bone density loss becomes so great that bones are fractured easily.

Weight-bearing exercise such as walking, stair-stepping, and weight lifting have been found to minimize bone loss and even to increase bone density in some cases. A diet rich in vitamins and minerals, especially calcium, contributes to maximal bone density through the mid-20s and then helps to minimize losses from the 30s on. A more extensive discussion on preventing osteoporosis appears later in this chapter.

Immune Function

A decline in immune response with age is a very important biomarker. This leaves us more susceptible to infections of all kinds and also to cancer. Certainly, nutrition is crucial in maintaining immune function, as the body cannot form immune bodies without the necessary resources that nutrients provide. In addition, exercise seems to enhance immunity, especially if it is done regularly. Immune bodies are supposed to attack and destroy all foreign invaders and abnormal cells such as cancer cells. Several recent studies involving thousands of people have shown that exercise decreases the risk for cancer, especially colorectal, breast, and lung cancers.

Intellectual/Brain Function

A most common attribution to aging is "slowing down," especially in terms of reaction time and intellectual function. Although the transmission speed of nerve impulses does decline about 10% with age, exercise seems to minimize this loss, or at least its impact. For example, older people who exercise have much better reaction times than their sedentary counterparts.

In terms of intellectual function, again both exercise and nutrition play vital roles in maintaining blood flow of oxygen and nutrients to the brain. To function at its best, the brain must have adequate oxygen and nutrients all of the time. To date, most of the physiological evidence of the impact of exercise on brain function comes from animal studies. These studies show increases in speed of nerve conduction, in memory and learning, in neurotransmitters (brain chemicals that transfer impulses among and between brain cells), and in blood supply. All of these increases enhance intellectual function. Evidence exists that older people who exercise tend to perform better than sedentary peers on tests of cognitive function. Keeping the brain stimulated via exercise, problem solving, creative expression, and the like seems to be critical in maintaining intellectual acuity.

Aside from providing stimulation, exercise is a major stress-reduction technique. Therefore, anyone who exercises regularly also gets regular doses of stress reduction, which in itself can help a person think more clearly.

STAYING ALIVE

Exercise has a huge impact on staying alive, as shown graphically in Figure 3.1. Men and women alike have markedly lower mortality rates when they are at least moderately fit, even if they are smokers, have high blood pressure, or have high blood cholesterol. Spending just 1000–2000 calories per week doing anything active—playing ping-pong, strolling through the park, washing the car—will increase your chances significantly of staying alive, and the impact of this becomes more powerful the older you get.

FIGURE
3.1

The effect of various levels of fitness on death rate. By looking at this graph, you can compare the mortality rates of persons with varying levels of fitness. For example, in comparing all-cause deaths for men, you can see that men who have a low level of fitness (a) have a relative mortality rate approximately three times that of men who have high levels of fitness (b).

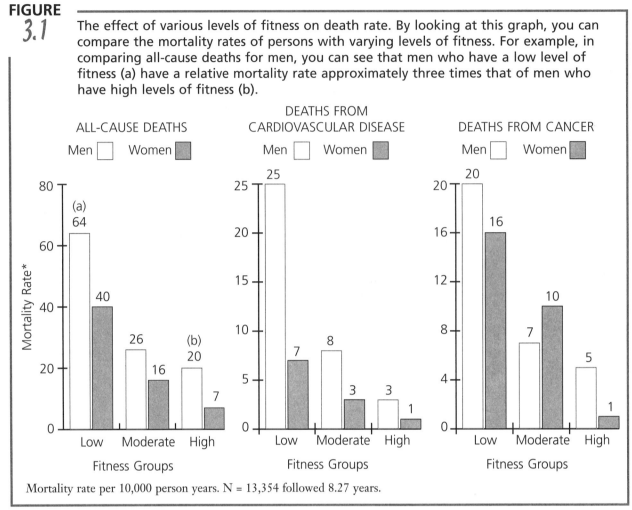

Mortality rate per 10,000 person years. N = 13,354 followed 8.27 years.

Adapted from *Exercise and Physical Fitness*, Gary A. Klug and Janice Lettunich. Dushkin Publishing Group, Guilford, CT, 1992 and S. Blair et al., "Physical Fitness and All-Cause Mortality." *JAMA*. Nov. 3, 1989, pp. 2395-2401.

Next to choosing not to smoke, no one behavior, no choice has more impact on staying alive than exercise does. Exercise also is the most influential behavior for maintaining vigor while one is alive.

Certainly, many other choices contribute to wellness, including practicing good nutrition, not using dangerous drugs, avoiding exposure to the sun, and protecting yourself from disease agents and the possibility of violent assault. There is no question, though, that the foundation of the Fountain of Youth is exercise, being active, "moving it," a lot or a little, but "moving it."

The impact of exercise on the body's ability to function versus typical aging changes is shown in Figure 3.2, which reflects the preceding discussion. The message is not that exercise prevents aging; at present, aging can't be prevented. Nonetheless, exercise can preserve and promote the vim and vigor that everyone would like to have to go along with those additional 25 years of life expectancy gained during this century.

USE IT OR LOSE IT

The body thrives on use. "Use it or lose it" is an appropriate expectation about aging. Explaining any functional decline you may observe or think you observe as "I must be getting old" is an attitude that's getting old itself. The new way of thinking is to "move it," to expand it, to become more, to grow, and to build a fountain of youth for yourself. As Dylan Thomas wrote, "Do not go gentle into that good night. Old age should burn and rave at close of day. Rage, rage against the dying of the light," or in the spirit of this discussion, "choose, choose to keep the light alive."

In Chapters 4, 5, 6, and 7 you will find more information about how to exercise to achieve the health benefits you want. The nutritional choices that can help minimize aging changes and decrease susceptibility to diseases are discussed in Chapters 8 and 9. Ways to protect yourself from disease, drugs, violence, and stress are presented in Chapters 10, 11, and 12.

FIGURE

3.2   Exercise as a counterbalance to aging.

EFFECT OF AGING		EFFECT OF EXERCISE
↓	1. Overall physical working capacity (ability of cells to use oxygen)	↑
↓	2. Muscle tone and strength	↑
↓	3. Flexibility	↑
	4. Cardiovascular efficiency	
↓	a. Heart-pumping capacity	↑
↓	b. Unobstructed and pliant blood vessels	↑
↓	5. Respiratory efficiency	↑
↓	6. Caloric expenditure	↑
↑	7. Susceptibility to cardiovascular disease	↓
↑	8. Susceptibility to intellectual decline	↓
↑	9. Susceptibility to cancer	↓
↑	10. Susceptibility to diabetes (adult-onset)	↓
↑	11. Weight/body fat	↓
↑	12. Reaction time	↓
↑	13. Stress (←) ▪ (→) Stress management	↑

Never Too Late

For those who are older or who already have experienced a life-limiting disease or catastrophe or disabling health problems and may think it is too late to start working on a Fountain of Youth, consider the following people, who prove otherwise.

Marcella in Cincinnati decided at age 86 to begin walking as a way to strengthen her cardiorespiratory system so she might be able to take fewer medications. At age 90 she takes no medications and walks 1-mile distances once or twice a day depending on the weather. To date, her best total distance for one year is 460 miles. She says this is the best she's felt in years.

Ed from Portland, Oregon, returned to his old sport of swimming at age 96, after a 75-year layoff! At age 101 Ed competes in Master's swimming competitions, and he usually wins in his age category!

Forty-five male patients, aged 62–82, who had had heart attacks or bypass surgery subsequently engaged in endurance training. After only three months they had increased their capacity to exercise by an average of 40%.

Diabetics in their 40s and 50s have been able to lower their average blood glucose levels in just seven days by walking briskly 30 minutes each day.

Seventy patients over age 64, all suffering from at least one chronic illness (arthritis, high blood pressure, heart disease, lung disease, and diabetes) attended three exercise sessions per week for four months and achieved significant increases in walking times, flexibility, and muscle strength.

A C T I V I T Y

IS YOUR BODY OLDER THAN YOU ARE?

Your medical age tells you how fast your body is aging. This four-part inventory allows you to find your medical age and compare it with your chronological age. You may be surprised to find your body is aging faster than the years are going by. You may be 37 but have a life expectancy like that of a 50-year-old person.

This inventory is an attempt to predict your life expectancy based on your lifestyle, your family history, and your present health. It compares these data to insurance actuarial tables for your age, sex, and race. But, since actuarial tables are based on norms and not on individuals, exceptions can always be found, like the 100-year-old who attributes his long life to strong cigars and stronger drinks.

If you learn your body is aging faster than it should, you may want to change your lifestyle to improve your chances for living a longer and livelier life.

Note: This inventory is not suitable for persons under 25 years of age or persons known to have coronary heart disease, cancer, emphysema, cirrhosis of the liver, or any similar established disease.

Instructions: If uncertain, leave blank. Place scores (given in parentheses) on lines provided in the + or − columns.

Total the + and − columns and subtract the lower number from the higher to find the total (+ or −) for all sections.

At the end of the appraisal, follow the instructions for calculating your medical age.

1 LIFESTYLE INVENTORY

	+ (plus)	− (minus)

Disposition. Exceptionally good-natured, easy-going (−3); average (0); extremely tense and nervous most of time (+6). ____ ____

Exercise. Physically active employment *or* sedentary job with well-planned exercise program (−12); sedentary with moderate regular exercise (0); sedentary work, no exercise program (+12). ____ ____

Home environment. Unusually pleasant, better than average family life (−6); average (0); unusual tension, family strife common (+9). ____ ____

Job satisfaction. Above average (−3); average (0); discontented (+6). ____ ____

Exposure to air pollution. Substantial (+9). ____ ____

Smoking habits. Nonsmoker (−6); occasional (0); moderate, regular smoking 20 cigarettes, 5 cigars, or 5 pipefuls (+12); heavy smoking, 40 or more cigarettes daily (+24); marijuana frequently (+24). ____ ____

Alcohol habits. None or seldom (−6); moderate with fewer than 2 beers or 8 oz. wine or 2 oz. whiskey or hard liquor daily (+6); heavy, with more than above (+24). ____ ____

Eating habits. Drink skim or low-fat milk only (−3); eat much bulky food (−3); heavy meat (3 times a day) eater (+6); over 2 pats butter daily (+6); over 4 cups coffee/tea/cola daily (+6); usually add salt at table (+6). ____ ____

Auto driving. Regularly less than 20,000 miles annually and always wear seat belt (−3); regularly less than 20,000 but belt not always worn (0); more than 20,000 (+12). ____ ____

Drug habits. Use of street drugs (+36). ____ ____

Subtotals

2 PHYSICAL INVENTORY

	+ (plus)	− (minus)

Weight. "Ideal" weight at age 20 was ____. If current weight is more than 20 pounds over that, score (+6) for each 20 pounds. If same as age 20, or less gain than 10 pounds (−3). ____ ____

Blood pressure. Under 40 years, if above 130/80 (+12); over 40 years, if above 140/90 (+12). ____ ____

Cholesterol. Under 40 years, if above 220 (+6); over 40 years, if above 250 (+6). ____ ____

Heart murmur. Not an "innocent" type (+24). ____ ____

Heart murmur with history of rheumatic fever. (+48). ____ ____

Pneumonia. If bacterial pneumonia more than three times in life (+6). ____ ____

Asthma. (+6). ____ ____

Rectal polyps. (+6). ____ ____

Diabetes. Adult onset type (+18). ____ ____

Depressions. Severe, frequent (+12). ____ ____

Regular* medical checkup. Complete (−12); partial (−6). ____ ____

Regular* dental checkup. (−3). ____ ____

Subtotals ____ ____

*"Regular" refers to well people who have thorough medical exams at a minimum according to this age/frequency: 60 and up, every year; 50–60, every 2 years; 40–50, every 3 years; 30–40, every 5 years; 25–30, as required for jobs, insurance, military, college, etc. More frequent medical checkups are recommended by other authorities. Dental exams: twice yearly.

(continued)

A C T I V I T Y

(CONTINUED)

3 FAMILY AND SOCIAL HISTORY INVENTORY

	+ (plus)	− (minus)
Father. If alive and over 68 yrs, for each 5 yrs. above 68 (−3); if alive and under 68 or dead after age 68 (0); if dead of medical causes (not accident) before 68 (+3).	____	____
Mother. If alive and over 73 yrs, for each 5 yrs. above 73 (−3); if alive under 68 or dead after age 68 (0); if dead of medical causes (not accident) before 73 (+3).	____	____
Marital status. If married (0); unmarried and over 40 (+6).	____	____
Home location. Large city (+6); suburb (0); farm or small town (−3).	____	____
Subtotals	____	____

4 FOR WOMEN ONLY

	+ (plus)	− (minus)
Family history of breast cancer in mother or sisters. (+6).	____	____
Examine breasts monthly. (−6).	____	____
Yearly breast exam by physician. (−6).	____	____
Pap smear yearly. (−6).	____	____
Subtotals	____	____

CALCULATIONS

	+ (plus)	− (minus)
Enter totals from Part 1	____	____
Part 2	____	____
Part 3	____	____
Part 4	____	____
Chart total (subtract the lower number from the higher number to find the total for all sections. Use the sign (+ or −) of the higher number).	____	____
Enter current age here.	____	____
Divide chart number by 12 and enter resulting amount with + or − figure here.	____	____
If the figure is +, add to your present age. If it is −, subtract from your present age. The resulting figure is your MEDICAL AGE.	____	____

NOW THAT YOU ARE AWARE of the factors that are hazardous or helpful to your health, you are in a better position to look at your lifestyle and see where changes need to be made, or to pat yourself on the back for taking such good care of yourself.

REMEMBER: You can't change what you inherited. You alone can't change your environment. But *only* you can change your personal health habits and lifestyle.

Adapted from *How To Be Your Own Doctor . . . Sometimes* by Keith W. Sehnert, with Howard Eisenberg. Grosset & Dunlap, New York. Used by permission.

CHRONIC DISEASES

The beginning of health is to know the disease.

Cervantes

Lifespan is the length of time the average person would live if there were no disease or accidents to cause premature death. That length of time is thought to be 85–90 years of age. Because some people live to almost 120 years, maximum life potential is thought to be somewhere around that time. Why then, with all the advancements in modern medicine, is average life expectancy only 75.7 years? What is killing people prematurely, and can anything be done about it? Since the discovery of antibiotics in the early 1940s, infectious diseases have almost disappeared from the list of major causes of death and disability in the United States. Chronic diseases have become the major hazards to our health and longevity. They can't be cured by pills and injections like most infectious diseases; in fact, they have no cures at present.

Chronic diseases develop slowly, often over many years. Once their symptoms appear, they generally become lifelong problems. Currently, the best way to eliminate or minimize their impact on life and health is to prevent or curtail their development. How to do this is not fully clear yet, but many so-called risk factors that seem to increase susceptibility to these diseases have been identified. Eliminating or avoiding as many of these risk factors as possible and thus strengthening functional capacity is the best prescription available today for chronic diseases. No medicine does this; instead, the prescription relies on individual action. In the following pages the behaviors that seem critical to protecting and preserving the quality and length of life are discussed.

Leading Causes of Death

A quick glance at Table 3.A, listing the top 15 causes of death in 1994, reveals that heart disease and cancer are by far the major killers, accounting for exactly 55.6% of all deaths in the United States. Of these two, heart disease stands out as our number one killer, exceeding cancer by more than 1⅓ times. Two other entries among the 15 leading causes of death are blood vessel diseases: stroke and

TABLE

3.A   Leading causes of death in United States, 1994.

ORDER		% OF ALL DEATHS
. . .	All causes	100.0
1	Diseases of heart	32.1
2	Malignant neoplasms, including neoplasms of lymphatic and hematopoietic tissues (cancer)	23.5
3	Cerebrovascular diseases (stroke)	6.8
4	Chronic obstructive pulmonary diseases and allied conditions	4.5
5	Accidents and adverse effects	3.9
. . .	Motor vehicle accidents	1.8
. . .	All other accidents and adverse effects	2.1
6	Pneumonia and influenza	3.6
7	Diabetes mellitus	2.4
8	Human immunodeficiency virus infection (AIDS)	1.8
9	Suicide	1.4
10	Chronic liver disease and cirrhosis	1.1
11	Homicide and legal intervention	1.0
12	Nephritis, nephrotic syndrome, and nephrosis	1.0
13	Septicemia	0.9
14	Atherosclerosis	0.8
15	Certain conditions originating in the perinatal period	0.6
. . .	All other causes	14.5

Data from U. S. Department of Health & Human Services, *Monthly Vital Statistics Report*, Vol 43 #13 (DHHS Pub # (PHS) 96-1120) Oct. 23, 1995.

atherosclerosis, the latter being the most common form of hardening of the arteries. These two diseases accounted for 7.6 percent of all deaths. Although not among the top 15 causes of death, hypertension (.5 percent) and other arterial diseases (1.2 percent) together cause another 1.7 percent of deaths. Thus, heart and blood vessel disease, commonly referred to as cardiovascular disease (CVD), together caused 41.4 percent of all deaths in 1994. That's almost half of all deaths and in numerical terms, that's almost one million. A little-known but important fact about these one million deaths from cardiovascular disease (CVD) is that almost one-sixth, or about 160,000 deaths, occur at ages under 65.

In comparison, cancer causes 23.5% of all deaths, or about 536,860. This number is certainly significant and far exceeds other individual causes of death, but it stands a distant second to CVD in prematurely shortening life. As shown in Table 3.B, however, during the first two-thirds of life, cancer exceeds heart disease on the list of the five leading causes of death.

Why do so many people develop and die from cardiovascular disease and cancer? How do some manage to escape these fates? The answers are not yet clear, but we do know that personal habits and characteristics singly or in combination increase the risk of developing and dying from these diseases. Fortunately, as you will see, some of these risk factors, as they are called, can be reduced or eliminated by individual decision.

Because cardiovascular disease and cancer are the two primary causes of death in the United States, we will explore these diseases in more depth in this chapter, focusing on ways to minimize their presence in our lives. The discussion of cardiovascular disease will be more extensive, however, as it is the number one cause of death in this country and as many of the behaviors that decrease risk of CVD also decrease risk of cancer. Acquired immunodeficiency syndrome (AIDS), the leading cause of death for people aged 35 to 44 and the second leading cause of death for people aged 25 to 34, is covered in Chapter 10.

Cancer

The term **cancer** refers to a large number of diseases that are characterized by the development, uncontrolled growth, and spread (often referred to as metastasis) of abnormal cells. If this growth is not checked, eventually these abnormal cells literally "hog" so much of the nutrient and oxygen supply that normal cells can no longer survive, and death ultimately occurs.

The percent of cancer deaths in 1995 from its various forms is shown in Figure 3.3. By far the most prominent killer is lung cancer, taking an estimated 157,400 lives per year. About 60% of these victims are men, although the number of women dying from lung cancer has been increasing steadily over the years. In 1987, for the first time ever, lung cancer became the number one cancer killer of women, just as it is for men. The large number of male smokers and the increasing number of female smokers explain the prominence of this cancer and the death rates by gender. Cancer of the colon and/or rectum, called colorectal cancer, is the second biggest cause of cancer death and accounts for approximately 55,300 deaths per year. Colon cancer is responsible for the large majority of these deaths. For women, however, annual deaths from colorectal cancer (over 28,000) make it the *third* largest killer. Breast cancer holds second place for women, taking about 46,000 lives each year. For men, prostate cancer is the second biggest killer, causing about 40,000 deaths per year. Colorectal cancer ranks third for men, causing some 27,200 deaths per year.

Although cancer is most noted as a cause of death, it also disables. Not all who develop cancer

TABLE
3.B   Leading causes of death in United States by age group, 1994.

Age group (yrs)	1–14	15–24	25–34	35–44	45–54	55–64	65–74	75–84	85+
Rank order cause of death									
1	accidents (11.7)	accidents (39.0)	accidents (30.7)	HIV disease (44.6)	cancer (143.1)	cancer (430.3)	cancer (882.5)	heart disease (2120.6)	heart disease (6521.3)
2	cancer (2.9)	homicide (21.6)	HIV disease (28.2)	cancer (40.3)	heart disease (109.7)	heart disease (327.6)	heart disease (817.7)	cancer (1375.8)	cancer (1786.8)
3	homicide (1.7)	suicide (14.9)	suicide (16.0)	accidents (30.7)	accidents (27.3)	COPD* (47.0)	COPD* (162.8)	stroke (484.9)	stroke (1609.0)
4	heart disease (1.1)	cancer (4.8)	homicide 15.4	heart disease 30.4	HIV disease (25.9)	stroke (46.2)	stroke (137.6)	COPD* (360.9)	pneumonia & influenza (1043.2)
5	HIV disease† (0.8)	heart disease (2.4)	cancer (12.4)	suicide (15.4)	stroke (17.5)	diabetes (36.7)	diabetes (83.5)	pneumonia & influenza (237.9)	COPD* (512.8)

*Chronic obstructive pulmonary disease.
†Includes "under 1 year" mortality rates.

Note: Numbers in parenthesis indicate the age-specific death rate per 100,000 population based on 10% sample of deaths.

Source: *Monthly Vital Statistics Report*, 43(13). (DHHS Pub #(PHS) 96-1120), Oct. 23, 1995.

die. Today about 2 of 5 people who develop cancer will be alive 5 years after diagnosis. Sixty years ago this rate was only 1 of 5. Currently, more than 8 million living Americans have a history of cancer; 5 million of these were diagnosed 5 or more years ago and have no signs or symptoms today. The remainder still have some evidence of cancer. Thus, cancer also has earned the label of major disabling disease.

Risk Factors for Cancer

The major risk factors for cancer are given in Table 3.C. Not all apply to every form of cancer. The nonmodifiable risk factors for cancer are heredity, gender, race, and age. Modifiable risk factors include smoking and chewing tobacco, exposure to sunlight, diet, exposure to industrial agents and radiation, obesity, stress, and physical inactivity. Of these, tobacco use, exposure to sunlight, and dietary practices have been ranked by specialists as the three most significant factors for development of cancer.

FIGURE
3.3

Cancer cases and deaths — 1995 estimates.

Cancer Deaths by Site and Sex

Male	Female
Lung 95,400 – 33%	Lung 62,000 – 24%
Prostate 40,400 – 14%	Breast 46,000 – 18%
Colon & Rectum 27,200 – 9.4%	Colon & Rectum 28,100 – 11%
Pancreas 13,200 – 4.6%	Ovary 14,500 – 5.6%
Lymphoma 12,820 – 4.4%	Pancreas 13,800 – 5.3%
Leukemia 11,100 – 3.8%	Lymphoma 11,330 – 4.4%
Stomach 8,800 – 3%	Leukemia 9,300 – 3.6%
Esophagus 8,200 – 2.8%	Liver 6,500 – 2.5%
Liver 7,700 – 2.7%	Brain 6,000 – 2.3%
Bladder 7,500 – 2.6%	Uterus 10,700 – 4.1%
Brain 7,300 – 2.5%	Stomach 5,900 – 2.3%
Kidney 7,100 – 2.5%	Multiple Myeloma 5,000 – 2%
Other 15%	Other 15%
All Sites 289,000	All Sites 258,000

Source: *Cancer Facts & Figures*, American Cancer Society, NY, 1995.

TABLE 3.C   Major risk factors for various types of cancer.

NONMODIFIABLE	MODIFIABLE	
Heredity	Tobacco use	— Chewing, smoking, and exposure to smoke
Gender		
Race	Sunlight	— High exposure
Age	Diet	— High intake of alcohol, fat, and foods cured with salt, smoke, or nitrate; low intake of fiber and foods rich in vitamins A and C
	Occupation	— Exposure to industrial agents such as nickel, chromate, asbestos, vinyl chloride, pesticides
	Radiation	— High exposure
	Obesity	
	Stress	
	Physical inactivity	
	Exposure to passive smoking	

From *Cancer Facts and Figures*, American Cancer Society, New York, 1994.

Smoking. Approximately one-third of all cancer deaths are attributed to smoking. That means about 170,000 deaths per year could possibly be prevented if people were to stop smoking.

According to the American Cancer Society, overall cancer mortality actually would have declined 14% over the last 40 years if lung cancer deaths were eliminated. Instead, cancer mortality has risen during this time. Lung cancer deaths have increased approximately 96% in men and 451% in women.

Smoking is considered responsible for 87% of these lung cancers. It's easy to see why stopping smoking and/or avoiding exposure to secondary smoke, or passive smoking, are extremely important choices for protecting yourself from cancer.

Sunlight exposure. Approximately 39% of all new cancer cases each year are skin cancers. That's about 800,000 new cancers. Almost 96%, or 765,900 of these skin cancers are highly curable, which certainly is comforting. Malignant melanoma, however, which accounts for the other 4%, is a very serious skin cancer, responsible for primarily 77% of all skin cancer deaths. The incidence of malignant melanoma has increased 88% since 1973.

Excessive sun exposure is considered to be a major factor in the development of almost all skin cancers, including melanomas. Using sunscreens and wearing protective clothes, especially between 10:00 A.M. and 3:00 P.M. when the sun's rays are the strongest, are ways you can protect yourself from skin cancer. Because sunburns during childhood

are associated with increased risk of melanoma, protecting children from the sun is especially important. The "artificial sun" from tanning booths, by the way, is not 100% safe, as some advertising claims. Ultraviolet rays from any source are dangerous with repeated exposure. The long-term question is "Is a great tan really worth the risk of skin cancer?"

Diet. Dietary practices have been linked to various cancers for a long time. Current studies continue to reinforce previous findings regarding the associations of high-alcohol, high-fat, and low-fiber intake with cancer. New dietary guidelines recommend fruits and vegetables high in antioxidants and other potentially protective substances.

Three or more alcoholic drinks per day increase the risk for cancers of the mouth, larynx, throat, esophagus, and liver. This risk is increased if drinking is accompanied by smoking. New research also suggests a link between alcohol and breast cancer. Several studies have reported a 50% increase in the risk for breast cancer even with just two drinks per day. It appears that alcohol can increase estrogen production, which, over the long term, may increase the risk for breast cancer. This link requires further study before the role of alcohol will become clear, if one exists. For women who are considering beginning drinking or who are evaluating current drinking habits, however, this association deserves some thought.

High-fat diets have been linked to a number of cancers but notably to three of the four top causes of cancer deaths in the United States: colon, breast, and prostate cancers. This is also notable because the average American eats a high-fat diet with more than one-third of daily calories coming from fat. Animal fat, in which saturated fat dominates, seems to be the culprit. Red meat, more than dairy products or fish, has been implicated. Current thinking about the fat–cancer association is that a high-fat diet may not be a cause as much as a contributor to tumors that become aggressive or recurrent. Cutting back on fat in your diet and eating less red meat are choices you can make to protect yourself from cancer.

Low fiber intake has been linked to colon cancer in 29 of 37 studies. Basically, studies have shown that people who eat the most dietary fiber are 40% less likely to develop colon cancer than those who eat the least fiber. Fiber speeds the transit of potentially cancer-causing wastes through the colon and also reduces concentration of these wastes in the colon by increasing the size of stools.

Including more fiber in your diet definitely seems to be protective. This means eating more fruits, vegetables, and grains. Fruits and vegetables, in turn, seem to offer additional protection against cancer via antioxidants such as vitamins C and E, and beta-carotene, as well as folacin, indoles, isoflavones, and a myriad of other substances now being examined. Which of these substances truly offers protection will become clear only with future research. It is abundantly clear, however, that people who consume diets high in fruits and vegetables have a lower risk for cancer, particularly of the lung, colon, prostate, bladder, esophagus, and stomach.

Exposure to chemicals and radiation. Exposure to chemicals or sources of radiation in the environment has been linked to various forms of cancer. The degree of risk depends on the amount of exposure, length of time, and sometimes other lifestyle factors such as smoking. For that reason, clear evidence regarding the specific risk of any particular chemical has been difficult to establish. For example, breast cancer has been linked to exposure to DDT and PCB in some studies but not in others.

For self-protection, the best choice currently seems to be to limit exposure to known environmental carcinogens such as nickel, chromate, asbestos, vinyl chloride, arsenic, aflatoxins, X-rays, radon and ultraviolet radiation (sun). Until evidence regarding electromagnetic radiation (from microwaves, radios, computers, and so on), toxic wastes and pesticides (at human consumption levels) clearly shows a connection to cancer, our choices are either to ignore these environmental factors or to be careful, but not paranoid.

Obesity. Obesity is clearly associated with the development of some cancers. Specifically, being 40% or more overweight increases the risk of developing cancer of the colon, breast, prostate, gall bladder, ovary, and uterus. The mechanism by which obesity increases vulnerability to these cancers is yet unknown. We do know a lot about weight control, however. (See Chapter 7 for a complete discussion.)

Stress. Growing evidence suggests that high levels of stress also may increase the risk of developing cancer via depression of the immune system. However, some experts believe more data is needed to establish this relationship firmly.

Physical inactivity. Associations between low levels of fitness and incidence of cancer, in particular colon, lung, and breast cancer, have been reported by researchers in the United States and Japan. In both countries, thousands of people were followed for 8 to 21 years, making this new finding particularly noteworthy. Further evidence for the impact of exercise comes from Los Angeles County, California, where the exercise habits of 1,000 women 40 years of age and younger (child-bearing years) were compared with incidence of breast cancer. The risk of breast cancer was 60 percent lower for women who exercised an average of four hours per week. It was 30% lower for women who exercised one to three hours per week. The types of exercise these women reported included individual and team sports, dance or exercise classes, swimming, jogging, and working out at the gym.

The theorized mechanisms of the influence of exercise include altering hormone production, decreasing percent of body fat (either by increased muscle or decreased fat) and reducing stress. Very likely, older women could also experience these exercise benefits, although confirmation of this will await further studies.

The Goal: Early Detection of Cancer

Whereas minimizing the risk factors will help reduce the chances of developing cancer, early detection is the key to surviving it. To detect cancer early, every individual needs to know the warning signs. The seven warning signs of cancer are:

1. Change in bowel or bladder habits
2. A sore that doesn't heal
3. Unusual bleeding or discharge
4. Thickening or lump in breast or elsewhere
5. Indigestion or difficulty in swallowing
6. Obvious change in wart or mole
7. Nagging cough or hoarseness

If you have one of these warning signs, you need to see your doctor or nurse practitioner.

It is also very important to be examined and tested (screened) for specific cancers as recommended by the American Cancer Society and the National Cancer Institute. Early detection screening procedures are particularly important for two reasons: (1) Many people who do not have any of the known risk factors develop cancer, and (2) early detection procedures usually find cancers before warning signs occur.

The specific risk factors, warning signs, and recommended early detection procedures for cancers of the lung, colon/rectum, breast, and prostate are give in Table 3.D. Together these cancers result

TABLE 3.0 Risk factors, warning signs, and early detection procedures for leading causes of cancer.

CANCER SITE	ESTIMATED # OF DEATHS FOR 1995	RISK FACTORS	WARNING SIGNS	EARLY DETECTION PROCEDURES
Lung # 1 cause of all cancer deaths	Total = 157,400 Male = 95,400 Female = 62,000	Smoking, especially 20+ years Exposure to sidestream smoke Exposure to industrial substances (e.g., arsenic and asbestos, especially if smoker) Radiation exposure in occupation, medical treatment, or environment Residential radon exposure, especially if smoker	Persistent cough Sputum streaked with blood Chest pain Recurring pneumonia or bronchitis	Usually not detectable until advanced stages when warning signs occur
Colorectal *(Colon & rectum)* # 2 cause of all cancer deaths # 3 cause of cancer death for men, # 3 cause for women	Total = 55,300 Male = 27,200 Female = 28,100	Personal or family history of polyps of the colon or rectum Inflammatory bowel disease High-fat and/or low-fiber diet	Rectal bleeding Blood in stool Change in bowel habits	Digital rectal exam, annually after age 40 Stool blood slide test, annually after age 50 Proctosigmoidoscopy, every 3–5 years after age 50
Breast # 3 cause of all cancer deaths # 2 cause of cancer deaths for women Not significant cause of death for men	Total = 46,240 Male = 240 Female = 46,000	Over age 40 Personal or close family history of breast cancer Never had children Late age of first live birth Obesity — 40% above normal weight Early age of menarche Late age of menopause	Persistent breast changes (e.g., lump, thickening, swelling, dimpling, skin irritation) Pain, tenderness of the nipple, nipple discharge	Monthly breast self-examination for women after age 20 Professional breast exam every 3 years for women 20–40, yearly for those over 40 A screening mammogram by age 40 Mammogram every 1–2 years for women age 40–49, yearly for women 50 and older
Prostate # 2 cause of death for men	Male = 40,400	Over age 65 Being NW European or North American Being African-American Possibly dietary fat Industrial exposure to cadmium	Weak or interrupted flow of urine Inability to urinate or difficulty in starting/stopping urine flow Need to urinate frequently, especially at night Blood in urine Burning sensation when urinating Continuing pain in low back, pelvis, upper thighs	Annual rectal exam after age 40 Annual prostate-specific antigen (PSA) blood test at age 50 and over Possibly prostate ultrasound for high-risk men

Source: From *Cancer Facts and Figures*, American Cancer Society, New York, 1995.

in over half of all cancer deaths. Fortunately, there are good early detection procedures for colorectal, breast, and prostate cancers. No good early detection procedure is available for lung cancer; not smoking or stopping smoking as quickly as possible remain the best protective actions.

Three additional detection procedures can be done at home: breast self-examination, testicular self-examination, and skin self-examination. FYI 2 and FYI 3 show how testicular and breast self-examinations should be done each month. FYI 4 explains the monthly skin self-examination procedure.

You can do many things to protect yourself from cancer. You can choose behaviors that minimize your risk of developing cancer, and you can take the recommended actions to detect it early when it is most treatable. We *can* fight cancer, and more and more people are doing so successfully.

Several of the risk factors for cancer are the same as those for cardiovascular disease: smoking, dietary fat, obesity, stress, and lack of exercise. These modifiable, lifestyle-related risk factors are further discussed in the next section of this chapter on CVD and also throughout the book in the chapters on exercise, diet, and stress management. As you will see, you can make many choices that provide protection from both CVD and cancer.

Cardiovascular Disease

As reported earlier in this chapter, over 59 million Americans, more than one in five, are afflicted with some form of heart or blood vessel disease. Of all deaths each year, almost half are caused by cardiovascular disease. Because it is so lethal, so prevalent, and so hazardous to the length and quality of our lives, this special section on CVD is offered to clarify exactly what these diseases are, how they develop, and what can be done about them.

The potency of various forms of CVD in causing death is identified in Figure 3.4. In the category of heart disease—disorders of the heart and its blood vessels—heart attack is by far the biggest enemy, causing 51.9% of all the deaths from CVD. In second place, but far behind heart attack statistically, is stroke (cerebrovascular disease). As a result of this blood vessel disorder, not enough blood is available to the brain. This leads to dysfunction of the body parts controlled by the affected area of the brain. Stroke accounts for over 15.5% of all deaths from cardiovascular disease.

Heart attack and stroke also fit into the category of major disablers. About 1½ million people have heart attacks each year. Of these, about 1 million survive. The approximate number of heart attack victims still living to date is over 6 million. Likewise, of the approximately half a million people who have strokes every year, about 356,360 survive. More than 3 million survivors of stroke are living today. Although some of these survivors do regain their former quality of life, many are left with disabilities and faced with the task of redefining the term "quality."

Hypertension, better known as high blood pressure, is responsible for 3.9% of deaths from cardiovascular disease, far fewer deaths than caused by heart disease and stroke. Yet, high blood pressure far exceeds heart disease and stroke combined in the number of people living with the condition. More than 50 million Americans have high blood pressure; the combined number of living victims of stroke and heart disease is approximately 14 million. For this reason, high blood pressure is considered more of a disabler than a major cause of death. Even so, high blood pressure is one of the leading causes of heart disease and stroke and is a threat to life and to quality living.

The CVD Process

Although heart attack, stroke, and high blood pressure are the primary manifestations of CVD,

---

Testicular Self-Examination Procedure

Your best hope for early detection of testicular cancer is a simple three-minute monthly self-examination. The best time is after a warm bath or shower, when the scrotal skin is most relaxed.

Roll each testicle gently between the thumb and fingers of both hands. If you find any hard lumps or nodules, you should see your doctor promptly. They may not be malignant, but only your doctor can make the diagnosis.

Following a thorough physical examination, your doctor may perform certain X-ray studies to make the most accurate diagnosis possible.

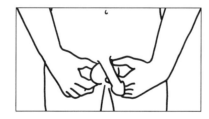

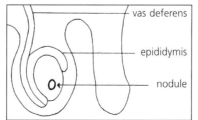

Source: American Cancer Society. "For men only: Testicular cancer and how to do a TSE (a self exam)," No. 2093–LE. New York: Jan. 1990.

Breast Self-Examination (BSE) Procedure

1 In the Shower:

Examine your breasts during bath or shower; fingers glide over wet skin, making it easy to concentrate on the texture underneath.

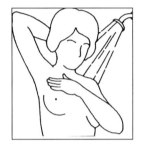

Use the sensitive pads of the middle three fingers and a massaging motion. Move gently over every part of each breast including up into the armpit. Use right hand to examine left breast, left hand for right breast. Check for any lump, hard knot or thickening.

2 Before a Mirror:

Inspect your breasts with arms at your sides. Next, raise your arms high overhead. Look for any changes in contour of each breast such as a swelling, dimpling, puckering, scaling or discoloration of the skin or changes in the nipple.

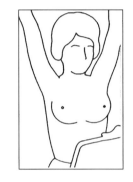

Then rest palms on hips and press down firmly to flex your chest muscles. Bend slightly towards your mirror as you pull your shoulders and elbows forward. You are looking for any change in the shape or contour of your breasts.

Also try clasping hands behind your head and pressing elbows forward to flex the chest muscles. Watch closely in the mirror, looking for any changes.

If you notice any changes, see your doctor without delay. Most breast lumps or changes are not cancer, but only your doctor can make the diagnosis.

3 Lying Down:

To examine your right breast, put a pillow or folded towel under your right shoulder—this distributes breast tissue more evenly on the chest. Place right hand behind your head. If your breasts are large, you may need to use the right hand to hold the breast.

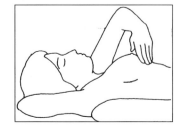

With left hand, fingers flat, use a firm touch and massaging motion to feel for lumps or changes in the breast tissue.

Completely feel all parts of the breast and chest area. Examine the breast tissue that extends toward the shoulder and the tissue between the breast and the armpit.

If using the circular or clock method, begin at the outermost top of your right breast for 12 o'clock, then move to 1 o'clock and so on around the circle back to 12. A ridge of firm tissue in the lower curve of each breast is normal. Gradually work toward the nipple.

Now slowly repeat the procedure on your left breast with a pillow under your left shoulder and left hand behind your head. Compare what you feel in one breast with the other.

BSE REMINDERS

✓ Regularity
Examine the same time each month, a few days after your menstrual period when your breasts are least likely to be lumpy, tender or swollen. If you do not have menstrual periods, BSE should be done on the same day of each month.

✓ Complete Coverage
Examine all of the breast and chest area to cover breast tissue that extends toward the shoulder and up into the armpit. Allow enough time for a complete exam. Compare what you have felt in one breast with the other.

✓ Consistent Pattern
Use the same pattern to feel every part of the breast tissue. Choose the method easiest for you.

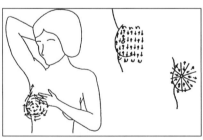

✓ Use of Finger Pads
Use the sensitive pads of the middle three fingers of one hand to examine the opposite breast. Feel for lumps or changes using a massaging motion.

✓ Adequate Pressure
Press firmly enough to feel different breast textures.

Source: "How to Examine Your Breasts," by the American Cancer Society. Reprinted with permission.

Monthly Skin Self-Exam

1. Look for any pale, waxlike, pearly nodule or any red, scaly patch.
2. Look for any molelike growths that increase in size, change color, or break open and bleed easily.
3. Look for moles with the "ABCD" warning signs of melanoma (see illustration).
4. Look for any lesions or sores that do not heal quickly or fully.

Consult your dermatologist *immediately* if any of your moles or pigmented spots exhibit:

Normal mole.

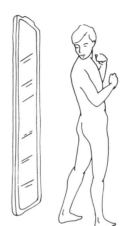

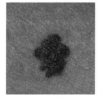

A. **ASYMMETRY**. One half does not match the other half.

1. Examine your body front and back in the mirror, then right and left sides, arms raised.
2. Bend elbows and look carefully at forearms and upper under arms *and* palms.

B. **BORDER IRREGULARITY**. The edges are ragged, notched or blurred.

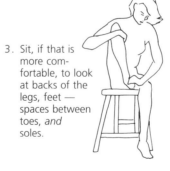

3. Sit, if that is more comfortable, to look at backs of the legs, feet — spaces between toes, *and* soles.

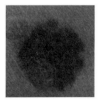

C. **COLOR**. The pigmentation is not uniform. Shades of tan, brown, and black are present. Red, white and blue may add to the mottled appearance.

D. **DIAMETER GREATER THAN 6 MILLIMETERS**. Any sudden or continuing increase in size should be of special concern.

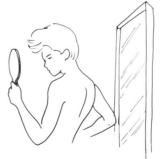

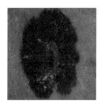

Change in the surface of a mole—scaliness, oozing, bleeding or the appearance of a bump or nodule.

4. Examine back of neck and scalp with the help of a hand mirror, part hair (or use blow dryer) to lift it and give you a closer look.

the most common condition is **arteriosclerosis,** the hardening and narrowing of the arteries that occurs gradually with the passage of time. It happens to a greater or lesser extent to everyone. The most common form of arteriosclerosis is **atherosclerosis,** the gradual accumulation of fat on blood vessel walls. This is the major condition underlying cardiovascular disease. It seems to begin early in life, developing quietly until midlife or later, when it shocks its victims to attention with a heart attack or stroke. Atherosclerosis can become severe earlier than midlife, as autopsies of young American soldiers in the Korean War revealed. These young men, only 18–22 years of age, already had developed extensive fatty deposits on their blood vessels. Men are especially prone to early development of this condition.

In atherosclerosis the walls of arteries become thickened and rough, and the passageway narrowed, all because of fatty deposits, especially cholesterol, calcium, and other cellular debris. When sufficiently hardened into place, this is called fatty plaque. This process can continue to the point of completely occluding or blocking an artery or, at least, narrowing the blood vessel channel so much that movement of blood is difficult, possibly depriving tissues in that area of oxygen. This is called **ischemia,** meaning inadequate blood flow in a certain body area. It usually is accompanied by a great deal of pain. When ischemia exists in the heart, the pain is called **angina pectoris,** meaning pain in the chest. This is a major warning sign for heart disease.

Fatty plaque develops most frequently at points where the arteries branch and blood flow is turbulent. The rough surface of the plaque can cause the blood to clot, obstructing the

FIGURE
3.4 Estimated deaths from cardiovascular diseases in United States by major type of disorder, 1992.

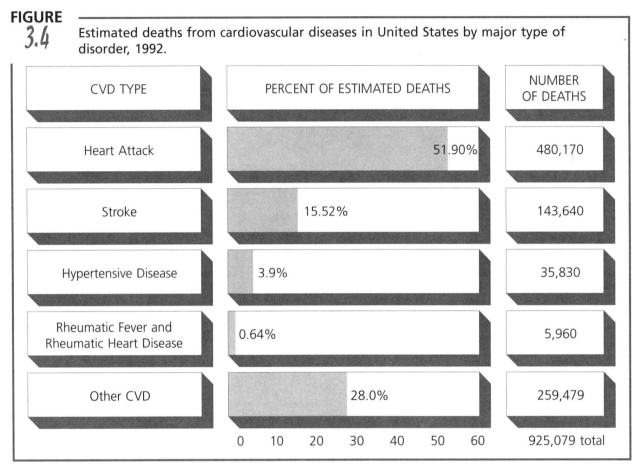

CVD TYPE	PERCENT OF ESTIMATED DEATHS	NUMBER OF DEATHS
Heart Attack	51.90%	480,170
Stroke	15.52%	143,640
Hypertensive Disease	3.9%	35,830
Rheumatic Fever and Rheumatic Heart Disease	0.64%	5,960
Other CVD	28.0%	259,479
	0 10 20 30 40 50 60	925,079 total

Data from *1995 Heart and Stroke Facts*, statistical supplement, American Heart Association, Dallas, 1995.

artery further. A blockage of this sort is called a **thrombus.** It can form quickly, causing sudden, total blockage of an artery. When this happens, the tissue supplied by the artery can't get any oxygen and will become nonfunctional and die if the oxygen supply is not restored quickly. A clot forming in and blocking an artery in the heart is called **coronary thrombosis,** a heart attack. If the clot blocks the coronary artery long enough to cause tissue death, the heart attack is called a **myocardial infarction,** which means death of heart muscle tissue.

The heart does have a back-up network of small blood vessels that may open up as major arteries become blocked gradually or suddenly. If developed adequately, this collateral system can prevent heart damage even if the major coronary arteries do become occluded. This system does not always develop adequately, though. The main stimulus for developing collateral circulation seems to be inadequate tissue oxygenation, or ischemia. Because exercise places more energy demands on the heart and, therefore, on blood flow requirements, some have suggested that regular vigorous exercise might induce collateral circulation. Researchers, however, have failed to confirm this as a consistent benefit of exercise. Vigorous exercise may enhance development of collateral circulation in some people, but there is no guarantee of this result.

Coronary thrombosis is the most common form of heart attack. This same process can occur in the brain, where it is called **cerebral thrombosis,** one form of stroke. Actually a thrombosis can occur anywhere in the body, but these two sites, as statistics show, are the most lethal.

A clot also can form at one spot, be dislodged by the constant flow of blood, and float through the vascular system until it becomes lodged in a vessel too small for it, thereby blocking the vessel. This floating clot, called an **embolism,** can cause the same damage as a thrombus. **Aneurysm** is the term used to describe a section of blood vessel that has bulged or ballooned outward due to tissue injury and/or weakness. Both fatty deposits and high blood pressure (discussed later in this chapter) can cause this extremely dangerous condition to develop. If an aneurysm in the brain or heart ruptures or hemorrhages, the result would be a stroke or heart attack. Figure 3.5 provides illustrations of a thrombus, an embolism, and an aneurysm.

The Role of Cholesterol

Why does all of this happen? What causes atherosclerosis? The answer to these questions isn't complete at this time, but some pieces of the puzzle have been identified. Most clearly connected with atherosclerosis is a high level of fat in the blood, particularly the form of fat called **cholesterol.** It is carried in the blood in combination with several other types of fat and protein. These fat and protein packages are called **lipoproteins.**

Several different lipoprotein carriers of cholesterol have been identified. These are shown in Figure 3.6. One form is called **low-density lipoproteins,** or **LDLs.** This form of lipoproteins is made in the liver for distribution to body cells and contains a large amount of cholesterol. High levels of LDLs are associated with increased atherosclerotic risk of cardiovascular disease. The lower the level of LDLs in the blood, the better. The best way to minimize LDLs in the blood seems to be to eat as little fat as possible, especially saturated fat and cholesterol. Eating more foods rich in antioxidants and soluble fiber is also helpful. In addition, weight training seems to lower LDLs from 5 to 30% in people with high cholesterol levels. The impact for people with normal cholesterol values, however, may not be notable; more studies are needed. Data from the long-term Framingham Heart Study also suggest that exercise and weight loss can help to lower LDLs. How to get more antioxidants and fiber into your diet is discussed in Chapters 8 and 9.

Very low-density lipoproteins, VLDLs, are another form of lipoprotein produced in the liver. These contain even more fat than LDLs, but very little of that fat is cholesterol. Consequently, LDLs are of greater concern. High levels of VLDLs are also undesirable, because about half of these are reformulated eventually into LDLs.

A third form of lipoprotein made by the liver is **high-density lipoprotein,** or **HDL.** This form of lipoprotein actually seems to minimize atherosclerosis. Unlike LDLs and VLDLs, HDLs carry unused cholesterol back to the liver for reuse or disposal. The

FIGURE 3.5 Blood vessel disorders.

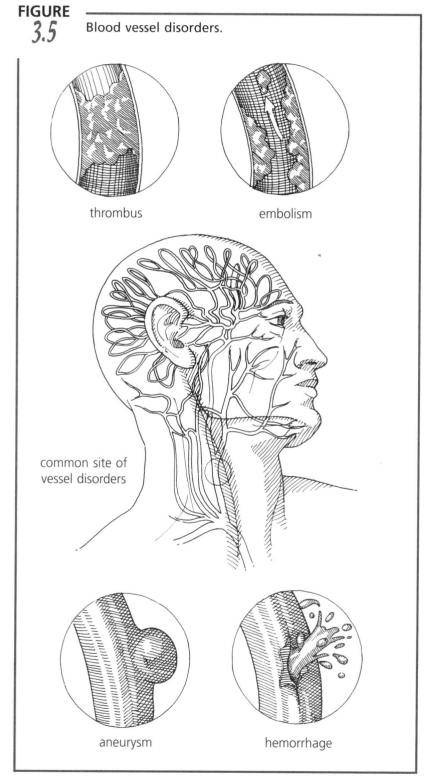

thrombus

embolism

common site of vessel disorders

aneurysm

hemorrhage

FIGURE
3.6   Types of cholesterol-carrying lipoprotein.

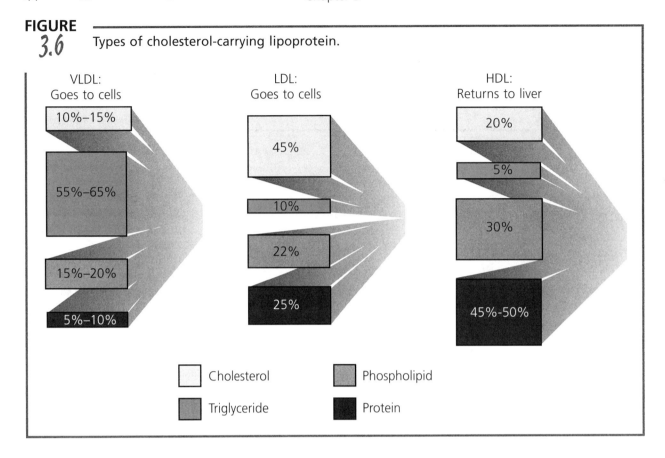

more HDLs in the blood compared to LDLs and VLDLs, the less is the risk of life-threatening atherosclerosis. The best way to raise HDL concentrations in the blood is by frequent, vigorous exercise, although even mild exercise such as gardening or walking on a regular basis can help. Weight training also boosts HDLs some 5 to 10%. Data from the Framingham Heart Study suggest that every milligram increase in HDL decreases the risk of CVD by 2 to 3%. The best way to have naturally higher levels of HDLs is to be a woman. The average level of HDLs for females is 55 mg/dl;* the average for males is 45 mg/dl. Smokers tend to have lower than average HDLs, as do people who carry excess body fat around the waist versus the hips (the apple-shaped body versus the pear-shaped body).

Last, but by no means a substitute for exercise, consuming one or two alcoholic beverages a day increases HDL (this is per day—not 7–14 drinks saved up for Saturday night!). Any more than this actually increases the risk of CVD, cancer, and many other health problems. For women the risks of even small amounts of alcohol may be too great. Alcohol is a potential cause of defects in an unborn child and also may increase the risk for breast cancer.

Because drinking alcohol poses so many potential problems for anyone, drinking is not considered a wise approach to risk reduction for CVD. Nondrinkers are not encouraged to begin drinking just to increase HDLs. Exercise offers a much safer way to accomplish this, and it is just as effective or more so. People who do drink can benefit in terms of HDLs, but *only* if their drinking does not exceed one or two drinks a day.

Some people have high levels of LDLs and VLDLs in their blood because of an inherited tendency to overproduce these substances. Others, who suffer from diabetes, hypothyroidism, and kidney disease, also have high LDLs and VLDLs. All of these people are especially prone to atherosclerosis and probably need to take cholesterol-lowering drugs. Regardless of the reasons—diet, genetics, or secondary diseases—high levels of fat in the blood mean increased risk for atherosclerosis and CVD. Fortunately, there are many choices we can make to reduce this risk.

Risk Factors for Cardiovascular Disease

The four major risk factors for CVD are high blood cholesterol level, high blood pressure, smoking, and physical inactivity. The fortunate thing

*mg/dl = milligrams

about these risk factors is that they are all modifiable: their potential for damage can be increased or decreased depending upon the choices a person makes. In fact, of the 11 risk factors shown in Figure 3.7, only four—heredity, gender, age, and race—cannot be modified.

High blood cholesterol and high blood pressure. As just discussed, high blood cholesterol is prominent in the development of atherosclerosis. For every 1% decrease in total blood cholesterol, there is a 2% to 3% increase in risk of heart attack. High blood pressure also contributes to development of atherosclerosis. It can even damage the heart muscle and blood vessels directly, to the point of insufficiency and hemorrhage. For every one-point drop in diastolic (lower, resting) pressure, the risk for heart attack decreases 2 to 3%. Thus, controlling blood cholesterol and blood pressure levels can reduce CVD risk significantly. (A detailed discussion of high blood pressure is presented in the last section of this chapter.

Smoking. Another risk factor for CVD, cigarette smoking facilitates development of both atherosclerosis and high blood pressure, probably by lowering the HDL level, causing arteries to constrict, and by decreasing the amount of oxygen available to cells from the blood. (The carbon monoxide in smoke is about 210 times more able to combine with the hemoglobin in red blood cells than is oxygen, and thus reduces the oxygen in the smoker's blood.) Indeed, smoking is considered the single most damaging behavior to health and life. Between 20 and 40% of all deaths from cardiovascular disease are directly attributable to smoking. In addition, an estimated 37,000–40,000 nonsmokers die each year because of exposure to other people's smoke. The good news is that three years after quitting smoking, the risk for heart attack is similar to that of people who have never smoked.

Physical inactivity. The link between physical inactivity and CVD has become increasingly clear. For more than 30 years, epidemiological data have shown lower rates of CVD in physically active people. As mentioned previously, the effects of exercise that may help reduce the risk for CVD include elevation of HDLs, loss of excess body fat and weight, reduction of elevated blood pressure, possible stimulation of collateral blood circulation, increased pumping capacity of the heart, and decreased potential for clots to develop. As these benefits are basically the opposite of conditions that seem to promote or characterize the CVD process, including regular physical exercise in one's life is considered the most powerful risk reduction tool we have, next to stopping smoking. Sedentary people who begin a regular exercise program can reduce their risk for heart attack by 35 to 55%.

FIGURE 3.7   Risk factors for cardiovascular disease.

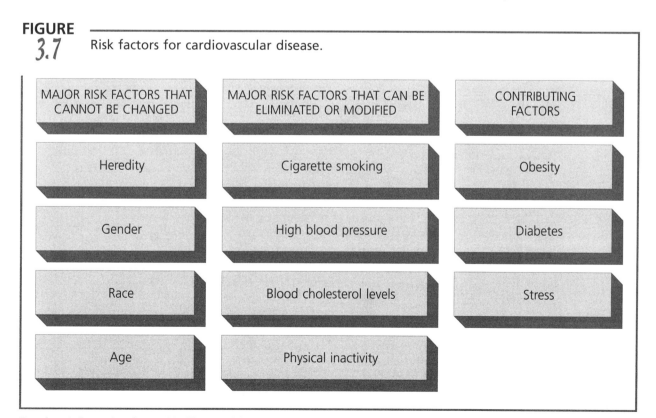

MAJOR RISK FACTORS THAT CANNOT BE CHANGED	MAJOR RISK FACTORS THAT CAN BE ELIMINATED OR MODIFIED	CONTRIBUTING FACTORS
Heredity	Cigarette smoking	Obesity
Gender	High blood pressure	Diabetes
Race	Blood cholesterol levels	Stress
Age	Physical inactivity	

Based on information from *1994 Heart and Stroke Facts,* American Heart Association, Dallas, 1994.

Other risk factors for CVD. Less potent risk factors for CVD are diabetes, obesity, and stress, the so-called contributing factors. Unmanaged diabetics have continuously high fat levels in the blood and, as a result, the incidence of heart attack and stroke is two to six times higher for diabetics. Fortunately, *adult-onset diabetes* usually is controllable by exercise, weight loss, or drugs, in some combination.

Overweight/obesity is recognized as a contributing factor to diabetes and high blood pressure as well as to CVD. Currently, one in three Americans is overweight or obese, a weight status that doubles the risk for CVD. The more overweight, the greater the risk for CVD, so losing even a small amount of weight can be helpful. As noted previously, extra weight around the waist area (the apple-shape) presents more risk for CVD than extra weight elsewhere. To check your "apple" or "pear" status, refer to the activity at the top of this page.

For some time, *stress* has been associated with CVD. At first, the Type A personality was thought to be the link. Type A people have been described as competitive, having a sense of time urgency, striving for achievement, inclined toward aggressiveness or hostility, and suppressive of feelings of fatigue. Most recently the anger-hostility component of the Type A personality has been suggested as the major problem. People who suppress anger seem to be at higher risk for CVD and other illness.

The amount of control or power a person has, or believes to have, has emerged as a major link to high blood pressure and heart attack. For example, when risk factors such as age, race, education, and smoking are controlled statistically, people at the bottom 10 percent of the job scale (performance pressure but no power) have four to five times the risk for heart attack as those at the top 10% of the job scale (performance pressure and a lot of power).

Data from the Framingham Heart Study show that middle-aged men and women who scored highest on a stress scale over a 20-year period were twice as likely to develop high blood pressure as their calmer counterparts. The stress test used in this study is presented as an activity. You might want to check if your current stress experience could be leading you toward high blood pressure. Fortunately, stress management has become a rather well-developed discipline, and you can learn to reduce feelings of stress or deal with them more effectively. Some of the techniques are described in Chapters 11 and 12.

As mentioned earlier, some risk factors for cardiovascular disease are nonmodifiable, things you

A C T I V I T Y

ARE YOU AN "APPLE"?

1. Measure in inches the smallest part of your waist and the widest part of your hips.
2. Divide your waist measurement by your hip measurement.

   .9 or above indicates an apple shape for men.

   .8 or above indicates an apple shape for women.

   An apple-shaped body increases the risk for CVD significantly.

   Results below .9 (men) and .8 (women) are not associated with increased risk of CVD.

can't change. These include heredity, gender, age, and race. Because everyone will find one or more of these risk factors applicable, this situation may seem alarming. Even though you can't change who you are or how old you are, however, you can reduce or eliminate risk factors that *are* modifiable, and thus minimize your overall risk for CVD.

If your parents or other relatives have developed or died from CVD, the inherited tendency to develop those conditions increases. High blood cholesterol levels and high blood pressure are examples of cardiovascular problems that can be related to family history.

In terms of *gender*, the death rate from heart attacks in men is almost 2.5 times that for women between 15 and 45 years of age. Even after menopause, when their death rate from heart attack increases, women don't catch up with men until age 75. The female's higher level of HDL may account for at least some of this disparity.

Race is another variable. The incidence of moderate to severe high blood pressure for African Americans is two to three times higher than for Caucasians. The reason is unknown, but research is beginning to target this factor.

The final nonmodifiable risk factor is age. The longer you live, the more likely you are to die from cardiovascular disease. This is easy to understand, given the atherosclerotic process described earlier. Nonetheless, 45% of all heart attack victims are under the age of 65; 5% are under 40 years of age. One of every five deaths from heart attacks also occurs before age 65. Thus, *young* does not mean *safe* where this risk factor is concerned.

The risk of developing these conditions can be curtailed. How you can do this is discussed in the remaining chapters. That this might be worth your time and effort is suggested by the recent decline

A C T I V I T Y

FRAMINGHAM HEART STUDY STRESS TEST

Answer yes or no:

_____ Are you often troubled by feelings of tenseness, tightness, restlessness, or inability to relax?

_____ Are you often bothered by nervousness or shaking?

_____ Do you have trouble sleeping or falling asleep?

_____ Do you feel you are under a great deal of tension?

_____ Do you often have trouble relaxing?

_____ Do you often have periods of restlessness so you cannot sit for long?

_____ Do you often feel that difficulties piling up are too much for you to handle?

The more times you answer "yes" to the above items, the higher your stress level. In a recent study of middle-aged working men and women, the chance of developing high blood pressure was double for those answering "yes" to at least five of these questions. More studies are needed to determine if this finding holds true for all age groups. You might wish to check your results here by taking the stress tests offered in Chapter 11.

in deaths from heart disease and stroke, the first downward trend ever recorded. The decline is attributable partly to advanced medical techniques, but researchers also have noted that Americans are smoking less, controlling their blood pressure better, exercising more, and lowering their blood cholesterol levels.

As you can see, several of the risk factors for CVD are the same as those for cancer. Smoking, dietary fat, obesity, stress, and lack of exercise are those over which we have some control. Choosing to modify your behavior in these areas decreases your risk for both CVD and cancer. These lifestyle-related risk factors are discussed further in the remainder of the book.

Normalcy Checks for Your Cardiovascular System

How can you determine your status in relation to cardiovascular disease? Are you heading for a heart attack, or are you fairly well-protected from that potential fate? You can calculate your risk by rating your own behavior and personal characteristics using Lab 6, "What's Your Risk of Heart Attack?", in Appendix 9. Actually measuring some of the physiological functions known to indicate cardiovascular risk might give you more precise information. Some of these "normalcy checks" can be self-monitored; others require medical assistance.

The rate and rhythm of your heartbeat is one indicator of heart function. A doctor or nurse practitioner can best evaluate these, but you can at least monitor your pulse rate regularly. Several ways to take your pulse rate are explained in Chapter 5. The average heart beats about 70 times per minute, and the normal range is 60–80 beats per minute. Thus, the heart beats about 100,000 times per day, pumping more than 4,300 gallons of blood throughout the body.

An average heart rate below 60 beats per minute is called **bradycardia,** which simply means a slowed heart rate. People who engage in regular, vigorous exercise are likely to have bradycardia because the heart is stronger than average and can pump more blood with each beat. Thus, the trained heart doesn't have to work so hard to do the job. People who don't exercise regularly and vigorously and have an average heart rate lower than 60 beats per minute may have inherited the tendency or may be in trouble with cardiovascular disease. One sign of the latter is failure of the heart rate to increase appropriately with exercise or emotion. Low heart rate combined with extreme fatigue or faintness, or both, brought on by even mild exercise signals a visit to the doctor.

An average heart rate of 100 or more is called **tachycardia,** a faster heart rate than normal. This may be an inherited trait, but the three most frequent causes of tachycardia are fever, nerve reflexes that stimulate the heart, and toxic conditions in the heart, such as lack of oxygen, overuse of stimulants such as caffeine and nicotine, lack of sleep, anxiety, or some other debilitating condition. Besides increasing the heart rate, these toxic conditions may cause some irregularity in the heart rhythm, called **dysrhythmia.**

Usually the heart maintains a steady rhythm, although deep breathing can cause some fluctuation. Many people who experience dysrhythmia have no detectable cardiovascular problem. Therefore, prudence, not panic, is in order if you detect this in your own pulse rate. Nonetheless, tachycardia and dysrhythmia can be indicators of cardiovascular disease and should be checked by a physician.

Physicians usually use a stethoscope to listen to the heartbeat, but they also could record heartbeat and its rhythm pattern on graph paper. This is called an **electrocardiogram,** or **ECG.** This graph can pinpoint specific areas of the heart that might not be receiving adequate oxygen or might be damaged. Each person's ECG recording has its own unique but normal features, some of which might be considered abnormal for most people. Thus, a baseline ECG should be done *before* experiencing some sort of cardiovascular symptoms. Electrocardiograms taken at rest might be quite normal whereas the exercising ECG is abnormal. Exercise ECGs are not done routinely, however, and they are expensive. You should discuss the need for this test with your physician if you have had any shortness of breath, chest pain, or abnormal heart rhythms while exercising.

Having your blood pressure checked regularly is another normalcy check. You will need some trained assistance to do this, but it can be obtained easily. Free blood pressure screenings are offered frequently in most communities. These screenings usually are announced in newspapers or on television or radio. The health department, Red Cross, Heart Association, local hospital, and senior centers usually have information on where and when screenings might be offered. Some stores, usually pharmacies, have self-testing machines, and you can even purchase blood pressure testing devices to use at home. These usually are easy to use and may give digital readings or printouts, but unless these devices are calibrated properly, their results may not be accurate. If you buy a home unit, make sure it's accurate. Take it with you when you have your blood pressure checked by a trained person at one of the free screenings or at your doctor's office.

The normal standard and ranges for blood pressure and those indicating you are at risk are given in Table 3.E. Systolic readings of 140 or higher and diastolic readings of 90 or more suggest high blood pressure and warrant medical follow-up. An explanation of these pressure readings is provided in the next section.

Monitoring the level of fat in your blood, especially the total amount of cholesterol you have and how much of that is in the form of total cholesterol, HDLs, and LDLs, is an important normalcy check. You can't do this without trained help, and only you can seek that assistance. A fee is charged for this test because it

entails chemical analysis of a sample of your blood. Some hospitals and other health-care organizations now are offering these tests at health fairs for a reduced price.

Average blood cholesterol levels for Americans have dropped from an average of 220 mg/dl in the early 1980s to 205 mg/dl today. That is a significant drop considering that each 1% decrease in cholesterol is associated with a 2% decline in risk for heart attack. Even so, experts estimate that half or more of Americans have cholesterol levels that are too high, putting them at risk for CVD. The National Cholesterol Education Program (NCEP) has the goal of identifying these Americans and directing them (as well as the rest of us) to appropriate medical care or into cholesterol-lowering behaviors. Blood levels of total cholesterol, HDLs, and LDLs that are considered "desirable" or "risky" for CVD are listed in Table 3.F. The blood testing schedule recommended by the NCEP is shown in Table 3.G.

Knowing your total cholesterol, HDLs, and LDLs means you can reduce or regulate them to your benefit through diet, exercise, weight loss,

TABLE 3.E Normal and elevated blood pressure readings.

	SYSTOLIC	DIASTOLIC
Stage 4 hypertension	210 and above	120 and above
Stage 3 hypertension	180–209	110–119
Stage 2 hypertension	160–179	100–109
Stage 1 hypertension	140–159	90–99
High normal	130–139	85–89
Normal	Below 130	Below 85
Lowest risk for CVD	Below 120	Below 80

Key:

High normal—in danger of becoming hypertensive; exercise, diet, and lose weight to stop further increases.

Stage 1 hypertension—Mild risk for CVD; lose excess weight, exercise, and reduce sodium (salt) for 6 months before considering medication.

Stages 2 and 3 hypertension—Moderate to severe risk for CVD; exercise, control diet, and lose weight; in addition, medication is essential.

Stage 4 hypertension—Severe risk for CVD; dangerous condition. Prescribed medication is imperative in addition to all other measures.

Source: *Fifth Report of Joint National Committee in Detection, Evaluation and Treatment of High Blood Pressure*, NIH Pub. # 93–1088, 1993, available from U. S. Government Printing Office, Washington, DC.

smoking cessation, or with prescribed medications, if necessary. The decline in average blood cholesterol levels suggests that Americans are taking those measures in greater numbers. Not knowing, of course, leaves you without any information regarding the level of protection your current lifestyle is providing and if you need to change anything. You can't tell what your blood cholesterol levels are by how you feel. Beginning the recommended blood testing program is an important action to take now.

TABLE 3.F Classification of adult blood cholesterol levels for risk of cardiovascular disease.

CHOLESTEROL COMPONENT	BLOOD VALUES	RISK CLASSIFICATION
Total Cholesterol	Less than 200 mg/dl	Desirable
	200–239 mg/dl	Borderline High/At risk
	Above 240 mg/dl	High/High Risk
HDLs	60 mg/dl or more	Desirable/Protective
	35 or less mg/dl	At risk
LDLs	Less than 130 mg/dl	Desirable
	130–159 mg/dl	Borderline High/At risk
	160 and above	High/High risk

mg/dl = milligrams per deciliter

Source: USDHHS (1993). *National Cholesterol Education Program Second Report of the Expert Panel on Detection, Evaluation, and Treatment of High Blood Cholesterol in Adults (Adult Treatment Panel II)*, National Institutes of Health, National Heart, Lung, and Blood Institute, NIH Pub. No. 93-3096. Washington, DC: U. S. Government Printing Office.

TABLE 3.G Recommended testing schedule for blood cholesterol.

Test for Total Cholesterol and HDLs every 5 years	All adults as long as both values are Desirable
Retest for Total Cholesterol and HDLs every 2 years	If Total Cholesterol is Borderline High but HDL is higher than 35
Immediate test for Total Cholesterol, HDLs and LDLs (Complete lipoprotein profile)	If Total Cholesterol is High & HDL is greater than 35
	If Total Cholesterol is Borderline High or High and HDL is less than 35, especially if there are two or more CVD risk factors (smoking, HBP, diabetes, family history of early heart attack, or if male 45 years or older or if female, 55 years or older)
	If Total Cholesterol is Desirable but HDLs are lower than 35, if male 45 years of age or older, or female 55 years or older

Note: For Desirable, Borderline High, and High values, consult Table 3.F.

Source: USDHHS (1993). *National Cholesterol Education Program Second Report of the Expert Panel on Detection, Evaluation, and Treatment of High Blood Cholesterol in Adults (Adult Treatment Panel II)*, National Institutes of Health, National Heart, Lung, and Blood Institute, NIH Pub. No. 93-3096. Washington, DC: U. S. Government Printing Office.

Major Causes of Disability

Chronic diseases can interfere with the quality of life, causing millions to suffer pain and disability. Most prominent as causes of disability in America are high blood pressure, diabetes, osteoporosis, arthritis, and low back pain. If you find you are susceptible, you might consider the recommendations for protecting yourself. Signs and symptoms of each problem are presented, along with a discussion of customary diagnostic and treatment procedures. You may be able to lessen the severity of any of these problems by early detection and treatment.

High Blood Pressure

Blood pressure is simply the force exerted by the blood against blood vessel walls. On each beat, blood is ejected from the heart and the pressure rises. The level to which it rises is called **systolic pressure.** Between beats the pressure drops slightly; this is called **diastolic pressure.** An air pressure cuff called a *sphygmomanometer* is used to measure these pressures. The units of measure are millimeters of mercury (mmHg).

Systolic pressure normally ranges between 110 and 140 mmHg, and diastolic pressure between 70 and 90 mmHg. The standard norm is 120/80. Blood pressure readings below these ranges usually are not harmful unless dizziness or fainting occurs, which indicates that the blood pressure is so low that blood cannot be pushed upward to the brain in adequate amounts. This eventuality requires medical treatment.

Lower than normal blood pressure in the absence of these symptoms is no cause for worry. It simply means the heart doesn't have to work as hard to circulate an adequate supply of blood for you.

When the arteries that carry the blood from the heart to the cells become narrowed by fatty deposits on the vessel walls or lose their ability to expand to accommodate the blood being pumped by the heart, blood cannot flow through them easily. The heart then must pump more forcefully to push the blood through the arteries, and this creates greater pressure against the blood vessel walls and within the heart itself. If this elevates the blood pressure above 140/90 consistently the individual has high blood pressure. One elevated blood pressure reading is not enough to make this judgment; two or more elevated readings over a period of at least three days are needed before diagnosing high blood pressure.

The danger that high blood pressure creates for the heart and blood vessels can be visualized quickly by recalling the effect of water rushing against stone, such as a waterfall. Over time, the water actually wears grooves in the stone. If the flow is fast enough and hard enough, it may even cut through the rock, breaking it apart. Huge sections of broken-off rock lie at the bottom of Niagara Falls, for example. Constant high blood pressure likewise wears away at the walls of blood vessels and the heart. This tissue injury may become the site of fatty deposits or become a weak spot that balloons out and eventually bursts, causing a hemorrhage. As discussed earlier, aneurysm is the term used to describe a section of blood vessel that has bulged or ballooned outward (see Figure 3.5).

In addition to the wearing or eroding effect, high blood pressure causes the heart, which is a muscle, to become enlarged just as any muscle does when it's subjected to higher than normal work loads. A slightly enlarged heart may be able to do its work quite well, but one that is much enlarged becomes overextended and has difficulty meeting the demands of pumping blood against high pressure.

Why does high blood pressure occur? The answer isn't clear yet. In fact, 90 to 95% of the cases of high blood pressure are called "essential hypertension," meaning "cause unknown." The other 5 to 10% of cases can be attributed to some other underlying disease such as a kidney abnormality. Whatever the cause(s), about one in four Americans has high blood pressure. For African Americans the incidence is two to three times higher than for Caucasians. Thus, race is one of the risk factors for high blood pressure. Increasing age, lack of regular exercise, being overweight, stress, and heredity are also risk factors. Eating too much salt also may increase blood pressure, but this does not seem to be the case for all people. Most recently, an inadequate intake of calcium and potassium has become recognized as possibly facilitating high blood pressure, especially when salt intake is high.

About half of the people who have high blood pressure don't know it. The disease often has no symptoms, although it can produce frequent headaches and feelings of fatigue. Unfortunately, high blood pressure will do its damage regardless of whether symptoms are present. The blood pressure check is a quick and painless process. Once discovered, almost all cases of high blood pressure can be controlled. Normal blood pressure levels can be attained through diet, exercise, and weight loss, or through medications. These measures usually must continue for the remainder of one's life.

Diabetes

Like cardiovascular disease, diabetes has more than one form. Type I, insulin-dependent diabetes, generally affects children and young adults. These people are unable to produce needed amounts of a hormone called insulin. Type II, non-insulin-dependent diabetes, usually occurs in adults over the age of 30 who are overweight. Type II diabetics usually can produce insulin, but the body cannot use it effectively. Type II, or adult-onset diabetes, is the predominant form of diabetes, accounting for approximately 90% of the diabetic population.

Type I diabetes appears suddenly and acutely; Type II develops gradually and may go undetected for a long time. Thus, although an estimated 7 million people are known to have diabetes, an additional 7 million may have it and not know it. Combined, these estimates indicate that diabetes affects about 1 in 20 Americans.

Diabetes is called a metabolic disease because it affects the way the body uses or metabolizes glucose, the digestive end product of foods containing sugars and starches (such as, pasta, potatoes, rice, and cereals). If not enough insulin is available to help move the glucose into cells, it accumulates in the blood. Then, despite the best efforts of the kidneys, whose job it is to make sure that only waste, not nutrients, passes out of the body in urine, the high blood sugar levels may overwhelm it and sugar will end up in the urine. Elevated blood sugar and sugar in the urine are prominent indicators of diabetes.

At this point a second means by which cells can obtain energy begins to operate at an accelerated rate: The body begins to utilize large amounts of fat, a process that produces acids called *ketones*.

These acids also begin to accumulate in the blood and urine. If this process continues long enough without intervention, the diabetic person will lose consciousness and die because the blood has become acidic beyond the body's tolerance.

Diabetes is a serious disease in and of itself, causing about 55,110 deaths annually. You may recall from Table 3.A that it ranks seventh in leading causes of death. When the classification is "diabetes and its complications," however, it becomes the fourth leading cause of death, accounting for some 150,000 lost lives. Diabetes is considered a major disabler rather than a major killer here because these complications are most frequently cardiovascular in nature. Diabetics are two to six times more likely than nondiabetics to have heart attacks and strokes, and 50 to 100 times as likely to have problems with peripheral vascular disease (disease of blood vessels other than in the heart and brain), which sometimes causes gangrene. Because of this, diabetes accounts for half of all the foot and leg amputations performed annually. The high blood fat levels that occur because of the faulty glucose metabolism are one of the primary reasons for the severe cardiovascular complications. In addition to all of this, diabetes is the leading cause of new cases of blindness between ages 25 and 74. It also markedly increases the risk of kidney disease and the frequency of birth defects.

Diabetes is obviously a disease worth avoiding when possible, or detecting and controlling otherwise. Avoiding Type I diabetes is difficult because the cause is unknown. Detection is not difficult because the symptoms are severe; they include frequent urination, excessive thirst, extreme hunger, dramatic weight loss, weakness, and nausea. Controlling Type I diabetes requires daily insulin and careful attention to diet and exercise.

Avoiding Type II diabetes may be possible by controlling weight. An estimated 80%–90% of people diagnosed with Type II diabetes are overweight at the time of diagnosis. Excess body fat seems to decrease cell sensitivity to insulin. On the other hand, exercise increases it. Thus, regular exercise has a double impact with regard to Type II diabetes. It (a) facilitates the body's ability to use insulin and (b) helps to control body weight and fat. Many cases of Type II diabetes might be prevented by regular exercise and weight control. This becomes especially important because none of the other risk factors for Type II diabetes is modifiable. These factors include having diabetic relatives (heredity), being female, being African American or Hispanic or American Indian, and being over 30 years of age.

Symptoms of Type II diabetes can include any of those listed for Type I plus recurrent or hard-to-heal skin sores, recurring gum or bladder infections, drowsiness, blurred vision, itching, and tingling or numbness in hands or feet. These symptoms tend to occur gradually, however, and may be ignored or not recognized as potentially serious. Controlling Type II diabetes may require insulin, but frequently weight loss and management combined with a careful diet and regular exercise are sufficient. Simple as they sound, these measures typically require many changes in long-term habits, which may be difficult. The symptoms or warning signs of Type I and Type II diabetes are highlighted in FYI 5.

Osteoporosis

In 1965 the estimated incidence of osteoporosis was between 12 and 14 million people, about the same as for diabetes. Yet, few people were familiar with the term osteoporosis, much less the disease process, though they may have known that old people had brittle bones that were easily broken or bent, sometimes resulting in a "dowager's hump." Even most doctors accepted this process as an inevitable part of aging. Today the situation is quite different. The estimated incidence of the disease has increased to about 24 million as the older

Warning Signs for Type I and Type II Diabetes

TYPE I
(usually occur suddenly)

frequent urination
excessive thirst
extreme hunger
dramatic weight loss
irritability
weakness and fatigue
nausea and vomiting

TYPE II
(usually occur less suddenly)

any of the Type I symptoms
recurring or hard-to-heal skin,
    gum, or bladder infections
drowsiness
blurred vision
tingling or numbness in hands
    or feet
itching

Source: From *Diabetes Facts and Figures*, American Diabetes Association, Alexandria, VA, 1994.

population has grown in number. As a result, osteoporosis is in the news, on TV, and on people's minds, especially women's minds. Four times as many women as men have osteoporosis, so this fear is well-founded. But men certainly should be aware that osteoporosis is not just a women's disease. One of five osteoporosis victims is male.

The term *osteoporosis* describes the outcome of the disease—porous, empty-looking bone—rather precisely. This result seems to be caused by an imbalance between the rate of bone resorption and bone building. Most people are not aware that bone is a dynamic tissue; it constantly is being restructured, broken down, and reformed. At some time around age 35 the bone rebuilding process begins to fall behind the rate of bone resorption. As a result, bone density and mass start to decline. The rate of loss is greater for women, and this is compounded by the fact that the peak bone mass for women is also much less than for men.

The form of osteoporosis just described is called *senile* ("old age") *osteoporosis*. It affects both men and women, usually over 70 years of age, and typically results in hip fractures. As you might expect from the above description of the disease, women have twice the rate of hip fractures as men. Broken bones are not the only problem osteoporosis presents, however. In older people, hip fractures are often the precipitating event to an overall decline in health.

Post-menopausal osteoporosis affects women only and results from the loss of estrogen following menopause. Besides being a sex hormone, estrogen supports bone growth. This type of osteoporosis affects primarily the spine, causing disintegration of the vertebrae and the classic stooped posture called "dowager's hump." The rate of bone loss following menopause becomes accelerated for 10–15 years and then is thought to slow considerably. Nevertheless, by then the resulting posture collapse may be evident in highly susceptible and untreated women.

Risk factors for osteoporosis are summarized in FYI 6. Being female, Caucasian or Asian, with a slight build (low weight), having a family history of osteoporosis, and undergoing early menopause are risk factors that can't be changed. Nonetheless, calcium intake, alcohol consumption, smoking, and physical inactivity can be modified,

with great success. The skeletal condition scoliosis also can be treated.

Some experts believe that diet and exercise constitute the best means of preventing osteoporosis. Increased calcium intake seems to help in building a bigger bone mass to start with and also in retarding bone loss. Arriving at age 35 with the biggest, strongest bone mass you can grow is one of the best protective strategies. Minimizing intake of substances such as alcohol and caffeine, which enhance calcium excretion, is another helpful measure. Not smoking or stopping smoking is also important because smoking lowers the estrogen content of the blood. Weight-bearing exercise such as fitness walking and exercises using weights seem to be especially valuable.

The negative effect of weightlessness on bone density has been known for some time. Astronauts have been found to lose 3 to 4% of heel bone density within a mere two to three weeks in space. Individuals confined to bed can lose 1% of heel bone and spinal density per week! In favor of weight-bearing exercise, researchers at the University of Wisconsin found that tennis players may have 20 percent greater density in the lumbar spine area (low back) than swimmers do. In another four-year study, women 35–65 years of age who exercised three times per week, 50 minutes per session, retained 75% more arm bone than nonexercising women. Their workout consisted of a 10-minute warm-up, 30 minutes of aerobics, and a 10-minute cool-down period using arm weights.

Weight training by itself has been shown to increase bone density between 2 and 8% over a

Risk Factors for Osteoporosis

Nonmodifiable risks

Age: 45 or older
Female
Race: Caucasians and Asians
Slight build
Low weight
Family history of osteoporosis
Early menopause (before age 45)

Modifiable risks

Low calcium intake
High alcohol consumption (more than two drinks a day)
Smoking
Scoliosis (curvature of spine)
Lack of physical activity
Long-time use of cortisone-type drugs

year. In this case, an effective program would be three workouts per week for 20–30 minutes, ultimately reaching 80 percent maximum effort.

As a caution, overexercising to the point of menstrual cessation, which can happen in severely strenuous training programs, means loss of estrogen and thus bone loss. In one study of young female long-distance runners who had ceased menstruating, bone content of the runners was comparable to that of 52-year-old women. In sum, weight-bearing exercise, but not to excess, seems to be a wise choice to minimize bone loss.

In addition to exercise, **hormone replacement therapy (HRT)** greatly minimizes bone loss in post-menopausal women. Recent studies show that the bone density of post-menopausal women under the age of 75 who are taking estrogen may be as much as 11% higher than that of women who are not taking estrogen. Beyond age 75, the comparison lessens to a difference of 3%, although at least some of this decline is attributed to women who stopped taking estrogen in their later years. When HRT is stopped, bone loss resumes immediately and, some evidence suggests, at an accelerated rate.

Estrogen probably is the single best protector of post-menopausal bone. In addition, studies now are showing that estrogen seems to protect post-menopausal women from cardiovascular disease by keeping blood levels of HDLs (good cholesterol) higher, and thus minimizing fatty deposits on blood vessel walls. Other recent reports indicate that the occurrence of Alzheimer's disease is as much as 40% lower among women who take estrogen.

Although the Osteoporosis Panel created by the National Institutes of Health has endorsed HRT, its use is not without risk. As noted, estrogen has to be taken continually to get its benefits. This means a woman needs to take estrogen from menopause on, possibly 25 to 35 years or more. No one knows the effect of such long-term estrogen intake. Also, HRT may be inappropriate for women with a history (or even a family history) of breast or endometrial cancer, uncontrolled hypertension, thrombophlebitis (inflammation of a vein with formation of blood clots), or fibroid tumors. The combination of progestin and estrogen curtails the risk of endometrial cancer for women who have a uterus.

The bottom line with HRT seems to be that each woman needs to consult with her doctor about her own risk/benefit ratio regarding HRT. In general, the benefits of HRT seem great for the post-menopausal woman, but for some, the risks could be greater.

Detecting osteoporosis before its victims have had bone fractures is progressing into a well-developed science. Although X-rays have not been able to detect bone mineral losses until they have reached 20 to 30%, the newer Dual Energy X-ray Absorptiometry technique (DEXA) is capable of measuring bone mineral density with a high degree of accuracy. This makes it possible to monitor bone mineral status and undertake preventive or corrective therapy before osteoporotic fractures occur. Unfortunately, as DEXA screening (and other similar screening techniques called SPA and DPA) is considered "preventive medicine," many insurance policies will not pay for the test, and therefore it is not available to everyone.

Arthritis

Arthritis is the number one crippling disease in the United States. More than 40 million people have one or more of its forms. Of the more than 100 forms, only three occur with notable frequency: osteoarthritis, rheumatoid arthritis, and gout. Osteoarthritis is by far the most common, causing painful problems for an estimated 16 million Americans. Rheumatoid arthritis, generally a severe form, affects nearly 2½ million people. Slightly fewer than 2 million people, mostly men, have gout. Because of the predominance of osteoarthritis, it is the main focus of this discussion.

The term **arthritis** literally means inflammation of the joint, even though that is not the major symptom in all forms of arthritis (osteoarthritis being a prime example). As shown in Figure 3.8, the ends of the bones in a joint are covered with cartilage that provides a smooth gliding surface between the bones and protects the bone ends from damage. Ligaments and tendons hold the bones together and allow movement in the correct directions. All of these tissues are enclosed in a capsule lined with a special lubricating tissue called the synovial membrane. All forms of arthritis damage this structure, each in its own way. The outcome is a joint that is stiff and painful to move and even touch, sometimes swollen and inflamed, and, ultimately, permanently damaged.

Osteoarthritis has been called a "wear and tear" disease. Everyone who lives long enough develops this problem to some extent, although not everyone will have serious symptoms. Women are affected about twice as often as men. Those who are overweight, who have some imperfections in joint structure, and who have subjected their joints to more than the usual wear are the most likely to develop symptoms of osteoarthritis. Usually, symptoms begin slowly and don't appear before age 40, but severe injury or overuse can hasten the onset.

Basically, osteoarthritis involves a wearing away of the cartilage pads covering the ends of the

FIGURE
3.8 Normal joint structure and joint with osteoarthritic damage.

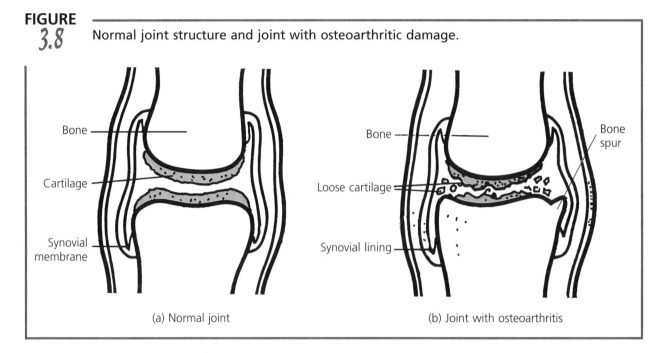

(a) Normal joint   (b) Joint with osteoarthritis

bones in the joint, leaving them unprotected, to be ground away with movement. Because of the irritation, the bone ends may thicken and develop bony growths called "spurs," causing additional irritation. All of this can precipitate considerable pain, especially upon movement. At this point the tendency is to not move the joint. This in turn causes the muscles around the joint to weaken, leaving the joint stiff and hard to move. The weight-bearing joints—hips, knees, feet, neck, and low back areas of the spine—are the most frequent problem sites, although fingers, thumbs, and big toes sometimes show wear, too.

Diagnosing arthritis is often based solely on medical history, symptoms, and general physical condition, although sometimes X-rays and tests of joint fluid may be done to determine the extent of damage and joint involvement. The symptoms that might tell you to take action to save joints from severe damage are listed in FYI 7. The most common of these are joint swelling and morning stiffness, recurrent pain and tenderness in joints, and inability to move a joint normally. If any of these symptoms persists longer than two weeks, a physician should be consulted.

Because so many people have arthritic pain, arthritis "cures" probably constitute one of the biggest quack industries. From copper bracelets to special foods, vitamins, and minerals, a myriad of "cures" exists. In truth, arthritis has no known cure. In lieu of a cure, however, a treatment regimen can be relatively successful if it is followed carefully. Treatment generally calls for a combination of medication, rest, exercise, and methods of joint protection.

The most widely used treatment medication is aspirin, which, in addition to being a pain-reliever, also is an effective anti-inflammatory agent. Other anti-inflammatory medications may be prescribed, but often they are no more effective than aspirin and cost more. Corticosteroid drugs (substances similar to cortisone, a natural body hormone) can offer marked relief from inflammation, but their long-term use can produce serious side effects, so physicians try to use them sparingly.

Regular exercise is extremely important in controlling osteoarthritis. Without it, joints become increasingly stiff and hard to move, and muscles become weak, making the joint even more susceptible to injury. The type of exercise referred to here is gentle exercise; it does not include marathon jogs or strenuous bouts of weight lifting. Gentle exercises increase and maintain joint flexibility and muscle strength without over-stressing the joint. Examples of these exercises are presented in Appendices 1 and 3. Exercise that causes a lot of pain is too much, too hard, and potentially damaging for arthritics and anyone else.

For that matter, carrying too much body weight can be just as stressful to a joint as overexercising it. Weight control, then, is another way to minimize and control arthritis problems.

Low Back Pain

Low back pain is the most common cause of occupational and domestic disability. Eighty percent of Americans will have trouble with low back pain at some time. It is second only to upper respiratory illness as the major cause of office visits to

FYI

Warning Signs for Arthritis

Swelling in one or more joints
Early morning stiffness
Recurring pain or tenderness in
  any joint
Inability to move a joint normally
Obvious redness and warmth
  in a joint

Unexplained weight loss, fever, or
  weakness combined with
  joint pain
Symptoms such as these that last
  more than two weeks

Source: *Arthritis Information: Basic Facts and Answers to Your Questions.* Arthritis Foundation, Atlanta, 1993.

physicians. Low back pain usually affects people between 25 and 60 years of age, but no one is immune. In most cases low back pain without treatment resolves itself within three days to eight weeks.

With so many people affected by low back pain, why don't we hear more about it? Chances are that you have heard about it, only in different terms. Many people use the term *lumbago*, which simply means "pain," to describe a back problem. Others may say their "back is out," they have a "slipped disc," or they have "sciatica." Of these, **sciatica** is the only correct term. It refers to pain in the sciatic nerve, which runs through a large part of the spinal column and into the leg. If this nerve is pressed or squeezed by the spine in some way, severe pain can result. Regarding the other references used to describe back pain, backs don't "go out" and discs don't "slip." In the former case, an actual injury has occurred. More often than not, a muscle has been strained or torn as a result of sudden movement or forceful exertion while the spine is out of alignment. Because so many people have poor posture, this is not rare. The latter condition is not a slipped disc but, rather, a disc (the cushion or pad between vertebrae) that is being squeezed out of shape by abnormal pressure from the spine, or one that actually has ruptured under this pressure.

Pain in the back, most often the low back area, is the main symptom. Other symptoms may be muscle weakness in the extremities (arms and legs), numbness and tingling in the feet or hands, and morning stiffness. Low back pain also can be symptomatic of diseases of the kidney, pancreas, abdomen, or bowel, and of osteoporosis. To have disc abnormalities without back pain is quite possible, as is back pain without any observable reason.

The two conditions that seem to cause most low back problems are: (a) spinal misalignment or poor posture which causes the pelvis to tilt out of position, and (b) weak postural muscles, essentially back, hamstring, and abdominal muscles. Thus, a position such as bending forward to pick up something can be harmful to discs, ligaments, and muscles in the back. In these positions the spine is out of alignment with the body, and weak or overstretched muscles won't be able to support it, especially if any sort of sudden or extra force is exerted.

Faulty posture, then, is the major cause of low back pain. Although poor posture most often is the result of habit and improper weight distribution, it can be inherited. For example, **scoliosis,** a sideways curvature of the spine, is thought to be inherited in most cases. Primary indications of scoliosis are a tilting pelvis and a difference between length of legs, but unless these are noticeable, only X-ray can detect the condition. For many, this condition may not be severe enough to cause great pain, but for others discomfort may be great.

Two other common abnormal curvatures of the spine are related primarily to improper weight distribution and habit. A weight imbalance might be caused by overweight, such as with a "pot belly," but it also can be created by wearing high heels. The abnormal curvature associated with these conditions is called *lordosis*, or swayback. A woman who is nine months pregnant is one of the best illustrations of this condition. The other abnormal curvature, called *kyphosis*, usually is associated with rounded shoulders and a sunken chest. Tall girls often adopt this posture in an attempt to minimize their height.

Diagnosing the immediate source of back pain is not always easy. Often the main clue is what you were doing when pain became severe, if it was sudden in onset, or related to the kinds of work and postures that you've engaged in for years. X-rays may be of some help in detecting degenerative problems in the spine. Special forms of X-ray—the CT scan and magnetic resonance imagery (MRI)—are particularly useful in searching for disc problems. Also, the normality of nerve conduction can be tested by means of an electromyograph.

The best immediate treatment for acute low back pain is spinal manipulation. Osteopaths and chiropractors have training in this technique.

Relief, however, is likely to be short-term. Hot baths or heat may help by relieving muscle tension. Cold is also useful as a pain reliever. The best long-term treatment for low back pain is exercise aimed at strength deficiencies in postural and lifting muscles—the quadriceps, glutei, abdominals, hamstrings, and back muscles. These exercises also constitute one of the best ways to prevent low back pain. Controlling stress and tension as well as body weight are additional measures to help prevent back problems. Finally, maintaining good posture when standing, sitting, and lifting probably is the only way to take full advantage of the benefits offered by the other preventive measures.

DO YOU HAVE A CHOICE?

Almost daily, researchers are finding yet another way that the development, or at least the extent of development, of the major chronic diseases can be minimized by what you do. A summary of the risk factors for these diseases is presented in Table 3.H.

Everyday choices about what to eat, whether to exercise, and how to handle the stress in life are most critical. Indeed, you can do something in one or more of these areas to limit the development or severity of each of the diseases discussed in this chapter.

Table 3.I summarizes the potential impact of your daily choices—what to eat, whether to exercise, how much stress to expose yourself to, how to handle stress—on the diseases that shorten or interfere with our lives. The information in this table should be encouraging to those who wish to have at least some control over the quality of their lives. Many other factors are involved in the development of these diseases about which little is known. Thus we cannot determine comprehensive protective actions. Although freedom from disease cannot be guaranteed, choosing to follow current health guidelines can most certainly minimize your risk and reduce the severity of the major chronic diseases discussed here. You can select a course of action to protect yourself.

TABLE 3.H Modifiable and nonmodifiable risk factors for major chronic diseases.

RISK FACTOR	CVD	CA	HBP	DIABETES	ARTHRITIS	LBP	OSTEO
Nonmodifiable							
Heredity	•	•	•	•	•		•
Race	•	•	•	•			•
Age	•	•	•	•	•		•
Gender	•	•	• (oral contraceptive)	•	•		•
Modifiable							
Smoking	•	•	•				•
HBP	•						
High blood fats	•		•				
Diabetes	•		•				
Obesity	•	•	•	•	•	•	
Lack of exercise	•	•	•	•		•	•
Stress	•	•	•		•	•	
Diet	•	•	•	•	• (gout only)		•

Key: CVD = Cardiovascular disease; CA = Cancer; HBP = High blood pressure; LBP = Low back pain; Osteo = Osteoporosis; • = Factor applicable to this disease

TABLE
3.1   Impact of behavior choices on aging and disease.

CHOICES	EFFECT ON BODY FUNCTIONS*	IMPACT ON AGING/DISEASE**	
Reduce and manage stress	↑ Effectiveness of immune response ↑ CV efficiency ↑ Cellular functioning ↓ Muscle tension/anxiety ↓ Blood fat/stress-related hormones ↓ Intracellular destruction	↓ CVD ↓ Cancer ↓ Diabetes ↓ Aging	↓ HBP ↓ Arthritis ↓ LBP
Recommended exercise: aerobic strength and flexibility	↑ CV efficiency/effectiveness ↑ Bone strength ↑ Metabolism/weight control ↑ Strength and flexibility ↑ Respiratory efficiency ↑ Cellular functioning ↓ Blood fat	↓ CVD ↓ Cancer ↓ Diabetes ↓ Aging	↓ HBP ↓ Arthritis ↓ LBP ↓ Osteo
Recommended dietary practices	↑ Weight/fat control ↑ CV efficiency/effectiveness ↑ Bone strength ↑ GI function ↑ Effectiveness of immune response ↕ Cellular functioning ↓ Blood fat	↓ CVD ↓ Cancer ↓ Diabetes ↓ Aging	↓ HBP ↓ Arthritis ↓ LBP ↓ Osteo

  * ↑ = improve/increase;
    ↓ = decrease;
** ↓ = prevent, delay, minimize

Key: CV = cardiovascular; CVD = cardiovascular disease; HBP = high blood pressure; LBP = low blood pressure;
GI = gastrointestinal; Osteo = osteoporosis

SUMMARY

Aging is defined as changes that occur during adulthood as a result of the passage of time. The basic trend of these changes, in terms of body functioning, is gradual decline, with some functions aging more rapidly than others. Changes in muscle mass and strength, body fat, BMR, aerobic capacity, glucose tolerance, blood cholesterol, blood pressure, immune function, and intellectual capacity are considered major biomarkers of aging. Susceptibility to disease tends to increase with age also.

Nonetheless, as much as half of the decline in function generally attributed to aging may actually result from disuse. Current research suggests that by following a program of regular vigorous exercise and consuming a quality diet, a person 60–70 years of age could have the functional capacities or biological age of someone 20–30 years younger. Exercise and diet also are significant factors in combating susceptibility to disease. In addition, managing stress constructively seems to minimize immune system dysfunction and susceptibility to

disease. The extent to which one experiences loss of function with age, then, is determined, at least in part, by daily choices in the areas of exercise, diet, and stress management.

Chronic diseases have become the major threat to the health and longevity of Americans. Cardiovascular disease and cancer together account for over 65% of all deaths in the United States. Cardiovascular disease is by far the most prominent of these, being responsible for almost 42% of all deaths. High blood pressure and diabetes are also noteworthy as causes of death, but they affect the greatest number of people as risk factors for heart disease and as disabling conditions. Additional major causes of disability for Americans are osteoporosis, arthritis, and low back pain.

As the number one killer/disabler of Americans, cardiovascular disease (CVD) warrants special attention. The gradual accumulation of fat on blood vessel walls, called atherosclerosis, is the most common underlying cause of cardiovascular problems. When this condition becomes severe enough, ischemia and thrombus can occur, both of which can result in heart attack and stroke. High cholesterol levels in the blood, especially in the form of low-density lipoproteins (LDLs) are associated most prominently with the development of atherosclerosis. Smoking and high blood pressure are also high on the list of risk factors for cardiovascular disease. As fatty deposits on blood vessels can be detected only with complicated, expensive, and potentially dangerous procedures, monitoring basic indicators of cardiovascular functioning can be critical to health and life itself. These basic indicators include heart rate and rhythm, ECG, blood pressure, and blood fat levels, especially cholesterol in its various forms.

Chronic diseases develop slowly, often over many years, but once their symptoms appear, they usually become lifelong problems. Currently the best way to minimize their impact on the quality and length of life is to avoid or limit exposure to factors known to increase susceptibility to these diseases. Although some risk factors, such as heredity, gender, age, and race, are not modifiable, others can be influenced directly by lifestyle choices. Modifiable risk factors include smoking, high blood pressure, high levels of fat in the blood, diabetes, lack of exercise, obesity, diet, and stress.

In terms of aging and chronic diseases, how you choose to live today can have a major influence on how you will live in the future.

CHOICES IN ACTION

Several laboratories are associated with the material in this chapter. Labs 6–8 in Appendix 9 ("What's Your Risk of Heart Attack?," "Cancer: Assessing Your Risk," and "Are You at Risk For Diabetes?") will allow you to assess your risk for these major conditions. Most important, these assessments will suggest what you can do to lower your risk of being limited by these major challenges to your health and quality living.

If you completed the activity "Is Your Body Older Than You Are?" in this chapter, you determined your body's age relative to your chronological age. One of the most potent factors affecting body age and longevity is the amount of exercise you choose to engage in. Lab 9, "Exercise, Health, and Longevity," gives you the opportunity to determine if you are spending enough calories in one week doing active things to maximize your potential length of life. Lab 10, "What Am I Using/What Am I Losing?," provides a worksheet for recording how much you exercise various parts of the body critical to your "get up and go" potential. Use these worksheets to see how well you are doing to maintain and/or repair that biological vigor you would like to have with each successive year.

REFERENCES

"A Lifelong Program to Build Strong Bones." 1993. *University of California, Berkeley Wellness Letter* 9(10): 4–5.

Albanes, D., et al. 1989. "Physical Activity and Risk of Cancer in the NHANES 1 Population." *American Journal of Public Health* 79(6): 744–750.

"Alcohol: A Fine Line for Health." 1994. *Johns Hopkins Medical Letter, Health After 50* 6(8): 4–5.

"Alcohol, Heart Disease, and Mortality." 1989. *Harvard Medical School Health Letter* 14 (May): 7.

American Cancer Society. 1995. *Cancer Facts and Figures–1995 (No. 5008.95).* Atlanta: ACS.

American Cancer Society. 1990. *For Men Only: Testicular Cancer and How to Do TSE (A Self-Exam) (No. 2093-LE).* New York: ACS.

American Cancer Society. 1992. *Special Touch: Mammography, Clinical Exam, Monthly Breast Self-Exam (No. 2095-LE OR).* New York: ACS.

American College of Sports Medicine. 1992. *ACSM Fitness Book.* Champaign, IL: Leisure Press.

American Diabetes Association. 1992. *Diabetes Facts and Figures.* Alexandria: Author.

American Diabetes Association. 1994. *Diabetes Facts.* Alexandria: Author.

American Heart Association. 1994. *Heart and Stroke Facts.* Dallas: Author.

American Heart Association. 1995. *Heart and Stroke Facts: 1995 Statistical Supplement.* Dallas: Author.

"Are We in the Middle of a Cancer Epidemic?" 1994. *University of California, Berkeley Wellness Letter* 10(12): 4–5.

Arthritis Foundation. 1993. *Arthritis Information: Basic Facts and Answers to Your Questions* (No. 400). Atlanta: Author.

Arthritis Foundation. 1990. *Arthritis Information: Exercise and Your Arthritis.* Atlanta: Author.

Blair, S. N., et al. 1992. "Physical Activity and Health: A Lifestyle Approach." *Medicine, Exercise, Nutrition, and Health* 1: 54–57.

Blair, S., et al. 1989. "Physical Fitness and All-Cause Mortality. A Prospective Study of Healthy Men and Women." *Journal of the American Medical Association* 262: 2395–2401.

Blum, C. B., et al. 1987. "Role of Dietary Intervention in the Primary Prevention of Coronary Heart Disease." *Cardiology* 74: 2–21.

"Breast Cancer and Pollutants." 1994. *American Health* (July/Aug.): 25.

Chase, J. A. 1992. "Outpatient Management of Low Back Pain." *Orthopaedic Nursing* 11(1): 11–20.

"Cholesterol: Making Sense of the New Guidelines." 1994. *Johns Hopkins Medical Letter, Health After 50* 6(4): 4–6.

"Cholesterol: New Advice." 1993. *University of California, Berkeley Wellness Letter* 10(3): 4–6.

Cooper, K. 1988. *Controlling Cholesterol.* New York: Bantam Books.

"Cutting Your Risk of Colon Cancer." 1994. *Consumer Reports on Health* 6: 55–58.

Deyo, R. A., et al. 1992. "What Can the History and Physical Examination Tell Us About Low Back Pain?" *Journal of the American Medical Association* 268(6): 760–765.

Evans, W., and I. Rosenberg. 1991. *Biomarkers.* New York: Simon & Schuster.

Fiatarone, M. A., et al. 1990. "High-Intensity Strength Training in Nonagenarians: Effects on Skeletal Muscle." *Journal of the American Medical Association* 263(22): 3029–3034.

Fiatarone, M. A., et al. 1994. "Exercise Training and Nutritional Supplementation for Physical Frailty in Very Elderly People. *New England Journal of Medicine* 330(25): 1769–1775.

Fernhall, B. 1988–1989. "About Exercise and Longevity." *ARAPCS Newsletter* 10: 1–2.

Food and Nutrition Board. 1989. *Diet and Health: Implications for Reducing Chronic Disease Risk.* Washington, DC: National Academy Press.

"Foods May Reduce Your Risk of Lung Cancer." 1987. *Tufts University Diet and Nutrition Letter* 4(February): 12.

Friedman, M., and D. Ulmer. 1984. *Treating Type Behavior and Your Heart.* New York: Alfred A. Knopf.

Grundy, S. M. 1987. "Dietary Therapy for Different Forms of Hyperlipoproteinemia." *Circulation* 76: 523–528.

Guralnik, J. M., et al. 1989. "Predictors of Healthy Aging: Prospective Evidence from the Alameda County Study." *American Journal of Public Health* 79: 703–708.

Gurtz, T. W., et al. 1987. "'Salt-Sensitive' Essential Hypertension in Men: Is the Sodium Ion Alone Important?" *New England Journal of Medicine* 317: 1043–1048.

Hagberg, J. M. 1987. "Effect of Training on the Decline of VO_2 Max with Aging." *Federation Proceedings* 46: 1830–1833.

Hagberg, J. M., et al. 1989. "Effect of Exercise Training in 60- to 69-Year-Old Persons with Essential Hypertension." *American Journal of Cardiology* 64: 348–353.

Hamm, V. P., et al. 1993. "Life-Style and Cardiovascular Health Among Urban Black Elderly." *Journal of Applied Gerontology* 12(2): 155–169.

Harris, T., et al. 1989. "Longitudinal Study of Physical Ability in the Oldest-Old." *American Journal of Public Health* 79: 698–702.

Henry, H., et al. 1985. "Increasing Calcium Intake Lowers Blood Pressure: The Literature Reviewed." *Journal of the American Dietetic Association* 85: 182–185.

"How Can You Tell if You're Having a Heart Attack?" 1988. *University of California Berkeley, Wellness Letter* 4(May): 8.

Kasch, F. W., et al. 1990. "The Effect of Physical Activity and Inactivity on Aerobic Power in Older Men." *Physician and Sportsmedicine* 18: 73–83.

"Keeping Cancer at Bay with Diet." 1994. *Johns Hopkins Medical Letter, Health After 50* 6(2): 1–3.

Klug, G. A., and Lettunich, J. 1992. *Exercise and Physical Fitness.* Guilford, CT: Dushkin Publishing Group.

LaCroix, A. Z., et al. 1993. "Maintaining Mobility in Late Life. *American Journal of Epidemiology* 137(8): 858–869.

Liebman, B. 1990. "The HDL/Triglyceride Trap: An Interview with Wm. Castelli." *Nutrition Action Newsletter* 17: 5–7.

Markovitz, J. H., et al. 1993. "Psychological Predictors of Hypertension in the Framingham Study: Is There Tension in Hypertension?" *Journal of the American Medical Association* 270(20): 2439–2444.

McClung, M. 1990. "Improved Bone Density Testing with Dual-Energy X-Ray Absorptiometry." *Contemporary OB/GYN* (Oct): 1–6.

Murray, R. F. 1991. "Skin Color and Blood Pressure: Genetics or Environment?" *Journal of the American Medical Association* 265(5): 639.

National Osteoporosis Foundation. 1989. *Boning Up on Osteoporosis: A Guide to Prevention and Treatment.* Washington, DC: Author.

"Osteoporosis: No Sex Discrimination." 1994. *Johns Hopkins Medical Letter* 6(1): 3, 8.

"Our Readers Ask: Does Lifting Weights Help Fight the Bone Loss of Osteoporosis?" 1994. *Johns Hopkins Medical Letter, Health After 50* 5, (Jan.): 8.

Paffenbarger, R. S., et al. 1986. "Physical Activity, All-Cause Mortality, and Longevity of College Alumni." *New England Journal of Medicine* 314(10): 605–613.

Paffenbarger, R. S., et al. 1993. "The Association of Changes in Physical-Activity Level and Other Lifestyle Characteristics with Mortality Among Men." *New England Journal of Medicine* 329(8): 538–545.

Pak, C., et al. 1994. "Slow-Release Sodium Fluoride in the Management of Postmenopausal Osteoporosis." *Annals of Internal Medicine* 120(8): 625–632.

Piscopo, J. 1985. *Fitness and Aging.* New York: John Wiley and Sons.

President's Council on Physical Fitness and Sports. 1993. "Physical Fitness and Healthy Low Back Function." *Physical Activity and Fitness Research Digest* 1(3): 1–6.

"Rating Your Risks for Heart Disease." 1994. *University of California, Berkeley Wellness Letter* 10(8): 4–5.

"Rethinking the Diabetic Diet: The 'Rules' Ease Up." 1994. *Tufts University Diet and Nutrition Letter* 12(6): 3–6.

Severson, R., et al. 1989. "A Prospective Analysis of Physical Activity and Cancer." *American Journal of Epidemiology* 130(3): 522–529.

"Should You Take Estrogen to Prevent Osteoporosis?" 1994. *Johns Hopkins Medical Letter, Health After 50* 6(6): 4–5.

Steinberg, D. 1987. "Lipoproteins and the Pathogenesis of Atherosclerosis." *Circulation* 76: 508–514.

Steinmetz, K. A., et al. 1994. "Vegetables, Fruit, and Colon Cancer in the Iowa Women's Health Study." *American Journal of Epidemiology* 139(1): 1–13.

"Stress: The 'Type A' Hypothesis." 1992. *Harvard Heart Letter* 2(5): 1–4.

Tenebaum, G. 1992. "Physical Activity and Psychological Benefits." *Physician and Sportsmedicine* 20: 179–183.

"The Alcohol/Breast Cancer Connection." 1994. *University of California, Berkeley Wellness Letter* 10(6): 1–2.

Topp, R., et al. 1993. "The Effect of a 12-Week Dynamic Resistance Strength Training Program on Gait Velocity and Balance of Older Adults." *Gerontologist* 33(4): 501–506.

U. S. Department of Health and Human Services. 1995. "Annual Summary of Births, Marriages, Divorces, and Deaths: United States, 1994." *Monthly Vital Statistics Report* 43(13): 1–31.

U. S. Department of Health and Human Services. 1993. *The Fifth Report of the Joint National*

Committee on Detection, Evaluation and Treatment of High Blood Pressure. (National Institutes of Health, National Heart, Lung, and Blood Institute, NIH Pub. No. 93-1088). Washington, DC: U. S. Government Printing Office.

U. S. Department of Health and Human Services. 1993. *National Cholesterol Education Program Second Report of the Expert Panel on Detection, Evaluation, and Treatment of High Blood Cholesterol in Adults (Adult Treatment Panel II)* (National Institutes of Health, National Heart, Lung, and Blood Institute, NIH Pub. No. 93-3096). Washington, DC: U. S. Government Printing Office.

U. S. Department of Health and Human Services. 1993. *Research Highlights: Arthritis, Rheumatic Diseases, and Related Disorders.* Washington, DC: National Institutes of Health.

Vaitkevicius, P. V., et al. 1993. "Effects of Age and Aerobic Capacity on Arterial Stiffness in Healthy Adults." *Circulation* 88: 1456–1462.

Whitney, E. N., and S. R. Rolfes. 1993. *Understanding Nutrition.* St. Paul: West Publishing.

Wolf, M. S., et al. 1993. "Blood Levels of Organochlorine Residues and Risk of Breast Cancer." *Journal of National Cancer Institute* 85(8): 648–52.

General Guidelines
for Fitness

✓ What is *fitness,* and what
aspects of fitness relate to
health? To performance?

✓ Why should you know
about overload, progression,
and specificity in training?

✓ How should you organize a typical
exercise session to achieve maximum
benefit?

✓ What should you do if you experience
sore muscles, tendinitis, or other problems
that commonly result from training?

✓ How should you alter your workout
when exercising in the heat? In the cold?
Or if the humidity is high or the air is
polluted?

The term *physical fitness* can mean a variety of things. To a runner, fitness may mean the ability to run 10 kilometers in a given span of time. To a nonathletic person, fitness may mean a trim appearance. To the student, it may refer to both of the above or possibly to the strength or speed needed in a favorite sport. Is the term *fitness* used correctly in all of these contexts? What precisely does fitness mean? This chapter addresses these questions and provides general guidelines for exercising correctly. In addition, we discuss common fitness injuries and environmental problems that you may encounter while training and offer suggestions to help you personalize a fitness program to fit your individual needs.

FITNESS DEFINED

In the broadest sense, **physical fitness** is the capacity to meet the demands of modern-day life with relatively little strain. A physically fit person is able to work and play with ease because of regular and continuing preparation for activity. If an emergency arises, or even a day of nonroutine activity such as skiing or hiking, this individual has the capacity to stretch farther than usual and rise to the occasion. Evidence increasingly confirms that fit people take fewer sick days from work, cutting down on medical expenses. They are more productive, and their quality of life is better than that of unfit people. The economic implications of fitness are enormous if you imagine the number of members of our workforce who potentially could benefit from increased fitness.

To be prepared for any eventuality may sound like an idealistic goal that the average person cannot attain. Before attempting to answer this and other questions, we will describe the components of fitness and discuss several important generalizations about methods to improve fitness.

COMPONENTS OF FITNESS

Fitness encompasses such a wide variety of elements that breaking it into the components shown in Table 4.A is useful. **Health-related fitness** refers to components that are related to health and well-being. These include: (a) cardiorespiratory fitness, (b) body composition, (c) strength and muscular endurance in the major muscle groups, particularly in the abdominal region, and (d) flexibility of the low back and hip region. The remaining components—power, speed, agility, and flexibility in other regions of the body—are components of **performance-related fitness.** All of the health-related components contribute to both health and physical performance. Because the focus of this book is on the aspects of fitness that have significance for everyone, not just the athletically inclined, we will devote more time to the health-related fitness components than to the performance-related fitness components.

Health-Related Fitness

Cardiorespiratory Fitness

Cardiorespiratory fitness refers to the combined abilities of the respiratory and circulatory systems to provide adequate oxygen to muscles during continuous, rhythmic exercise for extended periods of time. Sports events that depend heavily on this component include running, cycling, cross-country skiing, and swimming long distances. Cardiorespiratory fitness also is important for hiking, jogging, and walking, except that in these activities the individuals usually are not taxing themselves maximally. Cardiorespiratory fitness is said to be the most important component of fitness because evidence suggests that activities that promote this form of fitness are associated with a lower incidence of death from all causes (particularly atherosclerosis), with favorable changes in blood lipid profile and enhanced collateral circulation in the heart, as well as other positive changes. The term **aerobic fitness** often is used interchangeably with cardiorespiratory fitness. In Chapter 5 the importance of cardiorespiratory fitness and how it can be measured, improved, and maintained will be discussed in detail.

Body Composition

Body composition refers to the relative amount of fat in the body compared to other tissues. More

TABLE 4.A The components of fitness.

HEALTH-RELATED FITNESS	PERFORMANCE-RELATED FITNESS
Cardiorespiratory (aerobic) fitness	Flexibility of other parts of the body
Body composition	Power
Strength and muscle endurance (particularly in the abdominal muscles)	Speed
Flexibility of the lower back and hip region	Agility

precisely, **fat weight** refers to the weight of all fat deposits in the body and **fat-free weight** to the weight of all the other tissues combined, including muscle, bone, and the various organs. Excess fatness or obesity puts an individual at greater risk for many cardiovascular diseases, for diabetes, and for many other health problems. The topics of weight control and weight loss, as well as methods of measuring body composition, are discussed more fully in Chapter 7.

Strength and Muscle Endurance

Strength is the capacity of a muscle group to exert force under maximal conditions. The greater this capacity, the greater a person's strength is said to be. **Muscle endurance** refers to the ability of a muscle to engage in repetitive exercise for long periods with little fatigue. Sufficient strength and muscle endurance in the major muscles of the body is important in many aspects of health. It can make the difference when it comes to survival in emergencies. Recreational pursuits often require the use of many body parts, particularly the upper body. In daily activities an individual often is required to lift, hold, or carry objects of various sizes, shapes, and weights. Being able to do so without undue stress and strain and without injury can make a big difference in your health and your freedom to do what is asked of you and what you choose to do.

Women typically have relatively lower levels of strength in their upper body than they do in their lower body. This suggests that women in general should engage in a program of regular upper body exercise with a special focus on strength.

Evidence suggests that lower back problems are related strongly to low levels of strength and muscle endurance in the abdominal muscles. The abdominals are one group of **antigravity muscles,** among others, that are responsible for maintaining an upright posture (Figure 4.1). When the abdominals become weak, they permit the pelvic girdle to tilt forward, which puts pressure on the spinal nerves in the lower back region. A protruding belly (Figure 4.2) is evidence of poor alignment in this region, and possibly excessive abdominal fat, and it places the lower back at considerable risk for injury when doing even simple tasks such as bending over.

Flexibility of the Lower Back and Hip Region

Flexibility is the ability of body segments to move through a range of motion. Poor flexibility of the

neck flexors

spinal extensors

abdominals

iliopsoas

gluteus maximus

hamstrings

quadriceps femoris

gastrocnemius and soleus

tibialis anterior

Source: J. N. Barham and E. P. Wooten, *Structural Kinesiology*. Copyright © 1973. All rights reserved. Reprinted by permission of Allyn & Bacon.

spine, particularly in the lower back region, combined with a poor range of motion in the hips, including the tendons and ligaments supporting muscles such as the hamstrings (see Figure 4.1), is also strongly implicated in problems of the lower back region. As mentioned in Chapter 3, low back pain represents one of the most significant ways that individuals become temporarily or chronically disabled. In Chapter 6 we present methods for evaluating flexibility, strength, and muscle endurance and suggest ways to improve each of these fitness components.

FIGURE

4.2   The "protruding belly syndrome" arises from weakened abdominal muscles and/or excessive abdominal fat and allows the pelvic girdle to tilt forward, placing the lower back region at greater risk for pain and injury.

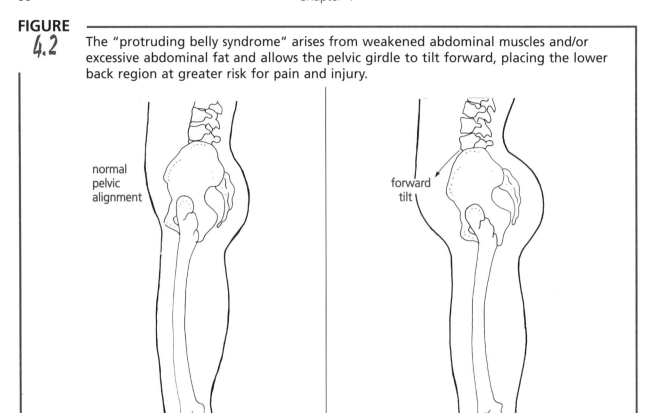

normal pelvic alignment

a.

forward tilt

b.

Performance-Related Fitness

Flexibility in Other Regions of the Body

Having sufficient flexibility throughout the body is an important aspect of fitness. Having a wide range of motion, especially when coupled with sufficient strength and endurance, can permit you to move freely and easily and to perform more fully whatever activity you choose.

Power

Power is the ability to exert force explosively. For example, when softball players throw the ball as fast as they can, the effect on the ball is a combined function of force and speed. The greater the force applied, and the faster the force applied (i.e., the less the time required to generate the force), the greater the power. In many athletic events power is a primary requirement if one is to attain a high level of achievement, but the nonathletic individual has little need for this fitness component. Training to improve power is discussed briefly in Chapter 6.

Speed and Agility

Speed and agility are fitness components that involve moving the whole body as rapidly as possible. Whereas speed usually refers to rapid movements in a straight line (such as in sprinting), agility is the ability to change directions of movement rapidly (such as when a volleyball player moves in a fraction of a second from spiking the ball over the net to diving to retrieve the ball if it is blocked suddenly). The nonathletic person has little need for a high level of speed or agility. If you are interested, however, training procedures for each are discussed briefly in Chapter 6.

GENERAL PRINCIPLES OF FITNESS

If you wish to improve your fitness, regular training is required. **Training** is a process of regular activity directed toward building up or maintaining any of the components of fitness. It does not imply a spartan-like, regimented commitment of several hours of sweat and toil each day. Nor does it require you to "live half your life in a smelly gym." For some, especially those who are athletically inclined, training does involve a large investment of time and effort because the goal of reaching one's limits or of achieving a given level of performance is often unattainable without such a commitment. For most individuals, however, training takes the form of a regular time several days each week devoted to moderate, submaximal exercise that is enjoyable. It is not a "grit your teeth and bear it" type of experience.

The type of training that will elicit optimum benefits is different for each fitness component. For each of the training methods, however, several general principles must be applied if you wish to realize some gain for your efforts. These principles include *the overload principle, the principle of progressive exercise, and the specificity principle*.

Overload Principle

In the most simple terms, the **overload principle** states that exercising a body part or system regularly beyond its normal limits will cause that system to adapt positively and become more able to withstand stress. The term *overload* refers to the process of using a stressor or some stimulus that taxes the body part in question. *Body part* can apply to a single muscle or a group of muscles or to entire systems such as the oxygen transport system, in which the coordinated efforts of the circulatory and respiratory systems deliver oxygen to exercising muscles to enable the production of energy. The overload stimulus can take very different forms depending on what body part or system is being overloaded—from lifting weights for improved strength to slow jogging for increased ability to mobilize and use fat as a fuel.

A related phenomenon is that, with few exceptions, the beneficial changes that accrue from training are *reversible* when the training is reduced or stopped. The rate of decline in function is typically about as rapid as the rate of improvement from added training.

Often, many systems are improved by a given type of overload exercise. For example, if you were to go to a swimming pool and swim steadily several laps of the front crawl, your arm-pulling muscles would be overloaded by the repetitive pulling action against the water. After weeks and months of this type of exercise, the strength and muscle endurance of these muscles would improve. Beyond that, your heart and lungs and the blood vessels leading to all the muscles engaged in swimming the crawl would become more able to perform their specific functions. Within the active muscles, changes would be occurring that improve the capacity to produce energy during exercise. The net effect of all of these latter changes would be improvement in cardiorespiratory fitness.

The overload principle should not be confused with what often is called "no pain, no gain"—a myth that continues to be passed along by word of mouth in gymnasiums and locker rooms. In truth, pain at any time in exercise indicates that you should stop, determine what is wrong, and, if necessary, seek medical attention. To say that benefits from exercise will not accrue unless you train vigorously, in effect overloading yourself at or near your limits, is incorrect. Setting an appropriate level of overload will result in appropriate gains.

Certainly, working hard will stimulate training benefits, presuming you are not at risk *and* presuming you are sufficiently fit to tolerate that level of overload. This is precisely what athletes do in preparing themselves for competition and peak performance. The average person, however, should not train hard, because there is no reason to do so and there are plenty of reasons that argue against taking that approach. In addition to the reasons already mentioned are the risk of inducing injury and the psychological distress that inevitably accompanies such training. In short, the benefits do not outweigh the risks.

Details as to the length of time required before a given overload will result in noticeable changes and other related questions are discussed in Chapters 5, 6, and 7. Another general principle, that of progressive exercise, works hand-in-hand with the overload principle.

Principle of Progressive Exercise

Again in most simple terms, training to improve fitness must involve incrementally increasing the overload stimulus as adaptations occur. This is called **progressive exercise.** Progressive increments of the overload stimulus maintain the relative degree of stress to the system at an appropriate level to continue its overload effect, regardless of fitness status. If the progressive exercise principle is not employed, the improvements will be small and performance soon will level off.

A weight-lifting example is used to illustrate why this is true. Suppose Suzanne decides to begin working on her upper body strength by going into the local weight room. After several days of learning about the weight room and getting some instruction on which exercises she may choose from, she finds that she can do seven repetitions of the bench press exercise using 60 pounds of weight

FIGURE

4.3 Principle of progressive exercise illustrated through bench press.

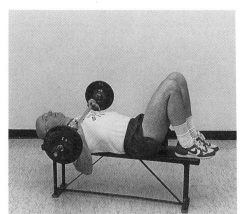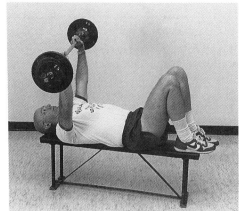

before she is unable to continue because of fatigue. So she sets herself up on a routine of doing seven repetitions, three days per week, and leaves it at that. If she were to continue in that manner over the course of several weeks and months, she would find that the strength and endurance of the muscles used in bench pressing would increase. Eventually, however, she would stop improving, and her strength and muscle endurance would plateau at the new levels they had attained.

If Suzanne desires greater improvements in either strength or endurance, she will have to raise the overload stimulus. She might do this in one of several ways. She could do more repetitions in keeping with her improved capacity, continuing onward to eight, nine, 10 or more repetitions before reaching failure instead of stopping at seven. Or she could do another set of seven repetitions after a rest period and later build that up to three sets per day. Alternatively, at some point she could raise the resistance to 70 pounds and later to 80 pounds. And, of course, she could do any combination of the above.

The point is that, after training at a given level for a certain period of time, the stimulus becomes less of an overload because the system has adapted. For the system to continue to be overloaded at a similar level, the stimulus must be increased. This periodic raising of the overload stimulus should continue until the individual attains the desired goal or until what is needed becomes unrealistic.

The process of making progressive steps in overload during an aerobic training program is described in Figure 4.4. The progression depicted in this figure can be used as a model for developing a similar progression for any other form of training. At the beginning of a training program, we advocate a starter fitness program that involves smaller increments in overload, to allow the body parts adequate time to adjust to being overloaded. This may last four to five weeks, and certainly long enough for the muscles, joints, and other body parts not to feel overworked. Once this initial period has passed, progressive increments can be made in slightly larger jumps, usually every two or three weeks. Eventually, a maintenance period is reached in which progressive increases in overload no longer are necessary. In some cases evidence suggests that the amount of exercise required to maintain a given level of fitness is less than that required to increase fitness. More discussion on this topic is found in Chapters 5–7.

If you are athletically inclined, or wish to attain a certain level of performance by a given date, the harder you work, the faster your improvement will be. This is true for any type of training and at any level, as long as you do not exceed your fitness status so much that you are unable to recover between training days. **Overtraining**—excessive exercise that leads to poorer performance—is fairly common in athletics and can lead to injury or illness. Other signs of overtraining include sleep disturbances, excessive fatigue, and frequent illness such as colds or flu. The solution is the one that common sense would suggest: Ease off in the training.

In applying what might be called the "harder you work" rule, one reaches a point of diminishing return, as illustrated in Figure 4.5. For example, suppose John was a devoted cross-country skier who decided to double his training from 30 minutes per day to 60 minutes per day. Although his cardiorespiratory fitness likely would increase as a result, the gain likely would be less than twice that he had achieved previously. The same would be

FIGURE 4.4 Progression in aerobic training has been found to be most successful if a 4–5 week, gentle, starter fitness program is undertaken first. Thereafter, increases in exercise should occur every 2–3 weeks until a level is reached that can be maintained indefinitely. For each decade after 30, increase time by 40% to allow for adaptation.

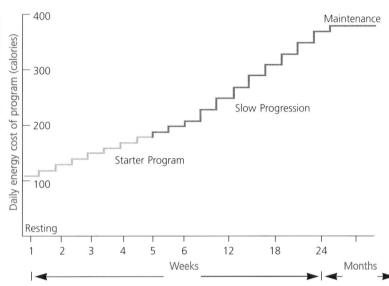

Source: M. L. Pollock, J. W. Wilmore, and S. M. Fox, *Health and Fitness Through Physical Activity*. Copyright © 1978. All rights reserved. Reprinted by permission of Allyn & Bacon.

FIGURE 4.5 Law of diminishing return.

Source: Used by permission from H. A. deVries, *Physiology of Exercise*, 4th ed. (Dubuque, IA: Wm C. Brown, 1986), p. 294.

true if he decided to ski at a faster pace than before, to overload his cardiorespiratory system, although admittedly it would be difficult for him to double his initial speed. The point is that potential gains operate on a changing "effort-scale": The greatest gains occur initially, with the least amount of effort; as the effort increases, the gains also increase, but to a lesser and lesser degree.

A related phenomenon, also illustrated in Figure 4.5, is that improvements are related inversely to initial fitness. Individuals with the lowest level of initial fitness will be able to increase their capacity to the greatest degree, all else being the same. Further, as you train and experience improvements from your efforts, additional improvements become more and more difficult to achieve. Again, there seems to be a point of diminishing return, whereby training-induced gains approach zero after a long period of time. Although each person has different limits, which seem to be determined largely by genetic predispositions, little has been explored on this question. These limits seem to differ for different components of fitness. For example, strength has been known to improve from training to a much greater extent than has cardiorespiratory fitness.

Principle of Specificity

The **principle of specificity** states that training outcomes are specific to the type of training that is done. It applies to all types of training. Let us say, for example, that you decide to develop your upper body strength by doing certain weight-lifting exercises. Over time your strength will improve, but only in those specific muscle groups and only when they are used in the specific ways that you train them. Thus, if you had been using the vertical press exercise, in which you lift a barbell over your head, you would find it easier to put heavy objects up on the top shelf or to handle anything heavy above your head. But if you were asked to carry something heavy, such as a big box, in front of you, your greater strength will not be of much assistance because it involves different muscles or some of the same muscles used in different ways.

Consider the specificity principle as it applies to training the cardiorespiratory system. Although many forms of aerobic exercise are available from which to choose, and although each places similar demands on the heart and lungs, each different exercise involves muscle groups different from the others. Thus, if you are a trained runner, you may be able to swim a long distance more easily than if you were not trained as a runner, but your ability to engage in aerobic exercise in the water will not have been enhanced as much as your capacity to do endurance exercise while running.

The athlete must pay close attention to the specificity principle because training programs for athletes should be designed to elicit the greatest gains in performance in relation to time spent training. Training procedures must overload the body parts or body systems in ways that are similar to how they will be used while performing. To the extent that the procedures are followed, training is likely to result in the greatest possible improvement, all else being the same.

For the average individual with specific goals, the specificity principle also can be used to devise a training program that will be cost-effective. To illustrate, suppose you were interested in being able to pull yourself up over a ledge. Strength training the specific pulling and pushing muscles of the arms and chest as they mimic this move would be more appropriate than a general weight-training program emphasizing muscle strength in a variety of muscle groups.

If your goals are not limited to certain types of performance then, in light of the specificity principle, you might elect to engage in a variety of activities for training. In this manner you can overload many body parts and many systems in different ways. Such a comprehensive program also could involve training different fitness components. If you look at individuals who are fit, you will be able to find those who are relatively fit in one area and relatively unfit in another. By contrast, a comprehensive training program involves training the whole body for use in a variety of ways.

THE EXERCISE SESSION

An exercise session always should begin by warming up and finish by cooling down. Within the actual workout, the arrangement of various parts of the training session can vary. You may wonder whether the order in which you do various parts of your exercise program matters. For example, if you plan to lift weights and run, should you begin with the weights and then go running, or should you do this the other way around? These and other questions are discussed in this section on the specifics of the exercise session.

Warm-Up

The **warm-up** (Figure 4.6) is a process of preparing the body gradually for more vigorous activity. Just as you never should start your car when it is cold and immediately "floor it," for fear that you

FIGURE 4.6 The warm-up.

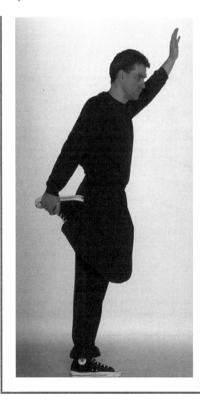
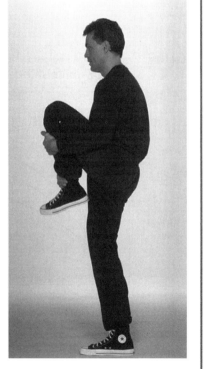

might damage parts that need adequate lubrication or heat to work properly, the same applies to exercising your body. *You should never begin vigorous activity without a warm-up.* The muscles, joints, and organs are designed in marvelous ways to enable you to do many things, but they require proper care and treatment, and this includes proper warm-up.

Proper warm-up is important for at least three reasons:

1. Evidence has demonstrated that presumably healthy hearts can develop unusual patterns of electrical activity called dysrhythmias if vigorous activity is not preceded by a warm-up. With prior warm-up, the same vigorous activity is much less likely to cause an electrical disturbance. Certain dysrhythmias are particularly dangerous to the heart, so this is one of the most important reasons warm-up is recommended as a preventive measure.

2. During vigorous activity such as jogging/running, the muscles and joints of the lower extremities are subjected to large forces, which can lead to injury. Warming up reduces muscle **viscosity,** which is the resistance to movement. It also causes the cartilage and other tissues within the joints to absorb fluid. Both changes reduce the likelihood of injuring these tissues.

3. Warming up increases performance. This is particularly helpful for explosive tasks such as jumping, throwing, and sprinting. Prior to beginning any explosive, all-out activity, warming-up is absolutely necessary, not only as an aid to increased performance but also to reduce the possibility of injury.

Warm-up should begin with general activity involving the whole body, gentle exercise such as walking, followed by a specific warm-up of the specific muscles and joints in question, using light activity. A basic rule is to build gradually upward with the intensity of exercise. The length of warm-up time may vary, but 5–10 minutes usually is more than adequate.

Before engaging in aerobic activity, warm-up often is accomplished by beginning with the same activity, except at a slow pace. Thus, if you plan to begin swimming (or jogging), start by swimming (or jogging) slowly for 5–10 minutes. Walking is always a good activity to precede jogging/running.

Workout

What type of exercise should you incorporate into the workout? How hard should you work, for how long, and how often? The answers to these questions depend on your personal goals and your starting point. In any case, a workout that focuses on developing the components of health-related fitness can serve as a basis for discussion on this topic. An adequate and relatively comprehensive workout consistent with the 1990 position of the American College of Sports Medicine can be accomplished in 50–65 minutes using the following guidelines:

Warm-up:	10 minutes
Workout:	
Strengthening/ flexibility Exercises	10–15 minutes
Aerobic exercise	20–30 minutes
Cool-down:	10 minutes

The details of a workout such as the one outlined (and illustrated in Figure 4.7) may vary depending on your specific goals and needs. For example, a 45-minute workout period certainly would be too long for a beginner, and adjustments

FIGURE 4.7   The workout.

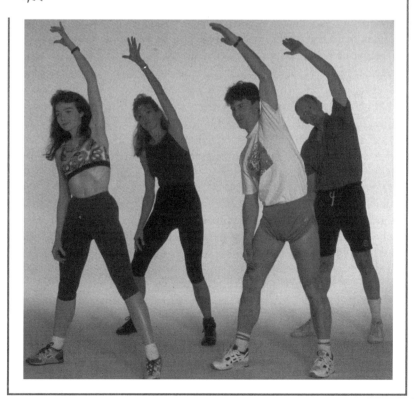

would have to be made. This outline simply provides a framework to consider when formulating your own workout. Specific recommendations for improving the various fitness components are offered in Chapters 5, 6, and 7. These chapters provide the information necessary for you to develop a fitness program that addresses your personal circumstances and preferences.

When integrating several types of training into one workout, you may wonder which parts of your exercise routine to do first. For example, let's suppose you are interested in developing your upper-body strength by working out with weights, but you do not want to let your already well-established, 30-minute aerobic exercise period slip. Should you lift weights and then do your aerobic workout, or the other way around? Is combining two different types of training together in the same workout harmful?

Unfortunately, little concrete evidence is available on which to base recommendations regarding these questions. Some evidence suggests that strength training does not interfere with the benefits of cardiorespiratory exercise, and vice versa. Experienced coaches and athletes who face this problem often use an approach dictated by what works best. If you are better able to lift weights after your aerobic workout, do the activities in that order, or vice versa. Certainly your decision should take into account which part of the total workout you deem most essential. By placing the most essential part of your workout into a place of prominence, where you are less likely to be plagued by residual fatigue or other carryover that detracts from the quality of training, you are maximizing your potential for positive changes.

Cool-Down

Following vigorous activity should be a **cool-down** period, in which the exerciser continues to remain active at a slow pace until the body has recovered substantially. One guideline for determining how long to cool down is a check of the heart rate, which should drop below 110–120 beats per minute. Under most circumstances this is accomplished with 5–10 minutes of gentle activity that gradually trails off.

Reasons for cooling down before heading to the shower include three factors related to health and to comfort.

1. It has long been known that **epinephrine** and **norepinephrine** (also called adrenalin and noradrenalin) are hormones secreted more heavily under stress, including exercise. More recently, levels of these hormones have been shown to continue to rise for a few minutes following exercise. Such high hormone levels stimulate the heartbeat, and researchers believe this is part of the reason the period immediately after exercise is one of the most dangerous to people with heart disease. With the continued but light activity of a cool-down period, these hormone levels can be brought down gradually rather than allowing the heart to be subjected to great stress at the same time as the skeletal muscles are recovering.

2. Cool-down prevents blood from pooling in the lower extremities. Pooling is a problem particularly when doing upright activity such as running and cycling, in which the large leg muscles have been active. Following such exercise, blood continues to be pumped to these tissues, and without continued muscular activity that pumps this blood back toward the heart, a substantial amount of blood can pool in these regions, leaving little blood in the upper extremities. The effect is a light-headed feeling, which in extreme cases can even lead to fainting.

3. Cooling down hastens recovery. Odd as it may seem, evidence shows that recovery from vigorous activity is more rapid following an active cool-down.

COMMERCIALIZATION OF FITNESS

As a consumer, you probably feel somewhat overwhelmed by the endless number of products generated by the fitness industry and by the choices you must make between competing products. Books written by celebrities who are marketing primarily their looks and fame compete with books written by knowledgeable professionals whose goals are increased health and fitness. Spas and health clubs whose main objective seems to be selling memberships compete with other establishments whose goal is to serve the needs of the public well. You must choose sources of information, services, and clothing and equipment that carry implications for social status. As with many products and services, the best-marketed fitness products usually prove to be the most successful. Unfortunately, these are not necessarily the products with the best overall quality.

Choosing Health Fitness Products and Services

Faced with a myriad of products and services, your best bet is to read consumer-oriented literature and be as educated as possible, to ask questions of those who seek to sell you a product, and to gauge the responses against what others have told you and against what you already know. In this regard, the American College of Sports Medicine recently commissioned a book with the goal of increasing the standards of health/fitness facilities, and the Association for Fitness in Business commissioned a book designed to improve the standards of employee health promotion programs. Both were written by competent professionals whose concern is to serve the interests of the consumer.

Whenever shopping for services, it is wise to ask about the training and experience of the service-giver, including a question as to whether he or she is certified and, if so, by what organization. Even the question of certification is difficult to answer satisfactorily because more than fifty organizations offer training and certification. Some of these are reputable and nationally recognized organizations; others are not. As the Latin phrase *caveat emptor* tells us, "Buyer beware!"

Selecting Activity Shoes

If you decide to purchase a pair of activity shoes, you will have to choose from a tremendous assortment of styles and features, and the costs will range from the barely reasonable to the exorbitant. Is the most expensive pair the one to get?

To help you in this selective process, we offer a few generalizations. First, make sure that you choose a running shoe, a walking shoe, a basketball shoe, an aerobics shoe, or a court shoe, depending on the type of activity you will engage in most frequently. Choose a shoe with a width that properly fits the width of your feet. The "last" of the shoe is the form on which a shoe is built, and is readily observable by looking at the sole. The straighter the last, the more support it will provide along the inner edge of the foot. If your experience tells you that you need such support, you should choose a shoe with a straighter last. Then look for a shoe with a reputation for a durable midsole and a durable outsole. The *midsole* refers to the cushioning layers between the upper part of the shoe and the outsole, which is the part that hits the ground.

In addition to the above generalizations, the choice of which shoe to purchase depends on a number of other factors, including your height and weight, and in the case of running, the number of miles you run per week, whether the shoes are to be used for training or racing, and, most important, the nature of *your* foot mechanics as your foot strikes the ground. Technically, determining which shoe is best for you, considering all these requirements, requires that you have a biomechanical analysis done by a competent professional, using slow-motion photography while you wear each of the shoe models that fit. Only then can you determine which shoe is best for your needs. This method of choosing shoes usually is not employed, of course. Clearly, determining what is best for you is not simple.

A practical suggestion is to ask for assistance and information from a competent salesperson. Considering your objectives, price, safety, comfort, and cosmetic features, you should buy a shoe only if it fits well when you mimic the types of movements you intend to be doing while wearing the shoe.

Selecting an Exercise Video

Many exercise videos now are available in the marketplace, including many featuring celebrities or fitness "stars." Similarly, exercise programs on television have long been a resource for people who wish to exercise in the privacy of their home. Unfortunately, not all resources feature exercises that are safe. If you contemplate purchasing a video, the following generalizations may help you purchase an appropriate one:

1. Choose a video designed for someone of your age and fitness level and one that permits you to regulate your pace. Too often videos give the expectation that you must keep up with the leader.

2. Do not choose videos that involve exercises that put you at risk (see "Exercises to Avoid," in Appendix 2).

3. Avoid videos that involve bouncing while stretching, as this can lead to muscle strain.

4. Avoid videos that feature "high-impact aerobics" (exercises in which both feet leave the floor at the same time). These exercises give a more jolting workout, which can result in injuries. "Low-impact aerobics" and "step aerobics" are safer, particularly for the beginning exerciser.

COMMON PROBLEMS RELATING TO EXERCISE

An individual commonly begins an exercise program with good intentions only to develop some type of injury because of improper exercise techniques. This can be discouraging. If properly treated and responded to, however, many injuries can be overcome without major inconvenience. In this section we discuss several common injuries and their treatments.

Muscle Soreness

The muscular pain you feel a day or two after doing some form of strenuous exercise to which you are not accustomed is by far the most common fitness-related injury. Muscle soreness subsides gradually and, in most cases, is gone within four to six days. Recent evidence suggests that this soreness is caused by damage to the muscle cells or connective tissue that runs through muscle. The ways in which this damage alters the normal physiological activity within the muscle are not well understood, but in one way or another, nerve endings are stimulated and pain is the result.

Muscle soreness is not to be confused with the weakness and "burning" feeling you may experience when you exercise a muscle heavily and become fatigued. This immediate muscle fatigue itself is not fully understood, but it seems to be related partly to the build-up of a byproduct of heavy exercise called **lactic acid.** Lactic acid does not seem to be implicated in the muscle soreness that appears one to three days following exercise, however, because it disappears from the muscles during the recovery period, usually within an hour or two.

Because fit and unfit individuals alike become sore following any form of strenuous exercise to which they are not accustomed, muscle soreness cannot be avoided. Still, an adequate warm-up before and cool-down after engaging in vigorous activity should reduce its severity. Another suggestion for minimizing muscle soreness is to build up slowly in your exercise program, never subjecting your muscles to excessive strain to which they are not accustomed. Fortunately, once muscles begin to adapt to the stress of vigorous exercise, they do not become sore again unless they are used in different ways, in which case they are subject to new areas of soreness.

Once you are sore, the best method to reduce the severity seems to be low-level muscular activity. Unfortunately, the pain will not disappear totally following exercise. As with most musculoskeletal injuries, damp heat—as in a hot bath or whirlpool—can be used to stimulate local circulation. This also will hasten healing time.

Strains and Sprains

Injuries to muscles are called strains, whereas injuries to ligaments are called sprains. Sprains can occur in the ligamentous tissues that connect muscles to bones or cartilage. Muscle strains (commonly called "pulled muscles") are severe tears to the muscle fibers and surrounding tissues. They often occur in the quadriceps and hamstring muscles on the front and back of the leg, respectively, or in the muscles of the groin, probably because of the large forces that these muscles are able to generate. They also occur in the muscles of the back as a result of improper lifting techniques and inadequate strength.

The treatment for strains and sprains is rest and intermittent application of ice and pressure and elevation of the affected area to minimize hemorrhage. After a few days, provided there is no pain during activity, a gradual rehabilitative exercise program can begin. The program should emphasize full range of movement following application of cold to the affected area. Medical assistance certainly should be sought if the injury is severe or recovery does not take place in the expected manner. Resting and avoiding vigorous activity until recovery is complete are vital to avoid reinjury.

Tendinitis and Other Overuse Syndromes

Tendinitis is inflammation of the connective tissue that attaches the muscle to the bone. It results from overuse or overstretching. The usual symptoms are pain during movement, tenderness to touch, and weakness, particularly when stretching. Tendinitis commonly occurs in the Achilles tendon in runners and in the shoulders of swimmers.

Treatment involves rest, massage, anti-inflammatory medication, repeated applications of cold, moist heat, and gradual stretching two or three times per day. Qualified personnel also use muscle stimulation, ultrasound, and phonophoresis to treat tendinitis. Cold can be applied by using icepacks for 15–20 minutes at a time. Moist heat can be applied through a warm shower, a hot tub or bath, or a damp, warm cloth under a hot water bottle, for up to 20–30 minutes.

Shin splints is a term used to describe pain in the front of the lower leg. The causes are various, and treatments are tied to the underlying cause.

Self-Monitoring Signs of Injury

Learning to tell the difference between ordinary types of fatigue and discomfort that accompany training from those that foretell injury will help prevent serious injury and prolonged recovery. Excessive fatigue or lack of enthusiasm are signs that training is too rigorous for your current level of fitness. The remedy is to reduce how hard and how often you train and the rate of progression in your training.

Acute pain indicates that a body part has been injured and you should seek medical evaluation to determine the cause and remedy. Pain that increases gradually with successive activity is a sign of chronic irritation or injury and should be heeded. Activity should be curtailed or reduced. If the problem is severe or if it does not dissipate with rest, medical evaluation should be sought.

Caring for Injuries from Exercise

The objective in responding to injuries is to reduce excessive pain, swelling, and inflammation that might retard the process of healing. The first step is to *rest* for a day or more, depending on the severity of the injury. *Ice* or other cold application should be applied to the injured body part to reduce bleeding, swelling, inflammation, and pain. Chipped ice packed in plastic bags is the simplest approach. Ice packs should be applied for 20–30 minutes at a time at intervals depending on the severity of the injury.

Compression by wrapping the injured body part with an elastic wrap helps to reduce swelling. Compression can be combined with ice packs but should not cut off circulation. *Elevating* the injured body part will decrease blood flow and excessive pressure in the injured area. *Heat* can be used to increase blood flow but normally should not be applied until two or three days after an injury because it may induce leakage or swelling. *Anti-inflammatory medication* such as aspirin or ibuprofen is useful in rehabilitating from injury but normally should not be used within the first few days of an injury, as the inflammatory response promotes healing.

ENVIRONMENTAL CONSIDERATIONS

The environment plays an important role in the pursuit of fitness because a mild, sunny day and an attractive setting in which to exercise are rare luxuries. More often than not, it is cold, wet, humid, hot, or smoggy, and you must adapt to the environmental conditions at hand. In the following section we offer some general guidelines about what to do in less than desirous conditions, including selecting appropriate clothing.

Heat, Humidity, and Fluid Requirements

Body temperature must be regulated closely within narrow limits to maintain health. Exercise causes the core temperature to rise, particularly if the exercise is vigorous and sustained for long periods. This effect is accentuated dramatically if the exercise is performed in a warm or hot environment. The immediate effect of this rise in temperature is for the body to initiate several heat-loss mechanisms, including: (a) redirection of blood toward the surface of the body, causing the skin to appear red or flushed, and (b) secretion and evaporation of sweat. This evaporative process cools the surface of the body and the blood passing through it, and this helps maintain core temperature within tolerable limits.

Several factors influence the evaporative process. These include air currents, environmental temperature, humidity, and clothing. The greater the air currents, the more easily sweat will evaporate. Also, as temperature goes up during the day, the relative humidity drops. These two changes tend to offset each other to some extent. As temperature increases, the thermal load on you will rise, but as relative humidity drops, the evaporative process is enhanced. The overall effect on you depends on which change is greatest.

Unless you choose to exercise inside an air-conditioned gym, you cannot control the weather, but both temperature and humidity are still partly under your control as an exerciser. You can choose to exercise in places and at times of the day when the temperature and humidity are least hostile, such as in the early morning or in the evening, thereby reducing the threat to your health and well-being. You can choose to reduce the intensity or duration of your exercise, or both. You also can choose the amount and type of clothing you wear while exercising. Any time you are in danger of becoming overheated, you should adjust your clothing appropriately to allow for the greatest possible heat loss. This may mean taking off clothing and choosing clothing that "breathes" (allows water vapor to pass outward through it). Cotton is a good example of a material that breathes well.

Any garment that prevents or restricts the passage of air over the large surfaces of the body and head never should be worn during exercise in the heat or even in mild temperature, because of the danger of overheating. This is true especially of rubber suits, which still are used occasionally as a means of losing weight rapidly. These suits effectively eliminate evaporation; in an attempt to counteract this, the body releases excessive amounts of sweat. The effect is dehydration of the body, which can be a major threat to health if carried to extremes.

To offset the evaporative water loss, fluids must be replaced irrespective of thirst sensations. Under extreme conditions, waiting for thirst to dictate when to drink can be dangerous because thirst mechanisms are slow to respond. Ideally, fluids should be replaced as they are lost. This entails drinking 1 cup or more of a fluid-replacement beverage every 15 minutes during continuous exercise. Because this still may result in dehydration, you should prehydrate before exercising in hot weather by drinking up to 2½ cups of a fluid 2 hours before starting, and again drinking up to 1½ cups of a fluid 15 minutes before beginning. A simple method of determining whether you are dehydrated is to weigh yourself immediately before and after exercise; drink 2 cups of fluid for every pound of body weight lost during exercise.

Although some commercially prepared drinks are satisfactory as replacement fluids, others, such as soft drinks, contain 10%–12% sugar or more. Such a high sugar content has been found to be detrimental when replacing fluids in the heat. Fluids containing 6%–8% sugar are tolerated more easily and can be a useful source of supplemental energy in prolonged exercise without interfering with fluid-replacement mechanisms.

Some evidence suggests that fluid-replacement beverages that contain a small amount of sodium and other electrolytes are helpful in maintaining thirst mechanisms, reducing the output of urine, and maintaining proper fluid balance under conditions of prolonged exercise in the heat. According to this evidence, these beverages, particularly when cooled, are superior to cool water in helping to maintain hydration. Beverages that contain alcohol or caffeine should be avoided because they add to dehydration and increase the production of urine.

If the core temperature rises too high because of inadequate cooling, *heat exhaustion* and an even more dangerous condition called *heat stroke* can result. Both are dangerous, and first-aid should be administered immediately. Proper first aid consists of the following:

1. Resting the individual in a cool environment with clothing removed.

2. Giving cold fluids to drink.

3. In the case of heat stroke, in which body temperature is dramatically elevated, immediately cooling the individual by whatever means are available—cold shower, hose, cool water, pool.

4. Notifying an emergency vehicle and local hospital of a possible heat casualty.

Heat cramps are involuntary muscle contractions, usually in the muscles of the calf, thigh, or abdomen, as a result of exercise in a hot environment. The cramps, which can be quite painful, are thought to result from a sodium and potassium imbalance in the muscle. Treatment includes rest, fluid, and electrolyte replacement. Usually, salting of food coupled with a balanced diet is sufficient to restore electrolyte balance and correct this problem.

Cold

Cold temperature, particularly if accompanied by wind that exaggerates the wind-chill factor, presents another problem for the exerciser. Just as excess heat must be eliminated so core temperature does not rise precipitously, the core temperature must be protected from dropping when the body is threatened by heat loss. Because exercise creates a warming effect, you can tolerate colder temperatures while exercising. Certain body parts, however, tend to be more vulnerable than others, and they warrant protection. These include the hands and the head, the latter giving off a large proportion of the total heat that is lost. These parts of the body should be covered adequately in cold temperatures.

The remainder of the body should be covered with one or more layers of clothing that can be removed as comfort dictates. If wind is a factor, a garment that is impermeable to wind, with sleeves and a collar that can be cinched up, is particularly helpful. The lungs seem to be in no danger from exercising in cold temperatures. Comfort should always be considered, though.

Air Quality

Most people live in an urban environment where air pollutants are emitted into the air in large quantities. Some pollutants, such as carbon monoxide, limit the ability to do aerobic exercise by reducing the oxygen-carrying capacity of the blood, an effect evident in smokers, whose lungs are exposed routinely to large quantities of this pollutant. Other pollutants, such as ozone, cause eye irritation, chest tightness, and pain, which interfere with aerobic exercise.

The effect of pollutants depends on their concentration and on the length of time you are exposed. Their impact, too, is partly a function of how heavily you breathe. On high-pollution days you would be wise to avoid times of day when pollutant levels are likely to be highest and exercise at times when levels are likely to be lowest. Often,

Quick Tips: Increasing Exercise Motivation

1. Develop exercise plans that meet your needs and interests. Make exercise as pleasurable as possible.
2. Identify the benefits and liabilities (costs) of becoming active.
3. Set realistic goals for yourself.
4. Write a contract with yourself to exercise, and have a friend read and sign it.
5. Keep records of your progress.
6. Anticipate impediments to exercise, and develop contingency plans before they are needed.
7. Give positive rewards to yourself when you are successful.
8. Build positive social support for your exercise habits.
9. Evaluate and reevaluate yourself regularly. Do not be afraid to change your plans or modify your strategies. Be flexible and adaptable.

EXERCISE MOTIVATION: A CLOSER LOOK

Only you can know what is best for you. Only you can make the decision of whether you want to be fit. Only you can muster the necessary commitment to follow through. Perhaps you already have made a commitment to fitness, or perhaps you are considering making a decision to be fit. The following suggestions are intended to assist you if this is the case.

1. *Match strategies with your interests, skills, personality, income level, level of fitness, and other personal circumstances.* Because time for regular exercise competes with other needs and interests (work demands, time with family/friends, time to take care of everyday needs, and so on), rearranging your life to allow time for regular exercise will require planning and forethought. No single prescription will work for everyone. Trust yourself to chart your own best path toward improved fitness.

2. *Choose a mix of activities you find pleasurable and satisfactory.* The role of enjoyment in exercise should not be underestimated, because sustaining the commitment to anything is difficult if it does not bring you pleasure. You are more likely to succeed in developing and maintaining the habit of regular exercise if it meets your needs in some important way.

3. *In written form, clarify your perception of the benefits of becoming active versus the liabilities.* At a later date, reexamine this list to see if and how things may have changed.

4. *Set clear and realistic goals for yourself and state them in measurable terms.* For example: "Next week I plan to walk 15 minutes on Monday, Thursday, and Saturday mornings before I eat breakfast." This is superior to a more loosely defined goal such as, "I will get out and walk next week." To check whether your goals are realistic, show them to a friend to get some feedback.

5. *Write a contract with yourself, and have a friend read and sign off on the contract.* This is an excellent way to assure success. (Chapter 2 has a more thorough discussion of self-contracts including a sample contract.)

6. *Keep records of your progress, perhaps through an activity diary.* Seeing in retrospect where you began can be highly reinforcing. Keeping track of what you do will help bring to consciousness the many ways in which activity can be incorporated into your life.

7. *Anticipate ahead of time how you will contend with impediments (such as poor weather or unexpected time conflicts).* If you can anticipate an alternative way to accomplish your planned exercise, you likely will be more successful if your plans have to change. You probably will feel better about yourself for having done so, too.

8. *Reward yourself for success.* The importance of building self-confidence is not to be underestimated. Because change often takes considerable time, rewards can be powerful tools for staying with your goals until you experience the natural satisfaction that comes from success. Rewards should be positive, be contingent on success, and be a mixture of tangible (gifts to yourself) and intangible (taking time to do something you love to do).

9. *Social support can be of great help.* For example, plan to exercise with a friend, join a group where you will meet people who have similar goals, or take a class. Avoid social influences that are contrary to your goals.

10. *Reevaulate your goals and strategies regularly.* The passage of time is always a threat to successfully continuing a new habit. Also, you will change as you make progress, and adjusting your plans based on changing circumstances may be necessary. Be flexible and adaptable. Work for success.

but not always, pollution is highest in mid to late afternoon and lowest in early morning.

MAKING A DECISION ABOUT FITNESS

What would be required to be physically prepared for all eventualities? Is it cost-effective in terms of time and effort? How much exercise should you get to avoid gradually getting fatter or having greater risk of cardiovascular disease? What would it take to be able to backpack without undue fatigue or ski without having to pace yourself or quit early? The behavior patterns that make up your current lifestyle are determined partly by the answers you have given to questions such as these in the past. The answer you give today and tomorrow will determine your behavior on these issues in the future, for what becomes of you is a matter of personal choice.

For some people, the time required to train is not worth the gain. For others, the effort is too much to put themselves through regularly. Many believe a high level of fitness is not really necessary in day-to-day life. Or they find they have too many things to think about regarding health and fitness, so they avoid dealing with any of it.

If you decide to engage actively in developing and maintaining fitness, the range of choices open to you is wide. It encompasses not only the components of fitness but also various forms of exercise, as well as how long, how hard, and how often to exercise.

Attaining a high level of fitness at one time in your life does not protect you from the negative effects of sedentary living *unless you maintain your fitness by working on it regularly*. The pursuit of fitness requires ongoing commitment. Even those who are diligent in this regard have no guarantees of health, because aging is unavoidable and many chronic diseases have multiple causes, some of which allow choices and some of which do not.

People who are most successful at developing a lifestyle that includes a commitment to fitness are those who have incorporated fitness activities into their interests and individual circumstances. If their daily schedule requires them to rise and depart early, they make time for exercise during the day, perhaps during lunchtime or right after work. If they find it difficult to exercise regularly during the week, they do so on the weekends and pick up the slack by doing one or two workouts during the work week. If they enjoy tennis or racquetball more than jogging, they join a club that offers those facilities and make arrangements ahead of time for games with suitable partners. They take opportunities to engage in exercise, such as walking instead of driving short distances, or choosing the stairs instead of the elevator, or working in the garden on a nice day. In short, they seek out rather than avoid exercise whenever and wherever the opportunity presents itself, and they do so in ways that bring enjoyment into their lives in keeping with their interests and preferences.

In the final analysis, it comes down to personal choice. People who are fit made a decision to engage regularly in developing and maintaining fitness, and they continue to reaffirm that decision. Those who are committed find ways to follow through, to stay with it over the long haul.

As you consider what is being discussed in this book on the topic of exercise, you have to formulate your own decision. If you decide to attain and maintain fitness, the specifics of tailoring the forms of exercise to your needs and interests will be helpful to you. The next few chapters present the tools and basic knowledge that you can use to individualize a fitness program in light of your personal needs.

SUMMARY

The capacity to meet the demands of modern-day life with little strain is what physical fitness means in its most general terms. More specifically, physical fitness can be broken down into components, some of which are related more closely to health and others of which are related more closely to physical performance. The components of health-related fitness are cardiorespiratory fitness, body composition, strength, muscle endurance, and flexibility of the lower back and hip region. Performance-related fitness components are flexibility in other regions of the body, power, speed, and agility. Physical performance also is influenced strongly by the health-related components of fitness.

By taxing yourself within appropriate limits, you can improve any of the fitness components. This overload must be regular and must include progressive increments in workload if fitness is to improve. Maintaining any improvements you achieve requires continued exercise without further increments in workload. The extent of improvement is determined partly by genetic factors but also is influenced by how hard you are willing to work and your initial level of fitness. To achieve a specific goal relating to exercise or to physical performance requires training in ways that specifically mimic the intended outcome.

Exercise sessions always should begin with a 5–10 minute warm-up and end with a cool-down of sufficient duration to allow substantial recovery. Injuries such as muscle soreness, muscular strains and sprains, and tendinitis, as well as many relating to poor posture, often can be prevented. Their occurrence requires a prompt and specific therapeutic response.

Excessive heat and humidity can accelerate fluid losses of the exercising person. To prevent heat exhaustion and heat stroke, adjustments should be made in clothing, fluid replacement, and how much exercise you do. When exercising in the cold, appropriate clothing should be worn to prevent excessive heat loss, especially from the hands and head. If air pollutant levels are high, exercise should be avoided or the amount of exercise reduced. Individualizing your exercise to fit your talents, circumstances, and interests, especially if you find ways to make it enjoyable, will help you adopt and maintain regular exercise habits. The choice is yours.

References

American College of Sports Medicine. 1992. *ACSM's Health/Fitness Facility Standards and Guidelines*, edited by N. Sol and C. Foster. Champaign, IL: Human Kinetics Publishers.

Association for Fitness in Business. 1992. *Guidelines for Employee Health Promotion Programs*. Champaign, IL: Human Kinetics Publishers.

Barham, J. N., and Wooten, E. P. 1973. *Structural Kinesiology*. New York: Macmillan.

Brumick, T. 1986. "On Your Feet." *Runners World* 21: 13–15.

Coleman, E. 1988. "Sports Drink Update." *Sports Science Exchange* 1(5).

deVries, H. A. 1994. *Physiology of Exercise*, 5th ed. Dubuque, IA: Wm. C. Brown.

Fox, E., Bowers, R., and Foss, M. 1993. *The Physiological Basis for Exercise and Sport*, 5th ed. Madison, WI: W. C. Brown and Benchmark.

Fox, E. L., and Mathews, D. K. 1981. *The Physiological Basis of Physical Education and Athletics*, 3d edition. Philadelphia: Saunders College, pp. 270–273.

Jones, B. H., Reynolds, K. L., Rock, P. B. and Moore, M. P. 1993. "Exercise-related Musculoskeletal Injuries: Risks, Prevention, and Care." In *ACSM's Resource Manual for Guidelines for Exercise Testing and Prescription*, 2d edition, edited by J. L. Durstine, A. C. King, P. L. Painter, J. L. Roitman, L. D. Zwiren, and W. L. Kenney. Philadelphia: Lea & Febiger.

Jones, B. H., Rock, P. B., and Moore, M. 1988. "Musculoskeletal Injury: Risks, Prevention and First Aid." In *Resource Manual for Guidelines for Exercise Testing and Prescription*, edited by S. N. Blair et al. Philadelphia: Lea & Febiger.

Kendall, H. O., Kendall, F. P., and Wadsworth, G. E. 1971. Muscles: Testing and Function, 2d ed., Baltimore: Williams and Wilkins.

Nadel, E. R. 1988. "New Ideas for Rehydration During and After Exercise in Hot Weather." *Sport Science Exchange* 1(3).

Pollock, M. L., Wilmore, J. W., and Fox, S. M. 1978. *Health and Fitness Through Physical Activity*. New York: MacMillan.

Pollock, M. L., Wilmore, J. H. 1990. *Exercise in Health and Disease*. 2d ed. Philadelphia: W. B. Saunders.

Raven, P. B. 1980. "Effects of Air Pollution on Physical Performance." In *Encyclopedia of Physical Education, Fitness, and Sports: Training, Environment, Nutrition, and Fitness*, edited by G. A. Stull and T. K. Cureton, Jr. Salt Lake City: Brighton Publishing.

Rejeski, W. J., and Kenney, E. A. 1989. *Fitness Motivation*. Champaign, IL: Life Enhancement Publications.

Wiseman, D. C. 1982. *A Practical Approach to Adapted Physical Education*. Reading, MA: Addison-Wesley.

The Heart of the Matter

Cardiorespiratory Fitness

✔ Why is cardiorespiratory fitness said to be the most important component of fitness for good health?

✔ Do you know your cardiorespiratory fitness level?

✔ What tests can you use to determine your cardiorespiratory fitness, and what precautions should you take?

✔ To improve your cardiorespiratory fitness, what type of exercise do you need to do? How often, how hard, and how long should you exercise?

✔ How do factors such as initial fitness and age affect the degree of improvement you will gain from training? What about genetic differences?

✔ How can you motivate yourself to exercise regularly?

If you want to optimize your health status, regular exercise offers a variety of benefits. This chapter begins with evidence linking cardiorespiratory fitness to health, cardiovascular disease, and aging. Methods to assess your cardiorespiratory fitness status are then presented, followed by an overview of the guidelines to follow in developing and maintaining this type of fitness.

THE RELATION OF PHYSICAL ACTIVITY AND CARDIORESPIRATORY FITNESS TO HEALTH AND AGING

Recent surveys suggest that only 22% of Americans engage in regular physical activity at the level recommended for health benefits in *Healthy People 2000*. Some 54% of Americans are minimally active, and 24% are completely sedentary. Even though participation in regular physical activity has increased since the late 1960s, it seems to have leveled off.

For a number of years discussion among experts has centered on how much exercise is enough. Previously it was thought that health benefits would accrue only in individuals who trained vigorously enough to improve their cardiorespiratory endurance. It has come to be recognized that gentle forms of exercise such as walking and easy cycling provide considerable health benefits even at moderate levels. The term "physical activity" is used to distinguish this level of exercise from more rigorous forms of endurance training.

It has been shown that three 10-minute walks during the day have approximately the same positive impact on fitness in sedentary elderly people as one 30-minute walk. This and other evidence suggest that a program of moderate physical activity is likely to create important health benefits. Among these benefits is a reduction of risk for cardiovascular disease (CVD). In addition, regular physical activity seems to provide some protection against adult-onset diabetes, high blood pressure, depression, certain forms of cancer, and osteoporosis.

Health benefits from vigorous forms of aerobic endurance training are well documented in individuals of all ages (Table 5.A). Aerobically fit individuals have stronger hearts, lower resting heart rates, and better developed vascular systems.

Aerobically fit people also have greater work capacity, enabling them to take part in physical activities at a lower percent of their maximal capacity than if they were unfit. They tend to have less body fat, more lean tissue, and more favorable blood lipid profiles, including slightly lower VLDL and LDL levels and higher HDL levels (refer to Chapter 3 for a discussion of these forms of cholesterol).

Many of the typical reasons for the decline in work capacity with age can be minimized by maintaining gentle aerobic activity. Aerobic exercise is used as a treatment for people who have CVD and its risk factors, such as diabetes, hypertension, and obesity. Coronary patients in cardiac rehabilitation programs have demonstrated remarkable improvements in their ability to return to normal life through supervised aerobic exercise.

Studies have demonstrated that the incidence and severity of CVD are lower among people who engage in regular physical activity and who train aerobically. Evidence also demonstrates that these people as a whole live longer; death rates from all causes are lower.

Benefits from regular activity and from endurance training are considerable and within reach of anyone with a goal of improving his health. Without doubt, some activity (and training) is better than none. And more activity (and training) is better than less.

ASSESSING YOUR CARDIORESPIRATORY FITNESS

Before embarking on a training program designed to improve your cardiorespiratory fitness, you should determine your current fitness status. This will enable you to measure improvement from your training by charting your progress along the way. A record can provide considerable motivation! A complete assessment of your current health status is important for another reason, too: People sometimes are unaware of preexisting conditions that might put them at risk when doing vigorous exercise, and a thorough examination should reveal any possible problems.

What preexisting conditions should concern you? If you have symptoms of cardiovascular disease, such as chest pain or shortness of breath, or a previous history of CVD, you are strongly advised to complete a medical evaluation before beginning an exercise program. The evaluation would include both a resting and an exercise electrocardiogram (ECG) on a "graded exercise test." A medical evaluation also is recommended if you have one or more of the following conditions:

1. blood pressure of 160/90 or above on at least two separate occasions (or if you are taking antihypertensive medication)

TABLE 5.A   Effects of endurance training on physiological functions.

ORGAN/SYSTEM	CHANGES IN YOUNGER AND MIDDLE-AGED ADULTS	CHANGES IN OLDER ADULTS
Resting values		
oxygen consumption	no change	
blood pumped from heart/min.	no change	
heart rate	decrease	decrease
blood ejected from heart/beat	increase	
blood pressure	no change/decrease	decrease
work of heart	decrease	
muscle capillary density	increase	
size of deepest breath	increase	increase
blood volume	increase	
hemoglobin volume	increase	
*Submaximal values**		
oxygen consumption	no change/decrease	
blood pumped from heart/min.	no change	no change/increase
heart rate	decrease	decrease
blood ejected from heart/beat	increase	no change/increase
blood pressure	decrease	
work of heart	decrease	decrease
Maximal values		
oxygen uptake	increase	increase
blood pumped from heart/min.	increase	
heart rate	no change/decrease	no change
blood ejected from heart/beat	increase	
oxygen unloaded to tissues	increase	
ventilation capacity	increase	increase
blood pressure	no change	
work of heart	no change	
ability to do endurance exercise	increased	increased

*Measured at the same absolute workload before and after training.

From *Exercise in Health and Disease* by M. L. Pollock, J. H. Wilmore, and S. M. Fox III. Copyright © 1984 by W. B. Saunders, Philadelphia. *Physiology of Exercise*, 4th edition, by H. A. deVries. Copyright © 1986 by Wm C. Brown, Dubuque, IA.

2. serum cholesterol of 240 mg/dl or above
3. cigarette smoking
4. diabetes mellitus
5. a family history of coronary or other athero-sclerotic disease in your parents or siblings prior to age 55

If conditions such as these are not present, the risks to most apparently healthy persons for beginning an exercise program of moderate to vigorous intensity are relatively slight.

The term *vigorous exercise* is defined as an intensity of exercise that an untrained person could not sustain for more than 15 minutes continuously. *Moderate exercise* is defined as exercise that is well within your current capacity and that can be sustained for at least 60 minutes. Above age 40 years in men and 50 years in women, it is recommended that before beginning a vigorous exercise program,

a person should have a medical exam, including a graded exercise test. Moderate exercise programs are relatively safe for apparently healthy persons of all ages.

In a *graded exercise test* (GXT) the individual is required to exercise in gradual increments on a treadmill or a bicycle ergometer (a tool for measuring work capacity) until unable to continue or until symptoms warrant terminating the test. Normally the individual has chest electrodes attached to an electrocardiograph, which monitors the electrical events of the heart at all levels of exercise to determine whether exercise at similar levels on the field is safe. Occasionally the amount of oxygen the individual consumes also is measured during a GXT by analyzing the contents of the exhaled air. By measuring the amount of oxygen consumed under conditions of maximal exercise, the *maximum oxygen intake* of the individual can be determined. This commonly is referred to as the individual's maximum *aerobic capacity*, or $\dot{V}O_2$ max. Most authorities agree that an accurate measure of aerobic capacity is the best single measure of cardiorespiratory fitness.

Another frequently used term is the **anaerobic threshold,** the level of exercise intensity that just avoids a rapid rise of lactic acid in the blood. Lactic acid, a byproduct of incomplete metabolism of carbohydrates, is associated with muscle fatigue. Its role is a subject of great controversy, but if you have a large build-up of lactic acid, you clearly will be forced to slow down or even stop exercise because of the resulting fatigue. The anaerobic threshold typically is in the range of 60%–70% of $\dot{V}O_2$ max in the average person. One of the most important characteristics of elite distance runners is a high anaerobic threshold.

Detailed descriptions of GXT procedures and how to measure $\dot{V}O_2$ max and anaerobic threshold will not be given here, but we will describe tests of cardiorespiratory fitness that can be administered easily and without expensive equipment. If you need further information about the more technical tests, your personal physician can refer you to a place where you can obtain a GXT. Many well-equipped human performance or exercise physiology laboratories can do tests of $\dot{V}O_2$ max and anaerobic threshold.

Tests of Cardiorespiratory Fitness

Submaximal Tests

Several methods can be used to estimate cardiorespiratory fitness submaximally. The term **submaximal** refers to a test that does not require you to push yourself to the limits of your exercise tolerance. Submaximal tests do not provide direct or exact measurements of aerobic capacity; instead, they allow you to *estimate* your cardiorespiratory fitness. The tests require you to count how many times your heart beats in response to a standard amount of exercise, which allows you to *predict* your aerobic capacity. Although predictions are accurate when applied to large groups of individuals, they are not exact when applied to an individual. Error also can result if the testing procedure is not followed accurately. The size of the error is commonly described by computing the *standard error of the estimate* when the test is first developed and validated. Because there is no easy way of determining the actual degree of error for you personally, it is safest to recognize that tests such as this provide only a rough approximation of aerobic

capacity. If you require a more exact determination, you will have to go to a laboratory that can measure $\dot{V}O_2$ max directly.

Despite the potential for error, general testing can be useful. If you compare your results *now* to your results *at a later date*, whatever improvements you make will be just as visible as if you had followed a more sophisticated testing procedure. The results may be off to an unknown degree in absolute value, but the error should remain constant over time and in a sense will be canceled out when you determine the degree of change that has occurred.

Step Tests

One of the more common step tests is the Queen's College Step Test in Appendix 9, Lab 14. This test has been used widely and is easy to administer. It involves stepping up and down at a fixed rate for 3 minutes and is particularly useful because it uses as the step the standard bleacher found in most schools and gymnasiums as the step bench.

Maximal Field Tests

The purpose behind a maximal field test is to determine the level of performance you can attain when pushed to your limits. The most commonly used test is the Cooper 12-Minute Run, which measures the greatest distance you are able to cover in 12 minutes (Appendix 9, Lab 16). The Cooper 1.5-Mile Run test is virtually the same except that it measures the time taken to cover 1.5 miles. This test evolved from research showing a high correlation between $\dot{V}O_2$ max as determined in the laboratory and the ability to run distances. Continued research has determined that this correlation is not as high as thought originally. One reason is that, although the ability to run distances is related strongly to aerobic capacity, it also is dependent on factors such as skill, a sense of the pace you can maintain, motivation, body composition, and the ability to avoid the rapid build-up of exercise-induced wastes and other byproducts that interfere with performance. People who can run long distances at a fast pace are not able to do so simply because of high aerobic capacity; they can do so for a variety of reasons. Nevertheless, because of its ease of administration to large groups and because it can be self-administered repeatedly requiring only a stopwatch, this test continues to be used widely as a screening test for cardiorespiratory fitness.

Maximal tests of this nature should be taken only by healthy people who have had a few weeks of preliminary training to precondition themselves. If you have not had the necessary preconditioning, you should defer taking this test until you have. Certainly, if you have any of the major risk factors or other contraindications for cardiovascular disease described earlier, you should have a thorough medical evaluation before taking this test.

Another field test, the Rockport Walk Test, has been developed for predicting $\dot{V}O_2$ max (Appendix 9, Lab 15). This test is based on the fastest time in walking a measured mile on a track.

Fitness Norms

Since tests of cardiorespiratory fitness make reference to norms, a few comments concerning the interpretation of these norms are in order. Comparisons to others do provide a basis for determining what is normal. That is why cholesterol counts, blood pressure, and blood glucose tests are flagged if they fall outside the normal range. But in the case of cardiorespiratory fitness (and all other components of fitness for that matter), some people tend to be overly concerned with where they are compared to others. Ironically, given the relatively low fitness level of most contemporary adults, the present norms may not even reflect a truly desirable level of fitness from the standpoint of optimal health!

No single level of cardiorespiratory fitness can be advocated as a desirable goal for everyone. People score differently on most tests because of genetics alone. If you wish to compare yourself to others, norms are available for all tests describing what category or percentile ranking you hold in relation to the sample of people on which the norms were based. It is unlikely that everyone can attain the 90th percentile or the "excellent" category on a given test—even by training hard—simply because of inherent individual differences. Therefore, one suggestion is to score as high on the norms as permitted by the time and interest you are willing to put into regular exercise.

As has been pointed out already, on some tests the norms pertain only to certain segments of the population, such as college-age adults. None of the norms has been developed from all segments of society, including the various ethnic groups. None considers education, socioeconomic, or demographic differences. Therefore, even if you are a college-age adult, for example, the norms for a given test may not truly describe where you fall relative to all others of your same age. Perhaps the safest generalization is that if you follow the recommended guidelines for developing cardiorespiratory fitness in the next section, whatever level of fitness you attain on a given test is appropriate for you.

In your quest for fitness, comparisons between yourself and others are really irrelevant under most circumstances. The only person who matters is you. True, most of us like to know where we stand compared to others, particularly if we think we're better than most. Unless you are competing as an athlete, however, or have some other job-related performance requirement that requires you to achieve a certain standard of fitness, the best comparison you can make is to yourself. By knowing your fitness status at a given point in time and then rechecking it periodically, you can determine how well you are doing—whether you are making progress, holding your own, or losing ground.

This is analogous to the comparisons we make in other areas of our lives: We step on the scale periodically to check our body weight and go to the doctor periodically to check our health status. Imagine how silly it would seem if an individual were to ask his physician every time he had a checkup whether his cholesterol count, blood glucose, or blood pressure were in the 90th percentile compared to others and, upon discovering they were not, he pushed himself competitively toward achieving that goal within a few months.

DEVELOPING THE HABIT OF REGULAR ACTIVITY

If you are a healthy, nonathletic individual interested in moving toward the habit of regular physical activity, your goal should be to accumulate 30 minutes or more of moderate-intensity physical activity most days of the week. Some easy methods to incorporate more activity into your daily routine include walking up stairs, walking part of the way to or from work, walking while taking a break at work, and gardening. One specific way to do this is to walk 2 miles briskly most days of the week. Of course, your activity can include planned exercise sessions, but it does not have to be formalized. Also, it can be broken up into several segments spaced throughout the day.

If you currently do no physical activity, you can begin by incorporating just a few minutes of activity into your day and slowly build upward from there. People who have irregular activity habits should strive to be more consistent. Exercises that develop and maintain muscular strength and flexibility are encouraged as well. Appendix 3 offers excellent exercises to accomplish such a goal, and these require no special equipment.

DEVELOPING CARDIORESPIRATORY FITNESS

General Guidelines

When beginning an exercise program, several preliminary considerations should guide your behavior. In accordance with the principle of progression discussed in Chapter 4, your preliminary efforts should not raise your activity level abruptly above what you have been doing previously. Experience has shown that abrupt approaches to activity are counterproductive and also may lead to musculoskeletal injuries, excessive fatigue, or, in extreme cases, increased risk of heart attack. (This latter risk applies mostly to middle-aged and older individuals who have not had a medical evaluation and clearance before beginning an exercise program.)

When choosing an activity, you should consider your interests, abilities, objectives, and circumstances. Setting realistic goals for yourself, both short-term and long-term, will help you adhere to the program you set up. The activities you choose should be compatible with your lifestyle and your financial means. You should enlist the assistance of others who can help you. This includes choosing exercise leaders who are knowledgeable and can help motivate you, as well as companions who have similar interests and capacities for exercise. Social support is a powerful stimulus for successfully beginning and maintaining regular exercise habits.

One important component of any exercise program designed to improve cardiorespiratory fitness and assist with weight control is the amount of energy expended during the exercise program. Evidence suggests that for males who are successful in maintaining an adequate level of fitness and body weight, the total caloric expenditure from exercise amounts to 900–1500 calories per week, or 300–500 calories per exercise session. Equivalent values for females are 700–1200 calories per week, or 225–400 calories per exercise session. To assist you in determining the caloric cost of various activities, Appendix 4 contains a list of common activities and exercises. Instructions for how to compute caloric costs and more information on the role of exercise in weight control are found in Chapter 7.

A general description of warm-up and cool-down procedures was provided in Chapter 4. With respect to beginning endurance exercise, your warm-up should be specific to the type of exercise you plan to do during your training and should gradually increase in intensity. It may include light stretching exercises (see Chapter 6). The duration of warm-up should be 5–10 minutes. The cool-down period also should be at least 5–10 minutes, depending on how hard and how long you exercised. It should consist of light exercise that gradually tapers off in intensity toward full rest. You should avoid standing still immediately, especially if you have been doing upright exercise with your legs, because of the danger of blood pooling in your lower extremities, creating a lightheaded feeling or worse effects. Following cool-down is a good time to do strengthening exercises and more extensive flexibility exercises because your body parts and joints are warm and respond better to stretching.

For healthy, nonathletic individuals who are interested in developing and maintaining cardiorespiratory fitness, the essential ingredients of an exercise program must take into account the type of exercise (the mode), the frequency of exercise (how often), the intensity of exercise (how hard), and the duration of exercise (how long). A summary of the generalizations that can be made from the completed research on these topics can be found in Table 5.B.

Mode of Exercise

Evidence suggests that any large-muscle, rhythmic exercise is an appropriate mode for improving cardiorespiratory fitness. The **mode** is simply the type of exercise selected. Large muscles should be involved because this form of exercise places a large overload on the cardiorespiratory system. Small-muscle exercise, such as working with the upper body in carpentry, will cause the heart rate

TABLE 5.B Guidelines for developing and maintaining cardiorespiratory fitness.

PARAMETER	GUIDELINE
Mode of exercise	Any large-muscle, rhythmic exercise (e.g., walk, jog, run, swim, cycle, row, hike, cross-country ski, endurance games)
Frequency of exercise	3–5 days per week
Intensity of exercise	50%–85% of maximum heart rate reserve or 60%–90% of maximum heart rate
Duration of exercise	20–60 minutes per day

Source: American College of Sports Medicine. 1990. "Position Stand: The Recommended Quantity and Quality of Exercise for Developing and Maintaining Cardiorespiratory and Muscular Fitness in Healthy Adults." *Medicine and Science in Sports* 22(3): 265–274.

to increase modestly but will not put a sufficiently large overload on the heart to force it to increase its ability to pump blood. The exercise should be *rhythmic* because *static exercise*—which entails little or no movement, as in carrying a heavy load with the arms—puts an excessive strain on the heart. (Although static exercise is safe for healthy hearts, it puts anyone with potential heart disease at greater risk than rhythmic exercise because it raises blood pressure and heart rate very high.)

Examples of appropriate rhythmic activities are walking, jogging, running, swimming, cycling, rowing, cross-country skiing, aerobic exercises, rope-skipping, and hiking. In recent years aerobics has become a popular mode of exercise. High-impact aerobics classes that involve rapid jumping and bouncing movements can lead to orthopedic injuries over time. Instead, low-impact aerobics (Figure 5.1) and step aerobics (Figure 5.2) classes are preferable.

Intermittent activities or activities with low energy cost have little effect on increasing cardiorespiratory fitness. These include activities such as moderate calisthenics, golf, gardening, and weight-lifting. Depending on how they are played, many games such as tennis, basketball, racquetball, handball, and soccer also can be appropriate for developing cardiorespiratory fitness. Under most circumstances, this sort of game has frequent breaks, which reduce potential usefulness as a rhythmic tool, but by modifying these games, the range of appropriate activities from which to choose is widened considerably.

Imagine that Jamal is a 35-year-old former college tennis player who has been a part of the business world for the last 12 years, only to find himself overfat and underfit. Having long ago discovered that if he has to run to keep in shape, he doesn't keep it up because he dislikes running, Jamal decides to take up tennis again. To assure himself of an adequate workout, he and his regular tennis partner agree to play tennis on a competitive level, and they also agree to continue moving actively between rallies. For example, instead of walking to pick up the balls, they both jog easily as necessary, in effect keeping themselves in motion. By modifying their game-playing in this way, Jamal and his partner have made their game of tennis more aerobic than it would have been otherwise. In effect, they have ensured continuous large-muscle, rhythmic exercise for the 45–60 minutes they play each day.

Frequency of Exercise

The relationship between **frequency of exercise,** or how often one exercises, and improvements in cardiorespiratory fitness (holding all else constant)

FIGURE 5.1   Low-impact aerobics.

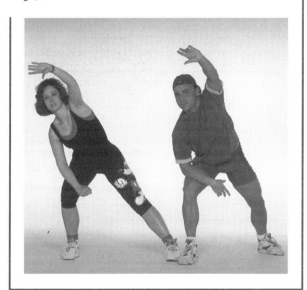

FIGURE 5.2   Step aerobics.

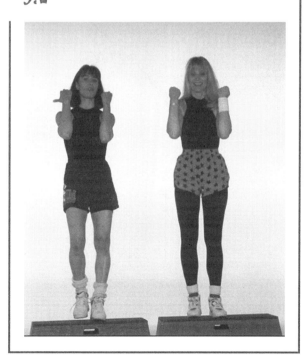

is illustrated in Figure 5.3. As you can see, optimal benefits are obtained when exercise is performed regularly three to five days per week. Benefits can be attained from exercising as few as two days per week, but this requires exercising harder than when you exercise more frequently. Evidence indicates that in some cases—running, for example—exercising more than five days per week results in a greater incidence of injury than exercise done less often. These data are depicted by the dashed line in Figure 5.3.

Most people who exercise three days per week space the exercise sessions to every other day. Though this is not absolutely necessary, allowing a day between exercise sessions permits full recovery and distributes the exercise relatively evenly throughout the week. Exercising three days in a row, however, seems to be just as effective at improving cardiorespiratory fitness as sessions spread throughout the week. Therefore, if your schedule dictates that you exercise both weekend days plus one day during the work week, don't worry.

This information also should help if you have a regular exercise schedule that has to be interrupted temporarily. For instance, many regular exercisers feel distressed when they miss their usual activity on vacation days and fear they will lose some of their hard-earned fitness or will not expend enough calories. One simple solution is to exercise a few additional days before and after the trip to make up the difference.

Depending on your initial state of fitness, the intensity at which you plan to exercise, and the total duration of exercise, increasing the frequency of exercise is one way to expend additional calories. Perhaps more important, by exercising frequently, you address what is perhaps the most important issue of all: *establishing regular exercise habits*. For example, suppose Valerie wishes to begin an exercise program. Her initial state of fitness being relatively low, she begins with a walking program instead of a jogging program, at first walking 15 minutes two days per week, then progressing to one-half hour per day five days per week within a month. (An alternative for Valerie might be to walk 15 minutes twice a day if that fit her schedule better.)

Depending on how fast she walks and how much she weighs, by walking five days per week for 30 minutes, Valerie may expend as much as 750 calories of energy per week in her activity program. This is less than the recommended amount of 900–1500 calories per week, but certainly closer to that target than when she was sedentary. And despite her low fitness, Valerie has demonstrated to herself that she can begin to exercise regularly without undue stress and strain. As her fitness improves, Valerie eventually may progress with her activity, perhaps adding periods of walk-jog-walk into her routine and eventually moving into periods of continuous jogging as she is able, all of which will increase her fitness and add to her total caloric expenditure.

Intensity of Exercise

Target Heart Rate

Intensity of exercise refers to how hard you need to work to obtain some benefit. In practical terms that can be measured, research indicates that the optimal range of intensities for developing cardiorespiratory fitness is to maintain a heart rate

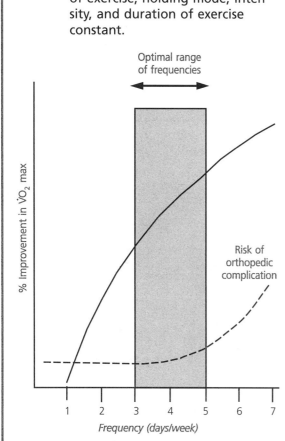

FIGURE 5.3 Improvement in $\dot{V}O_2$ max and the risk of orthopedic complication as a function of different *frequencies* of exercise, holding mode, intensity, and duration of exercise constant.

Source: Modified by permission from "Exercise Testing and Prescription," by H. K. Hellerstein and B. A. Franklin, in *Rehabilitation of the Coronary Patient*, edited by N. K. Wenger (New York: John Wiley & Sons).

How to Measure Your Heart Rate

Each heartbeat causes the heart to eject blood, giving rise to a pulse wave that is transmitted throughout all arteries. This pulse wave is what is commonly measured because of the direct correspondence between pulsations and heartbeats (Figure 5.4). Many people measure their pulse at the carotid artery by pressing their fingers near their throat, just under their jaw (a). Evidence suggests, however, that the heart actually may slow down because of pressure at this location. A better method is to find your pulse by pressing gently with your fingers (and not your thumb) at the radial artery near your wrist (b). By counting the number of pulsations in 10 seconds and multiplying by 6 to convert it to a minute rate, you will obtain a good indication of your heart rate. You also can count your pulse at the temple (c).

The easiest time to measure resting heart rate is before getting up in the morning, provided, of course, that your heart rate has not been elevated by an abrupt alarm. This measure should be taken several times and averaged to determine the most representative value for you.

When measuring your pulse after exercise, you should start counting within 5 seconds of stopping, because the heart rate begins to decline immediately. If you wait longer, your measurement will not reflect accurately how fast your heart was beating during exercise. If you do begin counting within 5 seconds of stopping and measure for only 10 seconds, you can obtain an accurate estimate of the rate at which your heart was beating during exercise. A 10-second count is better than a 6-second count because it allows for a lower error if you miss a beat.

Maximum heart rate can be determined by several methods. If you have completed a maximal exercise test to evaluate your fitness status, the highest heart rate you achieved on that test usually is a good estimate of maximum heart rate. Another method is to measure your heart rate immediately after a bout of heavy exercise (e.g., after the 12-minute run). Heart rate under these conditions can give a good indication of your maximum heart rate, but unless you are fit enough to take such a test safely, you should not do so. If neither of the above conditions applies to you, the most common procedure is to predict maximum heart rate as follows:

predicted maximum heart rate = 220 − age

For example, the predicted maximum heart rate of a woman at age 23 is: 220 − 23 = 197 beats per minute. Although this will enable you to obtain a rough estimate of your maximum heart rate using average values obtained on people of differing ages, research has shown considerable individual differences using such an estimate. The standard deviation is ± 10 beats per minute, which means 68% of the individuals of any age have a true maximum heart rate within 10 beats of their predicted maximum heart rate. Another 27% may fall within 20 beats per minute of their predicted maximum heart rate. Simply said, this prediction formula gives only a rough approximation of true maximum heart rate. It should be used only until you are able to obtain a more accurate measure of your true maximum heart rate using one of the other methods described.

FIGURE 5.4 Measuring pulse at three locations.

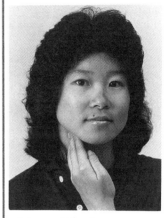

(a) carotid artery

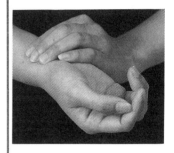

(b) radial artery

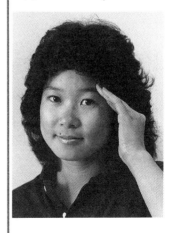

(c) temple

between 60% and 90% of the maximum heart rate, or between 50% and 85% of the maximum heart rate reserve (Figure 5.5). **Heart rate reserve** is defined as the difference between your resting heart rate and your maximum heart rate. **Resting heart rate** is the rate at which your heart beats under truly resting conditions. **Maximum heart rate** is defined as the fastest rate that your heart can attain under conditions of maximal exercise. Figure 5.6 shows the method for calculating a target heart rate using both methods.

The region of heart rates that falls between the 50% and 85% HRR level is often referred to as the training-sensitive zone (see Figure 5.7). In effect, training at any intensity that causes the heart rate during exercise to fall within the training-sensitive zone is appropriate if you wish to improve or maintain cardiorespiratory fitness.

Because maximum heart rate declines with age, target heart rates at the 50%–85% levels decline as well. This means that as you get older, you do not have to raise your heart rate as high during exercise to obtain a training effect. This declining target heart rate zone is illustrated by the downward slant of the training-sensitive zone in Figure 5.7. (Resting heart rate does not decline with age.)

You may wonder what will happen if you do not achieve these limits for one reason or another. If you exercise in such a way that your heart rate does not reach your 50% target heart rate level, you simply will not receive as much of a training effect as if you had worked harder. This may be an entirely appropriate strategy for you if you are trying to develop regular exercise habits gradually and you find vigorous exercise unpleasant. Over time and with practice you are likely to find yourself able and willing to exercise harder, thereby bringing your heart rate into the training-sensitive zone. A gradual approach toward improving your fitness always is preferable to an abrupt approach, and you should feel encouraged to set your own pace toward achieving that goal.

At the other end of the spectrum, if you exercise so hard that your heart rate exceeds the 85% level, probably nothing will happen except that you will be placing all your bodily systems under greater strain and your fitness will not improve any faster. If you are healthy, you may become more fatigued and less inclined to adhere to such an exercise routine. You may even be less inclined to exercise the next day. If you have risk factors or latent cardiovascular disease, this intensity of exercise will put you at greater risk for an injury or a heart attack.

Is it better to work closer to the 50% or the 85% target heart rate level? As long as you exercise within the training-sensitive zone, you apparently will receive optimal benefits. You will have to push yourself harder to achieve the 85% target heart rate than if you worked at the 50% level, though. The best strategy depends on your initial state of fitness and on the duration of the exercise session. Individuals should exercise at the lower level of intensity if they are

FIGURE 5.5 Improvement in $\dot{V}O_2$ max and risk of cardiovascular complication as a function of differing *intensities* of exercise, holding mode, frequency, and duration of exercise constant.

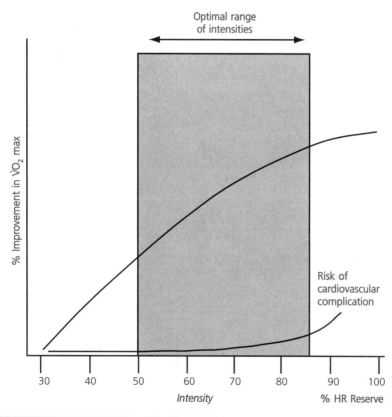

Modified from "Exercise Testing and Prescription," by H. K. Hellerstein and B. A. Franklin, *Rehabilitation of the Coronary Patient*, edited by N. K. Wenger (New York: John Wiley and Sons).

FIGURE 5.6

Calculating target heart rate.

Method 1: Calculating target HR at 60% and 90% of max HR*

Assume max HR	= 200 beats/minute
.6(200)	= 120 beats/minute
.9(200)	= 180 beats/minute

Method 2: Calculating target HR at 50% and 85% of heart rate reserve (HRR)

Assume max HR* = 200 beats/minute and resting HR** = 70 beats/minute

HRR	= 200 − 70	= 130 beats/minute
50% of HRR	= .5(130)	= 65 beats/minute
85% of HRR	= .85(130)	= 110.5 beats/minute
Target HR @ 50% HRR	= 70 + 65	= 135 beats/minute
Target HR @ 85% HRR	= 70 + 110.5	= 180.5 beats/minute

* Max HR = the fastest heart rate (in beats per minute) that you can achieve during heavy exercise. If it is not known, it can be estimated as follows: Max HR = 220 − age in years.

** Resting HR = heart rate (in beats per minute) under truly resting conditions, taken before arising in the morning.

FIGURE 5.7

The training-sensitive zone as a function of age. Maximum heart rate and heart rates within the training-sensitive zone decline with age. Resting heart rate does not.

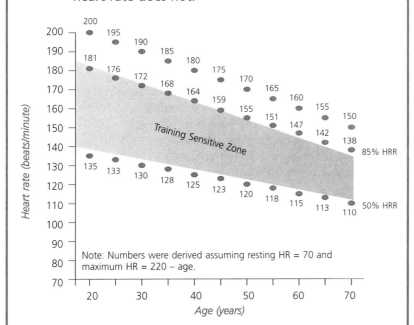

Note: Numbers were derived assuming resting HR = 70 and maximum HR = 220 − age.

Source: Modified by permission from *Nutrition, Weight Control, and Exercise*, 2d edition, by F. I. Katch and W. D. McArdle (Philadelphia: Lea and Febiger, 1983).

less fit or if they plan to exercise for a longer time. More will be said about both of these topics later.

Perceived Exertion Scale

Another way to monitor the intensity of exercise involves measuring the **rate of perceived exertion (RPE)** during exercise. This method is close to what many regular exercisers do naturally once they become experienced. They exercise at a pace that feels comfortable and that they know is vigorous enough to accomplish their goals. The rate of perceived exertion is a measure based on all the sensory information received from the muscles, joints, and various internal organs, as they all affect the person at the same time. Some evidence suggests that RPE is an even better predictor of maximum work capacity than is heart rate.

The scale for measuring RPE is seen in Figure 5.8. To use this scale, simply determine the number that best describes how hard the exercise feels, using the scale of 6 to 20 and the adjectives adjacent to the scale. For example, if while swimming the crawl steadily for 20 minutes, you felt like it was mildly vigorous, you might rate the exercise as a 12 or a 13 ("somewhat hard" or below). On the other hand, if it was difficult to maintain your pace, your RPE score might have been a 17 or an 18 ("very hard" or above). A guideline for using perceived exertion that is roughly equivalent to your training-sensitive zone is to exercise at a pace that falls between 12 and 16 on the RPE scale (between "somewhat hard" and "hard").

Duration of Exercise

Evidence suggests that for optimal improvements in cardiorespiratory fitness, exercise should last between 20 and 60 minutes per day. **Duration** refers to total amount of exercise time per session and does

FIGURE
5.8

The Borg Perceived Exertion Scale allows you to rate the difficulty of an exercise according to your perceptions.

6	
7	Very very light
8	
9	Very light
10	
11	Fairly light
12	
13	Somewhat hard
14	
15	Hard
16	
17	Very hard
18	
19	Very very hard
20	

"Perceived Exertion: A Note on 'History' and Methods," by G. A. V. Borg, *Medicine and Science in Sports* 5(1973): 90-93. © American College of Sports Medicine. Used by permission.

not include the time taken to enter the locker room or to finish dressing after a shower! The relationship between duration of exercise and improvements in $\dot{V}O_2$ max (holding intensity and frequency of exercise constant) is seen in Figure 5.9. Exercise shorter than 20 minutes, though not likely to cause as much of an increase $\dot{V}O_2$ max, nevertheless will cause some improvement. Evidence suggests that as few as 6 minutes of aerobic exercise per day can be beneficial. Exercise lasting longer than 60 minutes per day results in additional benefit but to a lesser degree.

At least for people involved in jogging/running programs (the programs for which data exist), the rate of injury rises sharply after 45–60 minutes of exercise. The dotted line in Figure 5.9 represents this phenomenon.

Intensity and duration are related directly. The harder you exercise, the less time you have to spend to achieve a given benefit. Or, if your exercise intensity is lower, you can achieve the same benefit

by working longer. This is important for anyone beginning an exercise program, because it means you do not have to exercise extremely hard to do yourself some good. You can accomplish your goals by working submaximally for a longer time. By working intensively for a short period, you may even be doing yourself some harm in the long run. The psychological stress of intensive exercise (similar to that experienced by many athletes during competitive training) is so much greater than in submaximal exercise that most people will not continue the pace very long—certainly not over the course of a lifetime. So, even discounting the potential injury problems and other risks, gentle exercise of longer duration seems most appropriate.

Does exercise have to be continuous to be effective? Although the evidence suggests that the total duration of exercise time has to conform to the range of 20–60 minutes per day, it does not indicate that this exercise must be done all at one time. When the total caloric expenditure is held constant, the effect of continuous exercise is no different than two or three shorter bouts of slightly more intensive exercise. So, for example, you could jog twice a day for 10 minutes and expect approximately the same benefit as if you were to jog once a day for 20 minutes.

Total caloric expenditure is a critical variable in determining the effects of an exercise program on cardiorespiratory fitness. Caloric expenditure is a function of the total work accomplished, which itself depends on a number of factors such as body weight, intensity, and duration of exercise. The greater the total work (caloric expenditure), the greater the improvement in fitness likely will be. For more on the caloric cost of exercise and related topics, see Chapter 7.

Guidelines published by the American College of Sports Medicine for developing and maintaining fitness in healthy adults suggest that, as a minimum, an exercise program should cause you to expend 300 calories per session.* If you wish to achieve this goal, some rough generalizations regarding how hard and how long you would have to exercise are:

40–50 minutes of moderate-intensity exercise at 60%–80% heart rate reserve

20–30 minutes of moderately high-intensity exercise at 80%–90% heart rate reserve

---

*The recommended guideline of expending at least 300 calories of energy in an exercise program is based largely on data in which males served as subjects. Because men on the average are taller and heavier than women, and energy expenditure in exercise is partly a function of body weight (the greater the weight, the greater the energy expenditure), we can estimate that the number of calories an average woman should expend to accomplish the same gains, assuming all else is equal, will be less. A tentative guess might be 250 calories. These are generalizations based on averages; if you know you are noticeably different from your peers in weight, for example, you need to adjust these estimates upward or downward accordingly, regardless of your gender.

FIGURE 5.9

Improvement in $\dot{V}O_2$ max and risk of orthopedic complication as a function of differing *durations* of exercise, holding mode, frequency, and intensity of exercise constant.

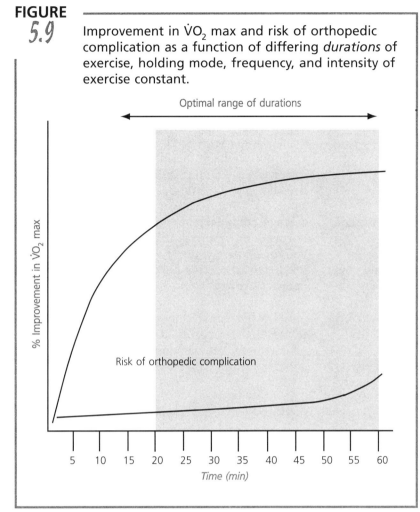

Source: Modified from "Exercise Testing and Prescription," by H. K. Heller-stein and B. A. Franklin, *Rehabilitation of the Coronary Patient*, edited by N. K. Wenger (New York: John Wiley and Sons, 1978), p. 185.

15–20 minutes of high-intensity exercise at greater than 90% heart rate reserve

As mentioned earlier, high-intensity exercise is not recommended for the average person. Again, exercise of moderate intensity and longer duration is a satisfactory, and even preferred, method of improving cardiorespiratory fitness.

When beginning an exercise program, the participant should not feel bound by the guideline of 20–60 minutes of exercise per day. At first the duration of exercise should be lower—perhaps as little as 5 minutes per day—and then slowly progress upward. It depends on what the person can do comfortably. An alternative would be to begin with a longer duration but keep the intensity of exercise relatively low. Again, progressing slowly and in small steps enhances the chances of maintaining a regular exercise routine.

Integrating Mode, Frequency, Intensity, and Duration of Exercise

Having discussed each of these aspects of training separately, we again emphasize their interrelationship. All the aspects of training (mode, frequency, intensity, and duration) must be present to a sufficient degree for noticeable improvements in cardiorespiratory fitness to occur. If a given training program is inadequate in one area or more, the effect will be to reduce the total benefit drastically, even if all other aspects are adequate.

Suppose Henry and Lester are college roommates. Henry always has too many things going for him, and he never seems to have enough time to do anything he starts. Lester, on the other hand, is methodical, almost plodding in his approach to life. Henry and Lester sign up for a college fitness class together, but as soon as the term gets under way, it becomes clear that each is approaching the class in his own unique way. Henry figures he can just as easily work out on his own time as go to class, so he schedules a chemistry lab on two of the three afternoons the fitness class meets. After two weeks of missing class and not fitting in his alternative workout, he decides that he will just run a little harder and longer on the one day he does come to class, thereby making up the difference. In contrast, Lester always gets to class late. Accordingly, by the time he finishes his warm-up on a typical day in class, usually less than 5 minutes of actual exercise time remains before he has to cool down and move on to his next class.

Henry and Lester both have failed to include all the components of exercise to a degree sufficient to achieve marked improvement, even in a 15-week term. Both chose an appropriate mode of exercise (jogging). Henry worked out with sufficient intensity and duration to do himself some good, but he failed to do so often enough to achieve the improvements he desired. Lester's problem was not the frequency or the intensity of his exercise; it was the short duration. As a result, he improved only slightly, again much less than would have been the case had he met the recommended levels in all areas. For optimal (or even modest) improvements in cardiorespiratory fitness, the recommended guidelines must be met in mode, frequency, intensity, and duration *together*.

FACTORS AFFECTING PERFORMANCE AND IMPROVEMENT

Initial Fitness

Your rate of improvement after beginning an exercise program is dependent on your initial state of fitness (Figure 5.10). The poorer your cardiorespiratory fitness when you begin, the more easily you will be able to achieve noticeable improvements, all else remaining the same. If your ability to do endurance exercise is low to begin with, you will be able to improve without undue effort and likely will be reinforced for your efforts. On the other hand, if your initial state of fitness is higher to begin with, not only will your improvements likely be smaller, but they will come only through more intensive, longer, and more frequent exercise.

Genetics

In cardiorespiratory or any type of fitness, the role that initial fitness plays is connected partly to genetics. Whatever your genetic endowment, the farther you are from achieving your limits, the more easily you will improve. As you approach your limits, further improvements become more difficult, as shown in Figure 5.10. Certainly this is not encouraging news, but it seems to be a fact of life.

The role of genetics is understood poorly at present, but the differences between people in terms of cardiorespiratory fitness seem to be attributable to genetic endowment to a much greater extent than they are to training. Let's suppose an elite athlete and an average, sedentary individual differ 100% in $\dot{V}O_2$ max. Because evidence indicates that, through training, you can improve your $\dot{V}O_2$ max by about 15%–25%, this means the remaining differences between elite and average probably are related to genetics.

Because of the differences derived from genetic endowment, having a high $\dot{V}O_2$ max in itself does not provide an accurate picture of fitness status. Results of any testing must be interpreted with respect to your genetic make-up as well as how much exercise you do.

For example, people with "great genes" can have a high $\dot{V}O_2$ max or even high ability to perform endurance exercise easily (e.g., a former endurance athlete performing a 12-minute run test) and yet be unfit. *Compared to their own potential*, they may be unfit because they do not exercise sufficiently, but when compared to others of more average potential, they may score near the top in norms. The reason is that most norms that allow you to compare yourself to others have been developed by measuring heterogeneous samples of people. Because most heterogeneous samples do not contain many people who are genetically gifted, when those who are gifted compare themselves to these norms, they are at the top of the scale, sometimes with no training at all. This is another example of "unfair but true!"

Age

As indicated, a given amount of training in older individuals results in improvements in cardiorespiratory fitness similar in *relative value* to those

FIGURE 5.10

Improvements in VO$_2$ max as a function of *initial fitness and genetics*. Assuming monthly increments in training, larger improvements occur the lower the initial state of fitness. Smaller improvements occur the closer you get to your genetically determined limit.

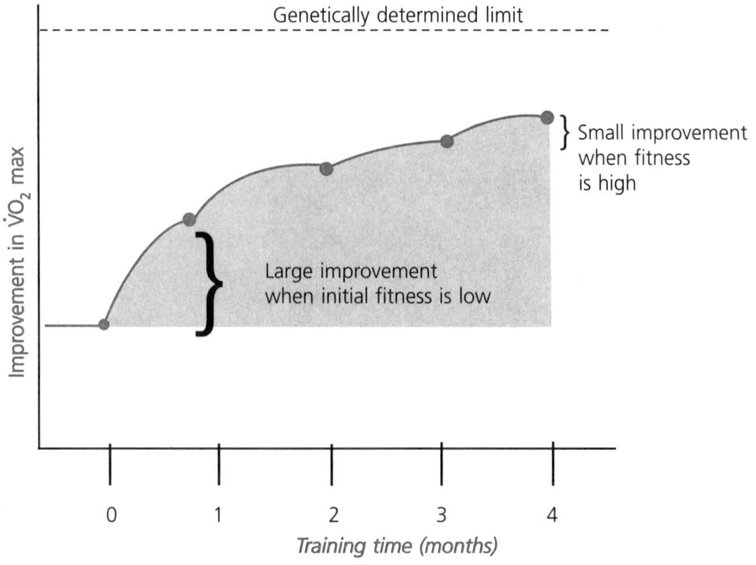

younger individuals attain. The improvements are smaller when expressed on an *absolute scale*. In addition, the rate of improvement is slower. The improvements that become visible in a young adult after several weeks of training might be seen in an older individual only after several months of training. This may be attributable partly to a more gentle approach to training used with older, sedentary individuals, particularly those over age 60.

As noted earlier, cardiorespiratory training can result in drastic improvements in the functional status of older individuals, enabling them to perform at a level similar to that of many sedentary individuals 20–30 years younger. Evidence, however, does not indicate that fitness can stop the aging process. Although the level of function can be raised by training, the rate of decline seems similar in the sedentary and the well-trained. Declines seem to accelerate after age 60, but again it is not clear whether this is a result of true aging or a decline in the total amount of regular exercise. Even for the most active people, the amount of exercise seems to decline more rapidly after age 60.

Gender Differences

Most of the research that has led to the generalizations regarding mode, frequency, intensity, and duration of exercise has been done using men as subjects. This is because, until the last 20–25 years, the number of women participating in aerobic exercise was considerably smaller than the number of men. The studies that have been done indicate that women tend to adapt to cardiorespiratory training in a manner similar to men. Many gender differences are found, however, in performance and physiological function. These changes become apparent after puberty. Typically, the differences arise from the larger stature and body mass of most males compared to most females.

Data comparing the sexes on several variables are seen in Table 5.C. When comparing the sexes in $\dot{V}O_2$ max per unit of fat-free tissue (thereby removing the effect of body fat), gender differences are reduced considerably. Reasons for the remaining differences include smaller volume and maximal pumping capacity of the heart, smaller blood volume, and lower oxygen-carrying capacity in blood in females compared to males.

Disability

Developing and maintaining cardiorespiratory fitness is also of concern to people who have disabilities, either permanent or temporary. Depending on the cause of the disability and on how long it will last, fitness strategies will vary. For someone who is temporarily in a leg cast that allows walking on crutches, for example, the mere task of walking from here to there to meet the normal needs of contemporary living usually places sufficient physical stress on the upper body to provide sufficient exercise. Those with more permanent disabilities can engage in wheelchair activities. Road races often include paraplegic competitors whose upper bodies are developed superbly from miles of aerobic wheelchair training. A number of activities that can be done in the water, from simple swimming to water exercises and water games, provide an alternative medium for engaging in physical activity while weight-supported. The references include approaches for adapting activity for people with special needs.

TABLE 5.C Gender differences in circulatory and oxygen transport systems.

| | REST | | | | | | MAXIMUM | | | |
| | HEART RATE (BEATS/MIN) | | SYSTOLIC BLOOD PRESSURE (MM HG) | | DIASTOLIC BLOOD PRESSURE (MM HG) | | HEART RATE (BEATS/MIN) | | MAX $\dot{V}O_2$ (ESTIMATED) (ML/KG/MIN) | |
Age	Male	Female	Male	Female	Male	Female	Male	Female	Male	Female
20–29	63	65	121	112	80	75	194	188	39.1	30.2
30–39	63	68	120	114	80	76	189	184	37.0	30.2
40–49	62	66	121	118	80	80	182	177	35.7	26.7
50–59	63	67	128	122	82	80	173	170	32.9	24.5
60+	62	64	131	130	81	80	162	153	29.0	21.8

Source: Data from the Cooper Clinic Coronary Risk Factor Profile Charts, by M. L. Pollock, J. H. Wilmore, and S. M. Fox, *Exercise in Health and Disease* (Philadelphia: W. B. Saunders, 1984), pp. 418–427.

Exercise and Pregnancy

The safety of exercise during pregnancy, to both the developing fetus and the mother, has been of considerable interest. The evidence to date suggests that regular, gentle exercise done three days per week at a heart rate equal to or below 144 beats/minute for 40 minutes or less, seems not to be associated with adverse effects to the mother or fetus. In fact, regular exercise of the type described is associated with increased maternal fitness and physical capacity. Effects on weight gain during pregnancy, maternal self-image, physical well-being, labor, and recovery from labor are less well understood.

Guidelines by the American College of Obstetricians and Gynecologists recommend avoiding more strenuous, competitive activities as well as vigorous activities done in hot, humid weather and during illness. Very low-intensity activity and slow progression are best, especially for women who have led sedentary lives. Pregnant women should follow the warm-up and cool-down procedures described in this chapter. Further, although the literature does not suggest that exercise during pregnancy is associated with an increase in musculoskeletal injury or complaints, the guidelines warn against jerky and bouncy movements, activities that require jumping and jarring motions, and rapid changes in direction. The guidelines also warn against doing exercise in the supine (on the back) position after the fourth month, and doing any exercise in which the breath is held or the body temperature is raised more than 2 degrees Fahrenheit.

Fluid replacement is important, as is a caloric intake that not only meets the extra needs of pregnancy but also of the exercise performed. If any unusual symptoms appear, activity should be stopped and the physician consulted.

Motivation

For one reason or another, many people do not exercise regularly. Among them, some would like to exercise regularly and may dedicate themselves to, and later abandon, new exercise regimes. If this description fits you and you would like to follow through on a lasting exercise/fitness program, motivation is paramount. Throughout this chapter we have offered a number of suggestions addressing the issue of motivation. First, you should feel free to exercise at a lower intensity when beginning, rather than thinking you must achieve a target heart rate at the 50% to 85% level right away. The goal is to develop some form of regular exercise that you will be motivated to continue for the rest of your life. Another suggestion is to modify endurance games you enjoy (such as tennis or basketball) so you can do what pleases you and develop or maintain cardiorespiratory fitness at the same time. The bottom line is to do whatever is necessary in an exercise program to make your exercising experience as *comfortable and pleasant as possible.*

Someone once described an exercise program as "something that a mesomorph thinks up for an endomorph" (translation: "something that a person with a muscular, fit body thinks up for a person with a round, fat body"). Although that may have been the case at one time, *your exercise program should be designed by you and for you.* If exercising with others helps you keep at it, look for exercise companions. If you like the outdoors and the time alone, choose an exercise setting like that. Only you know how you feel. With careful choices you can make your exercise as pleasant as possible and move from the ranks of the sedentary to the ranks of the fit.

MAINTAINING CARDIORESPIRATORY FITNESS

Once a satisfactory level of cardiorespiratory fitness is achieved, how much exercise is required to maintain that status? One option is simply to continue at the same exercise level thereafter. As discussed earlier, less exercise may be required to maintain your cardiorespiratory fitness than is needed to improve it. Thus, if you have been exercising five days a week, and you drop down to only three days per week, all else remaining the same, your fitness status may not decline substantially.

Unfortunately, few longitudinal studies have followed individuals for more than a few months after reductions in regular exercise. This means it eventually may be shown that if a reduction were carried out over a year or more, a small loss in fitness would occur.

Therefore, the wisest conclusion at present is to maintain your exercise habits within the guidelines discussed in this chapter for achieving an improvement. As long as you continue using an appropriate mode, frequency, intensity, and duration of exercise, the only reason for your fitness to decline will be from true aging. If the amount of exercise you do declines substantially, however, your cardiorespiratory fitness will decline as well.

SUMMARY

Physical activity and regular aerobic exercise have been shown to bring about a number of favorable effects in adults of all ages, including reducing the risk of cardiovascular disease. Regular activity also is associated with a longer life, independent of other influencing factors. When first beginning an aerobic exercise program, you should determine whether you have any medical condition that might put you at greater risk during exercise. Initial fitness status can be assessed in a variety of ways. Some of these are sophisticated and expensive; others are relatively simple and just as effective if used on a periodic basis for comparing yourself to yourself.

If you wish to improve your health, a goal should be to accumulate 30 minutes or more of moderate-intensity physical activity most days of the week. If you wish to improve your cardiorespiratory fitness, you should engage in any form of large-muscle, rhythmic exercise, three to five days per week, 20–60 minutes per day, at an intensity of 50%–85% of heart rate reserve. The methods of building up to this level of exercise depend on individual differences, including initial fitness, genetics, age, and gender. Specific warm-up and cool-down procedures should be followed. Most important, making your exercise experience as comfortable and pleasant as possible will greatly enhance your motivation.

REFERENCES

American College of Obstetricians and Gynecologists. 1985. *Exercise During Pregnancy and the Postnatal Period* (ACOG Home Exercise Programs). Washington, DC: ACOG.

American College of Sports Medicine. 1990. "Position Stand: The Recommended Quantity and Quality of Exercise for Developing and Maintaining Cardiorespiratory and Muscular Fitness in Healthy Adults." *Medicine and Science in Sports* 22(3): 265–274.

American College of Sports Medicine. 1991. *Guidelines for Exercise Testing and Prescription* (4th ed.). Philadelphia: Lea and Febiger.

American College of Sports Medicine. 1992. *ACSM Fitness Book.* Champaign, IL: Leisure Press.

Blair, S. N. 1985. "Physical Activity Leads to Fitness and Pays Off." *Physician and Sportsmedicine* 13(3): 153–157.

Blair, S. N. 1993. "1993 C. H. McCloy Research Lecture: Physical Activity, Physical Fitness, and Health." *Research Quarterly for Exercise and Sport* 64(4): 365–376.

Blair, S. N., Kohl, H. W. III, Paffenbarger, R. S., Clark, D. G., Cooper, K. H., and Gibbons, L. W. 1989. "Physical Fitness and All-Cause Mortality." *Journal of the American Medical Association* 262: 2395–2401.

CHOICES IN ACTION

Several laboratory exercises in Appendix 9 have been developed to help you work with the concepts discussed in this chapter. Lab 11 assists you in obtaining baseline measurements of heart rate and blood pressure. Lab 12 helps you calculate your target heart rate during cardiorespiratory exercise. Lab 13 provides a simple warm-up and cool-down routine for you. Labs 14–16 provide assistance in performing various tests of cardiorespiratory fitness that you can use in obtaining baseline measurements on yourself, as well as follow-up measurements.

Boone, T., Frentz, K. L., and Boyd, N. R. 1985. "Carotid Palpation at Two Exercise Intensities." *Medicine and Science in Sports and Exercise* 17(6): 705–709.

Bokovoy, J. L., and Blair, S. N. 1994. "Aging and Exercise: A Health Perspective." *Journal of Aging and Physical Activity* 2: 243–260.

Borg, G. A. V. 1973. "Perceived Exertion: A Note on 'History' and Methods." *Medicine and Science in Sports* 5: 90–93.

Clapp, J. F., Rokey, R., Treadway, J. L., Carpenter, M. W., Artal, R. M., and Warrnes, C. 1992. "Exercise in Pregnancy." *Medicine and Science in Sports and Exercise* 24(6, supplement): S 294–300.

Cooper, K. H. 1982. *The Aerobics Program for Total Well-Being: Exercise, Diet, Emotional Balance.* New York: M. Evans.

deVries, H. A., and Housh T. J. 1994. *The Physiology of Exercise.* 5th ed. Madison, WI: W. C. Brown and Benchmark.

Drinkwater, B. L. 1984. "Women and Exercise: Physiological Aspects." *Exercise and Sports Sciences Reviews* 12: 21–51.

Durstine, J. L., and Haskell, W. L. 1994. "Effects of Exercise Training on Plasma Lipids and Lipoproteins." *Exercise and Sport Sciences Reviews,* edited by J. O. Holloszy. 22: 447–521.

Fox, E. L., and Matthews, D. K. 1981. *The Physiological Basis of Physical Education and Athletics* (3d ed.). Philadelphia: Saunders College.

Hellerstein, H. K., and Franklin, B. A. 1978. "Exercise Testing and Prescription." In *Rehabilitation of the Coronary Patient,* N. K. Wenger (Ed.). New York: John Wiley.

Jetté, M., Campbell, J., Mongeon, J., and Routhier, R. 1976. "The Canadian home fitness test as a predictor of aerobic capacity." *CMA Journal* 114: 680–682.

Kasch, F. W. et al. 1988. "Changes in Aerobic Power of Men, Ages 25-70 Years." *Physician and Sportsmedicine* 16(1): 117–124.

Katch, F. I., and McArdle, W. D. 1991. *Introduction to Nutrition, Exercise, and Health,* 3rd ed. Philadelphia: Lea and Febiger.

Kline, G. M., Porcari, J. P., Hintermeister, R., Freedson, P. S., Ward, A., McCarron, R. F., Ross, J., and Rippe, J. M. 1987. "Estimation of VO$_2$ Max from a One-Mile Track Walk, Gender, Age, and Body Weight." *Medicine and Science in Sports and Exercise* 19(3): 253–259.

LaPorte, R. E., Dearwater, S., Cauley, J. A., Slemenda, C., and Cook, T. 1985. "Physical Activity or Cardiovascular Fitness: Which is More Important for Health?" *Physician & Sportsmedicine* 13(3): 145–150.

Lokey, E. A., Tran, A. V., Wells, C. L., Myers, B. C., and Tran, A. C. 1991. "Effects of Physical Exercise on Pregnancy Outcomes: A Meta-analytic Review." *Medicine and Science in Sports and Exercise* 23(11): 1234–1239.

McArdle, W. D., Katch, F. I., and Katch, V. L. 1993. *Exercise Physiology* (3rd ed.). Philadelphia: Lea and Febiger.

Morris, J. N., Chave, S. P. W., Adam, C., and Sirey, C. 1973. "Vigorous Exercise in Leisure-Time and the Incidence of Coronary Heart Disease." *Lancet* 1: 333–339.

Paffenbarger, R. S., and Hyde, R. T. 1980. "Exercise as Protection Against Heart Attack." *New England Journal of Medicine* 302: 1026–1027.

Paffenbarger, R. S., Hyde, R. T., Wing, M. B. A., and Hsieh, C. C. 1986. "Physical Activity, All-Cause Mortality, and Longevity of College Alumni." *New England Journal of Medicine* 314: 605–613.

Pollock, M. L., Wilmore, J. H., and Fox III, S. M. 1984. *Exercise in Health and Disease.* Philadelphia: W. B. Saunders.

Public Health Service. 1990. *Healthy People 2000: National Health Promotion and Disease Prevention Objectives* (DHHS Publ. No. PHS 91–50212). Washington, DC: U. S. Government Printing Office.

Robertson, L. D., Cunningham, M., Changsut, R., Himmelsbach, J. and Koenig, P. "Statistical and Practical Issues Affecting the Acceptability of Timed and Untimed Conditions for a New Abdominal Fitness Test. *Human Movement Studies* 14: 255–268.

Rohm-Young, D., and Steinhardt, M. A. 1993. "The Importance of Physical Fitness Versus Physical Activity for Coronary Artery Disease Risk Factors: A Cross-Sectional Analysis." *Research Quarterly for Exercise and Sport* 64(4): 377–384.

Shephard, R. J. 1983. "The Value of Exercise in Ischemic Heart Disease: A Cumulative Analysis." *Journal of Cardiac Rehabilitation* 3: 294–298.

Smith, E. L., and Zook, S. K. 1986. "The Aging Process: Benefits of Physical Activity." *Journal of Physical Education, Recreation and Dance* 57: 32–34.

"Summary Statement: Workshop on Physical Activity and Public Health." 1993. *Sports Medicine Bulletin* 28(4): 7.

Winnick, J. P. 1990. *Adapted Physical Education and Sport.* Champaign, IL: Human Kinetics, Publishers.

Wiseman, D. C. 1994. *Physical Education for Exceptional Students: Theory to Practice.* Albany, NY: Delmar Publishers.

Able Bodies
Flexibility, Strength, and Muscle Endurance

✓ How do flexibility, strength, and muscle endurance enhance quality living?

✓ How can you tell if you have adequate flexibility? Strength? Muscle endurance? How can you increase these components of fitness safely and effectively? Are some methods superior? Unsafe?

✓ What effects, if any, do procedures such as circuit training and interval training have on fitness?

✓ How should you train to improve your power, speed, and agility, which you may need for participation in a particular sport?

✓ How can you build muscle? Are anabolic steroids safe for this purpose?

If you wish to attain optimum function, all-around fitness is necessary. Having good *flexibility* in all of your muscles and joints enables you to move freely without restriction. Adequate *strength* and *muscular endurance* will reduce the fatigue from daily tasks, and you will look better and feel better about yourself. You also will be better prepared in the event of an emergency. This chapter contains a discussion of these components of fitness and the role they play in overall function, and provides guidelines for how to measure, develop, and maintain status in each of these areas.

THE PROCESS OF DEGENERATION

The term **hypokinetic degeneration** refers to *a degenenerative process resulting from too little movement*. When movement is restricted, many bodily functions deteriorate. In extreme cases, such as with prolonged bedrest, the following have been documented to occur to some degree:

1. *Muscle atrophy.* Gradual loss of muscle tissue results in loss of strength and loss of ability to do aerobic exercise.

2. *Loss of flexibility.* Without regular movement, the connective tissue that makes up the tendons and ligaments shortens and becomes resistant to stretching.

3. *Osteoporosis.* This degenerative disease (described in Chapter 3) involves the loss of proteins and minerals from bones, making them considerably more susceptible to fractures.

4. *Cardiovascular and respiratory malfunctions.* In bedridden people, resting heart rate tends to rise while the ability of the heart to eject blood per beat drops. Aerobic capacity declines dramatically, and the person is unable to maintain adequate blood pressure when upright. Blood volume decreases, and blood clots may develop in the veins. The lungs become congested with fluids, and bronchial obstructions can develop. Pneumonia is fairly common in bedridden people.

5. *Bladder and bowel malfunction.* Being immobile often leads to difficulty in eliminating urine and feces.

These dramatic malfunctions have been observed in people who are confined to bed for a long time. These conditions are found wherever old people reside: in nursing homes and retirement communities. Also, as anyone who has had a cast can attest, muscle atrophy sets in rapidly when a limb is immobilized. Many people of all ages have

these problems, and they do not set in overnight. The same degenerative process can take place, though to a lesser extent, in people who sit day after day at their jobs or at home.

WORKING AGAINST DEGENERATION

Virtually all the degenerative processes associated with hypokinetic degeneration can be prevented or alleviated by engaging in regular exercise. Postsurgical patients used to be kept bedridden for days or weeks; today these people are encouraged to get up and move as soon as they are able, because people respond better when they move around. *People who are active are healthier.* They feel better, look better, and perform better. Regular exercise can and does play an important part in maintaining a higher quality of living for most people.

An interesting illustration supports this point. As we get older, grip strength normally declines, particularly after we reach the age of 60. In a group of men whose job duties required them to use their hands vigorously on the job, this decline in grip strength was not evident. Even for the men who were in their 60s, grip strength was similar to that of younger counterparts, presumably because they continued to use their strength. Imagine what the world would be like if people were to remain vigorously active all their lives? Now imagine what you will be like when you retire, and what you will want to experience and do with your time.

Another health problem that affects a great number of adults is low back pain, as discussed in Chapter 3. Based on clinical evidence, fitness experts, physical therapists, kinesiotherapists, and orthopedic surgeons have long linked the incidence of low back problems to lack of exercise. The rationale is that weak muscles are fatigued easily and cannot support the spine and pelvis in proper alignment. In an upright position the abdominal muscles and the spinal extensors in the lower back are designed to stabilize the spine and pelvis and keep it from tilting forward into the "swayback" position (see Figure 4.2 in Chapter 4). If the abdominal muscles are weak, the pelvis tilts forward into the abnormal swayback position, putting greater stress on the vertebral column and compressing the space through which nerves pass to and from the spinal cord.

Another contributing factor is tight muscles at the back of the leg (hamstrings), which attach to the lower pelvis. Tight hamstrings inhibit the natural forward tilt of the pelvis when bending forward at the waist or stretching, thereby reducing mobility and increasing the possibility of strain, spasm, and pain.

This raises the general question of posture and the role that flexibility and strength play in overall postural problems. Whenever one or another body part is out of alignment, it places greater strain on other muscles to compensate against the pull of gravity and keep the body upright. As a result, these muscles are more susceptible to fatigue, spasms, and chronic pain. Over long periods, the muscles, tendons, and ligaments accommodate the misalignment with more permanent changes in structure, which makes attempts at correction more difficult.

FLEXIBILITY
Measuring Flexibility

Being able to assess your current flexibility accurately, in a manner that can be repeated at a later date, is important. You may wish to determine where you are in relation to others. As we have stressed, assessing yourself when you first begin a fitness program is wise so you can monitor your progress periodically. This will help you gauge the level of progression to follow. The record also will be a motivational tool because you will be able to see how much you improve over time.

Flexibility in each person can vary widely from one part of the body to another. The most commonly used test of flexibility is the *sit-and-reach test*. This test has many versions, all of which provide essentially the same type of information: your ability to bend forward from the waist. Although the test is designed to measure flexibility of the lower back and posterior leg regions, evidence suggests that it may not truly measure flexibility in the lower back. Until a simple alternative test is developed, however, the sit-and-reach test continues to be the best choice available. Test results from the sit-and-reach test cannot be generalized to other types of flexibility.

In the version of the test developed by the national YMCA for use in its fitness programs, no specialized equipment is needed, although special sit-and-reach benches make it easier to evaluate yourself. (You will have the opportunity to perform the sit-and-reach flexibility test in Lab 17.)

Developing and Maintaining Flexibility

Stretching Principles

To improve your flexibility, you should use exercises that cause you to move through your whole

range of motion. This can be accomplished in two common ways. One involves doing exercises that are dynamic or bouncy, such as jumping jacks, alternate toe touches, and side bends. This is called **ballistic stretching.** Another form, **static stretching,** involves exercises in which you stretch while holding yourself in a fixed position. An example is reaching forward to touch your toes while sitting on the ground with your feet extended ahead of you.

Both ballistic and static stretching techniques are effective in improving flexibility. Caution should be taken, however, when stretching ballistically, because of the possibility of overstretching, which may cause soreness or injury. For this reason, static stretching is considered the safer technique. Ballistic exercises probably are safe if they are done easily and not vigorously, as in a gentle warm-up routine in which you move around easily to loosen your muscles and joints.

When using static stretching techniques, begin by holding each stretch 5–10 seconds; then, with practice, eventually work your way up to 15–30 seconds or more for each stretch. Repeat each stretch one to five or more times, depending on your time and interest. The overall routine should be done three to five days per week. You never should stretch to the point of pain or burning discomfort. Rather, you should move to the limits of your range of motion, using comfort as a guide, and then stretch slightly beyond and hold it there. When stretching, you should try to relax the muscles being stretched. For the most effective results and the least likelihood of injury, *you should warm up adequately before doing any stretching.* Stretching when not warmed up, or using vigorous stretching as a warm-up, may be injurious to your muscles and joints.

Research in rehabilitation has generated another technique for improving flexibility, called **proprioceptive neuromuscular facilitation,** or **PNF.** PNF techniques typically involve working with a partner. First you move your limb and the to-be-stretched muscle to the point of initial limitation in its range of motion. Your partner then holds your limb in this position and resists any movement while you maximally contract and then relax the stretched muscle. Finally, your partner moves the affected limb and muscle to the point where you again feel limitation. On the basis of limited research to date, PNF seems to be as effective as static stretching in increasing range of motion.

Factors That Limit Flexibility

The resistance you feel when stretching comes predominantly from connective tissue. Connective tissue binds muscle fibers together into bundles, surrounds muscles in sheaths, connects muscles to bones (via the tendons), and connects bones together (via the ligaments). This connective tissue has elastic properties that resist stretching. With time and practice it will stretch in response to applied pressure. Within reasonable limits, this deformation is the desired goal when undertaking a flexibility program.

Other factors also can limit flexibility. For example, resistance from skin, excessive fat, large muscles that interfere with a full range of motion, and even one's bone structure can limit improvement in flexibility. As with any type of training, the longer you work at stretching, the greater the changes will be. A word of caution, however: Excessive flexibility may be a hindrance in some cases, particularly if the support structures are weakened or loosened so as not to protect the joint from injury from the normal stresses accompanying vigorous activity. Therefore, you should not work on flexibility if a joint and the surrounding muscles and tendons already provide great range of motion.

Sample Stretching Routines

Appendix 1 presents a safe exercise routine designed to promote a healthy neck and back. The exercises promote flexibility and strength of the spine and related body parts. Clinical evidence suggests that low back pain can be related in part to poor flexibility in the hamstring muscles at the back of the upper leg. The hamstring stretch exercise (see photograph (d) in Appendix 1) should be of special interest in preventing and treating this condition.

Many common stretching exercises, when done repeatedly for long periods, have been linked to structural injury or chronic pain. Appendix 2 presents common exercises to avoid because they are associated with a higher risk of injury.

Additional Mild Flexibility Exercises for other parts of the body are included in Appendix 3.

STRENGTH AND MUSCLE ENDURANCE

Measuring Strength

Strength is defined as the capacity of a muscle or muscle group to exert force under maximal conditions. Several methods can be used to measure strength, all of which are very different from one another. As a result of these differences, strength is defined operationally in different ways, depending on the measurement procedure used.

Static Strength

Static strength is measured using special devices called *dynamometers* and *tensiometers*, which you push or pull against in a fixed position. The most common of these devices is the grip dynamometer (Figure 6.1; Lab 18). Tests of static leg extension strength or static strength of most other muscle groups require specialized equipment and techniques that are not as widely available. Measuring static strength is of somewhat limited value because it has been shown that static strength varies within the same muscle group according to the joint angle. You do not have just one static strength in a given muscle group; you may have many, depending on the position in which you measure the strength. Therefore, taking a single measurement of static strength will not provide an overall indication of your strength status because no single measurement is highly representative of the large number of strength scores you could generate if you were to take the time to do so.

Isokinetic Strength

Isokinetic strength is the peak force (or "peak torque," as it is called) you are able to exert while pushing against an isokinetic machine. To measure your strength, you push against a movable lever on the machine with a body part such as your lower leg, moving it through the full range of motion. The isokinetic machine is set to allow only one speed of movement at a time, regardless of how hard you push against it. Because these machines are expensive, they are not widely available and are found mostly in rehabilitation clinics. No widespread norms have been developed using isokinetic machines, so if you have a chance to be measured,

FIGURE 6.1 Grip dynamometer for measuring static grip strength.

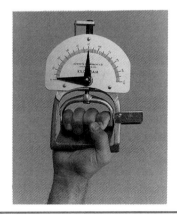

the best method is to compare your strength score to a score recorded for you at an earlier or later date.

Dynamic Strength

Dynamic strength is the heaviest weight that can be lifted correctly just one time. This is called the **1 repetition maximum** (1 RM) (see Lab 18). Because weights are available in most gyms and fitness establishments, determining 1 RM is the most practical way to measure strength. Typically, a trial-and-error approach is used to determine 1 RM, waiting one to three minutes between trials.

A note of caution is warranted. Experts disagree as to the safety of doing 1 RM tests unless you are conditioned properly and skilled in using correct techniques. A conservative approach is not to attempt it until you have engaged in regular resistance training for a minimum of several weeks.

Recommended standards for dynamic strength in several different muscle groups are given in Table 6.A. These standards may not be representative of all segments of the population (e.g., athletes), but they are suggested as appropriate goals for the average person. It is recommended that all the tests in the table be used to assess strength, because an overall strength profile is preferred; however. If there is time for only one test, however, it should be the bench press exercise, which has been shown to have the highest correlation to the whole battery of tests. The bench press exercise is pictured in Appendix 3.

Measuring Muscle Endurance

Typically, *absolute* muscle endurance and *relative* muscle endurance are measured dynamically, using either free weights or weight machines (see Lab 19).

Absolute muscle endurance is determined by counting the number of correctly completed repetitions one can do with a standard weight before being unable to continue. For example, suppose you decide to count the number of lifts you can do in the arm-curl exercise (in which you lift a weight upward to your chest with your arm flexors) using 40 pounds. If you can do 15 repetitions before being unable to continue, that will be your muscle endurance score. As you might surmise, muscle endurance measured in this manner is related highly to your dynamic strength. The greater your strength, the greater your absolute muscle endurance.

Relative muscle endurance is measured by taking some fraction of the 1 RM score (usually 70%) and determining the number of correctly executed repetitions one can do. For example, if your 1 RM score is 110 pounds for a certain exercise, the product of .70(110), or 77 pounds, is the weight you would use to determine your relative muscle endurance. If you cannot adjust the weight this accurately, you can use a 70- or 75-pound weight as an alternative. Standards for measuring muscular endurance using this method have not been developed, but on the basis of limited experience, a rough goal for the recreational exerciser is

TABLE 6.A — Strength standards recommended for four weight-lifting exercises.

BODY WEIGHT (LB)	BENCH PRESS		STANDING PRESS		CURL		LEG PRESS	
	Male	*Female*	*Male*	*Female*	*Male*	*Female*	*Male*	*Female*
80	80	56	53	37	40	28	160	112
100	100	70	67	47	50	35	200	140
120	120	84	80	56	60	42	240	168
140	140	98	93	65	70	49	280	196
160	160	112	107	75	80	56	320	224
180	180	126	120	84	90	63	360	252
200	200	140	133	93	100	70	400	280
220	220	154	147	103	110	77	440	308
240	240	168	160	112	120	84	480	336

Note: Data collected on Universal Gym apparatus is based on 1 RM. Information collected on another apparatus could modify results. Data expressed in pounds.

Source: M. L. Pollock, J. W. Wilmore, and S. M. Fox, *Health and Fitness Through Physical Activity.* Copyright 1978. All rights reserved. Reprinted by permission of Allyn & Bacon.

to be able to do twelve to fifteen repetitions in a given exercise using this method. For a competitive athlete, twenty to twenty-five repetitions is a reasonable goal.

Relative muscle endurance also may be measured by taking a fraction of your body weight to determine the load with which to measure yourself. In this case, muscle endurance is said to be relative to body weight rather than relative to strength. For example, you might take 40% of your body weight and count the number of repetitions you can do with this load. Alternatively, you might count the number of repetitions you can complete in a specific time, such as 60 seconds.

Another common method of measuring muscular endurance relative to body weight is through **calisthenics.** In calisthenic exercises your body weight serves as the resistance. Push-ups, sit-ups, and pull-ups are examples. If you use a calisthenic exercise as a test of muscular endurance (e.g., a push-up test), you actually are lifting a fraction of your body weight. In the case of the push-up, for example, the resistance is your body weight acting as if it were pivoting as a lever around your toes. The effect of the leverage in this case is to reduce the resistance to less than it would be if you had to lift your entire body.

Developing and Maintaining Strength and Muscle Endurance

General Principles

The general principles of warm-up, overload, and progression discussed in Chapter 4 are particularly applicable to this type of training because of the great stress placed on muscles, joints, and related connective tissue. Both a general warm-up, which raises your body temperature slightly, and a specific warm-up of the muscles that you will be training always should be done for 5–10 minutes before beginning this type of training. General warm-up can be accomplished by walking or doing light calisthenics, followed by light jogging. Specific warm-up can be accomplished by beginning with much lower resistances at first.

As with any type of training, properly applying the principle of progression will enable you to improve without subjecting yourself to excessive stress and potential injury. Your rate of progression will depend on your motivation to improve and how trained you are to begin with. A prudent and cautious approach is one in which you progress slowly rather than trying to set a world record in a few months. If you are training toward a specific goal, such as improved performance in a specific

athletic event, you also need to pay attention to the specificity principle and train in ways that mimic or imitate your performance (or parts of it) as much as possible. Otherwise, a general all-around training program that emphasizes the major muscle groups, particularly those of the upper body, is recommended for the average exerciser.

Exercises for Building Strength and Muscle Endurance

The Mild Resistive Exercises illustrated in Appendix 3, when done slowly, are safe for people of all ages and require little or no special equipment. For those with low initial fitness, these exercises will contribute modestly to the development of strength and muscle endurance and can be used as a preconditioning program before moving on to more rigorous training.

If your initial fitness permits you to begin at a higher level of training, the most practical method to build strength and muscle endurance is through dynamic exercises that typically involve lifting weights, although calisthenic exercises also are a form of dynamic exercise. Most beginners find it tolerable to start with loads that are about 50% of their 1 RM, doing a series of ten repetitions of a given exercise in a set and slowly building up to three or four sets per workout, 3 days per week. As fitness improves, you can begin slowly adding weight so you work with loads that equal 60% 1 RM, and then 70% and 80% 1 RM. The Dynamic Exercises in Appendix 3 illustrate common resistance exercises used for this purpose.

Often people mix exercise techniques together. For example, aerobics classes often include a portion of class time for aerobic exercise with supplemental hand weights or with flexible tubing or other stretchable material that offers resistance when stretched. The idea is to promote aerobic activity while also attending modestly to the development of muscular strength and endurance.

A special comment is warranted regarding abdominal exercises. Evidence has demonstrated that, compared to the more traditional curl-up exercise, in which you curl to the upright position to touch your knees, greater overload is placed on the abdominal muscles by doing a partial curl-up with the feet unsupported, the legs bent, and the hands at the side of the body, as illustrated in Appendix 1(j). This abdominal exercise is recommended particularly if you are interested in preventing low-back problems.

Another point is worth emphasizing. Improvements in strength and muscle endurance will be similar whether you use free weights or weight machines such as Universal or Nautilus, provided

A C T I V I T Y

BEGINNING 10-WEEK TRAINING PROGRAM FOR BUILDING STRENGTH/MUSCLE ENDURANCE

INTRODUCTORY COMMENT:

This program is a generic example and is not intended to be used by all people in the same manner. Individual preferences, interests, and needs should be considered in designing a program for yourself.

Exercises should be done 3 days/week and should be preceded by a general warm-up of 5–10 minutes (e.g., riding an exercise cycle at a light resistance + gentle stretching and unweighted movement of targeted body parts.)

PRECONDITIONING PROGRAM

Week 1:

Select 6–9 exercises, one each for the following body parts: chest, shoulder, arms (front and back); back, abdomen, thigh (front and back), and calf. Organize the exercises so the order proceeds from large to small muscle groups. Do one set of each exercise, allowing 60–90 seconds of rest between each set. Begin with a relatively light resistance that permits you to complete one set of 10 repetitions of the exercise comfortably.

Weeks 2–3:

Each week, add additional exercises up to 3 per body part. Choose exercises that involve new muscle groups or the same muscles used in a different manner. Also include other body parts (e.g., forearms, neck). Continue to do one set/exercise with resistances that allow you to complete 10 repetitions of the exercise comfortably.

CONDITIONING PROGRAM

Weeks 4–6:

a. Begin building up from one set toward the goal of three sets for each exercise in your program, adjusting the rate of build-up to reflect your exercise tolerance level. Continue to use loads that permit you to complete 10 repetitions of the exercise comfortably, but you may build up to where the last few repetitions are difficult. Allow 60–90 seconds between sets and 2–3 minutes of rest before beginning the next exercise.

b. At the end of this period, complete self-testing to determine your 1 RM and your muscle endurance score, using the procedures outlined earlier in this chapter.

Note: Max testing has been delayed until this point in the program because it is stressful and potentially could lead to injury from over-exertion. How much preconditioning is prudent before attempting such testing is a matter of debate. Including some initial testing is recommended, however, as a means of documenting improvement, adjusting workloads, and motivation. Periodic retesting also is recommended for similar reasons.

Weeks 7–10:

a. Once three sets/exercise has been reached, raise resistance so the third set is difficult to complete. You may not be able to finish the third set until your body

adapts to the higher resistance, so do as many repetitions as you can. Continue raising resistances periodically in this manner, depending on individual circumstances.

b. By 10 weeks, begin to use a "pyramid" approach to assist in achieving improvements. (Example: 4 sets: the first begins with lighter weights than you normally use (warm-up); on the second set, use the weights you normally lift; on the third set, use slightly heavier weights, causing the number of repetitions you can complete to drop; on the fourth set, use even heavier weights, with resulting drops in repetitions.)

c. Because these procedures are difficult to sustain week after week, a technique of cycling workouts referred to as "periodization" also is recommended. Periodization involves interweaving heavier and lighter workouts together within an overall upward progression of work and intensity. Experience suggests that improvements are accomplished more easily by raising intensity and/or number of repetitions in a workout intermittently rather than steadily increasing the difficulty of the workout. Larger periodization cycles lasting months often are devised to prepare for athletic competition. Smaller cycles, lasting one week, for example, also are used.

GENERAL COMMENTS:

1. This beginning weight-training program employs resistances that permit 10 repetitions/set and, as a result, will contribute to the development of both strength and muscle endurance together. If you wish to focus more on building strength, you should evolve gradually into using resistances that permit only 4–6 repetitions/set. Similarly, if you prefer muscle endurance to strength, resistances that permit more than 10 repetitions/set are superior.

2. Correct lifting technique should be maintained at all times when lifting weights. Inexperienced individuals sometimes lift quickly or use momentum to "cheat" their way past a difficult position, thereby allowing them to use heavier weights than they can handle safely. This can lead to injury.

3. As a precaution against accidents and possible injury, spotters should be used whenever lifting weights, particularly when you are working close to your maximum (as in testing or toward the end of a heavy set) in case you are unable to complete the exercise.

4. If you select calisthenic exercises instead of weight-lifting exercises, you should recognize that only calisthenics that do not permit more than 10–15 repetitions without fatigue likely will build strength (e.g., pull-ups). Most calisthenic exercises are suited to building muscle endurance relatively well (e.g., push-ups, curl-ups).

you use similar training procedures. Machines are handy in that the weights can be changed quickly to adjust to different people using the equipment. But they do not allow for significant adjustment in position to accommodate the different biomechanical needs of people of different sizes and leverage. Anyone can use free weights in any position, so they provide the most adaptability in this regard. But, because much time is required to change the weights on a barbell, they are not as easily adapted to the needs of large groups of people who all exercise in a short time. Machines and free weights are equally effective in similar conditions, and your choice should be based on your preference and circumstances.

If your focus is to be strictly on building strength using dynamic exercise, you should do a few repetitions with very heavy resistances. Translating this into more specific terms, it means doing three to six sets with sufficiently heavy weights so you cannot do more than two to ten repetitions in a set. This training is rigorous and should be undertaken only by well-conditioned and highly motivated individuals. It also should not be done more than 3 days per week for a given muscle group.

In contrast, if your goal is to build muscle endurance using dynamic exercise, you should do many repetitions with lower resistances. Specifically, this translates to three to four sets of ten to thirty repetitions, each with loads you can lift only ten to thirty times. Muscle endurance training should be done three days per week with a day of rest separating exercise sessions. Again, this training is rigorous and should be done only by those who are fit and highly motivated. Whenever weight-training with free weights for strength or muscle endurance, spotters should be used when the resistances begin to approach levels that you cannot safely handle.

Note that strength and muscle endurance both will be gained from the two types of training described. But strength is developed optimally with heavier weights and fewer repetitions, whereas muscle endurance is developed optimally with lighter weights and more repetitions. If you are interested in developing both at the same time, a good compromise is to work with three sets of 10 repetitions with loads you can lift only 10 times, 3 days per week.

Preliminary evidence suggests that you can maintain your strength and muscle endurance gains with fewer training sessions per week than are needed for improvements. Whereas three training sessions per week are required for increasing strength and muscle endurance, as few as one to two training sessions per week may be required to maintain yourself at that level, provided training intensity is maintained. This seems to be true over at least a 1–2 month period. Follow-up periods of longer duration using such a maintenance schedule have not been studied, though.

Before leaving the topic of building strength and muscle endurance, two other training methods—*static exercise* and *isokinetic exercise*—should be mentioned, as they can be used in this regard. For different reasons, neither of these is used as frequently as dynamic exercise.

Static Exercise

Static exercise involves doing a maximal (or near maximal) contraction against an immovable resistance for 5–10 seconds. For example, you could stand in a doorway and press outward with your arms on the doorjam. Research has demonstrated that strength will improve dramatically with such a procedure. It has one liability, however: Improvements occur only in the position in which you train. This means that in the example just cited, your strength in that position would improve quickly but your strength would not be much greater if you were to test yourself in a slightly wider doorway, causing your arms to be farther apart. This training is rather impractical because you would have to train a given muscle group in a variety of positions through its full range of motion to increase its overall strength in that range. Nevertheless, static exercises can be useful, particularly when equipment or time is limited or for reconditioning after an injury.

Static strength exercises also can aid dynamic strength. When lifting weights, one position or joint angle in the range of motion can be difficult to move past. This is referred to as the "sticking point." Static exercise at this joint angle can improve strength at the sticking point and thereby increase the ease with which the weight can be lifted through its full range of motion.

Isokinetic Exercise

Isokinetic exercise makes use of isokinetic machines. As mentioned, isokinetic machines are designed to allow you to pull (or push) against them at a variety of speeds predetermined by setting the controls of the machine. Once the speed is set, no matter how hard you pull, the speed does not change. This type of training seems to combine the advantages of dynamic exercise (which allows you to move through your whole range of motion but does not equally overload your muscle in all positions; only the weakest position is overloaded optimally) and static exercise (which allows you to work maximally at all points in your range of motion but which does not involve movement).

Because of the high cost of isokinetic machinery, few people have opportunities to train in this manner. To reduce cost, some manufacturers have developed isokinetic-like machines which, although they do not hold speed of movement strictly constant, permit training that is similar to isokinetic training. When doing this training, doing one to five repetitions at slow speeds is recommended for developing strength, although optimal training procedures have not been developed yet. When training for power, explosive repetitions at faster speeds are recommended.

Factors Affecting Strength and Endurance Gains

Large individual differences seem to be present in the degree of improvement in strength and muscular endurance from training. In some, improvements in excess of 40% have been documented, with small increases continuing even after several years of training. In others, the improvements are smaller. Reasons for the differences are not entirely clear. Improved strength has been shown to be related partly to changes in the cross-sectional area of muscle. As a result of strength training, muscle fibers increase in size but not in number. These changes result from increases in protein synthesis within these trained muscle fibers, causing them to increase in cross-sectional area. Muscle, connective tissue, tendons, and ligaments also are strengthened by heavy resistance exercise.

Improvements in strength also seem to occur because of changes within the central nervous system. A number of lines of evidence suggest this conclusion, including the fact that the improvements in strength are proportionally larger than the increase in cross-sectional area of the muscle. These mechanisms seem to be particularly significant in elderly people, who improve from strength training with little muscle hypertrophy.

Contraindications and Safety Precautions

Not only does strength and muscle endurance training put a high strain on muscles and joints, but it also works the heart more than aerobic exercise does in one specific way: Exercises designed to build strength and muscle endurance tend to raise heart rate while also raising blood pressure. This combined effect of elevated heart rate and elevated blood pressure can put an excessive burden on anyone with a weak heart. This same effect definitely applies when training statically or doing any form of static contraction. It also is exaggerated when

doing intensive exercise with the smaller muscles of the body such as those in the arms (e.g., chopping wood, pull-ups).

Anyone with a weak heart because of past or continuing illness, and anyone with the primary risk factors for cardiovascular disease (hypertension, cigarette smoking, high-serum cholesterol) would be wise not to put great emphasis on training for strength or muscle endurance. Even if the above conditions do not apply to you, whenever lifting weights, you should avoid holding your breath and instead inhale and exhale slowly while exercising. Holding the breath while exerting oneself maximally is called the **Valsalva maneuver.** The effect is to raise your blood pressure and results in a lightheaded feeling. This should be avoided.

One last suggestion relates to the skill needed in working with heavy weights and some exercise machines. Lifts in which you raise anything above your head can be dangerous if you lose control. Lifts in which you use your lower back can increase the strain on this region and can cause injury if they are done incorrectly. We highly recommend that you seek instruction in proper technique and use spotters to assist you in certain lifts.

Gender Differences in Training

Although males and females typically differ in strength and muscle endurance, evidence suggests that the training procedures to develop these components of fitness are similar for both sexes. Because men tend to be larger in stature and body weight and because they tend to develop larger musculature during puberty than women do, their strength and endurance tend to be higher, although many individual women, particularly athletes, can outperform the average man in specific areas. Differences between the sexes are smaller in the legs than in the upper body, perhaps as a result of similar levels of habitual activity using the lower body. Nevertheless, dynamic training has been shown to create dramatic improvements in the strength and muscle endurance of many women, often without large changes in muscular size. Exercises that focus on improving the strength and muscle endurance in the upper body can be particularly useful as an aid in handling body weight.

A common fear among women is that by engaging in strength or muscle endurance training, they will "bulk up" and develop large, unattractive muscles. The available evidence suggests this is not the case in most women. Muscle **hypertrophy,** referring to growth of muscle tissue in size, seems to be related to the amount of the circulating male sex hormone testosterone. Beginning at puberty, testosterone levels are much higher in males than in females. This causes the typical increase in muscle mass and decrease in body fat at this age. Because testosterone levels continue to be much lower in females than males during adulthood, women seem to be able to engage in weight-training exercises without fear of significant hypertrophy. Individuals differ, however, and therefore musculature size in some women may increase from such training. Practically speaking, women who already have well-defined muscles are more prone to hypertrophy than those who do not.

Back Problems

As a result of the widespread prevalence of backache and other back-related problems, the National YMCA developed and implemented a program called *The Y's Way to a Healthy Back*. Over the years this program has been effective in reducing chronic discomfort in thousands of people. If you have back ailments, however, you should first see your personal physician for possible referral.

OTHER TYPES OF TRAINING
Circuit Training

Circuit training refers to a type of training in which several exercises are completed one after the other in a series. The exercises can vary from calisthenics to weight training exercises to running stairs, to stretching, and so on. The term *circuit weight-training* is applied when weight-lifting exercises are used. What distinguishes circuit weight-training from traditional weight-training is that each exercise is done for only a specified time (usually 20–30 seconds), and then the individual moves onto the next exercise "station" with only minimal rest. Usually the exercises are arranged so that no one body part or muscle group is stressed in adjacent stations, thereby permitting some recovery before the body part is taxed again.

Using circuit training, you can easily develop a relatively taxing exercise program that serves your unique needs. The circuits created can be general, focusing on all the major muscle groups of the body, or designed specifically to focus on a particular goal, such as improving strength in the shoulder region. By varying the number of repetitions, the length of time at each station, the amount of time between each station, and the number of times you complete the whole circuit, you can determine how hard you wish to work. In recent years *parcourse* facilities have become more widely available, usually adjacent to parks, golf courses, or other recreational areas. The parcourse is simply a variation of circuit training and usually is a multi-station exercise apparatus, often built of wood, offering a variety of self-directed strengthening/stretching exercises.

Research has demonstrated that you can improve your strength and muscle endurance significantly using circuit weight-training. Evidence also has shown, however, that even when individuals trained for 20–30 minutes per day, 3 days per week, the improvements in VO_2 max were only modest. This was true even though the participants remained active almost continuously throughout the training, allowing little rest between stations. Also, their training heart rates were maintained within their target heart rate zones (see Chapter 5) throughout the training. One would think that this training procedure would serve as sufficient stimulus for large improvements in aerobic capacity. Unfortunately, improvements in aerobic capacity were much less than those that typically occur from an aerobic program of similar duration—for example, jogging.

Fortunately, an easy adjustment in this training procedure can be made simply by doing 30–60 seconds of aerobic activity between each exercise station. This aerobic activity can be as simple as riding a stationary bicycle, jumping on a mini-trampoline, jumping rope, or running in place. Or one could run/jog/walk between stations, as is often the case when parcourse stations are arranged at various locations around a park. This modification is called **super circuit weight-training.** Research comparing super circuit weight-training with traditional circuit weight-training has shown that it creates much larger improvements in aerobic function. Super circuit weight-training has proven to be an excellent method for developing and maintaining an overall fitness program, one that is useful particularly for those who have difficulty exercising outdoors all year round. It can serve as an alternative for the winter months, when outdoor activities may be more difficult to do.

Interval Training

Interval training is a procedure involving periods of work interspersed with periods of rest or light exercise. It is often used as a means of gently increasing the total demands of exercise on an individual. A common example is a run/walk program. By running 20 yards and walking 20 yards, and so forth, individuals can raise their intensity of exercise compared to just walking the same distance. Gradually, as fitness improves, the running intervals can be increased in length and the walking intervals decreased correspondingly. Such a program is useful when people wish to exercise frequently and for an adequate length of time but cannot maintain a high level of intensity because of low fitness or other reasons.

The same approach can be used in a pool, on an exercise cycle, or with any form of aerobic exercise, for that matter. Another application of interval training, discussed next, is in training athletes for maximal performances that require great speed, agility, power, or some combination thereof.

PERFORMANCE-RELATED FITNESS

Power, speed, and agility were identified in Chapter 4 as components of performance-related fitness that are not associated directly with health. Some individuals may be inclined to improve these types of fitness, perhaps simply for the joy of reaching their limits in an all-around manner. This is especially true of the athlete. Many sports and games require performers to move themselves, an object, or an opponent rapidly, explosively, and with great power.

Power

Power involves the application of force and speed together. Those with the greatest power are not necessarily the strongest, although increasing strength helps improve power. Therefore, strength-training is one way to increase power. Because greatest power is achieved by maximizing force and speed together, another method that can be used to improve power is to add light resistance as an overload and train explosively.

For example, suppose Janis wants to jump higher so she can spike a volleyball over the net and not into it. She may choose simply to jump a lot as a means of increasing her jumping skill as well as her leg power. In this case, her body weight would serve as the overload resistance. She also could do rebound jumps by jumping off and back onto a 2-foot box or a bleacher. Called **polymetric training,** it often is used to increase the explosive leg power of sprinters, jumpers, and so on. (Creative variations could be explored to increase the explosive power of other parts of her body, such as her arms and shoulders, as well.) Another method Janis could use would be to do repeated squat-jumps with a weight vest or using some other form of light resistance as an overload. (A squat-jump means jumping from a position with the legs bent slightly.) The weight should not be so heavy that the individual cannot jump, however.

Speed and Agility

Speed refers to the capacity to move rapidly, usually in a straight line, as in sprinting. **Agility** refers to the capacity to change directions of movement rapidly, as in tennis, which requires starting, stopping, and changing directions of movement and body position in a variable manner. Both speed and agility are highly dependent on skill. Therefore, an excellent way to improve is to practice doing the event in a realistic manner and force yourself to move rapidly. For example, if you are interested in improving your agility and speed in tennis, you should play a lot of tennis and push yourself to move rapidly, especially when you are tired.

Another training method involves the interval training discussed earlier. The basic principle behind interval training for speed and agility is to repeat periods of near-maximal exercise interspersed with periods of rest or light exercise to facilitate partial recovery. The length of each exercise period and the length of each recovery interval can vary from 10 seconds to several minutes, depending on the intended application. For example, sprinters might do eight repetitions of a 200-yard run before taking a long recovery. Between each run, they would do light exercise such as walking for two or three times as long as they took to run the 200 yards. This would be followed by another 200-yard sprint and so forth, until a set of 6–10 had been completed. The length of the recovery interval and the speed of running should be adjusted so the performer can maintain a heavy rate of work and be working maximally or near maximally by the end of the set. After a long rest of 10–15 minutes, a second and a third set may be done.

This type of training is very difficult to do, especially when pushing to maximum. It is not recommended for any except the highly fit and the highly motivated. Variations can be created to incorporate the types of agility movements required in a specific game (such as tennis, racquetball, basketball). The basic procedures are similar in that periods of rapid activity are broken up with periods of rest or light activity. The length of each exercise bout and related rest intervals, of course, should be determined by the intended application and the specificity principle described in Chapter 4.

BUILDING MUSCLE

For a variety of reasons, many people are interested in building up their muscle mass. For some, the desire to build muscle becomes excessive, and many positive health practices may be sacrificed to attain as large and well-defined muscles as possible. Little scientific attention has been directed to the matter of how to accomplish these results effectively and safely, but any systematic overload to a muscle seems to result in some degree of muscle hypertrophy. The most commonly practiced method involves doing several sets of 10–20 RM loads. Competitive body builders typically take short rest periods of 10–60 seconds between such sets. The greater the total amount of work done, the more the overall gain that is likely to occur. The greatest gains probably will be seen in muscles that have the least amount of habitual overload. Also, larger muscles likely will have greater improvements on an absolute level.

For unknown reasons responsiveness to training varies widely. For some, particularly young males at or soon after puberty, heavy resistance training results in greater gains in muscle. In others of the same age and gender, it has a smaller effect. Women in general experience much less hypertrophy from strength training than men do, probably because of lower levels of male sex hormone. As men get older, their ability to increase the size of muscle through training seems to decline. One possible clue as to whether you are likely to be responsive to such training is to observe the degree of muscle development you have without training. If you are heavily muscled already, you may be more responsive than others, and vice versa.

Many body-builders and other athletes who require great strength, such as football players, shot-putters, discus-throwers, weight-lifters, and so forth, take illegal drugs called **anabolic steroids** to hasten and magnify the improvement they obtain from their training. Anabolic steroids are synthetically produced drugs that have growth-promoting properties similar to those of the male sex hormone testosterone. Research into the effectiveness of these drugs has demonstrated that some, but not all, males who took these steroids while in weight-training, gained weight (particularly fat-free tissue) and strength. The dosages used in this research, however, were significantly lower (for ethical and safety considerations) than the dosages reportedly being taken by many athletes in the field. The research also has been conducted over only 1–2 month periods, which are relatively short compared to the time spans during which many appear to be using these drugs.

A number of negative health consequences are associated with anabolic steroids. These include liver dysfunction, liver cancer, lowered high-density lipoprotein levels, more aggressive behavior, mood swings, hypertension, and testicular atrophy. Anabolic steroid use also has been associated with virilization in females, including deepening of the voice, increased facial and body hair, and clitoral enlargement. Some of these masculine changes are irreversible in women. Children also are particularly susceptible to the virilizing effects of these drugs. They may develop precociously on initial exposure to these drugs and later experience premature closing of the growth centers of their bones, resulting in overall stunting of growth. Long-term use of anabolic steroids has been implicated in the development of abnormal changes in the structure of muscle.

In view of the possible grave and life-threatening consequences posed by anabolic steroids, use of these drugs is strongly discouraged. Most international amateur athletic organizations prohibit athletes from using anabolic steroids, but enforcing the rules is difficult. Because the use of these drugs is so widespread, drug testing is becoming common.

SUMMARY

Maintaining flexibility, strength, and muscle endurance is important in maintaining a high quality of life and in preventing hypokinetic degeneration and low back pain. Flexibility will improve with gentle, dynamic, range-of-motion activities or through static stretching for 15–30 seconds, 3–5 days per week. Strength and muscle endurance will increase by contracting muscles repetitively against a relatively large resistance. Strength improvement requires performing a small number of repetitions with very high resistances. Muscle endurance improves from performing a large number of repetitions against lower resistance. Calisthenics, weight-lifting, and working on exercise machines are the most common forms of activity for this training. When equipment is not available, static exercises can be used to increase strength and muscle endurance.

Training procedures should be similar for both sexes. Circuit training may be used to increase strength and muscle endurance in many areas of the body and, with proper adjustment of exercises, to improve aerobic capacity. Power, speed, and agility will improve from specific, high-intensity training.

Finally, anabolic steroids are known to have numerous harmful health consequences and have been banned in many settings.

CHOICES IN ACTION

Now you can try for yourself some of the fitness tests discussed in this chapter. Lab 17 covers assessment of "Sit-and-Reach Flexibility." Lab 18 provides "Strength Tests," and Lab 19, "Endurance Tests." Each of these labs allows you to compare your results with the norm for your age and gender and gives a space for future measurements so you can log your progression.

REFERENCES

American College of Sports Medicine. 1984. "The Use of Anabolic-Androgenic Steroids in Sports." *Sports Medicine Bulletin* 19: 13–18.

Canadian Standardized Tests of Fitness: Operations Manual. 1985. Hull, Quebec: Fitness and Amateur Sport.

Clarke, D. H. 1973. "Adaptations in strength and muscular endurance resulting from exercise." *Exercise and Sports Science Reviews* 1: 73–102.

Corbin, C. B., and Noble, L. 1980. "Flexibility: A Major Component of Physical Fitness." *Journal of Physical Education and Recreation* 51: 23.

deVries, H. A. 1986. *Physiology of Exercise*, 4th ed. Dubuque, IA: Wm. C. Brown.

Domingues, R. H., and Gajda, R. S. 1982. *Total Body Training.* New York: Charles Scribner's Sons.

Fleck, S. J., and Kraemer, W. J. 1987. *Designing Resistance Training Programs.* Champaign, IL: Human Kinetics Books.

Fox, E., Bowers, R., and Foss, M. 1993. *The Physiological Basis for Exercise and Sport*, 5th ed. Madison, WI: W. C. Brown and Benchmark.

Gettman, L. R., and Pollock, M. L. 1981. "Circuit Weight Training: A Critical Review of Its Physiological Benefits." *Physician and Sportsmedicine* 9: 44–60.

Gettman, L. R., Ward, P., and Hagen, R. D. 1982. "A Comparison of Combined Running and Weight Training with Circuit Weight Training." *Medicine and Science in Sports* 14: 229–234.

Golding, L. A., Myers, C. R., and Sinning, W. E. (Eds.). 1982. *Y's Way to Physical Fitness (revised).* Rosemont, IL: YMCA.

Heyward, V. H. 1984. *Designs for Fitness.* Minneapolis: Burgess.

Jackson, A., and Langford, N. J. 1989. "The Criterion-Related Validity of the Sit and Reach Test: Replication and Extension of Previous Findings." *Research Quarterly for Exercise and Sport* 60(4): 384–387.

Kraemer, W. J., and Fleck, S. J. 1988. "Resistance Training: Exercise Prescription (part 4 of 4). *Physician and Sportsmedicine* 16(6): 69–81.

Kraus, H., Nagler, W., and Melleby, A. 1983. "Evaluation of an Exercise Program for Back Pain." *American Family Physician* 28: 153–158.

Lamb, D. R. 1984. *Physiology of Exercise.* New York: Macmillan.

Lemon, P. W. R. 1989. "Influence of dietary protein and total energy intake on strength improvement." *Sports Science Exchange* 2(14): 1–5.

Mayhew, J. L., and Gross, P. M. 1974. "Body composition changes in young women with high resistance weight training." *Research Quarterly* 45: 433–440.

Messier, S. P., and Dill, M. E. 1985. "Alterations in Strength and Maximal Oxygen Uptake Consequent to Nautilus Circuit Weight Training." *Research Quarterly for Exercise and Sport* 56: 345–351.

Petrofsky, J. S., and Lind, A. R. 1975. "Aging, Isometric Strength and Endurance, and Cardiovascular Responses to Static Effort." *Journal of Applied Physiology* 38: 91–95.

Pollock, M. L., Wilmore, J. W., Fox, S. M. 1978. *Health Through Physical Activity.* New York: Macmillan.

Pollock, M. L. and Wilmore, J. H. *Exercise in Health and Disease*, 2nd ed. Philadelphia, PA, W. B. Saunders, 1990.

Sapega, A. A., Quendenfeld, T. C., Moyer, R. A., and Butler, R. A. 1981. "Biophysical Factors in Range of Motion Exercise." *Physician and Sportsmedicine* 9: 57–65.

Svoboda, M., Kauffman, L., Robertson, L., Gilbert, G., Heyden, M., Althoff, S., Davis, R., Lehman, A. E., and Schendel, J. S. (Eds.) 1985. *Health and Fitness for Life Laboratory Manual*, 2d ed. Scottsdale, AZ: Prospect Press.

Wilmore, J. H., and Costill, D. H. 1988. *Training for Sport and Activity: The Physiological Basis of the Conditioning Process*, 3d. ed. Dubuque, IA: Wm. C. Brown.

Y's Way to a Healthy Back. 1976. New York: YMCA of the City of New York and National Council of YMCAs.

The Weight Control Challenge

✔ What is the relationship between body composition and quality living?

✔ How can you tell whether you are overfat?

✔ Are all methods of assessment equally accurate?

✔ How can you determine how much energy you consume or expend on the average?

✔ How can you lose fat without losing weight?

✔ Why is regular exercise effective in helping you maintain your weight at a certain level over the long run?

✔ What type of exercise should you choose to maintain recommended weight?

Y ou do not need great deductive powers to discover the importance of weight control in contemporary American society. In any given week the top ten best-selling books invariably include one or more on diet, exercise, nutrition, or related topics. Many of us are preoccupied daily with our body weight and devote a great deal of money, time, and energy to modifying and regulating our weight. This preoccupation with weight usually centers on the amount of visible fat on the body. In this chapter, we describe the nature, extent, and consequences of excess fat. We provide you with information that will enable you to obtain an approximate estimation of your fat content, methods of reducing fat if it is excessive, and avoiding accumulation of fat throughout your life.

DEFINITION OF TERMS

The term **obesity** refers to having an excess amount of fat. Being able to determine the point at which obesity begins has been of considerable interest to researchers, health professionals, and consumers alike. Still, no clear line of demarcation exists between obese and nonobese. Rather, fitness exists on a continuum, and the point at which obesity begins is an arbitrary one that experts continue to discuss and debate.

Overweight means having excess weight relative to the average person of the same sex and stature. Although being overweight often comes from having excess body fat, this is not always the case. For example, many professional football players are heavily muscled and weigh 30–40 pounds more than the average person of the same height.

Body composition is the proportion of body weight composed of fat and the proportion composed of fat-free tissues (e.g., muscle, bone, connective tissue). The most accurate methods for determining body composition are not generally available for use in population studies, so determining accurate standards is difficult at present.

Therefore, height/weight tables (Table 7.A) derived from the characteristics of life insurance policy holders (who may not be entirely representative of the American population as a whole) often are used. Keep in mind that these are only guidelines, not standards every individual must achieve. Ways to determine your own body composition are discussed later in this chapter.

Two other terms also require clarification. *Weight loss*, of course, refers to the loss of weight. Many people find themselves trying continually to

TABLE 7.A Normative body weights (ages 25 and over).

	HEIGHT	SMALL FRAME	WEIGHT (LBS.) MEDIUM FRAME	LARGE FRAME
Women	4'8"	88–94	92–103	100–115
	9"	90–97	94–106	102–118
	10"	92–100	97–109	105–121
	11"	95–103	100–112	108–124
	5'0"	98–106	103–115	111–127
	1"	101–109	106–118	114–130
	2"	104–112	109–122	117–134
	3"	107–115	112–126	121–138
	4"	110–119	116–131	125–142
	5"	114–123	120–135	129–146
	6"	118–127	124–139	133–150
	7"	122–131	128–143	137–154
	8"	126–136	132–147	141–159
	9"	130–140	136–151	145–164
	10"	134–144	140–155	149–169
Men	5'1"	104–112	110–121	118–133
	2"	107–115	113–125	121–136
	3"	110–118	116–128	124–140
	4"	113–121	119–131	127–144
	5"	116–125	122–135	130–148
	6"	120–129	126–139	134–153
	7"	124–133	130–144	139–158
	8"	128–137	134–148	143–162
	9"	132–142	138–152	147–166
	10"	136–146	142–157	151–171
	11"	140–150	146–162	156–176
	6'0"	144–154	150–167	160–181
	1"	148–159	154–172	165–186
	2"	152–163	159–177	170–191
	3"	156–167	164–182	174–196

Note: Based on the weights published by the Metropolitan Life Insurance Company in 1959, which were associated with the lowest mortality of those who were insured. They have been recalculated from the originally published tables to permit you to determine your height in bare feet and your weight without clothes. In 1983 these standards were revised upward because Americans in all weight categories had gained weight on average over that 24-year time period, even though evidence did not suggest the changes were healthful. Also, other factors that affect mortality, such as smoking, were not controlled for in revising the table upward. For this reason, the 1959 standards have been retained in this book as a reference. (Adapted from *Statistical Bulletin of the Metropolitan Life Insurance Co.* 40 (Nov.–Dec. 1959): 1–4.)

lose weight as a means of losing fat. Often, those who are successful at losing weight are unable to maintain the loss permanently. This usually happens because they are unsuccessful at transforming the method they used to lose the weight into a long-term plan that will enable them to maintain their weight at the new and lower level. *Weight control* refers to maintaining a stable body weight.

PROBLEMS ASSOCIATED WITH BEING OVERWEIGHT

Research continues to explore the many factors that govern the regulation of body weight and body fat. Although many essential principles have been firmly established, many more remain unclear. The complexity of the concept makes it difficult to establish firm guidelines that apply to all individuals. Even the issue of determining whether you are too fat is a matter of debate, as evidence now suggests that no single level of body fat separates good health from ill health.

According to a national sample, approximately one-third of U.S. adults of all ages (roughly 58 million) are overweight. The prevalence of being overweight is greater in the age group 40–70 years. Comparisons to a similar survey completed approximately 12 years earlier revealed an 8% increase in overweight adults during this time period. Translated, this suggests that, on average, adults weigh approximately 8 pounds more than they did just 12 years ago.

Reasons why this has occurred are unclear and alarming from a public health perspective. Being overweight clearly is implicated with a number of health problems. Evidence comes from large surveys of the U.S. adult population. For example, for those who are in the top 15% of their weight category across all ages, the risk of hypertension is 2.9 times greater than in the overall population; in younger adults (ages 20–44), it is 5.6 times greater than average. Further, the risk of having a high total cholesterol count (in excess of 250 mg/dl*) is 21 times greater, and the risk of diabetes is 2.9 times greater. All of these are primary or secondary risk factors for coronary heart disease (CHD), and, as we might expect, being overweight puts a person at greater risk for this disease as well. (Research has not been entirely clear regarding whether the effect of overweight on CHD is linked directly to its effect on other risk factors or is independent of those factors. The reasons for the discrepancies are unclear at present.)

Other negative health consequences from being overweight exist. The risk of cancer is higher. So also are the risks for gout, gallstones, respiratory insufficiency, congestive heart failure, and thromboembolic and vascular disease. Arthritis and low-back pain are exacerbated by being overweight. Overweight people are at greater risk in surgery, and their overall longevity is lowered. In sum, what can be said is that "excessive" weight has negative health consequences. Again, excessive weight arises from excessive fat in most people.

The situation is worsened because our culture is in many ways preoccupied with thinness. Thus, individuals who carry excess fat often are viewed negatively and may encounter prejudice, sometimes overt and sometimes subtle, in all walks of life. Clearly, being overweight has a negative impact on the quality and the quantity of life.

Eating Disorders

Before leaving the discussion of health problems associated with being overweight we note that two eating disorders have become increasingly evident in recent years: anorexia nervosa and bulimia. Both conditions seem to occur predominantly in females and relate to a distorted body image. Anorexia is most prevalent during the teenage years, and bulimia during the late teens and early to mid-twenties. Although they have several characteristics in common, these conditions are recognized as separate and distinct health problems.

Simply stated, **anorexia** is self-induced starvation. People with anorexia nervosa are characterized by an intense fear of becoming obese. Anorectics become so irrationally obsessed with having an emaciated figure that they refuse to maintain body weight within normal range and lose as much as 25% of their original body weight or more. They deny any impulse to eat or any enjoyment of food.

Bulimia is a syndrome characterized by binge eating, preoccupation with body weight, repeated efforts to lose weight, and sometimes by purging, vomiting, or excessive use of laxatives. Bulimic individuals are preoccupied with thoughts of food but may not exhibit abnormal body weight. Bulimics also engage in fasting behavior and usually have frequent weight fluctuations of 10 pounds or more as a result of alternating fasts and binges.

Recently a subclinical eating disorder called *anorexia athletica* has been identified in athletes, often female, who train heavily and are preoccupied with body shape and weight. Although these individuals may not be classified as anorexic or

---

*mg/dl = milligrams/deciliter

Anorexia Nervosa and Bulimia: What Can Be Done?

If you have a friend or relative whom you suspect has anorexia or bulimia:

- Locate professional help as soon as possible. Often, the best place is your local community mental health center.
- Because you cannot force someone to get help, share your concern with the person directly and honestly. Offer your support, and if the individual is willing, your assistance. You may have to be assertive by making the appointment and accompanying the person to the appointment to see the therapist.

Other resources for help include:

American Anorexia/Bulimia Association
418 East 76th St.
New York, NY 10021
(212) 734–1114

National Association of Anorexia
Nervosa and Associated Disorders
P.O. Box 2771
Highland Park, IL 60035
(708) 831–3438

National Anorectic Aid Society
1925 East Dublin-Granville Rd.
Columbus, OH 43229
(614) 436–1112

---

bulimic using strict definitions, they nevertheless exhibit unhealthy behaviors relating to body weight. Their adverse health consequences include a decline in performance, chronic fatigue, increased susceptibility to infection, poor healing and recovery from injury, anemia, electrolyte imbalances, endocrine abnormalities, osteoporosis, and many negative psychological disturbances.

The treatment goal for bulimics is to help them cope with their body image insecurities and other stresses in less destructive ways. For anorexics, treatment should involve psychological counseling, medical monitoring, and nutritional help. The anorexic's struggle often is related to low self-esteem, the struggle for control and independence, and fears relating to sexual development. The treatment goal is to overcome the denial that a problem exists and usually requires involvement of the entire family in the therapy, often for one to two years or more.

METHODS OF MEASURING BODY COMPOSITION

Body composition refers to the make-up of your body, the proportions of your body weight made up of fat and of fat-free tissues. Once you have determined your body composition, you will be better able to make decisions regarding weight loss and exercising. Hydrostatic weighing and skinfold fat measurement techniques are the two most common methods of determining body composition.

Hydrostatic Weighing

In the research laboratory the most widely used method for measuring body composition is called **hydrostatic weighing,** also referred to as "underwater weighing." In this technique the individual is weighed both on land and under water, and then, using an equation, the percent of body weight composed of fat is calculated. Adjustment for the amount of air left in the lungs after full exhalation is required. The procedure normally requires a half-hour or more, making its use impractical on a widescale basis. Measurement error for most people is ±2.5%–3% as compared to cadaver dissection studies, making this method more accurate than most other methods.

Skinfold Fat Techniques

Another measurement technique involves taking measurements of **skinfold fat** thickness at various sites on the body surface (Lab 21). The procedure has evolved over the years because of difficult questions regarding where to take measurements, what technique to use, type of caliper (the measuring tool) needed, and so on. The more fundamental problem of determining whether a set of measurements taken at standard sites truly reflects the total fat content of all types of people—considering differences in age, gender, fitness status, fat content, body size, and shape—is still being explored through research. Currently the best that can be said is that no *one* skinfold technique will be accurate given all the variations among people.

The measurement error using these procedures is typically ±3%–4% fat. The greatest accuracy in skinfold techniques will be possible if a trained technician using a reliable set of calipers takes the measurements.

Other Methods of Measurement

A number of alternative procedures for measuring body composition have been developed. These include circumference, ultrasound, arm X-ray, bio-electrical impedance, and computerized tomography. Most are not readily available. One in particular, **bioelectrical impedance,** involves measuring the resistance to a low level of electrical current passing through the body. It has been marketed as an easy and accurate alternative to more standard techniques such as hydrostatic weighing. The error associated with this technique is similar to that found with skinfold procedures (3%–4% fat units).

Two other indices should be mentioned. Evidence shows that high levels of fat in the abdominal region are associated with greater risk of cardiovascular disease compared to similar levels of fat in other regions of the body. The risk increases sharply when the **waist-to-hip ratio** (Lab 20) exceeds .9 in men and .8 in women, respectively. These standards are important markers by which you can monitor yourself.

The **body mass index (BMI)** is another measure used to determine relative risk from excess weight (Lab 20). The equation for determining body mass index is:

$$BMI = \frac{Wt}{Ht^2}$$

(where body weight is in kilograms (kg) and height is in meters (m), measurements are taken when barefoot and unclothed)

Although BMI is not a measure of body composition, it is highly correlated to percent of fat as determined by hydrostatic weighing. Most adults have a BMI between 20 and 25, and adults in the top 15% of their weight categories have BMIs in excess of 26, the point at which the health risk from obesity begins to increase.

COMPONENTS OF BODY COMPOSITION AND DESIRABLE FAT AND WEIGHT STANDARDS

Fat weight is simply your pounds of fat. Fat weight consists partly of **essential fat,** which refers to the minimum amount of fat needed for optimal health. Essential fat levels are thought to be 3%–5% fat for males and 8%–12% fat for females. (Females require a higher level of essential fat for reasons related to reproductive needs.) The part of

your fat weight that is not essential is called **storage fat.** Obesity is the state of having an excessive amount of storage fat.

Fat-free weight is an estimate of how much all the other tissues in your body would weigh if all the fat were removed. Of course, you should not aspire to attain a body weight equal to your fat-free weight. This actually is impossible, and efforts to achieve that goal will severely compromise your health status. The lowest body weight you can strive to achieve is equal to the sum of your fat-free weight plus your essential fat (Figure 7.1). Considering the margin of error in measuring body composition, even this weight probably would result in your being too lean, particularly if you were to get sick and need extra energy reserves.

How much fat is desirable? How can you tell if you are obese or not? Not enough objective data are available on a large enough sample of individuals to determine the point at which the risk from obesity accelerates. All that can be said is that many studies of young American men and women indicate that, on the average, women are 18%–30% fat and men 10%–20% fat. (Athletic groups typically are lower, with females 12%–22% fat and males 5%–13% fat.)

Because no clear evidence suggests that a single %fat value is optimum for all individuals, no single %fat value can describe the threshold of obesity. Rather, a range of body fat values is the best that can be provided for estimating obesity. Body fat values in excess of 30%–35% fat (females) and 20%–25% fat (males) are the current percentages used to signify the threshold of obesity. Obviously, differences in age and heredity factors must be considered when referring to these percentages.

People often are interested in calculating their target body weight at a desired %fat level. To do this, simply divide your lean body weight by the target %fat subtracted from 1.0.

For example, assume you weigh 150 pounds and were estimated as having 20% fat. Your fat weight would be 30 pounds (150 × .20 = 30). Therefore, your fat-free weight is: 150 − 30 = 120 pounds. Assume you wish to determine your target weight at 15% fat:

$$target\ weight = \frac{120}{1.0 - .15} = \frac{120}{.85} = 141.2\ pounds$$

ROLE OF ENERGY BALANCE IN WEIGHT CONTROL

The **caloric balance equation** describes the relationship between the amount of energy (in calories) you consume and the amount of energy

FIGURE 7.1   Components of body composition.

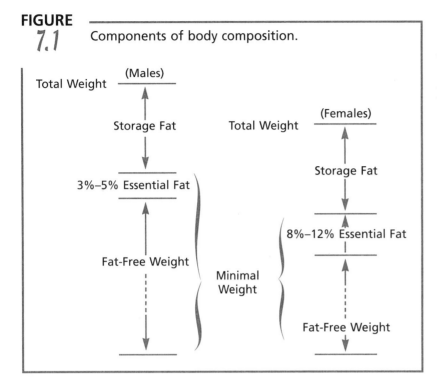

you expend. When energy intake equals energy expenditure, you are in a state of **energy balance.** As long as you remain in balance, your body weight will remain essentially the same. On a daily basis, a person may consume more calories than he or she expends, or vice versa, but as long as the total intake over several days equals the total expenditure, the net change in body weight or in body composition will not change. If caloric intake exceeds caloric expenditure, the person is said to be in positive caloric balance and the extra calories will be stored, mostly in the form of fat. If caloric intake is less than caloric expenditure, the additional calories are obtained from stored energy, again mostly in the form of fat.

Weight control is a process of achieving energy balance over the lifespan. For some this is easy. For countless others, however, the task is difficult and the long-term result is "creeping obesity," a gradual increase in body fat as the person grows older. Although a modest, gradual fat gain may be associated with health and longevity, excessive accumulation of fat may causes many health-related problems.

Often the imbalance is no more than a few calories, perhaps fewer than 25 calories per day on the average. Cumulatively, however, an imbalance of 25 calories/day would result in 2.6 pounds per year of added fat. Because most people who are overfat have perhaps 25–30 pounds of excess fat at most, and because in most cases this extra fat is acquired over 10–15 years, achieving energy balance does not involve making significant changes. For most people the imbalance is relatively small. For many, however, attaining lifelong energy balance is difficult and often leads people into taking extreme weight loss measures such as fasting or going on highly restrictive diets. To counteract these detrimental measures, we offer some information that you may find more useful in applying weight-control principles.

Energy

Of all the functions of food, one of the most important is the energy it provides. To be useful to your body, the energy contained in food first must be broken down, transformed into forms that are useful to your cells, and then transported to those cells. Because food typically is eaten in three or fewer meals (with occasional snacks), the supply of energy coming from the digestive process is not continuous. More energy than you can use at one time arrives in a big volume, followed by periods without any additional intake, sometimes as long as 12–18 hours. To compensate for this unsteady supply of energy, much of the food from a meal is converted into a usable form (fat) and stored in fat cells for later use as needed. (This is discussed in more detail in Chapters 8 and 9.) Thus, throughout the day the cells of the body receive a mixture of foodstuffs coming from the stomach and from various storage depots throughout the body. Foodstuffs from both sources serve the important function of providing energy for all life functions and for rebuilding and replacing cells.

Caloric Intake

The unit of measure used to equate energy from different foods is called the **calorie.*** The definition of a calorie is the amount of heat required to raise one kilogram of water one degree centigrade in temperature.

---

*Food energy actually is measured in kilocalories (Kcal). A calorie (spelled with a small "c") is technically only 1/1000 of a kilocalorie. Most Americans (even nutritionists), however, use the lowercased "calorie" to mean kilocalorie.

Caloric intake is defined as the number of calories of energy consumed in a 24-hour day, which means the sum of the caloric values of all the foods eaten in that period of time. In Table 7.B are step-by-step procedures for determining most accurately the total caloric values of two sample lunches. In brief, this involves weighing or measuring as precisely as possible all the foods you eat and then using the caloric values for each food (found in the *Nutritive Value of Foods*, published by the U.S. Department of Agriculture) to determine your total caloric intake. This can become quite a chore, but it is necessary if you wish to achieve the greatest accuracy.

Table 7.B describes the most practical method you can use to determine your caloric intake, but it is not without error. Given the difficulty of obtaining accurate measurements of the volume and weight of the food you eat, given the seemingly infinite variations in the content of most prepared foods, and given the large variations in calories in two samples of the same type of food (for example, the fat content of two 6-ounce steaks can vary considerably), these estimates require you to be meticulous to attain any reasonable level of accuracy.

Caloric Expenditure

Caloric expenditure is defined as the total number of calories a person expends in the form of heat and work in a 24-hour day. This also is difficult to measure precisely, for a number of reasons. Most important, there is no easy way of accurately measuring physical activity on a particular day given the great variety of things you might do. In an hour you may start and stop moving an untold number of times and change your pace a similar number of times. To calculate how much energy you expended, you would have to keep accurate records of the intensity and duration of each activity throughout a 24-hour period and then be able to translate this into units of energy expenditure. This task would be easier if each hour were spent at a relative steady rate of physical activity, but this rarely is the case.

The method typically used to obtain an approximate estimate of caloric expenditure involves keeping accurate activity records throughout the hours you are awake. By computing the calories you expend during your daily activities and adding this to the calories you use at your **resting metabolic rate (RMR),** you obtain an estimate of your total caloric expenditure. RMR is defined as the number of calories the body spends in a 24-hour period simply to maintain bodily functions under resting conditions. It represents the number of calories you would need to maintain yourself in energy balance if you were to lie in bed awake for a 24-hour period and were fed intravenously so you didn't even have to spend the energy required to digest your food.

Because measuring RMR is impractical and expensive to do routinely, a closely related measure called **resting energy expenditure (REE)** is estimated indirectly instead. Directions for estimating your REE and an example are provided in the accompanying activity. In Lab 25 you will have the opportunity to compute an estimate of total caloric expenditure for a 24-hour period.

A COMPREHENSIVE PROGRAM FOR WEIGHT LOSS

If you find yourself wishing to lose excess weight because you have too much fat, what approach should you use? Will you be able to maintain permanently any loss you achieve? Unfortunately, the vast majority of people who undertake a weight loss program are not successful at keeping the weight off. They are not successful at

TABLE 7.B Computations illustrating how to determine caloric value of two sample meals.

FOOD	MEASURE	WEIGHT (GRAMS)	(OUNCES)	NET CALORIES*
Lunch No. 1				
Turkey sandwich				
Italian bread	2 slices	60	2.12	170
lettuce	1 outer leaf	15	.53	—
mayonnaise (reg)	1 teaspoon	5	.18	33
turkey	2 pieces (white)	85	3	135
Skim milk	1 glass	245	81.67	85
Orange (peeled)	1 medium	120	4.24	60
			TOTAL	483 Cal.
Lunch No. 2				
Burger King Whopper	1 complete			606
French fries	1 serving			214
Vanilla shake	1 glass			332
			TOTAL	1152 Cal.

*Determined using the listed values in the *Nutritive Value of Foods* published by the U. S. Department of Agriculture.

A C T I V I T Y

ESTIMATING RESTING ENERGY EXPENDITURE (REE)

REE is similar to RMR except that REE includes the energy needed to digest food. Instructions for predicting your REE are as follows:

1. *Estimate your surface area:* Use Figure 7.2 and line up a straight-edge between your body weight and your standing height. By reading to the middle column, you will obtain an estimate of your surface area in square meters.

2. *Determine the average resting energy expenditure for your gender and age:* Refer to Figure 7.3.

3. *Determine your estimated REE:* Multiply the average REE by your surface area to obtain an estimate of your REE in calories per hour. When multiplied by 24, this will give you an estimate of your REE over a 24-hour day.

A sample calculation illustrating this whole procedure step-by-step follows. This technique is at best only an approximation; many factors including heredity, age, gender, amount of fat-free tissue, emotions, food, fever, and prior exercise cause individual differences in REE.

Sample calculation for determining resting energy expenditure

Name: Nat Holmes
Age: 32
Height: 71 inches
Weight: 177 lbs

1. Lining up a straight-edge on Figure 7.2 between Nat's height and weight, his predicted body surface area is:

    2.0 m^2

2. From Figure 7.3, the resting energy expenditure for a male aged 32 is:

    37 cal / m^2 / hour

3. Resting energy expenditure

    = (2.0 m^2) (37 cal / m2 / hr)
    = 74 cal / hr
    or

    $\dfrac{(74 \; \frac{cal}{hr})}{} \; \dfrac{(24 \; \frac{hr}{day})}{} = 1776 \; cal / day$

FIGURE 7.2 Nomogram to estimate body surface area from height and weight.

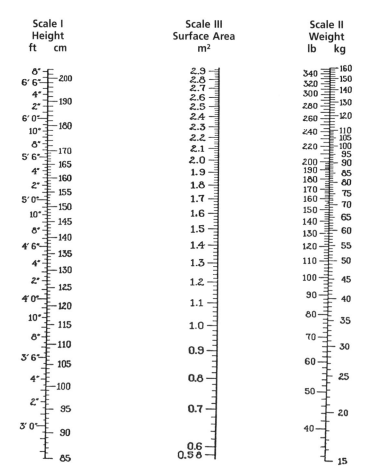

From *Clinical Spirometry* by Warren E. Collins, Inc., Braintree, MA, with permission. Dubois Body Surface Chart prepared by Boothby and Standiford of the Mayo Clinic.

FIGURE

7.3   Resting energy expenditure for men and women as a function of age.

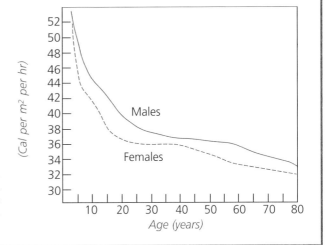

From *Nutrition, Weight Control and Exercise*, 2d ed., by F. I. Katch and W. D. McArdle (Philadelphia: Lea and Febiger, 1983). Used by permission of the authors. Data are from *Metabolism*, by P. I. Altman and D. S. Dittmer (Bethesda, MD: Federation of American Societies for Experimental Biology, 1968).

weight control. Before we address the reasons, we will present a comprehensive program for weight loss designed to ensure permanent changes in body composition.

The American College of Sports Medicine (ACSM) position stand on proper and improper weight loss programs includes these recommendations:

1. Weight loss should occur gradually and should not exceed 1–2 pounds of weight loss per week.

2. Weight loss should occur from a combination of a moderate diet and a regular aerobic exercise program.

3. Foods eaten on this diet should be balanced with respect to nutritional requirements and should be compatible with personal tastes. Caloric intake should be at least 1200 calories/day.

4. Aerobic exercise should consist of gentle, rhythmic exercise using large-muscle groups, done a minimum of 3 days/week, for at least 20 minutes/day, and at a low to moderate intensity to expend at least 300 calories per session. (Smaller persons, particularly women, may expend fewer than 300 calories/session and still obtain benefit.)

5. Behavior modification techniques should be employed to identify and eliminate dietary habits that lead to improper nutrition; these techniques will enable the individual to maintain the weight loss indefinitely.

The rationale for each item in these guidelines is as follows.

1. *Weight loss should not exceed 1–2 pounds/week.* One important reason is that modest changes are transformed more easily into permanent habits that can be maintained throughout life. What type of change will enable you to lose 1–2 pounds/week? Because one pound of fat contains 3500 calories of energy, a negative caloric balance of 500–1000 calories/day will help you accomplish this.

Consider this example. Daily caloric requirements for the average American female and male are approximately 2200 calories/day and 2900 calories/day, respectively. To lose 1 pound/week, an average woman would have to consume 1700 calories while still expending 2200 calories daily (2200 − 500 = 1700 calories). (The recommended 1700 calories is considerably higher than the number of calories the typical female consumes if she is on a diet.) Equivalent values for an average male to lose 1 pound/week are: 2900 − 500 = 2400 calories/day.

This example assumes that the individuals have elected to go on a diet only, rather than also adding moderate aerobic exercise to their programs. Because most Americans, especially those in need of weight loss, do not engage in regular aerobic exercise already, this diet-only approach does not take advantage of the long-term weight-control benefits that can be obtained through regular exercise in a weight-loss program.

Early in a program, we should note, pounds are lost more quickly because water is excreted along with fat losses. This means that initially you will be able to lose weight with less than the deficit of 3500 calories/pound that is needed when all the weight loss comes from fat. This is why losing weight seems to become more difficult after the first week or two.

2. *Weight loss programs should involve a moderate diet and regular aerobic exercise together.* There are many reasons for combining a moderate diet and

an aerobic exercise program. One is that a greater proportion of the weight loss comes from fat stores than when just dieting. Whenever you lose weight, just as when you gain weight, some of the loss (or gain) comes from fat stores, but some also comes from loss (or gain) of fat-free tissues. Research has shown that incorporating exercise into a weight-loss program helps reduce the loss of fat-free tissues and forces more to be lost from fat stores. A weight-loss program incorporating a moderate diet and an aerobic exercise program is outlined in Figure 7.4.

With a moderate diet coupled with exercise, you are likely to avoid a reduction in REE, which often arises from more severe caloric restriction. Apparently, with severe caloric restriction, your body doesn't know whether the dietary regime is likely to be long, arduous, and life-threatening (as in a famine) or whether it is just a temporary period of caloric restriction. Thus, your body reacts to severe caloric restriction by defending against any possibility: It *conserves* the amount of energy expended, lowering your REE.

This creates several consequences. First, your rate of fat loss will slow because total energy expenditure per 24-hour cycle is reduced. To continue achieving fat loss, you will have to restrict your caloric intake even further, which only continues the cycle. Second, if and when you attain your target weight and body composition, you will not be able to eat as much to maintain your weight at the new level because of your lowered REE. Thus, the chances of achieving weight control at the new level are sabotaged. What occurs is the "seesaw" effect that so many Americans experience—the recurring cycle of weight loss followed by weight gain, followed by another diet and resultant weight loss, and so on. The net effect is no real progress.

Two other consequences of cyclic dieting have been identified: (a) Weight is regained after a diet more rapidly than it was lost, and (b) equivalent weight loss in a subsequent trial is slower and more difficult. Both effects seem to occur because of enhanced food efficiency from dieting. Frequently,

---

FIGURE
7.4   Example of a weight-loss program following recommended guidelines.

Name: Melody	*Weight:* 150 pounds
	Height: 63 inches
	BMI: 27

Goal: Lose 1 pound/week

Program: If Melody were to add slow running at 12:00 minutes/mile, 5 days/week to her normal activities, her total added energy expenditure from the exercise would be as follows:

Rate of energy expenditure (from Appendix 4): .056 cal/min/lb
Body weight: 150 lbs
Duration: 30 minutes
Frequency: 5 days/week

Weekly caloric expenditure:

(.056 cal/min/lb) (150 lbs) (30 min) (5) = 1260 calories

Subtracting the energy expenditure for the activity she would have been doing (seated office work) during the same time period each day had she not exercised:

(.010 cal/min/lb) (150 lbs) (30 min) (5) = 225 calories

Net extra calories spent each week because of added exercise:

1260 − 225 = 1035 calories

Therefore, to lose 1 pound/week (remembering that 3500 calories = 1 lb fat), she would have to reduce her caloric intake by:
3500 − 1035 = 2465 calories
On a daily basis, this means:
$\frac{2352.5}{7}$ = 336 calories/day

So by jogging slowly for 30 minutes/day, 5 days/week and restricting her diet by 352 calories/day, Melody will lose fat at a rate of approximately 1 pound/week, assuming all else remains the same. When she achieves her target weight, she can increase her caloric intake to normal and perhaps even allow herself to consume extra calories. She will not regain the lost weight, provided she continues indefinitely with her exercise program.

several weeks or months after getting off a diet, people find themselves having gained back more weight (and fat) than they started with originally. They've lost ground. Eventually they may go on another diet, only to again find themselves losing ground once again. In effect, many people literally diet themselves into obesity.

Other negative health consequences associated with the body's attempt to conserve energy when exposed to repeated weight-loss cycles include:

- Deteriorated kidney function
- Increase in risk factors for cardiovascular disease
- Hypertension
- Altered fat distribution patterns
- Increased predisposition to develop gallstones
- Possibly lowered reproductive capacity

3. *Diet should be balanced and should contain at least 1200 calories.* The ACSM recommends that at least 1200 calories be consumed even during a weight-loss program, to assure a nutritionally sound diet at all times. Crash diets that provide fewer than 1200 calories restrict not only calories but also many other nutrients needed for proper health and function. (Chapters 8 and 9 describe nutritional requirements and guidelines in detail.) The only exception to this rule should be if you are on a medically supervised diet. Unfortunately, many individuals, including athletes who are concerned excessively with body composition, teens, and children who are still growing, put themselves on diets considerably more restrictive than a 1200-calorie diet. Growing persons, especially, need a healthy diet to assure proper development of bodily tissues, and crash diets put their health status in jeopardy. In addition, as noted, severe caloric restriction causes a reduced RMR. It also causes a significant loss of fat-free weight in addition to fat weight.

4. *Exercise should be low to moderate in intensity and at least 20 minutes/day and 3 days/week.* Research into endurance exercise programs indicates that individuals tend to lose fat when they exercise 3 or more days/week, for 20 minutes or longer, and at a low to moderate intensity sufficient to expend approximately 300 calories per exercise session. This therefore has become the basis for recommending how much exercise to do during a weight-loss program. As mentioned later in the chapter, lower intensity exercise uses fat as a fuel to a greater extent than does higher intensity exercise. By keeping the intensity down, you will be able to extend the duration of your exercise; and by maximizing duration, not only will fat utilization increase progressively, but total caloric expenditure will increase as well.

Although 300 calories/session is the recommended minimum number of calories to expend if body composition is to improve from an exercise program, this figure should be qualified: Most evidence on the topic of exercise and weight loss comes from research on men who, because of their greater size, use more calories per minute than women. If just as much evidence on women were available, a reasonable guess is that the minimum number of calories required per exercise session for a woman would be slightly lower than that required for a man, perhaps around 225–250 calories per session.

Though we have emphasized aerobic exercise thus far, this is not the only form of exercise that has an effect on body composition. Traditional forms of weight-training using procedures designed to increase strength and muscular endurance have been shown to reduce body fat and increase fat-free weight. Circuit weight training has been shown to have similar effects in previously sedentary persons. The mechanisms explaining these changes are not clear, but perhaps they relate to the effects of the exercise on raising fat-free weight, and hence REE.

Exercise can alter fluid balance in a short time through sweat losses, particularly if the climate is hot and humid. This dehydrating effect of exercise has given rise to a number of fraudulent gimmicks for rapid weight loss, including steam rooms, saunas, and rubber suits and similar garments. Such practices for weight loss are discouraged strongly.

One final point is worthy of note. Research has demonstrated a considerable variation among individuals in the amount of energy they expend while engaging in sedentary activities in a controlled environment. The differences in caloric expenditure were attributable to differences in "fidgeting" from one subject to another. Those who fidgeted a lot raised their REE by as much as 20% compared to those who remained still. This points strongly to the great variety of ways in which one can exercise throughout the day to expend more calories.

5. *Behavior modification techniques should be used.* Behavior modification techniques that identify and change poor nutritional habits and identify ways in which food is being consumed inappropriately (for example, as a pacifier for stress, as a source of pleasure when nervous) will improve the likelihood of maintaining the weight loss permanently. Also, behavior modification techniques can and should be applied to the task of developing lifelong exercise habits to ensure successful and permanent weight control once weight-loss goals are met.

Programs that employ behavior modification techniques have proven to have lower attrition rates, and they result in positive feelings and better maintenance of weight loss compared to programs that do not incorporate these techniques. The real test of whether a weight-loss program will be maintained permanently is whether losses are maintained one to two years later. This type of follow-up information is rarely available, however. The available information, for the better conceived and conducted programs, indicates that even for these programs the one-year success rates are exceedingly low. Of the individuals who join the program and lose weight initially, most regress or even exceed their previous weights. Understanding of the complexities of helping people achieve and maintain a desirable body composition has much room for improvement.

A number of suggestions taken from successful clinical programs on weight loss and weight control are outlined in FYI 2.

EXERCISE AND WEIGHT CONTROL

Beginning in early adulthood, the typical American adds roughly 1–1.5 pounds per year of excess fat through a combination of slow fat gain and slow loss of fat-free tissue. Because these two changes occur simultaneously, and because body weight may remain relatively unchanged, the fat accumulation is masked, causing people to conclude mistakenly that their body composition is unaltered. For these individuals or those who gain weight gradually with added years, regular, lifelong exercise is recommended highly.

Regular exercise is of great benefit to long-term control of body weight for a number of reasons, including the effect of regular exercise on body composition, fuel utilization, caloric expenditure, and appetite. Each of these factors is discussed more fully.

Exercise and Body Composition

One important connection between regular exercise and weight control relates to its effect on the composition of the body. An individual typically begins an exercise program only to discover that, although fitness improves, body weight does not change much. This is true particularly if the individual is not overfat to begin with, or if caloric intake increases to some extent after beginning the program. In reality, however, *body composition* changes. If the individual has been evaluated for body composition prior to beginning the program and then is remeasured later, results typically will indicate a loss of body fat coupled with a similar gain in fat-free weight, thereby rendering the total body weight unchanged.

Of course, individual results vary greatly because of differences in body make-up and the type, duration, and intensity of the exercise program. For example, if you choose a weight-lifting program as your fitness activity, you probably will gain more fat-free weight than if you spend the same amount of time in an aerobics class. (This is true for both males and females.) On the other hand, if you do not attend either to your weight-lifting or to your aerobics regularly, changes in your body composition likely will be much smaller, if any occur at all. Generalizations about the benefits and results of an exercise program, then, must be qualified: People differ in ways that as yet are poorly understood, and the results will depend partly upon factors unique to you.

One thing that does seem to be true, however, is that fat-free tissue expends more energy than fat tissue does. If, through regular exercise, you build up your fat-free tissue, hour-by-hour and day-by-day, you will expend more energy than if you were to have a larger proportion of fat and a relatively smaller proportion of fat-free tissue. The increase of daily energy expenditure will help tip the caloric balance equation in the desired direction and allow you to achieve weight control more easily.

Spot-reducing refers to attempts to reduce localized fat stores by exercising the specific body part where the fat is located. Research indicates that this does not work. Exercise stimulates mobilization of fat from deposits located throughout the body, not just from fat cells located over the exercising muscle. The only benefits likely to be obtained from this sort of exercise are improvements in flexibility, strength, and muscle endurance in the local body parts and related improvements in muscle tone.

Fuel Utilization in Exercise

The term **fuel** is used to refer to the foodstuffs the muscles use during various types of exercise. The three types of foodstuffs that contain energy are proteins, carbohydrates, and fats. For most circumstances a simple generalization can be made: Proteins are not used at all as fuels for muscular exercise. In prolonged exercise (such as marathon running) a small amount of the total energy production ($\leq$10%) comes from the breakdown of proteins. In all other types of exercise, however, the fuels the exercising muscles use come from a mixture of fats and carbohydrates. Before describing the factors that influence the proportion of fat

Losing Weight: Some Practical Suggestions

1. Because permanent and lasting changes are difficult, make them slowly.

2. Recognize and acknowledge that you may encounter internal and external constraints against losing weight. Obtain assistance in identifying and modifying your own constraints, if necessary. This assistance should precede or accompany weight loss. Examples of constraints are:
   - Poor social support for weight loss
   - Fear of failing
   - Fear of the consequences of success (for example, how will you feel if others find you more attractive with less fat?)
   - Fear of change
   - Low self-esteem issues that affect your weight-loss program (for example, "I don't deserve attention or love"; "I don't deserve to be treated well"; "I don't deserve to accomplish what I'd like to accomplish"; "If I do achieve what I want, there will be a dire consequence of one sort or another")

3. Restrict fat consumption severely, not only because of the energy density of fat but also because calories consumed from fat are stored more efficiently as fat than are calories consumed from other foods. The net effect of a high-fat diet is greater storage of fat. Reducing fat intake is the single most effective step in reducing caloric intake.

4. Learn more about yourself in the areas of what you eat, how much you eat, when you eat, how you eat, and why you eat. This will help you identify the appropriate steps to make a lasting difference.

5. To learn more about the foods you eat, including which foods are highest in visible and hidden fat, keep a food record for 3–7 days. Remembering all you eat is difficult unless you keep a running log and make entries as you consume food. Studies show that most people underestimate what they eat if they rely on recall—by as much as 44 percent, according to one study. Remembering to make food entries in your diary is easier if you:
   - Keep your records in a portable diary that you can keep with you.
   - Ask someone's help in reminding you to keep records.
   - Leave notes for yourself as reminders.
   - Jot down records on scratch paper and transfer them later if you forgot to bring the diary with you.

   In learning to estimate portion size, weigh and measure all foods you eat until you learn what standardized amounts look like.

6. In developing a physical activity plan, specify what you plan to do, for how long, what days and what times, where, with whom. Arrange for an exercise partner, if possible, so you can motivate one another. The activity you choose should be enjoyable and should allow you to increase the intensity and duration gradually. If you have been inactive to date, you may wish to choose walking.

7. A typical emotion-based eating episode is:
   - Something happens.
   - You think about it.
   - You experience emotional consequences.
   - You eat.

   Disrupt or alter any of these steps by avoiding the event, problem solving, or seeking an alternative outlet for the emotional reaction.

8. To deal with people who tend to sabotage your diet (or exercise) plans:
   - Avoid the saboteurs.
   - Tell them you are trying to lose weight and ask for their help.
   - Show your appreciation to those who respond helpfully.
   - Be consistent in your reactions and attitudes toward food.
   - Refuse the food they may offer that does not fit your diet, but compliment the cook.
   - Plan ahead by cutting back on what you eat before seeing the saboteur.
   - Seek alternative ways of relating to the saboteur without food.
   - Invite saboteurs to your home instead of visiting their home.
   - Prepare responses ahead of time, such as: "I really can't eat another bite"; "My doctor insists I lose weight"; "I really don't feel like eating anything right now."

Sources: *Lifesteps—Weight Management Leader's Guide*, by National Dairy Council, Rosemont, IL, 1985; and *Motivation Techniques: Practical Ways of Helping Our Patients Make Changes in Their Lives*, by H. M. Frankel and J. Staeheli (Portland, OR: Portland Health Institute), 1989.

and carbohydrate used as fuel, we will describe in more detail the differences between aerobic and anaerobic exercise.

Aerobic exercises rely on oxygen to liberate energy from fuel. Oxygen does not supply the energy; it simply is needed to complete the last step in a large number of biochemical reactions required to break down food and release the energy contained within it. This process occurs within all muscle cells in microscopically small structures called **mitochondria.**

Anaerobic exercises do not rely on oxygen for energy production (hence the term "anaerobic"). Instead they rely on immediate sources of energy found within the muscles or they derive energy from the partial (nonaerobic) breakdown of carbohydrate. The immediate sources of energy are in short supply and are thought to be able to sustain the energy requirements of the muscles doing heavy exercise for only 5–10 seconds. The anaerobic breakdown of carbohydrate results in the production of a byproduct called *lactic acid,* which is a significant contributor to muscle fatigue. The weakness you experience when lifting a weight 15–20 times to the point of failure, for instance, is thought to result in part from the build-up of lactic acid in your exercising muscles.

Anaerobic exercises tend to last for short periods, usually less than 2–3 minutes. Whenever you complete a task within 2–3 minutes, particularly if it is vigorous—running up a flight of stairs, carrying in a heavy suitcase from the car, running to catch up with a friend—you will rely primarily on anaerobic energy production. Depending on how long and how hard you push yourself, the fatigue will vary accordingly.

Aerobic exercises last longer than 2–3 minutes. Because they are sustained longer, they tend to be done at a more gentle pace and, as a result, are not as fatiguing as anaerobic exercises. Going for a walk, preparing a meal, and working in the garden are examples of aerobic activities. Jogging, cycling, and swimming—the types of activities suggested in Chapter 5 as suitable for cardiorespiratory training—are also aerobic activities. The latter tend to be more vigorous than the earlier examples. If you do them for long periods, they also tend to be fatiguing, particularly if you are not fit.

The fuel needs of an exercising person depend on a number of factors, including the following:

1. *Diet.* If your diet is high in fat content, you will use fat to a greater extent as a fuel, all else remaining the same. The opposite is true if you eat a diet that is higher in carbohydrate content. This certainly should not be interpreted as a recommendation to increase your fat intake, as a number of

health risks are associated with a high intake of dietary fat. More will be said on this matter in Chapters 8 and 9.

2. *Intensity of exercise.* In aerobic activities, fats and carbohydrates both contribute to the fuel requirements of the exercising muscles. Fats constitute the main source of fuel the muscles use in submaximal exercise, including activities during which you are at (or nearly at) rest. This fat comes from intracellular stores of fat within the muscles, as well as from fat stores within fatty tissue. The greater the intensity of aerobic exercise, the more carbohydrates contribute to the fuel needs of the muscles and the less fats contribute.

Any anaerobic exercise relies exclusively on carbohydrates as a fuel once the immediate forms of stored energy are used up, which, as mentioned earlier, occurs after 5–10 seconds of heavy exercise. Thereafter, carbohydrates are the only form of fuel that can be relied on for anaerobic energy production.

3. *Duration of exercise.* When aerobic exercise is continued at a given pace, fats contribute increasingly to fuel needs as duration of exercise increases. Thus, if you are able to keep up a jogging pace for 45 minutes, the relative contribution of fats will increase and be much greater toward the end of the workout than it was toward the beginning, all else remaining the same.

4. *Fitness status.* The more aerobically fit you are, the more you will be able to use fat in place of carbohydrate at a given level of exercise, all else remaining the same. This means that if you were to compare yourself under standardized conditions before and after 6 months of aerobic training, not only would a given level of exercise be much easier for you to perform because of your increased exercise capacity, but minute by minute you also would be using more fat and less carbohydrate to meet the energy demands of your muscles.

Why does this occur? Among the most important outcomes of aerobic training are structural and enzymatic changes in the trained muscles themselves. Mitochondrial surface area and density increase from aerobic training, yielding more of this specialized type of tissue where aerobic energy production occurs. Enzymes that facilitate the aerobic breakdown of fats and carbohydrates, but particularly those favoring fat utilization, also increase in concentration. The net effect is that fat is used as a fuel to a greater extent than it was in an unfit state.

An enhanced ability to use fat as a fuel not only will benefit you during your aerobic exercise sessions each day or week, but it will affect your fuel utilization at other times of the day as well—for example, while doing the tasks that make up your workday or while driving to and from work. This is useful for at least two reasons. First, the fat stores in the body are many times greater than the stores of carbohydrate, even if you are relatively lean. Being able to rely on fat to a greater degree spares the more limited supply of carbohydrate for use only when it is absolutely required. Second, by being able to use fat as a fuel to a greater extent under all conditions, the total amount of fat stores tend to be lower—a pleasant outcome if you are concerned with weight control.

Exercise and Caloric Expenditure

Another beneficial effect of regular exercise is that, when you exercise, you expend additional calories, which permits you to eat more food without the fear of gaining weight. The calories you expend during exercise are not the only additional calories spent. For as long as 1–2 hours after exercise, depending on the nature and extent of the exercise and on the climatic conditions, your body continues to recover and continues to expend calories. The total caloric expenditure during this recovery period is not large, but it nonetheless is part of your overall caloric expenditure. Evidence suggests that regular exercise training also causes an increase in REE. Genetic differences and variations in fitness seem to contribute to variability in response among individuals, however.

Losing weight by exercising, without any modification in diet, is relatively difficult. Some experts suggest that the number of calories spent in exercise is so small that the effort may not be worth the trouble. To illustrate how the calorie expenditure is determined, sample calculations taken from one of the activities listed in Appendix 4 (easy running at 12 min./mile) are provided in Figure 7.5. By adding 2 miles/day, 3 days/week of jogging into a previously sedentary routine, a 148-pound person would take 6.8 weeks to lose one pound of fat, a rate that most Americans probably would consider too slow. Although the immediate effects of the exercise are slow, however, if continued indefinitely, the caloric effects can be considerable simply because the caloric effects are cumulative. Over one year, 7.65 pounds of fat would be lost, all else remaining the same. Over 10 years

this amounts to 76.5 pounds; over 20 years, 153 pounds. Thus, over a long time, the effects of regular exercise can be a powerful means of losing fat and then of keeping fat levels under control. Between ages 20 and 40, the average individual gains 20–30 pounds of fat. If most 40-year-olds had maintained a regular exercise program (with emphasis on regular!) during the previous 20 years, many would not have gained the extra fat.

The calculations in Figure 7.5 are theoretical and simplified. They are offered merely to illustrate the potential impact of regular aerobic exercise on the challenge of weight control throughout life. In truth, the effect of regular exercise (or a consistent 500-calorie deficit, or a regular helping of more food than you require, such as an extra piece of pie), depends on a myriad of factors that are only beginning to become clear. For example, research has highlighted a strong genetic influence on an individual's response to excess caloric intake over time. Because of genetic factors, some people, when exposed to caloric excess, gain much more weight than others who are exposed to the same excess. Genetics undoubtably influences caloric expenditure similarly.

Even within the same individual, a given caloric deficit probably will have a different effect depending on whether it comes soon after beginning a weight-loss program or much later, by which time the body may have adapted itself to the

FIGURE 7.5 Potential caloric effects of regular exercise over time.

If a 148-lb person were to jog on the horizontal at a pace of 12:00 min/mile, the energy expenditure (from Appendix 4) is: .056 cal/min/lb Therefore, for 1 mile:

(.056 cal/min/lb) (12 min) (148 lb) = 99.5 cal

While sitting quietly, this same person expends .008 cal/min/lb. Therefore, during the same time period, the person would have expended:

(.008 cal/min/lb) (12 min) (148 lb) = 14.2 cal

The net extra cost of jogging 1 mile is therefore:

99.5 − 14.2 = 85.3 cal

Because 1 lb fat = 3500 cal, this means that

$$\frac{3500 \text{ cal/lb}}{85.3 \text{ cal/mi}} = 41.0 \text{ mi/lb fat loss}$$

If this person jogs 2 mi/day for 3 days/wk = 6 mi/wk

Therefore: $\frac{41 \text{ mi/lb fat}}{6 \text{ mi/wk}} = 6.8 \text{ wks/lb}$

which is equivalent to: $\frac{52 \text{ wks/yr}}{6.8 \text{ wks/lb}} = 7.65 \text{ lbs/yr}$

Over 10 years: (7.65 lbs/yr) (10 yrs) = 76.5 lbs
Over 20 years: (7.65 lbs/yr) (20 yrs) = 153 lbs

condition of being in deficit and managed to protect (or minimize) any further losses it incurs. Not only do people differ in these phenomena, but people differ within themselves over time. These differences also are likely to depend on prior history of weight cycling, composition of the diet, history of exercise, and body composition, to name a few possibilities.

Regardless of all the reasons individuals respond differently, if you manage to engage regularly in aerobic exercise, you will expend more calories than if you do not. As a result, you will be more successful in the lifelong challenge of weight control because these extra calories will come from the body's fuel stores, the major proportion of which is fat.

Exercise and Appetite

Contrary to what is commonly believed, adding regular exercise to your daily routine will not necessarily cause you to eat more. Evidence suggests that a moderate amount of regular exercise will not increase your appetite at all; it even may lessen your appetite slightly, especially if you exercise before a meal. In addition, evidence using lean persons suggests that when they eat a meal in close proximity to an exercise session, they expend more energy than if they partake in the meal and exercise session separately. This further supports the argument favoring exercise in a weight-loss program.

We should note, however, that this same accelerated energy expenditure accruing from the combination of meal and exercise has not been found to occur in obese persons. In fact, the energy expenditure that normally increases during and after a meal was reduced in obese people. This suggests that some people may be more prone to obesity than others because of this blunting of the normal increase in energy production as a result of a meal. The reasons for the difference remain unknown.

Reasons for Not Exercising

People give many reasons for not exercising even when they are aware they should. First, exercise requires a commitment of time and often money (for clothing, equipment, gym fees, lessons, and so on), precious commodities in contemporary American society. In addition, exercise leaves them tired and sweaty. Also, many are unwilling to take the real risks of injury. Further compounding the issue, our competitive, capitalistic marketplace offers hundreds of options from which to choose regarding agencies, instructors, books, testing facilities, and equipment, shoes, and clothing manufacturers. Although this diversity may allow you to find the combination that best fits your needs (provided you take the time and energy to investigate the var-

ious options), it also makes you vulnerable to fraudulent claims and offers. The only insurance against unsavory practices is to be as informed as possible as a consumer.

GAINING WEIGHT

Some people are naturally underweight. They seem not to be plagued by creeping weight gain. The reasons are variable and include a high basal metabolic rate, influences of heredity, nutritional disorders, and various medical and situational problems. Often these individuals wish to gain weight, particularly if they feel physically or emotionally at risk.

If you have no medical or health problems and wish to gain weight, the matter is one of increasing the number of calories consumed and modifying your caloric output so as to add weight in a healthful manner. Whenever embarking on a new regimen such as this, nutritional or medical problems should be ruled out by having a thorough physical exam.

The goal should be to add weight largely by increasing your muscle mass and not by increasing fat mass. (Some chronically undernourished individuals, we recognize, may indeed have to increase their stores of body fat. In these cases the matter is more one of ingesting additional calories from a nutritionally healthful diet.)

Set a reasonable goal in terms of how much weight to gain and how rapidly. In general, gaining one pound per week is reasonable and may even be too difficult for some individuals to accomplish. Next, estimate your average energy intake over a 3- to 7-day period. Also, estimate your average caloric requirement over a similar time period. With this baseline information about current habits, adjustments can be made in daily caloric intake to accomplish the goals. (Methods for estimating caloric intake and caloric requirement were described previously in this chapter.)

One pound of muscle tissue is approximately 70% water and 22% protein, and the balance consists of fat and carbohydrate. Unfortunately, to add one pound of muscle, it is not known how many extra calories are needed, nor is it known what form those calories should be in. A good estimate is that approximately 2500–3000 extra calories and about 100 grams of extra protein are needed. This translates into consuming 400–600 extra calories, including 15 grams of extra protein, per day above daily needs. The assumption is that your base diet meets but does not exceed daily requirements for calories and protein.

When adding extra protein to your diet, preferably it should not come in a form that also contains excessive fat, as is the case in fatty meats and most cheese. In most American diets protein intake already is well above the daily RDA (see Chapters 8 and 9), making expensive protein or amino acid supplements unnecessary. For example, approximately two glasses of skim milk per day will provide 16 grams of extra protein. Other foods high in protein and lower in fat content include egg whites and low-fat cheeses.

As always, sound nutritional principles should be followed when attempting to gain weight. Chapters 8 and 9 discuss principles of nutrition and eating healthfully. Other suggestions include eating nutritionally dense foods (those high in calories and nutrients), reducing intake of bulky foods that are filling but contain few calories, eating three or more balanced meals a day and one or more nutritional snacks, and avoiding much of an increase in fat intake, particularly saturated fats from animal products. Fat intake in the typical American diet is much too high. Unless intake of fats already is at or below the recommended level (less than 30% of total calories), increases in fat intake will not enhance health.

To maximize the probability of gaining muscle tissue, a weight-training program designed to build muscle should be instituted (see Chapter 6). For health benefits, an aerobic exercise program also should be undertaken, using principles described in Chapter 5. Including an aerobic program in the weight gain plan will increase caloric expenditure. The total number of calories expended, however, is relatively low, and caloric intake can be adjusted appropriately. All in all, the health benefits will far outweigh the costs.

SUMMARY

Some 30% of American adults are estimated to be overweight, and up to half of these are classified as obese. In addition to its negative social stigma, obesity is associated with health problems including higher risk for heart disease, cancer, and a higher overall death rate.

Determining your body composition is accomplished most accurately through hydrostatic weighing. Because it is not readily accessed, however, skinfold and bioelectric impedance techniques can provide a general estimate of your %fat.

Weight control is a function of energy balance, defined as the relationship between caloric intake and caloric expenditure. The recommended protocol for weight loss includes a moderate diet, in which no fewer than 1200 calories are consumed per day, in conjunction with regular physical activity. Weight loss should not exceed 1–2 pounds per week. Activity should consist of low- to moderate-intensity aerobic exercise for 20 minutes or more per day, 3–5 days per week.

As a method of bringing about lasting weight loss, dieting by itself is ineffective and may result in a decrease of REE, particularly with extreme dieting, in which case you also may fail to take in a sufficient amount of daily nutrients to meet nutritional requirements. Adding exercise to the routine may offset the loss in REE, and it does not increase appetite if done in moderation. In addition, exercise forces more of the weight loss to come from fat and not from loss of other tissues. Additional benefits of regular exercise for long-term weight control include a greater ability to use fat as a fuel (from aerobic training), overall improvement in body composition, and increased caloric expenditure, which assists in achieving long-term caloric balance.

Gaining weight is best accomplished by eating more calories than you expend and by adding a supplemental exercise program to build lean tissue.

CHOICES IN ACTION

Several labs have been developed to supplement the material discussed in this chapter. Labs 20 and 21 relate to assessment of body composition. Because fitness is an integral part of controlling body weight, Lab 22 will help you develop a personalized exercise prescription that focuses on cardiorespiratory fitness, flexibility, strength, muscle endurance, and body composition. Lab 23 provides a sample exercise log that you may adapt for any type of regular exercise you choose.

REFERENCES

American College of Sports Medicine. 1983. "Position Stand on Proper and Improper Weight Loss Programs." *Medicine and Science in Sports and Exercise* 15: ix–x.

Barrett-Connor, E. L. 1985. "Obesity, Atherosclerosis and Coronary Artery Disease." *Annals of Internal Medicine* 103(6, part 2): 1010–1019.

Beals, K. A., and Monroe, M. M. 1994. "The Prevalence and Consequences of Subclinical Eating Disorders in Female Athletes." *International Journal of Sport Nutrition* 4: 175–195.

Bjorntorp, P. 1985. "Regional Patterns of Fat Distribution." *Annals of Internal Medicine* 103(6, part 2): 994–995.

Bouchard, C., et al. 1990. "The Response to Long-term Overfeeding in Identical Twins." *New England Journal of Medicine* 322(21): 1477–1482.

Brehm, B. A., and Gutin, B. 1986. "Recovery Energy Expenditure for Steady State Exercise in Runners and Non-exercisers." *Medicine and Science in Sports and Exercise* 18: 205–210.

Brooks, G. A., and Fahey, T. D. 1995. *Exercise Physiology*, 2d ed. Mountain View, A: Mayfield Publishing. New York: John Wiley and Sons.

Brownell, K. D. 1988. "Yo-Yo Dieting." *Psychology Today* (January): 20, 22–23.

Brownell, K. D., Steen, S. N., and Wilmore, J. H. 1987. "Weight Regulation Practices in Athletes: Analysis of Metabolic and Health Effects." *Medicine and Science in Sports and Exercise* 19(6): 546–556.

Caspersen, C., Powell, K. E., and Christenson, G. M. 1985. "Physical Activity, Exercise and Physical Fitness: Definitions and Distinctions for Health-Related Research." *Public Health Reports* 100(2): 126–131.

Costill, D. C. 1985. "Carbohydrate Nutrition Before, During and After Exercise." *Federal Proceedings* 44: 364–368.

Council on Scientific Affairs. 1988. "Treatment of Obesity in Adults." *Journal of American Medical Society* 260: 2547–2557.

Dohn, G. L., Kasperek, G. J., Tapscott, E. B., and Barakat, H. A. 1985. "Protein Metabolism During Endurance Exercise." *Federal Proceedings* 44: 348–352.

Frankel, H. M. 1986. "Determination of Body Mass Index." *Journal of the American Medical Association* 225(10).

Frankel, H. M., and Staeheli, J. 1989. *Motivation Techniques: Practical Ways of Helping Our Patients Make Changes in Their Lives.* Portland, OR: Portland Health Institute.

Gollnick, P. D. 1985. "Metabolism of Substrates: Energy Substrate Metabolism During Exercise and as Modified by Training." *Federal Proceedings* 44: 353–357.

Gray, D. S. 1989. "Diagnosis and Prevalence of Obesity." *Medical Clinics of North America* 73(1): 1–14.

Holloszy, J. O. 1982. "Muscle Metabolism During Exercise." *Archives of Physical Medicine and Rehabilitation* 63: 231–234.

Horton, E. S. 1985. "Metabolic Aspects of Exercise and Weight Reduction." *Medicine and Science in Sports and Exercise* 18: 10–18.

"Is an Eating Disorder Developing in Your Family?" 1989. *Tufts University Diet and Nutrition Letter* 7(3, May).

"Is Fat More Fattening?" 1987. *Tufts University Diet and Nutrition Letter* 4(12).

Katch, F. I., Clarkson, P. M., Kroll, W., McBride, T., and Wilcox, A. 1984. "The Effects of Sit Up Exercise Training on Adipose Cell Size and Adiposity." *Research Quarterly for Exercise and Sport* 55: 242–247.

Katch, F. I., and McArdle, W. D. 1993. *Introduction to Nutrition, Exercise, and Health*, 4th ed. Philadelphia, PA: Lea and Febiger.

Kuczmarski, R. J., Flegal, K. M., Campbell, S. M., and Johnson, C. L. 1994. "Increasing Prevalence of Overweight Among U. S. Adults." *Journal of the American Medical Association* 272(3): 205–211.

Lifesteps—Weight Management Leader's Guide. 1985. Rosemont, IL: National Dairy Council.

Lohman, T. G. 1984. "Research Progress in Validation of Laboratory Methods of Assessing Body Composition." *Medicine and Science in Sports and Exercise* 16: 596–603.

McArdle, W. D., Katch, F. I., and Katch, V. L. 1991. *Exercise Physiology*, 3rd ed. Philadelphia: Lea and Febiger.

Metropolitan Life Insurance Co. 1959. *Statistical Bulletin* (Nov./Dec.): 1–4.

Metropolitan Life Insurance Co. 1984. "1983 Metropolitan Height and Weight Tables." *Statistical Bulletin* 64: 2–9.

National Institutes of Health. 1985. "Health Implications of Obesity" (Consensus Development Conference Statement). *Annals of Internal Medicine* 103(6, part 2): 981–982.

"New Weight Standards for Men and Women." 1959. *Statistical Bulletin* 40: 1–4.

Nutritive Value of Foods. 1981. U. S. Department of Agriculture, Department of Health and Human Services (Home and Garden Bulletin #72).

Washington, D.C.: Government Printing Office.

Oscai, L. B. 1981. "Exercise and Lipid Metabolism." *Nutrition in the 1980's: Constraints on Our Knowledge* (pp. 383–390). New York: Alan R. Liss.

Poehlman, E. T. 1989. "A Review: Exercise and its Influence on Resting Energy Metabolism in Man." *Medicine and Science in Sports and Exercise* 21(5): 515–525.

Poehlman, E. T., and Horton, E. S. 1989. "The Impact of Food Intake and Exercise on Energy Expenditure." *Nutrition Reviews* 47: 129–137.

Pollock, M. L., Wilmore, J. H. 1990. *Exercise in Health and Disease*. 2d ed. Philadelphia: W. B. Saunders.

Ravussin, E., Lillioja, S., Anderson, T. E., Christin, L., and Bogardus, C. 1986. "Determinants of 24-hour Energy Expenditure in Man." *Journal of Clinical Investigation* 78: 1568–1578.

Rodin, J., and Wing, R. R. 1988. "Behavioral Factors in Obesity." *Diabetes/Metabolism Reviews* 4: 701–725.

Schlesier-Stropp, B. 1984. "Bulimia: A Review of the Literature." *Psychological Bulletin* 95: 247–257.

Segal, K. R., Gutin, B., Nyman, A. M., and Pi-Sunyer, F. X. 1985. "Thermic Effect of Food at Rest, During Exercise, and After Exercise in Lean and Obese Men of Similar Body Weight." *Journal of Clinical Investigation* 76: 1107–1112.

Thompson, J. K., Jarvie, G. J., Lahey, B. B., and Cureton, K. J. 1982. "Exercise and Obesity: Etiology, Physiology, and Intervention." *Psychological Bulletin* 91: 55–79.

Webb, P. 1985. "Direct Calorimetry and the Energetics of Exercise and Weight Loss." *Medicine and Science in Sports and Exercise* 18: 3–5.

Willett, W. C., Stampfer, M., Manson, J., and Van Itallie, T. 1991. "New Weight Guidelines for Americans: Justified or Injudicious?" *American Journal of Clinical Nutrition* 53(5): 1102–1103.

Williams, M. H. 1992. *Nutrition for Fitness and Sport*, 3rd edition. Dubuque, IA: W. C. Brown.

Wilmore, J. H. 1983. "Appetite and Body Composition Consequent to Physical Activity." *Research Quarterly for Exercise and Sport* 54: 415–425.

The Daily Dilemma

What's Good to Eat?

✓ What nutrients do you need to be healthy?

✓ How much of these nutrients should you be eating—and does it matter that much if you don't meet these requirements?

✓ Are you, like most Americans, eating too much protein and fat and not enough carbohydrates?

✓ How can your diet affect your risk of contracting diseases such as cancer, heart disease, diabetes, osteoporosis, and even the common cold?

✓ Is herbal tea better for you than coffee? Wine better than beer? Mineral water better than soft drinks?

Good nutrition entails giving your body what it needs, when it needs it, and in the right amount to allow you to function in top form. This is no simple task, because the body requires quite a variety of things to function at its best. In addition to energy, the body needs building blocks, transport carriers, regulators, facilitators, cleansers, and lots of water. To meet these needs, you have to eat more than 45 different nutrients each day. Fortunately, you don't have to eat that many different foods to obtain these nutrients. Some foods, such as meat, milk, apples, oranges, and bread, contain many nutrients. Other foods, such as beer, soda pop, and pretzels, have almost none. The point is that no one food, or even a combination of several foods, can provide all the nutrients you need. No pill or capsule can do the job either. Only by consuming a variety of foods with certain qualities and in specific amounts can you meet the body's needs. Thus, variety, quality, and quantity are the key determinants of good nutrition. What foods have these qualities? How much of them do you need to eat, and how often? How much does it really matter if you don't pay attention to these issues? These are the questions addressed in the first part of this chapter.

The nutrients the body needs to be supplied with daily are called **essential nutrients** because the body can't function properly without them and it has no way to get them unless you eat them. The six main categories of essential nutrients are protein, carbohydrate, fat (also called lipid), vitamins, minerals, and water. The essential nutrients in each of these categories are listed in Table 8.A. Of these, only protein, carbohydrates, and fat provide energy or fuel for the body. The amount of energy these nutrients supply is measured in calories.*

Although it is a potential energy source, the main role of protein is to provide the structural components or building blocks for body tissues. Vitamins and minerals function primarily as regulators and facilitators or catalysts for the millions of chemical reactions within cells that keep the body functioning. Water forms the major part of every body tissue (you are more than 70% water). It also provides the medium by which materials are transported to and away from cells, and in which almost all body processes take place. The function(s) of the nutrient groups (except water) are summarized in Table 8.B.

The purpose of this chapter is to help you make informed choices about what you eat each day. Toward this goal, the special qualities of each of these essential nutrients will be discussed and the best food sources of each identified.

PROTEIN

The human body contains hundreds of different kinds of **protein,** all with highly specialized

TABLE 8.A Essential nutrients.

VITAMINS	MINERALS	PROTEIN	FAT	CARBOHYDRATE	WATER
Fat-soluble	Calcium	Amino acids	Linoleic acid	Glucose	
A	Phosphorus	Leucine	~~Linoleic~~ acid		
D	Sodium	Isoleucine	Linolenic		
E	Potassium	Lysine			
K	Sulfur	Methionine			
	Chlorine	Phenylalanine			
Water-soluble	Magnesium	Threonine			
Thiamin	Iron	Tryptophan			
Riboflavin	Selenium	Valine			
Niacin	Zinc	Histidine			
Biotin	Manganese				
Folacin					
Pyridoxine					
Vitamin B$_{12}$					
Pantothenic acid					
Ascorbic acid					

*Food energy is actually measured in kilocalories or Calories. A calorie (spelled with a small "c") is only 1/1000th of a kilocalorie or Calorie, but most Americans and even nutritionists simply use the term *calorie* to mean kilocalorie, as we will do in this text.

TABLE 8.B

Basic functions of major nutrient groups.

	FUNCTIONS		
	ENERGY SOURCE	GROWTH, MAINTENANCE, AND REPAIR OF BODY TISSUES	REGULATION OF BODY PROCESSES
Nutrient Groups	Carbohydrates Fats Proteins (Minerals)* (Vitamins)*	Protein (Minerals)* (Vitamins)*	Protein Minerals Vitamins
*Indirectly involved as catalysts for biochemical reactions			

functions. Typically, only muscle comes to mind in connection with protein, and, true, most protein is in muscle. Protein, however, also is a major structural component of every cell in the body. Table 8.C shows the distribution of protein among various body tissues. Protein also is used to make the antibodies in our blood and many of our hormones. It transports nutrients to and from cells, and the protein *hemoglobin*, which contains iron, carries oxygen. Special proteins called **enzymes** catalyze or facilitate the chemical reactions in cells that keep the body functioning.

Protein is made of nitrogen-containing components called **amino acids.** When you eat protein, the body digests it or breaks it down into some 22 different types of amino acids. These then are absorbed into the bloodstream and carried to the cells, where various amino acids are linked to

TABLE 8.C

Distribution of protein in the body.

TISSUE	% OF BODY PROTEIN (APPROX.)
Blood proteins (albumin and hemoglobin)	10
Fat cells of adipose tissues	3–4
Body skin	9–9.5
Bones	18–19
Muscles	46–47

Note: The values have been obtained from various sources and are presented in ranges to emphasize their variability in human bodies.

make the different proteins the body needs. Nine are called *essential amino acids* because the body cannot make them; they must be eaten. The body can make the other 13 amino acids as needed, even if they are not specifically consumed. The nine essential amino acids were listed in Table 8.A.

Any protein containing all nine of these essential amino acids in sufficient quantity for the body to use is called a **complete protein;** all others are **incomplete proteins.** They contain insufficient amounts of one or more of the essential amino acids. Consequently, the body will be able to use the amino acids supplied for building proteins only in relation to the amount of the "limiting" or insufficient amino acid(s). The situation is analogous to trying to make cookies when you have only one egg and the recipe calls for two. You can make only half the recipe. If you are about to leave on a 3-month vacation and can't store the rest of the ingredients, of which you have plenty, you will have to use them in another way or throw them out. Similarly, the body has no way to store amino acids. Those that can't be used to make protein are stripped of their nitrogen and used for fuel, or stored as fat if other sources of fuel (carbohydrate and fat) are sufficiently abundant. The nitrogen is eliminated through the urine.

The only way to ensure that the body can make all the protein it needs when it needs it is to supply it with complete proteins periodically throughout the day. Even when you eat enough protein, however, if the body receives insufficient calories for energy from its other fuel sources (carbohydrates and fats), it will use protein for energy instead of for building and repair, hormones, antibodies, and so on. It would be as if you weren't eating enough protein. In this sense, carbohydrates and fat are called "protein sparers."

Sources of Protein

All animals and animal products, except gelatin, provide complete proteins. These include meat, fish, poultry, eggs, and dairy products. Vegetables and grains also provide proteins, but in general these proteins are incomplete. Legumes are an exception; they are the richest sources of vegetable proteins and provide protein almost as complete as animal foods. Examples of legumes are lentils, peanuts, black-eyed peas, soybeans, chick peas, lima beans, kidney beans, pinto beans, black beans, and other types of dried peas and beans. Of these, soybeans and soybean products resemble animal protein most closely. Seeds and nuts are excellent vegetable proteins, too, but they also contain so much fat that their use as a major protein source is limited. All other vegetable and grain proteins are notably incomplete.

By eating certain combinations of vegetables and grains or by eating them with a source of complete protein such as milk, one can get complete protein without eating meat, poultry, or fish. Such protein combinations, called **complementary proteins**, provide the basis for the vegetarian diet. For example, by having milk with your cereal or toast, or by eating a combination of beans and rice, you can obtain a complete protein. On the other hand, toast and coffee (even whole wheat toast!) just won't fill the complete protein bill. If you decide to have some milk or yogurt a bit later, within two hours or so, you probably could still complement your toast into "completeness," but the best advice seems to be to eat them together.

The limiting amino acid(s) for various categories of vegetable and grain proteins are listed in Table 8.D. Combining legumes with grains and seeds seems to be the best overall recommendation for obtaining complete protein without eating animal products. Other combinations will accomplish this also, but a full discussion of vegetarianism is beyond the scope of this book. The point is that getting the protein the body needs requires some knowledge and planning, and even more so if you choose not to eat any animal products at all.

Some other conditions affect the body's ability to use the protein you eat. These include the amino acid pattern of the protein, its digestibility, availability of the vitamins and minerals needed to process it, and a sufficient intake of the "protein sparers," fat and carbohydrate, to prevent the protein from being used for energy. Vitamin and mineral needs will be discussed later in this chapter, and the protein-sparing effect of fats and carbohydrates has been mentioned already. The amino acid pattern and digestibility of proteins, however, deserve some explanation here. In brief, the more closely the amounts of essential amino acids in a protein you eat resemble the amounts in human protein, the more completely the protein can be used. This is called the biological value of protein. In this respect, egg is the best protein source, with a biological value of 100. It is followed by fish and dairy products, meats and soybeans, grains and nuts, in that order. But you can't use what you don't digest and absorb, and the body's ability to digest protein from different sources varies. Basically, the most easily digested proteins come from animal products, followed by soybeans, then other vegetables and grains.

Protein Requirements

Now that the quality of protein needed by the body has been defined, the final question is: How much protein do you need to eat? Your size and age help to determine the answer. Look again at Table 8.C, which shows the distribution of protein among various body tissues. Almost 90% of protein is located in lean or fat-free tissues. Obviously, a large-sized person, someone with big bones and muscles, needs more protein to maintain these tissues than a smaller person does. Also, during those times in life when these tissues are being built rapidly, such as during pregnancy, infancy, and childhood, a higher intake is needed compared to the amount needed merely to maintain existing tissue.

Thus, the amount of protein you need to eat is based on the amount of lean body tissue you have or are developing. For easier calculation, the

TABLE

8.D   Limiting amino acids in vegetable proteins.

VEGETABLE PROTEINS	LIMITING AMINO ACIDS			
	LYSINE	METHIONINE	THREONINE	TRYPTOPHAN
Most grains	✔		✔	sometimes (e.g., corn)
Most legumes		✔		✔
Nuts and seeds	✔			
Green leafy vegetables		✔		

Adapted from *Principles and Issues in Nutrition*, by Y. H. Hui (Belmont, CA: Wadsworth, 1985).

reference standard used is average body weight, the midpoint of the weight range for medium-framed people according to height. You can determine this value for yourself from the height/weight table provided in Table 7.A, Chapter 7. You can use the midpoint value for small- or large-frame people if you think you fit better in one of these categories *or* use your own body weight if it is within the given range. The important point is not to overestimate or underestimate your protein needs if you weigh more or less than recommended.

It is estimated that the average adult needs only .45 grams of protein per kilogram (2.2 lbs) of body weight. To allow for variation in individual need as well as in the quality of protein consumed, however, the official recommended intake for protein is .8 grams/kg, quite a generous allowance. This translates to .36 g/lb of body weight for adults 19 years of age and over.

The recommended protein intake for various age groups is given in Table 8.E, per pound and per kilogram. To find the amount of protein recommended for you to eat, you simply multiply your body weight (or the "average" body weight for your height) in pounds or kilograms times the unit given for your age. For a 58-kg (128-lb) female, this amounts to 46 grams of protein/day. For a 72-kg (160-lb) male, the recommended amount is 58 grams of protein/day. Given the generous safety margin built into this recommended

intake, however, it is estimated that 80% of the population actually could be quite healthy by consuming only two-thirds this amount! This recommendation applies to people who are basically healthy. Illness, prolonged bedrest, and injury can increase the body's need for protein.

How much do you have to eat to get 46 grams or 58 grams of protein? The answer is far less than the average American thinks. As you can see in Figure 8.1, a breakfast that includes one egg and one piece of toast provides 9 grams of protein. A peanut butter sandwich for lunch adds about 13 grams of protein. If you choose to have a *small*, 6-ounce steak (the petite cut in most American restaurants) on the same day, you will consume an additional 42 grams of protein. Just these foods alone total 64 grams of protein—6 grams more than the young adult male needs and 18 grams more than the young adult female needs! And this total doesn't even consider the protein in the foods that accompany the entree, such as vegetables, snacks, and dessert. Indeed, it is not difficult for the average American to consume 100 grams of protein a day, about twice the recommended amount. In fact, nutritional surveys show that the average protein consumption in America is 137% and 193% of the recommended amount for females and males, respectively. Average protein consumption compared to the recommended amount is shown in Table 8.F.

Overconsumption of protein presents several problems. Too much protein generally means not enough room for something else you need. In general, protein should comprise no more than 10 to 15% of our total calories; fat, 30% or less; and carbohydrate, 55% or more. For a woman consuming about 2000 calories/day, that translates to 200–300 calories from protein. Should she eat 100 grams of protein that contains 4 calories/gram, she would consume 400 calories, or 20% of her calories for the day in protein. If, like most Americans, she eats primarily animal products to obtain her protein, her intake of fat also is likely to be higher than recommended. Many animal sources of protein actually contain more fat calories than protein calories. Vegetable sources of protein, on the other hand, generally contain little if any fat but, rather, have large amounts of carbohydrate. The percent of

TABLE 8.E Recommended dietary allowance for protein.

AGE IN YEARS	GRAMS OF PROTEIN (PER POUND OR KILOGRAM OF IDEAL BODY WEIGHT)	
	G / POUNDS	G / KILOGRAMS
Infants		
0–0.5	1.0	2.2
0.5–1.0	.7	1.6
Children		
1– 3	.55	1.8
4– 6	.5	1.5
7–10	.45	1.2
11–14	.45	1.0
Adults		
15 and over	.36	.8
Pregnant women	.36 + 10g/day	.8 + 10g/day
Nursing women (1st 6 months)	.36 + 15g/day	.8 + 15g/day
(after 6 months)	.36 + 12g/day	.8 + 12g/day

From Food and Nutrition Board, *Recommended Dietary Allowances*, 10th ed. (Washington, DC: National Academy of Sciences–National Research Council, 1989).

FIGURE

8.1   Examples of protein contained in various meals.

	Example I	Protein (g.)		Example II	Protein (g.)

BREAKFAST	1 orange
	1 poached egg
	1 slice whole
	  wheat toast
	coffee
		1
		6
		
		3
		
		10 grams
				1 banana
				1 cup oatmeal
				1 slice white
				  toast
				1 cup milk
					1
					5
					
					2
					8
					16 grams

LUNCH	2 slices whole
	  wheat bread
	2 tbsp. peanut
	  butter
	1 cup milk
		6
		
		7
		8
		21 grams
				Quarter Pounder
				  with cheese
				Regular fries
				Milk shake
					30
					3
					9
					42 grams

SNACK	1/4 cup
	  sunflower seeds
		9 grams		1 cup
				  popcorn
					1 gram

DINNER	6-oz. steak
	1/2 cup mashed
	  potatoes
	1/2 cup spinach
	1 cup ice cream
		42
		
		2
		3
		5
		52 grams
				3 oz. broiled fish
				1/2 cup brown rice
				1/2 cup green
				  beans
				1 brownie
					17
					3
					
					2
					1
					23 grams

	Total protein = 92 grams			Total protein = 82 grams	

TABLE

8.F   Comparison of recommended (RDA) protein intake and average protein consumption per day by females and males.

FEMALES (AGE IN YEARS)	RDA* (GRAMS PROTEIN)	AVERAGE PROTEIN CONSUMPTION (GRAMS) AND % RDA*	
11–14	46	66	144%
15–18	44	63	143%
19–24	46	65	142%
25–49	50	65	130%
50–69	50	55	110%
70+	50	49	98%

MALES (AGE IN YEARS)	RDA* (GRAMS PROTEIN)	AVERAGE PROTEIN CONSUMPTION (GRAMS) AND % RDA*	
11–14	45	92	205%
15–18	59	122	207%
19–24	58	105	181%
25–29	63	105	167%
30–59	63	105	148%
60–69	63	79	126%
70+	63	69	110%

*Recommended Dietary Allowance

From: U.S. Department of Health and Human Services, *Nutrition Monitoring in the U.S.*, 1989.

calories from fat, protein, and carbohydrates for various sources of protein is shown in Table 8.G.

Americans typically get 34% or more of their daily calories in fat instead of the recommended 30% or less. One of the main reasons for this high fat intake is high consumption of animal protein, especially popular foods such as steak, hamburgers, hotdogs, bacon, eggs, cheese, and milk shakes. Even if the amount of protein consumed does not exceed recommended intake, eating a lot of foods like these can result in excessive fat intake, particularly saturated fats and cholesterol.

Crowded out of this picture are carbohydrates, found in fruits, vegetables, and grains. On the average, Americans consume 46% or less of total daily calories in carbohydrates, compared to the recommended 55% or more. Because fat contains 9 calories/gram compared to 4 calories/gram for carbohydrate, this high protein, high-fat, low-carbohydrate diet also can be a high-calorie diet. This is exactly the kind of diet associated with obesity, CVD, and cancer. High-protein and high-fat intakes also increase excretion of calcium, which can promote development of osteoporosis over time.

The bottom line for protein consumption seems to be to keep it in first place when it comes to quality and last place when it comes to quantity

(percent of calories). To do this means selecting complete or complementary proteins to eat and emphasizing low-fat sources such as fish, poultry, vegetables, and grains.

FATS

Fat has such a bad reputation today that it may be hard to think of it as an *essential* nutrient. Most people know this about fat: (a) They're not supposed to be eating as much as they do; (b) they're not supposed to be "wearing" as much as they do; and (c) they're supposed to be "watching" their cholesterol. These perceptions are basically correct, but you must eat *some* fat and have some body fat to function normally. The fact that many Americans typically exceed these needs accounts for our perception of fat as harmful. Excesses indeed are linked to major health problems and premature death. Saturated fat and cholesterol are particular culprits in this regard, although research suggests that other types of fat actually help to prevent or minimize these problems.

Dietary fat provides you with a concentrated source of energy and thus helps conserve protein for growth, maintenance, and repair. As noted previously, a gram of fat contains 9 calories, as

TABLE 8.G Percent of calories from protein, fat, and carbohydrates for selected sources of protein.

FOODS	TOTAL CALORIES	% PROTEIN	% FAT	% CHO
Almonds, 1/4 cup whole, shelled	212	10	79	11
Prime rib with fat, 3 oz	375	19	80	—
Sirloin with fat, 3 oz	330	24	74	—
Sirloin, fat trimmed, 3 oz	175	63	35	—
Cheddar cheese, 1 oz	115	25	74	trace
Egg, hard-boiled	80	30	67	3
Whole milk, 1 cup	150	21	48	31
Skim milk, 1 cup	85	40	trace	59
Hotdog, 8 per lb	170	16	80	2
Tuna, oil-packed, 3 oz	170	57	40	trace
Tuna, water-packed, 3 oz	117	90	6	trace
Chicken breast, with skin, 2.8 oz	160	65	30	3
Turkey, white meat (2 slices, no skin)	150	78	20	—
Kidney beans, 1 cup	230	25	4	71
Whole-wheat bread, 1 slice	65	15	5	80
Peanut butter, 1 tbsp	95	17	70	13
Spaghetti, 1 cup	190	15	3	82
Broiled hamburger, 3 oz (lean, 21% fat)	245	33	65	—
Salmon, broiled or baked, 3 oz	140	60	32	—
Halibut, poached, 3 oz	111	73	26	—

Note: All percentages are approximate.

compared to 4 calories/gram for carbohydrate or protein. In essence, you obtain more than twice as much energy from the same size intake. Without some fat in your diet, you cannot absorb vitamins A, D, E, and K, because they are soluble only in fat. In addition, fat increases the texture, aroma, and flavor of foods, making them more inviting to eat. Fat is said to have a high *satiety value* because you feel more satisfied when you've eaten a food with some fat, compared to lettuce or celery, for example. Because fat is digested rather slowly, it remains in the stomach longer and you feel fuller longer.

As a part of the body itself, fat provides padding to protect vital organs from injury. Fat beneath the skin serves as insulation against cold temperatures, and oils on the skin and hair give them a healthy sheen as opposed to a dried-out appearance. Fat is a constituent of hormones such as testosterone and estrogen. Without sufficient body fat, women may stop menstruating and thus lose the reproductive function. And of course, body fat stands as a ready fuel reserve whenever too few calories are consumed. It's your reserve fuel tank.

Types of Fat

Of the fat you eat, 95% is called **triglyceride** to describe its chemical make-up. It consists of three ("tri") fatty acids attached to a glycerol molecule,

like branches to a tree trunk. Our digestive process breaks apart this structure into individual fatty acids that can be absorbed into the blood.

The three different types of fatty acids are: saturated, monounsaturated, and polyunsaturated. These terms basically describe the chemical structures of the fatty acids. As shown in Figure 8.2, **fatty acids** consist of chains of carbon atoms with hydrogen atoms attached to them. When all of the possible attachment sites on each carbon atom are occupied by hydrogen atoms, the **fatty acid** is called **saturated.** If all the attachment sites are not occupied, the **fatty acids** are called **unsaturated. Polyunsaturated fatty acids** (PUFA) are missing many hydrogen atoms (at least four), and **monounsaturated fatty acids** have two hydrogen atoms missing (it is chemically impossible for only one hydrogen atom to be missing). In form, saturated fats are solid at room temperature and unsaturated fats are liquid.

The importance of being aware of these different forms of fatty acids is related to their link to heart disease. Diets containing a lot of saturated fat increase the risk of cardiovascular disease, whereas diets emphasizing polyunsaturated fats seem to provide some protection against cardiovascular disease. Monounsaturated fats may be even more protective. Even though most foods actually contain mixtures of all three types of fatty acids, saturated fats predominate in animal products, and mono- and polyunsaturated fats in vegetables, grains, and

FIGURE 8.2   Chemical structure of fatty acids.

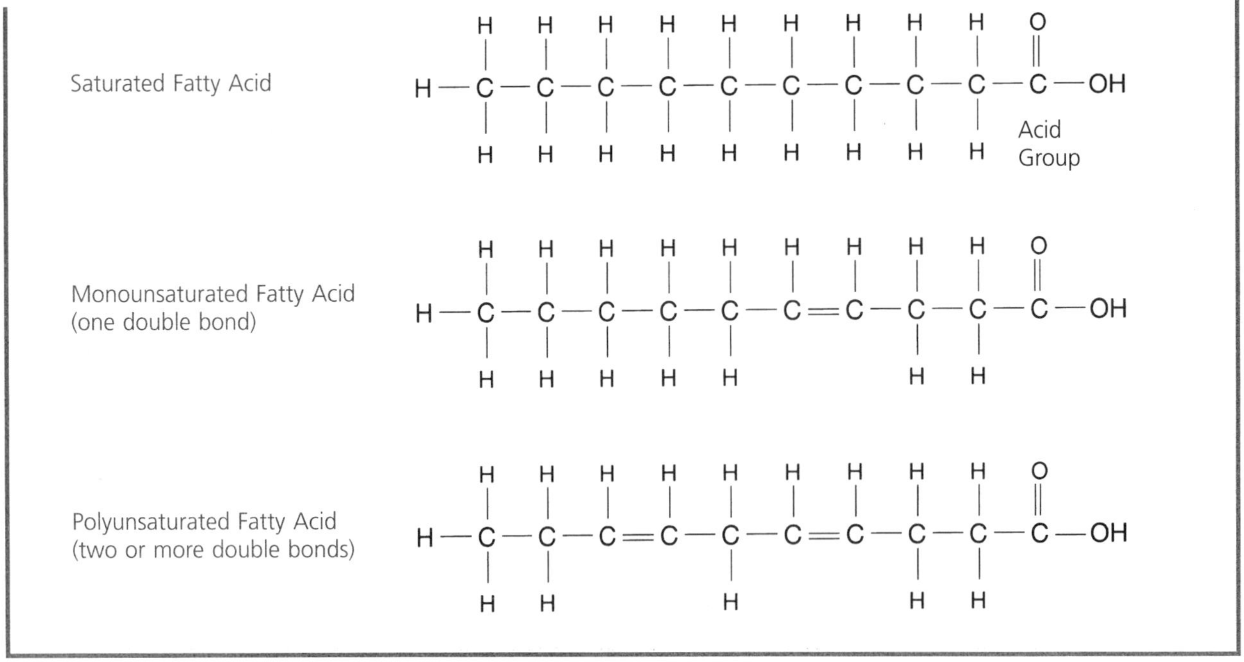

Saturated Fatty Acid

Monounsaturated Fatty Acid (one double bond)

Polyunsaturated Fatty Acid (two or more double bonds)

fruits such as the avocado. Most fruits have little or no fat at all.

Palm and coconut oils are natural exceptions to this general rule; they contain large amounts of saturated fats. An unnatural exception is hydrogenated or partially hydrogenated vegetable oil. If you use margarine instead of butter because it is a polyunsaturated fat, you may have been surprised to read that unsaturated fats are liquid at room temperature. Whether you buy margarine in cubes or in tubs, it is definitely not a liquid. The reason for this more solid, saturated appearance is that manufacturers have hydrogenated the vegetable oil to make it look and behave more like butter and to increase its shelf-life. (Polyunsaturated fats spoil more quickly than saturated fats, and hydrogenation retards this deterioration.) The reason **hydrogenation** makes vegetable oils appear and behave more like saturated fat is that it transforms polyunsaturated fat into saturated fat. Hydrogenation means "to add hydrogens." Thus, when the package label says the product contains hydrogenated vegetable oil, it really means saturated fat.

The term *partially hydrogenated* means that the vegetable oil is not fully saturated, but it certainly is much less polyunsaturated than a pure vegetable oil. It also contains a new type of fatty acid, a **trans-fatty acid** created during the partial hydrogenation process. Trans-fatty acids do not occur naturally in the body, and they may increase both total and LDL cholesterol and decrease HDL, as well as promote certain types of cancer. The evidence supporting these suspicions has been growing steadily, but many experts think it is not yet conclusive. Nonetheless, minimizing intake of trans-fatty acids seems like a wise choice at this point. Buying margarines or spreads that list water or liquid vegetable oil rather than partially hydrogenated oil as the first ingredient on the label is one way to minimize exposure to trans-fatty acids. Mixing soft butter with the same amount of safflower oil produces a spread with the same degree of polyunsaturation as margarine, but with no trans-fatty acids.

In addition to triglycerides, other types of fat in our food are *phospholipids* and *sterols.* You may have heard of a substance called *lecithin*, a natural emulsifier, that is supposed to dissolve the fat in your arteries. Lecithin is a phospholipid, and it does help to keep fats in solution in the blood; it also is an important cell membrane constituent. But the liver can make the lecithin the body needs; you don't need to eat it. The lecithin you do eat gets digested like other forms of fat before it can ever get into the bloodstream. For this reason, buying lecithin supplements to prevent atherosclerosis will benefit the health food store proprietor more than the consumer.

Cholesterol, the most recognized form of sterols, is best known for its prominence in the fatty deposits that accumulate on blood vessel walls. Cholesterol, however, is sufficiently necessary to body functioning that the liver makes about 1000 mg of it every day. The liver can make cholesterol from either saturated fatty acid or glucose. Thus, you do not have to eat any cholesterol at all. Nonetheless, average intake is between 320 and 450 mg/day, respectively, for women and men. The liver uses some of this cholesterol to make *bile*, which helps digest fats. Some cholesterol is used to make hormones. The rest is transported through the blood to cells, and some accumulates on blood vessel walls before reaching its destination. The cholesterol reaching the cells is used in many metabolic reactions and in parts of the cells' structure. The cholesterol that is not used is sent back to the liver.

As you will recall from Chapter 3, fats are transported through the blood by lipoproteins. The lipoproteins the liver makes to send to cells are called VLDLs (very low density lipoproteins) and LDLs (low density lipoproteins). Of these, LDLs are the prominent carriers of cholesterol. Thus, a high level of LDLs in the blood is considered a risk factor for developing fatty deposits on blood vessel walls. Diets high in saturated fats and cholesterol seem to promote high levels of LDLs. Some people, however, seem to have inherited a propensity toward high LDLs in the blood.

Cholesterol being transported from the cells back to the liver travels in the form of HDLs (high-density lipoproteins). People with high levels of HDLs in their blood seem less prone to developing fatty deposits on their blood vessels, and increasing HDLs in the blood may even result in some decrease in fatty deposits already formed. Regular vigorous exercise is the best way known to increase HDLs, although diets low in total fat but higher in unsaturated fats than saturated may help also. Women seem to have naturally higher levels of HDLs than men do.

Polyunsaturated fats from fish, especially a kind called omega-3, have been found to be particularly effective in reducing both cholesterol and triglyceride levels in the blood. Dr. William Castelli, director of the Framingham Heart Study in Framingham, Massachusetts, has flatly stated that eating fish two times a week could cut the incidence of heart disease in half. Even shellfish, once thought to be loaded with cholesterol, now are being recommended as "protective fare." Newer methods of measuring cholesterol in food have shown the cholesterol level of most shellfish to be lower than that of canned tuna or broiled chicken breast. Even shrimp and lobster, which have the highest cholesterol content of the shellfish, are only slightly higher in cholesterol than lean beef or lamb.

The cholesterol content of various types of fish is compared with chicken, pork, lamb, and beef in FYI 1. Cholesterol is found only in animal products. Of these, the very lowest sources are clams, fresh fish, oysters, and scallops. These also are very low-calorie sources of protein. By far the highest sources of cholesterol are eggs and organ meats such as liver and kidney.

The types of fish with the highest omega-3 oil content are listed in FYI 2. The fatter, higher-calorie fish (for example, salmon and tuna) are the best sources. The fat and calorie content in these fish is still low when compared to most meats, however.

The Body's Fat Requirements

As mentioned previously, Americans currently eat about 34% or more of their daily calories in fat compared to a recommended intake of 30% or less. It is also recommended that saturated fat intake be less than 10% of total calories, and Americans currently consume 12% or more of their calories in saturated fat.

The recommended intake of fat far exceeds actual need. The body needs only a small amount, 1%–2% of total calories, of the polyunsaturated fat called *linoleic acid*. Linoleic acid is called an essential fatty acid because the body cannot synthesize it; you must eat it. One to two tablespoons of vegetable oil, especially safflower, wheat germ, corn, or soybean oil, generally will supply the amount you need each day. The linoleic acid content of various oils is given in Table 8.H. Note the

How Much Cholesterol?

FOOD	PORTION	MG. OF CHOLESTEROL
Clams	3 oz	54
Fresh cod	3 oz	60
Oysters	3 oz	38
Scallops	6 oz	70
Canned tuna	3 oz	55
Crab	½ cup	67
Fresh pork	3 oz	76
Chicken, white meat, skinned	3 oz	76
Lean beef	3 oz	80
Lean veal	3 oz	86
Lean lamb	3 oz	83
Lobster	3 oz	70
Shrimp	3½ oz	147
Egg*	1 whole	274
Beef liver	3 oz	372
Chicken liver	1 each	126
Beef kidney	3 oz	425

*All of the cholesterol is in the egg yolk.

Seafood and Omega-3 Fatty Acids

SEAFOOD HIGH IN OMEGA-3 FATTY ACIDS

Anchovies
Sardines
Salmon
Albacore tuna (canned in water)
Mackerel
Sturgeon
Whitefish

SEAFOOD MODERATELY HIGH IN OMEGA-3 FATTY ACIDS

Bass	Haddock
Trout	Halibut
Catfish	Lobster
Cod	Perch
Crab	Oysters
Flounder	Pike
Shrimp	Scallops
Swordfish	Smelt

TABLE

8.H Linoleic acid content in various oils.

TYPE OF OIL	% LINOLEIC ACID
Safflower	74.5%
Sunflower	65.0%
Corn	58.7%
Soybean	58.0%
Cottonseed	51.9%
Sesame	41.7%
Peanut	32.0%
Canola	26.0%
Palm	9.3%
Olive	8.4%
Coconut	1.8%

very small amount of linoleic acid in palm, olive, and coconut oils compared to other types.

A small amount of the polyunsaturated omega-3 oil called *linoleic acid* is also though to be essential. An intake of 10%–25% of the recommendation for linoleic acid currently is suggested as adequate. Fish are the best sources of omega-3 fatty acids. FYI 2 lists fish species high and moderately high in omega-3s. Nevertheless, use of fish oil capsules is not recommended at this time by any major health or nutritional organization for several reasons:

1. Overconsuming omega-3 oil actually could create a deficiency of linoleic acid or vitamin E, or both.

2. Fish oil capsules could supply 200 or more calories per day in fat if taken as suggested.

3. Consumed in large enough amounts, omega-3 oil can increase susceptibility to stroke.

Eating a serving or two of fish a week to get the omega-3 you need seems a much safer practice.

The large difference between the recommended and needed amounts of fat reflects an attempt by scientists and nutritionists to be practical as well as safe. The Pritikin diet, in which fat accounts for only 10% of total calories, was proposed years ago as a powerful combatant against atherosclerosis. More recently, the Ornish Program, a 10% fat diet in combination with exercise, stress management, and elimination of caffeine and nicotine, reportedly has reversed arterial clogging in heart patients after just one year.

The Chinese, who have far fewer problems with heart disease and cancer than we do, traditionally have consumed a diet containing 10%–15% fat. Nonetheless, a diet this low in fat is not palatable for most Americans. We have grown accustomed to much higher amounts of fat in our

diet and the level of satiety that accompanies that. Therefore, even though current research suggests that consuming much less than 30% of daily calories in fat would be healthier, it doesn't seem likely that many Americans would follow that recommendation at this time. Decreasing the current 34+% intake of fat to 30%, however, is considered a strong step in the right direction.

The recommended intake of fat likely will be reduced even more in the future because of the connection between high-fat diets, heart disease, and cancer. As already noted, minimizing saturated fats in the diet seems particularly important to avoid or minimize atherosclerosis. Reducing cholesterol intake to 300 mg or less per day also is recommended. The primary intent of these measures is to lower blood levels of cholesterol, especially in the form of LDLs.

Using a tool called the **CSI**, the **Cholesterol–Saturated Fat Index,** you can estimate the combined influence of the cholesterol and saturated fat in any given food on blood cholesterol levels. This procedure is given in FYI 3.

Diets high in fat, either saturated or polyunsaturated, also seem to increase the risk of cancers of the colon, breast, prostate, and endometrium. The high fat content somehow may encourage development of carcinogens in the intestinal tract. High-fat diets generally are low in fiber, a nondigestible substance that helps move food through the intestines. This could result in a longer than usual passage time through the intestines and more opportunity for carcinogens to build up. Whatever the mechanism(s), eating a low-fat diet seems advisable in trying to avoid these types of cancer.

Choosing a low-fat, low-cholesterol diet means emphasizing consumption of vegetables, grains, and fruits. These have no cholesterol and are generally low in fat. Avocado, nuts, and seeds are the exceptions. These foods are high in fat content and should be eaten infrequently and in small amounts if a low-fat diet is your goal. Sources of animal products that are lower in fat, saturated fat, and cholesterol include fish, skim milk, and other low-percent fat dairy products. Limiting intake of meats such as beef, pork, and lamb, as well as butter and eggs, certainly will help your cause.

The long-term controversy about eating eggs warrants some additional attention. The cholesterol in an egg is very high, almost 260 mg. This is almost all of the 300 mg to which you are advised to limit yourself each day. Thus far, however, research has not been able to demonstrate firmly that eating eggs, even every day, raises blood cholesterol levels. Some studies support the contention that eggs increase blood cholesterol; others do not. Because eggs are such an excellent and economical

FYI

Calculating the Cholesterol–Saturated Fat Index

A new way to estimate the cholesterol-raising effect of food is to calculate the Cholesterol–Saturated Fat Index (CSI). Because this formula considers both of the dietary fats known to increase blood cholesterol, it offers a more precise evaluation of your diet as a risk for cardiovascular disease.

To compute the CSI, simply multiply the grams of saturated fat in food by 1.01 and the milligrams of cholesterol by .05 and add the two products together. The larger the result, the riskier the food!

For example:

A. 3-oz regular hamburger has 6.9 g saturated fat, 76 mg cholesterol

CSI = 6.9 g (1.01) + 76 mg (.05) = **10.77**

B. 3-oz water-packed tuna has 0.3 g saturated fat, 48 mg cholesterol

CSI = .3 g (1.01) + 48 mg (.05) = **2.7**

The CSI for the average American's daily diet ranges from 51–60 for women and children and 69–82 for men and teenagers. A healthier diet for your heart would yield a CSI of 16–19 for most women and children and 23–26 for men and teenagers.

---

source of protein, it seems premature to ban them from our diets. Until the evidence for or against eggs is clear, the best advice might be to limit consumption to four eggs per week.

CARBOHYDRATE

With overweight being of such concern in the United States today, why are nutritionists urging you to eat more carbohydrate foods such as potatoes, bread, and pasta? What exactly are carbohydrates, and why are you being encouraged to eat them?

Types of Carbohydrate

Carbohydrates are molecules of sugar linked together in complexes or in pairs or existing singly. Carbon, hydrogen, and oxygen are the elements that compose these molecules; hence the name carbohydrate. Single sugars and those in pairs are called *simple sugars*. Glucose, fructose, and galactose are the three forms of single-sugar molecules, also called *monosaccharides*. Glucose and fructose are found alone or in combination in all fruits, vegetables, grains, and milk; galactose is found only in milk. Paired combinations of these sugars are

called *disaccharides*. The three forms of disaccharides are *sucrose*, a combination of glucose and fructose; *maltose*, a combination of two glucose molecules; and *lactose*, a combination of glucose and galactose. Sucrose is common table sugar and its cousins, powdered sugar and brown sugar. Lactose is milk sugar; milk is the only nonplant source of carbohydrates. Maltose is the sugar that seeds contain to fuel germination. Plants generally use it all themselves while growing, but we can get some maltose from the malt in beer.

Complex carbohydrates or *polysaccharides* is the name used for combinations of dozens of glucose molecules. Starch and undigested fibers are complex carbohydrates. Of these, only starch provides nutrients; in fact, starch is the most abundant energy source in grain—such as wheat, rice, corn, rye, millet, barley, and oats—which is the basic food staple around the world. Beans and peas, especially dried beans, also are important sources of starch, as are tubers such as potatoes and yams. When carbohydrates are eaten, the body digests them into the basic units glucose, fructose, and galactose. The liver then converts fructose and galactose into glucose, the body's basic fuel source. Consequently, glucose is also called *blood sugar*.

Cellulose, hemicellulose, gums, and pectin are the types of complex carbohydrates that provide no nutrients for humans because we don't have the enzymes to digest them. Thus, fiber can't be called an essential nutrient, but few who understand its role in preventing constipation would say it's not important. As you will read later, fiber seems to be important in reducing the risk of several diseases including CVD and cancer. Whole grains, vegetables, and fruits all are sources of fiber.

The Body's Need for Carbohydrates

You are being advised to eat more carbohydrate for several important reasons. First, consumption of carbohydrate is *not* associated with increased risk of cardiovascular disease and cancer. In fact, the incidence of these diseases is lower among people whose diets are high in carbohydrates. The fiber and certain vitamins and minerals in carbohydrate foods may even help to prevent these health problems. As the only source of fiber in our diets, carbohydrates are especially important.

Eating foods high in carbohydrates helps with weight control, too. As noted previously, carbohydrates provide as many calories as protein, 4 per gram, but foods high in carbohydrate are much lower in fat than many sources of protein. Also, because the fiber in carbohydrate foods adds bulk but no calories to the food, you will tend to eat less *and* will get fewer calories. For example, a dish of gourmet ice cream is high in fat and might have 360 calories. You would have to eat three or four apples or bananas or almost five slices of bread, both primary sources of carbohydrate, to equal those calories. Although you might gladly eat a bowl of ice cream after dinner, you probably wouldn't consider eating that much fruit or bread. Therefore, choosing an apple or a banana will save more than 200 calories while providing about the same amount of food. An added bonus will be decreased intake of fat.

Most foods high in carbohydrates also contain large amounts of vitamins and minerals, especially if the foods are eaten raw or in their natural state. But sucrose or table sugar (and its various forms, brown sugar, powdered sugar, and raw sugar) is an excellent example of an "empty" carbohydrate. When the fructose and glucose of which it is composed were extracted from the sugar beets or sugar cane, none of the vitamins and minerals in those vegetables came with it. A teaspoon of table sugar is 5 grams of carbohydrate or about 20 calories, and that's it. You get nothing else from it.

This also applies to any other type of processed sweetener such as corn syrup, honey, maple syrup, and fructose. Molasses, the exception, does contain useful amounts of calcium, iron, potassium, and B vitamins. Honey has minute quantities of these nutrients, but nothing significant. (If you need extra calories in your diet because of a rigorous activity level, however, refined sugars and syrups certainly can provide them.) Refined or granulated fructose has no more nutritional value than table sugar. It is sweeter, however, and *if* you use less of it, you will save a few calories. On the other hand, if you consume fructose by eating fruit, a good natural source of both fructose and sucrose, you will be taking in substantial vitamins and minerals plus additional carbohydrate in the form of fiber.

Refined white flour is another example of a calorie resource deprived of nutrients in the manufacturing process. In this case, the calories provided aren't totally empty, but they certainly don't offer the nutritional quality of the original grain.

Even when white flour has been "enriched" by adding vitamins and minerals, it doesn't have nearly the nutrients contained in whole-wheat flour, especially stone-ground whole wheat. *Stone-ground* refers to the milling process that does the least damage to the nutrient content of the grain. In essence, then, when you eat foods that have lots of refined sugar and/or flour, you are taking in a lot of empty calories.

You can see, then, that pies, cakes, cookies, and doughnuts contain many empty calories. You should also recognize that many canned vegetables, fruits, and other products—even peanut butters—have added sugar, and that many cereals on the market are loaded with it. The refined sugar contents of numerous cereals and other foods are listed in FYI 4, with additional information provided in Appendix 7.

From the body's standpoint, carbohydrate provides the ideal fuel. You will recall that the body also can use fat and protein for fuel, but this is not the desired use for protein. Eating sufficient amounts of carbohydrate for fuel helps save protein for use in growth and maintenance of body tissue. Like fat, it is a protein-sparer.

Without a sufficient amount of carbohydrate in the diet, the body cannot utilize fat properly. When carbohydrate intake is inadequate, a toxic byproduct of fat metabolism, called *ketones*, increases in the blood. The kidney's job is to get rid of this substance, but if this process goes on too long and the quantities of ketones become too great, the blood becomes "poisoned" with this substance. This condition, called *ketosis*, is accompanied by feelings of fatigue, apathy, and nausea, plus loss of weight in the form of protein and water. At its extreme, ketosis can result in coma, brain and kidney damage, and even death.

If you have diabetes or know someone who does, you may recognize the process just described as the physiological problem diabetics face. Their problem is severe because no matter how much carbohydrate they eat, their body doesn't metabolize it properly. A nondiabetic person who consumes a low-carbohydrate diet (one popular approach to weight reduction) for any length of time faces the same physiological problems as the diabetic, although the situation is certainly easier to remedy. This also is the process that occurs during starvation. In effect, a low-carbohydrate diet sets up a "starvation syndrome" that has potentially dangerous consequences.

What is the least amount of carbohydrate you can eat before becoming a victim of the low-carbohydrate starvation syndrome just described? How much carbohydrate do you have to eat to get the protection from cardiovascular disease and

How Much Refined Sugar?

FOOD	PORTION	TEASPOONS OF SUGAR	CEREALS	TEASPOONS OF SIMPLE SUGAR PER SERVING
Peanut butter	1 tbsp	1	General Mills Fiber One	0.
Strawberry jam	1 tbsp	4	Nabisco Shredded Wheat	0.
Honey	1 tbsp	3*	General Mills Cheerios	.2
Applesauce, sweetened	½ cup	2	Kellogg's Corn Flakes	.4
Orange juice	½ cup	2	Ralston Wheat Chex	.6
Grape juice	½ cup	3⅖	Kellogg's Special K	.6
Canned peaches	2 halves, 1 tbsp syrup	3½	Kellogg's Rice Krispies	.6
Hot dog or hamburger bun	1	3	General Mills Kix	.6
Doughnut	1	3	General Mills Wheaties	.8
Doughnut, glazed	1	6	General Mills Total (multi-grain)	1.
Brownie, unfrosted	1	3	Kellogg's Healthy Choice	1.2
Fig newton	1	5	Nabisco 100% Bran	1.2
Oatmeal cookie	1	2	Quaker Life	1.2
Ice cream, regular	3½ oz	3½	Post Grape-Nuts	1.4
Chocolate milk	1 cup	6	Quaker Oat Bran	2.0
Sherbet	½ cup	9	Quaker Cap'n Crunch	2.4
Yogurt, sweetened fruit	1 cup	9	General Mills Lucky Charms	2.6
Custard pie	1 slice	10	Kellogg's Corn Pops	2.6
Pumpkin pie	1 slice	5	General Mills Trix	2.6
Apple pie	1 slice	7	Kellogg's Frosted Flakes	2.6
Hershey bar	1½ oz	2½	Kellogg's Fruit Loops	2.8
Fudge	1 oz	4½	Kellogg's Apple Jacks	2.8
Hard candy	4 oz	20	General Mills Cocoa Puffs	2.8
7-Up	12 oz	9	Quaker Cinnamon Life	2.84
Cola drinks	12 oz	9	Kellogg's Nutri-Grain	3.2
Orange soda	12 oz	11½	Kellogg's Granola	3.2
Root beer	10 oz	4½	Kellogg's Raisin Bran	3.4

*Actual sugar content, none added.

Survey of Cereals, November 1994.

cancer that a high-carbohydrate diet seems to offer? Does it matter what kind of foods you eat to get your carbohydrate? These are critical questions, and although not all of the answers are completely clear, sufficient information exists to provide the following guidelines.

Populations around the world who are less plagued by cardiovascular disease than Americans generally consume 60%–80% of their daily calories in carbohydrates.* The incidence of various forms of cancer also is lower among people with high carbohydrate intakes. Consequently, nutrition experts are recommending that Americans try to eat at least 55%–60% of their daily calories in carbohydrates.

For a male weighing 154 lbs (70 kg) who eats about 2700 calories/day, a 60% carbohydrate diet would mean consuming at least 400 g of carbohydrate, or 1600 calories. A woman who weighs 120 lbs (55 kg) and eats 2000 calories/day would have to eat at least 300 g or 1200 calories of carbohydrate. Currently, the average American eats only 46% of daily calories in carbohydrate, about 230 g for women and 310 g for men. As you will recall,

*The exception is the Eskimos, whose diet is extremely high in fat and low in carbohydrates. The fat they eat, however, comes almost entirely from fish and contains very high amounts of the polyunsaturated fatty acid omega-3, which seems to offer some protection against cardiovascular disease.

the average American also eats about 12% more fat calories than is recommended. In essence, Americans are shorting the "nutrient account" that seems to provide some protection from cardiovascular disease and cancer to invest more in the one most highly associated with both diseases—fat!

Replacing fats in your diet is not the only way carbohydrates seem to reduce risk from cardiovascular disease and cancer. Eating certain types of fiber can decrease blood cholesterol and triglyceride levels. *Pectin*, found in most fruits and many vegetables, and *gums*, found in beans and oats, are especially effective in this regard. Oat bran and rice bran are two popular sources of these soluble fibers. But the amount of oat bran/rice bran in any one muffin or bowl of cereal, by itself, would be unlikely to influence your blood cholesterol level. Wheat bran, the food most of us think of when we think of fiber, does not affect blood fat levels, as it is insoluble and is not absorbed from the intestinal tract. The cellulose and hemicellulose fibers contained in bran, cereals, whole grains, and vegetables exert their influence by keeping waste moving smoothly and quickly through the intestines. This is thought to decrease the risk of colorectal cancer. Fiber also tends to slow absorption of food from the gut, which is helpful to diabetics, who can handle small amounts of sugar over time much better than large quantities all at once. This slow absorption factor can be helpful in controlling weight, too, because fiber tends to make you feel full longer and on fewer calories.

The American Cancer Society is recommending that Americans increase their intake of fiber from a current level of 10–20 g to 25–30 g/day. Some experts think 40 or more g/day would be best. (Some vegetarians eat up to 60 g of fiber/day.) Fiber, however, can decrease absorption of some important minerals such as calcium, iron, and zinc. It also can cause gas, bloating, and diarrhea in some people. If you think it wise to increase your fiber intake given the previous information, increasing your intake gradually will help minimize gas and bloating, and not going overboard in your end goal will help curtail excessive mineral loss. Food sources for, and functions of, the various types of fiber are listed in Table 8.1.

Besides providing fiber, carbohydrates are excellent sources of vitamins A and C, which current evidence suggests may provide some protection against cancers of the larynx, esophagus, lung, and stomach. This evidence is sufficiently strong that the American Cancer Society is urging greater consumption of dark yellow and green vegetables and deep yellow-orange fruit. These colors are guides to good sources of carotenes and vitamin C in fruits and vegetables. (Carotenes are the plant precursors that the body uses to make vitamin A.)

TABLE 8.1 Types of fiber and where they are found.

	INSOLUBLE FIBER		SOLUBLE FIBER	
	CELLULOSE	HEMICELLULOSES	GUMS	PECTIN
Food Sources	Whole-wheat flour Bran Cabbage Young peas Green beans Wax beans Broccoli Brussels sprouts Cucumber skins Peppers Apples Carrots	Bran Cereals Whole grains Brussels sprouts Mustard greens Beet root	Oatmeal and other rolled oat products Dried beans Seaweed	Squash Apples Citrus fruits Cauliflower Green beans Cabbage Dried peas Carrots Strawberries Potatoes
What It Does	Mechanically smooths function of large bowel: Absorbs water, increasing stool and decreasing transit time. Helps constipation, and protects against diverticulosis, colon cancer, hemorrhoids, and varicose veins.		Influences absorption in stomach and small bowel: Binds with bile acids, thereby decreasing fat absorption and lowering cholesterol levels. Coats gut and delays glucose absorption, smoothing sugar surges for diabetics.	

Adapted from "Beyond Bran" by S. Lang, *American Health* 3:3 (May 1984): 64; and *Nutrition* by L. Smolin and M. Grosvenor (Philadelphia: Saunders, 1994).

Cruciferous vegetables such as broccoli, kale, brussels sprouts (all dark green, too), cauliflower, and cabbage are also being recommended not only because they provide carotenes and/or vitamin C, but also because they contain compounds called indoles and isothiocyanates, which seem to reduce the risk for stomach, colorectal, respiratory, and breast cancers. There is increasing evidence that vitamin E and the mineral selenium may also help to minimize the development of some cancers. At this time the American Cancer Society does not consider the evidence sufficient to recommend specific supplementation of the diet with special vitamins, minerals, or phytochemicals (nonvitamin and mineral substances such as the indoles, iso-thyocyanates, and flavonoids that are found in plants).

Preformed vitamin A is found in animal foods such as milk, cheese, butter, eggs, and meat. A serving of liver can provide six times the amount of vitamin A recommended for one day. The problem is the fat in these sources and, in particular, the cholesterol in liver. Because the strongest association of all between diet and cancer is a high-fat diet, the best sources of vitamins A and C would seem to be carbohydrates.

The recommendation to increase carbohydrate intake from 46% to 55% or more of daily calories also stipulates eating no more than 9%–10% of calories in refined sugars. In essence, we should eat at least 40% of calories in complex carbohydrates and about 6% in natural sugars from fruits, vegetables, and grains. Currently, Americans eat 18% of their calories in refined sugar and 6% in natural sugars, leaving 22% for complex carbohydrates.

Nutritionists are emphasizing complex carbohydrates because they are the source of fiber in the diet; refined sugars have none. Complex carbohydrates also contain many vitamins and minerals; refined sugars have none or insignificant amounts. As discussed previously, refined sugar offers only empty calories.

Although the average American consumes a little more than one-third pound of sweeteners every day, or about 134 lbs per year, such a high-refined sugar intake has not been linked to the development of any major disease or health problem. In a major study of diet and heart disease conducted in 37 countries under the sponsorship of the World Health Association, no link with refined sugars was found; fat, especially saturated fat, was the culprit. Sugar intake has not been tied to cancer either, but high-fat diets surely have.

Another misconception is that sugar causes diabetes. This is unproven. Diabetics cannot metabolize sugar properly and struggle against the physiological consequences, but what *causes* this problem remains unknown. Overweight, however, is an important risk factor for diabetes, and it often reflects a high-calorie, high-fat diet. We do know that diabetics must be careful about eating any carbohydrate food that produces a large increase in blood sugar or glucose. Although we used to think that only refined sugars did this, the situation clearly is not that simple. For example, complex carbohydrates such as potatoes and carrots seem to increase blood sugar more than rice, fructose,* and dried beans. On the other hand, ice cream does not seem to increase blood sugar adversely in some diabetics. In sum, even for diabetics, sugar does not seem as bad as was once thought.

Eating refined sugar is not problem-free, though. Carbohydrates containing sucrose are major culprits in tooth decay, especially sources of these that have a sticky texture. Most dentists advise limiting refined sugar intake. A diet high in sugar also may cause episodes of reactive *hypoglycemia*, which means having too little sugar in the blood. This occurs when a sudden and large increase in blood sugar (which follows ingestion of high-sugar foods) triggers release of more insulin than necessary. The excessive insulin drives too much glucose from the blood into the cells, resulting in a blood sugar level too low for proper brain and nerve function. If this happens to you, you will likely feel weak, dizzy, and anxious, and may experience lack of neuromotor coordination. A small percentage of people are hypoglycemic because of chronic overproduction of insulin, but most who experience this situation probably have overdone the sweets or waited too long between meals.

Three last issues involving sugar intake warrant comment.

1. The connection between *hyperactivity* in children and high sugar intake remains unsubstantiated. The biggest reason for minimizing refined sugar in your child's diet, and yours, for that matter, is to avoid empty calories and exposure to high-fat and high-calorie foods.

2. A connection may exist between consumption of lactose—the simple sugar natural to milk—and abdominal gas, pain, and diarrhea. Some adults, especially African American and Asian people, lack the enzyme to digest this sugar. Fortunately, this problem can be minimized by eating only small

Caution: Fructose is converted by the liver into glucose, which then must be metabolized, and the metabolism of glucose *is* the essential problem for diabetics. Studies indicate that indiscriminate use of fructose by diabetics could lead to a diabetic crisis.

amounts of dairy products at one time and eating products containing yeast or added enzymes capable of rendering lactose digestible. Examples of these foods are yogurt and lactase-treated milk.

3. To avoid calories, many Americans consume food with artificial sweeteners. Aspartame (marketed under the brand name *Nutrasweet*) and saccharin are the predominant ones currently in use. Saccharin has been around for a long time, more than 40 years, and still is used despite some legitimate concern that large intakes might lead to bladder cancer. Nevertheless, its popularity has waned significantly. Aspartame, a combination of two naturally occurring amino acids, phenylalanine and aspartic acid, now is the most popular artificial sweetener. So far no evidence suggests that it is harmful in any way except for people with phenylketonuria, a disorder characterized by inability to metabolize phenylalanine. Reports of headaches resulting from aspartame use have not been substantiated in controlled studies.

If calories are a problem, aspartame can be of some help. Although it contains the same number of calories as sugar, it is 180 times sweeter. One teaspoon of sugar has about 18 calories; the same sweetening power can be obtained from one-tenth of a calorie of aspartame. Because aspartame loses some of its sweetening power when heated or baked, its use is somewhat restricted, however. It currently is used primarily in cereals, soft drinks, puddings, gums, mints, and as crystals for table use. The best advice seems to be to use it if you want or think you need to, but do not overdo it. A 154-pound person would have to consume 100 packets of Equal (35 mg aspartame/packet), or 19½ diet sodas (180 mg aspartame/soda) a day to reach the limit of 50 mg/kg/day stipulated by the Food and Drug Administration (FDA) as safe.

With refined sugars you fill up on empty calories. With aspartame you fill up on fewer empty calories. Either way, you may miss out on important nutrients. Also, if the future brings other than good news about aspartame's impact on our health, moderate or minimal intake might be considered more than just a good choice.

Carbohydrates and Dieting

Because artificial sweeteners are used so frequently to allow consumers pleasure from sugary foods without weight gain, and because so many starchy foods such as potatoes and bread are viewed erroneously as fattening, some comment is needed about carbohydrates and dieting. The facts are these: You will gain weight if you eat more calories than you need from carbohydrate foods. It doesn't matter whether you eat potatoes, rice, pasta, and pancakes or apples, oranges, tomatoes, and broccoli. The same can be said for protein foods of any kind and for all foods high in fat. In essence, too many calories from any type of food can end up as extra pounds.

Carbohydrates have received a bad name largely because of the fat we consume in conjunction with them. For example, the gravy or sour cream plus bacon bits and cheese often added to potatoes may contain twice or more the calories of the potato itself. The same can be said for the butter on bread or pancakes. Nevertheless, many people equate carbohydrates with weight gain and think low-carbohydrate diets will lead to weight loss. Because fat has so many more calories than carbohydrate or protein, cutting back on fats rather than carbohydrates is the way to lose weight. In addition, excess calories from fat are stored more easily as fat than are excess calories from carbohydrates. It also would be safer and more effective because insufficient carbohydrate intake causes the body to fall into the starvation syndrome described earlier. Weight certainly can be lost by cutting out carbohydrates, but much of it will be in the form of protein and water rather than fat, which is hardly what the dieter desires.

To prevent the body from behaving as if it is starving, you must eat carbohydrates, a minimum of 60 g/day. To allow for individual differences, it is recommended that you eat no less than 100 to 125 g of carbohydrate per day to ensure proper metabolic functioning. And, as discussed, Americans actually are being encouraged to eat three to four times that much to decrease the risk of chronic disease. As it turns out, carbohydrates are essential for everyone, even dieters.

VITAMINS AND MINERALS

The essential nutrients called vitamins and minerals are substances the body needs to grow and to function properly, but they provide no calories for energy. Most vitamins and minerals have been identified when their absence in the body has resulted in a function abnormality referred to as *deficiency syndrome* or disease.

The amounts needed to prevent deficiency problems are extremely small. The units of measurement are milligrams (mg) or micrograms (mcg). A milligram is 1/1000th of a gram; a microgram is 1/1000th of a milligram. The recommended daily intake for vitamin B_{12}, for example, is 2 mcg. At 28 g/oz, an ounce of vitamin B_{12} would be enough for 14,000,000 people!

Even with the technological advancements over the years, we do not know how much of some of these substances people actually need, what they do in the body, or even if all of these substances have been identified yet. The gaps in knowledge generate much conjecture and controversy. Most nutrition and health authorities believe that if you eat a well-balanced diet containing a variety of foods, you will get all of the substances you need. This belief is based largely upon the rarity of deficiency diseases in the United States today. Others believe that the vitamin and mineral amounts needed to prevent deficiency aren't necessarily the same as the amounts needed for optimal health and well-being, or for preventing or minimizing susceptibility to diseases of all sorts, or for retarding the aging process. Consequently, you may feel bombarded with contradictory advice regarding vitamin and mineral supplements.

Some of this advice about vitamins and minerals is based on legitimate, but as yet inconclusive, research. Some is based on nothing more than personal experience. Undoubtedly you've heard testimonials such as, "I take this or that and it works for me." Unfortunately these personal observations fall far short of scientific evidence. Conjecture also is stimulated simply by the desire to make money by selling dietary supplements. Caught in the middle of all this are millions of people who do not want to spend money needlessly but who do want to protect themselves from illness and aging as much as possible. Until scientists can provide the answers to these controversies, the decision about what to take is yours to make. The following information about the vitamins and minerals for which need has been established should help you with these decisions. First, however, we offer some general guidelines for checking the validity of claims about vitamins and minerals and summarize them in FYI 5.

1. *Learn about vitamins/minerals, what they can and cannot do, and how much we seem to need.* Basic information is provided in this text. Additional reliable sources of information include the U. S. Department of Agriculture (USDA), the Food and Drug Administration (FDA), the U. S. Surgeon General, the American Dietetic Association (ADA), and the American Medical Association (AMA). Look in your phone book for the local numbers of these national organizations or government units. In addition, you can get free information and consultation from the nutritionists (registered dietitians) or nutrition education units at your local public health department, American Heart Association unit, and hospital. To find a registered dietitian in your locale, you can call the American Dietetic Association's Consumer Nutrition Hotline at 1-800-366-1655 weekdays from 10 A.M. to 5 P.M. EST. You can also read about vitamins and minerals in general nutrition textbooks obtainable at your local public or university library.

2. *Challenge the validity of claims about vitamins and minerals.* Does evidence exist for the claim, beyond personal observations and experiences? If so, did researchers compare the effectiveness of the

Guidelines for Determining the Validity of Claims for Vitamins and Minerals

1. *Learn about vitamins and minerals.*
   Reliable sources include:
   U. S. Department of Agriculture (USDA)
   Food and Drug Administration (FDA)
   American Dietetic Association (ADA)*
   American Medical Association (AMA)
   Certified physicians, nutritionists, and dieticians at your public health department, hospital, Heart Association, and university
2. *Challenge health claims for scientific evidence.*
   a. Any evidence beyond personal anecdotes?
   b. Effects of the vitamin/mineral compared with other treatments?
   c. Use of the vitamin or mineral as claimed safe? If risk, how great?
3. Investigate health experts and organizations making claims.
   a. What degrees do they hold?
   b. What experience do they have?
   c. Who funds them?
4. *Find out if you are deficient or at risk.*
   Dietary analysis by trained personnel
   Blood/urine tests
   Physical exam

*ADA Consumer Nutrition Hotline 1–800–366–1655

vitamin/mineral with a control treatment or substance (for example, a pill or placebo)? Is the dosage claimed to be effective actually safe? If risk exists, how high is it compared to the potential benefit? If no answers to these questions are forthcoming or if the answers are *no*, suspicion and caution are in order.

3. *Investigate the "health expert."* In the United States you are free to say just about anything about everything. You do not have to have a degree in nutrition to give advice about it. The initials Ph.D. after someone's name simply means the person has a doctorate or graduate degree in some field; it could be any area of study. One popular writer of diet books has a Ph.D. in radio communications! Find out what degrees or training an advocate for a certain supplement has before "buying" his or her claim. Institutes, foundations, and other organizations you haven't heard of should be checked out, too. The Institute for Vitamin Experimentation and Cancer Prevention (to the authors' knowledge, a fabrication) could be funded by the vitamin industry and may not even perform actual research.

4. *Find out if you are deficient or at risk of low-level intake of the vitamin or mineral.* Blood and urine tests are reasonably reliable indicators. Diet analyses can be helpful, too, if done carefully and analyzed by trained persons. These tests should be accompanied by a general physical exam. Self-analysis should be done only for a rough estimate of your dietary intake. The same goes for computerized analysis. In fact, a computerized analysis can be programmed purposefully for higher than recommended vitamin/mineral needs and may indicate deficiencies that do not actually exist. You should inquire about the source(s) of the standard the computer uses to rate your diet. The most accepted standard today is the Recommended Dietary Allowances (RDAs). Other techniques, such as hair analysis, simply aren't valid for predicting vitamin/mineral adequacy.

Vitamins

Vitamins are organic substances (derived from plant and animal life) that perform a myriad of functions in the body. Acting primarily as co-enzymes (assistants to enzymes), they help in processing other nutrients and in forming various substances and structures needed for proper functioning, such as hormones, blood cells, bone, membranes, and so on.

Currently 13 organic substances are known to be required by the body and must be consumed. These are the fat-soluble vitamins A, D, E, and K, and the water-soluble B and C vitamins. The B vitamins include thiamin (B_1), riboflavin (B_2), niacin

(B_3), pantothenic acid, pyridoxine (B_6), cobalamin (B_{12}), folic acid (folacin), and biotin. Some people proclaim other substances, such as choline, inositol, and PABA (para-amino-benzoic acid), as vitamins, but to date no deficiency syndrome has been related to these, and no dietary needs have been established.

The fat-soluble vitamins are carried into the body with the aid of fat in the diet and are stored in fat in the body. Because they can be stored, they do not have to be eaten each day unless you are eating only small amounts compared to the daily recommended intake. For example, you can get enough vitamin A in a week by eating one cooked carrot every other day. Because they can be stored, however, fat soluble vitamins can accumulate to toxic levels in the body if they are consumed in excess.

Water-soluble vitamins are not stored in the body to any great extent, although small resources are maintained. In general, these vitamins should be eaten daily to maintain adequate fluid concentrations, because they are being metabolized constantly and lost in urine and sweat. Consuming quantities of these vitamins in excess of body needs just results in vitamin-rich urine. Research, however, has indicated that megadoses—10 times or more the amount the body needs—can produce some undesirable and even harmful side-effects in some people.

The 13 fat- and water-soluble vitamins are listed in Table 8.J, along with their respective recommended daily intakes, main food sources, and basic functions in the body. Space doesn't permit a discussion of all of these, but some additional information is provided about vitamins A, C, and E because of their controversial association with cancer, heart disease, colds, aging, and so on.

Vitamin A

As previously stated, the American Cancer Society has suggested eating more foods containing vitamin A because diets high in this vitamin are associated with lower levels of cancer of the lung, larynx, and bladder. Specifically, you are urged to eat more dark green and yellow-orange vegetables because these provide the best sources of *retinoids*, in particular beta-carotene, which are precursors of vitamin A (substances converted to vitamin A in the body). The presence of these precursors in food, and not preformed vitamin A itself, has been associated with lower levels of cancer. Almost all *preformed* vitamin A is found in animal products (or in vitamin capsules).

At this point in time, there is no indication that people gain any benefit from consuming large

TABLE
8.1   Vitamins: A fact sheet.

VITAMIN	ADULT RDA*	SOURCES	WHAT IT DOES
A	800 RE (8,000 IU), women; 1,000 RE (10,000 IU), men *1 cup milk = 140 RE*	Milk, eggs, liver, cheese, fish oil. Plus fruits and vegetables that contain beta carotene. (You need not consume pre-formed vitamin A if you eat foods rich in beta carotene.)	Promotes good vision; helps form and maintain skin, teeth, bones, and mucous membranes. Deficiency can increase susceptibility to infectious disease.
Beta carotene (not a vitamin, but converted to vitamin A in the body)	No RDA; experts recommend 5-6 mg (milligrams) *1 medium carrot = 12 mg* *1 sweet potato = 15 mg*	Carrots, sweet potatoes, cantaloupe, leafy greens, tomatoes, apricots, winter squash, red bell peppers, pink grapefruit, broccoli, mangos, peaches.	Converted into vitamin A in the intestinal wall. As an antioxidant, it combats the adverse effects of free radicals in the body. Best known of a family of substances called carotenoids.
C (ascorbic acid)	60 mg *1 orange - 70 mg* *1 cup fresh O.J. - 120 mg* *1 cup broccoli = 115 mg*	Citrus fruits and juices, strawberries, tomatoes, peppers (especially red), broccoli, potatoes, kale, cauliflower, cantaloupe, Brussel spouts.	Helps promote healthy gums and teeth; aids in iron absorption; maintains normal connective tissue; helps in healing of wounds. As an antioxidant, it combats the adverse effects of free radicals.
D	5 mcg (micrograms), or 200 IU; 10 mcg, or 400 IU, before age 25 *1 cup milk = 100 IU*	Milk, fish oil, fortified margarine; also produced by the body in response to sunlight.	Promotes strong bones and teeth by aiding the absorption of calcium. Helps maintain blood levels of calcium and phosphorus.
E	8 mg, women; 10 mg, men (12-15 IU) *1 Tbsp canola oil = 9 mg* *1 Tbsp margarine = 2 mg* *1 oz peanuts = 2 mg* *1 cup kale = 6 mg*	Vegetable oil, nuts, margarine, wheat germ, leafy greens, seeds, almonds, olives, asparagus.	Helps in the formation of red blood cells and the utilization of vitamin K. As an antioxidant, it combats the adverse effects of free radicals.
K	60–65 mcg, women; 70–80 mcg, men *1 cup broccoli = 175 mcg* *1 cup milk = 10 mcg*	Intestinal bacteria produce most of the K needed by the body. The rest is supplied by leafy greens, cauliflower, broccoli, cabbage, milk, soybeans, eggs.	Essential for normal blood clotting.
B₁ (Thiamine)	1–1.1 mg, women; 1.2–1.5 mg, men *1 pkt oatmeal = 0.5 mg*	Whole grains, enriched grain products, beans, meats, liver, wheat germ, nuts, fish, brewer's yeast.	Helps cells convert carbohydrates into energy. Necessary for healthy brain and nerve cells, and heart function.
B₂ (Riboflavin)	1.2–1.3 mg, women; 1.4–1.7 mg, men *1 cup milk = 0.5 mg* *3 oz chicken = 0.2 mg*	Dairy products, liver, meat, chicken, fish, enriched grain products, leafy greens, beans, nuts, eggs, almonds.	Helps cells convert carbohydrates into energy. Essential for growth, production of red blood cells, and health of skin and eyes.
B₃ (Niacin)	13–19 mg *3 oz chicken = 12 mg* *1 slice enriched bread = 1 mg*	Nuts, meat, fish, chicken, liver, enriched grain products, dairy products, peanut butter, brewer's yeast.	Aids in release of energy from foods. Helps maintain healthy skin, nerves, and digestive system.
B₆ (Pyridoxine)	1.6 mg, women; 2 mg, men *1 banana = 0.7 mg* *1 cup lima beans = 0.3 mg*	Whole grains, bananas, meat, beans, nuts, wheat germ, brewer's yeast, chicken, fish, liver.	Vital in chemical reactions of proteins and amino acids. Helps maintain brain function and form red blood cells.
B₁₂	2 mcg *1 cup milk = 0.9 mcg* *3 oz beef = 2 mcg*	Liver, beef, pork, poultry, eggs, milk, cheese, yogurt, shellfish, fortified cereals, fortified soy products.	Necessary for development of red blood cells. Maintains normal functioning of nervous system.
Folacin (a B vitamin; also called folate or folic acid)	180 mcg, women; 200 mcg, men *1 cup raw spinach = 110 mcg* *1 pkt oatmeal = 150 mcg* *1 cup asparagus = 180 mcg*	Leafy greens, wheat germ, liver, beans, whole grains, broccoli, asparagus, citrus fruit and juices.	Important in the synthesis of DNA, in normal growth, and in protein metabolism. Adequate intake reduces the risk of certain birth defects, notably spina bifida.
Biotin (a B vitamin)	No RDA; experts recommend 30–100 mcg	Eggs, milk, liver, brewer's yeast, mushrooms, bananas, tomatoes, whole grains.	Important in metabolism of protein, carbohydrates, and fats.
B₅ (Pantothenic acid)	No RDA; experts recommend 4–7 mg	Whole grains, beans, milk, eggs, liver.	Vital for metabolism of food and production of essential body chemicals.

* These figures are not applicable to pregnant women, who need additional vitamins and should seek professional advice.

Excerpted from the University of California at Berkeley Wellness Letter. © Health Letter Associates, 1991. Used with permission.

amounts of preformed vitamin A. In fact, because vitamin A is a fat-soluble vitamin, consuming megadoses may be dangerous. Headaches, drowsiness, nausea, loss of hair, dry skin, and diarrhea can occur. More seriously, menstruation can cease in women, and bone substance can be lost in adults in general.

The amount of vitamin A you need to eat has traditionally been given in international units (IUs) rather than milligrams. This has been necessary because the different forms (precursors) of vitamin A don't all produce the same level of biological activity inside the body. Today, however, *retinol equivalent* (RE) is the preferred unit of measure because REs are more precise in estimating this biological activity. The recommended daily intake for men is 1000 RE. For women, it is 800 RE. (The body would need 5–6 mg of beta-carotene to make 800–1000 REs of vitamin A.)

Almost 30% of Americans have intakes significantly below the recommended intake for vitamin A. Given the important functions of this vitamin and its possible influence on cancer, it would seem prudent to assess the adequacy of your own intake and to make sure you are eating some of those recommended dark green and yellow vegetables at least every other day. Daily ingestion of more than 5000–10,000 RE of preformed vitamin A, however, may be toxic over time, so excessive doses of this vitamin should be avoided. There is no known toxicity for beta-carotene.

Vitamin C

Vitamin C, too, has been linked with reduced risk of cancer—stomach and esophageal cancers in particular. The evidence seems to support vitamin C ingestion as a preventive measure. Diets high in vitamin C may reduce the risk of cancer. No evidence suggests that vitamin C can cure cancer.

Not so widely known is the importance of vitamin C to the integrity of body tissues, both bone and soft tissue. For example, vitamin C is necessary for proper formation of the connective tissue called *collagen*, which forms that part of the bony structure in which calcium and other minerals are deposited. Collagen plays a critical role in maintaining and repairing body tissues in general; thus, so does vitamin C. In fact, extra vitamin C often is prescribed before and after surgery to facilitate healing of tissues. Vitamin C also enhances the absorption of calcium when the two are consumed together. All of this evidence emphasizes the importance of an adequate intake of vitamin C to minimize the degradation of bone and other tissues that comes with age.

Claims that vitamin C reduces blood cholesterol have not been substantiated by research efforts thus far, but some evidence indicates that vitamin C can minimize the symptoms of a cold. At the doses required, however, the risks might outweigh the benefits, especially because colds generally go away by themselves whether or not they are treated. In contrast to the recommended daily intake of 60 mg of vitamin C for nonsmokers, many proponents of vitamin C's cold-fighting capabilities recommend intake of a *minimum* 1000–2000 mg or 1–2 g. The thinking is that if this is more than you actually need, it simply will wash out of the body in urine. With vitamin C, however, this is not necessarily the case. Megadoses of C can interfere with copper metabolism, cause premature bleeding in pregnant women, cause kidney stones and, over time, increase the amount of vitamin C required to prevent scurvy, its primary deficiency disorder. In addition, some African Americans, Asians, and Sephardic Jews lack an enzyme needed to handle large doses of vitamin C and may develop a form of anemia by megadosing. Nevertheless, many researchers in the nutrition and health field are beginning to suggest that "adequate" vitamin C is a higher amount than the 60 mg/day currently recommended. Studies are ongoing to determine that.

Any decision to take supplements of vitamin C has to be weighed against the potential hazards just described. A safer way to get more than the recommended intake is to include many fruits and vegetables in your diet. An 8-ounce glass of orange juice, for example, provides almost twice the recommended daily intake. If you smoke, drink lots of caffeine-containing beverages such as coffee, tea, and colas, or take large quantities of aspirin, you may want to increase your intake of vitamin C because all of these practices diminish vitamin C supplies in the body. Actually, an increased intake of 100 mg/day of vitamin C has been specified for smokers; no recommendations exist for the other vitamin C–robbing circumstances.

Vitamin E

Vitamin E is popularly acclaimed for its power to slow the aging process, increase sexual potency, and prevent heart disease. All of these claims are gross misrepresentations of what actually is understood about this vitamin. Vitamin E is an *antioxidant*, as are vitamins A and C. Antioxidants curtail the incidence of oxidative reactions that degrade and destroy normal tissue. Some gerontologists believe that these oxidative reactions are responsible primarily for the loss of cells that underlies the aging process. Although increased longevity in cell cultures and in mice fed antioxidants has been reported, no data of this sort exist regarding humans. Some evidence is available, however, that vitamin E may decrease the risk of cancer, especially lung cancer. Evidence that vitamin E may protect against heart disease has been reported consistently. Consequently, some nutrition experts are recommending increased intakes.

The amount of vitamin E you need is not really known because the only deficiency syndrome identified in humans thus far is a type of anemia observed only in premature infants and adults who are unable to absorb fat properly. Consequently, average intake has become the recommended intake: 10 mg/day for men and 8 mg/day for women. Whether these amounts optimize healthy functioning has to be seriously questioned given current research.

With health food stores and other vitamin proponents recommending intakes up to 1000 mg/day based on proposed benefits largely unsupported by available evidence, it is important to know if danger exists in consuming these large quantities. Vitamin E is stored in body fat and thus, like vitamin A, has a potential toxicity level even though that level remains to be defined. Yet, current researchers have been testing dosages up to 800 mg/day with no adverse side-effects and, in fact, seemingly beneficial effects.

Antioxidants and Phytochemicals: Hype or Healthful?

There is no doubt about the answer to this question—the correct descriptor is healthful. How much of these substances called antioxidants and phytochemicals is healthful and how you should get them still requires some clarification. However, there are some basic recommendations to guide us until more information is available.

The most discussed antioxidant of late is **beta-carotene,** the plant precursor of vitamin A, along with vitamin C and vitamin E. As mentioned already, antioxidants curtail the oxidation reactions that destroy cells and tissues by generating unstable molecules called *free radicals.* Essentially, antioxidants "gobble up" free radicals and thus limit oxidative reactions and cell/tissue damage.

It now is thought that some cancers may result from this oxidative process by means of damage to genetic material, thus creating abnormal cells. Evidence also is emerging that free radical damage of blood fats carried by LDL cholesterol helps to begin the artery-clogging process of atherosclerosis. And free radicals generated by ultraviolet light

are thought to damage the fibers in the lens of the eye, resulting in cataracts.

Given these observations about free-radical damage, the body of literature is growing about antioxidants and their impact on cancer, heart disease, and cataracts as well as aging. Some of the data reported over the last 10 years regarding the potential for beta-carotene, vitamin C, and vitamin E to minimize the risk of heart disease and cancer follows.

The diets of 250,000 Japanese people were followed for 10 years. Those who ate the most beta-carotene had the lowest risk of cancer of the cervix, colon, lung, prostate, and stomach. In the United States, of 2,000 men followed for 19 years, those who ate the least beta-carotene had seven times more risk of lung cancer. The National Cancer Institute gave 30,000 cancer-free residents of Linxian County in China various combinations of supplements for 5 years. Those taking 25,000 IU of beta-carotene, 30 mg vitamin E, and 50 mcg of selenium were 21% less likely to die from stomach cancer.

Experimental doses of 600 mg of vitamin C have been reported to reduce "stickiness" of blood, which could decrease the risk of heart attack. Laboratory studies show vitamin C to be a potent blood scavenger of free radicals, helping to decrease oxidation of LDL cholesterol. Some association between vitamin C consumption and lower rates of cancer of the mouth, throat, stomach, colon, and rectum has been reported, but not consistently. More study is needed.

In terms of vitamin E, several large studies have shown an association between an intake of 100–250 mg of vitamin E and decreased risk of heart attack. One study followed 87,245 nurses who took 100 or more mg of vitamin E for 8 years, and another study followed 39,910 male pharmacists who took 100–250 mg of vitamin E for 2 years. Risk of heart attack was 34–37% lower for the nurses and pharmacists, respectively (more than 250 mg did not provide any more benefit in the pharmacist study). Of 35,000 Iowa women followed for 4 years, the highest consumers of vitamin E had one-third the risk of colon cancer. Reduction in the risk for oral, esophageal, and lung cancers also have been associated with vitamin E supplements. (Supplements were used in these studies. Unlike vitamin C and beta-carotene, which are fairly easy to get in large amounts from food, to consume 100 or more milligrams of vitamin E generally requires a supplement.)

Phytochemicals is a fairly new term and means, simply, the chemicals in plants (phytes). Phytochemicals number in the hundreds, perhaps thousands. Not a lot is known about them yet, but primarily they seem to inhibit cancer-producing substances or conditions in cells. Some of them also are antioxidants. Flavonoids, genisteins, indoles, isothiocyanates, lycopenes, and allium compounds are just some of the many phytochemicals you can consume each day *if* you eat lots of fruits and vegetables. Supplements of phytochemicals are not readily available, with the possible exception of garlic tablets (allium compounds). The sources of the phytochemicals named here are shown in FYI 6.

Sources of Selected Phytochemicals

PHYTOCHEMICAL	SOURCE
Flavonoids	Citrus fruit, tomatoes, berries, peppers, carrots
Genistein	Beans, peas, lentils
Indoles	Broccoli, cabbage family
Isothiocyanates (Sulforaphane)	Broccoli, cabbage, mustard, horseradish
Lycopenes	Tomatoes, red grapefruit
Allium compounds	Garlic, onions, leeks, chives

So what is the bottom line here? All nutrition and health authorities agree that eating a minimum of five to six servings of fruits and vegetables each day is really important, and *more* wouldn't hurt. Fruits and vegetables are the only sources of all the different phytochemicals. It could be that without them, vitamin C, beta-carotene, and vitamin E aren't as effective.

If you choose your foods carefully, you actually can eat some of the quantities of beta-carotene being used in current research studies (i.e., 30 mg). Vitamin C is much easier to get in larger quantities in your diet (e.g., up to 1000 mg). It really is not possible, however, to get the 100–800 mg of vitamin E currently used in research efforts by eating foods. Some of the best sources of beta-carotene, vitamin C, and vitamin E are given in FYI 7.

If you decide to try supplements, it is probably best not to exceed doses being tested currently: 15–50 mg beta-carotene, up to 1000 mg vitamin C, and 100–800 mg vitamin E. It is very important to keep in mind that vitamins (or any other substance) cannot be expected to undo damage caused by bad habits. Neither are they an adequate substitute when food intake is consistently below nutritional standards.

Minerals

Unlike vitamins, **minerals** are inorganic substances. They are not derived from living things but, instead, are inert elements that have been part of the earth since its beginnings. Twenty-one minerals are known to be essential to body functioning. These fall into two categories: macrominerals and microminerals. *Macrominerals* are needed in quantities of 100 mg or more. Calcium, phosphorous, sulfur, sodium, potassium, chlorine, and magnesium are macrominerals. *Microminerals* are needed in extremely small amounts, a few milligrams or less per day. For this reason, they sometimes are also called "trace" minerals or elements. Included in this category are iron, copper, zinc, fluorine, iodine, chromium, selenium, manganese, and molybdenum. Other minerals, including cobalt, tin, nickel, vanadium, and silicon may be essential, too, because they are contained in the body; however, deficiency syndromes have not yet been identified for these minerals.

Some minerals act as cofactors with enzymes just as vitamins do. Others are involved in regulation of body fluids, blood clotting, transmission of nerve impulses, maintenance of acid levels, muscle contraction, absorption of nutrients, oxygen transport, and so on. The list of functions is quite lengthy. Many minerals also are constituents of major body structures such as bone.

One might think that quite a lot is known about these minerals, but that is not the case. So far, recommendations for daily intake have been made for only seven minerals; for another seven, only "estimated safe and adequate" amounts have been stipulated. A minimum requirement has been set for two others. This situation is potentially dangerous for someone taking mineral supplements because minerals tend to be toxic at much lower levels than vitamins and toxicity levels for many minerals haven't been clearly established. In addition, an excess of one mineral can create a deficiency in another. As examples, too much zinc decreases the body's supply of copper and too much iron decreases zinc supplies.

If this seems complicated and confusing, you are right. Researchers are only beginning to learn how minerals interact with each other. This makes experimentation with mineral supplements a risky business. Even being well informed doesn't ensure

FYI

Sources of Beta-Carotene, Vitamin C, and Vitamin E

BETA-CAROTENE

Source	Portion	Amount (mg)
Carrot juice	1 cup	24.2
Sweet potato	1 medium	10.2
Dried apricots	10 halves	6.2
Carrot, raw	1 medium	5.7
Spinach	1/2 cup	4.9
Cantaloupe	1/3	4.8
Turnip greens	1/2 cup	3.9
Swiss chard	1/2 cup	2.2
Tomato juice	1 cup	2.2
Broccoli	1/2 cup	1.0

Adult recommendation (RDA) 5–6 mg = 800–1000 RE Vitamin A
Research studies 15–50 mg

VITAMIN C

Source	Portion	Amount (mg)
Red bell peppers	1/2 cup	95
Papaya	1/2 cup	94
Orange juice	6 oz	93
Navel orange	1 medium	80
Cantaloupe	1/3	75
Broccoli	1/2 cup	58
Brussel sprouts	1/2 cup	48
Grapefruit, pink	1/2	47
Sweet potato	1 medium	28
Baked potato	1 large	26

Adult recommendation (RDA) 60 mg
Research studies up to 1000 mg

VITAMIN E

Source	Portion	Amount (mg)
Sunflower seeds	1/4 cup	18
Sweet potato	1 medium	7
Sunflower oil	1 tbsp	6.5
Safflower oil	1 tbsp	4.5
Peanut butter	1/4 cup	4.0
Shrimp	3 oz	3.0
Canola oil	1 tbsp	2.5
Peanuts	1 oz	2.0
Salmon	3 oz	2.0
Cheddar cheese	1 oz	0.5

Adult recommendation 8–10 mg
Research studies 100–800 mg

safety because so little is known at present. The 15 minerals about which at least some information exists are listed in Table 8.K, along with estimated or recommended intake, food sources, and functions.

Calcium and iron are two minerals most often lacking in the American diet. Others, such as sodium and chloride (the combination of these yields table salt) are so abundant in our diets that deficiencies are unheard of. Instead, we seem to consume too much salt. Because of the health consequences and public attention associated with calcium, iron, and salt, some additional information about each of these might be helpful.

Calcium

Calcium has attracted a great deal of attention in the last few years, primarily because of a growing concern about osteoporosis (described in Chapter 3). With the goal of maximizing peak bone mass, which usually is not attained before age 25, the recommended intake of calcium for both sexes is 1200 mg from 11 to 24 years of age and 800 mg thereafter. Many physicians and nutritionists believe this recommendation is too conservative in view of current evidence. New guidelines from the National Institutes of Health regarding calcium intake are given in FYI 8. It is likely that official recommendations will be adjusted accordingly in the near future.

Additional pressure to increase calcium intake stems from studies that show high blood pressure to be more prevalent in adults who consume low amounts of calcium in comparison with those who eat the recommended amounts. Blood pressure levels have dropped beneficially in some people after taking calcium supplements.

TABLE
8.K   Minerals: A fact sheet.

MINERAL	ADULT RDA OR ESTIMATED INTAKE	FOOD SOURCES	WHAT IT DOES
Calcium	800 mg* (1200–1500 mg for older women, according to an NIH consensus report) 1 quart milk = 1250 mg	Milk and milk products, sardines and salmon eaten with bones, dark green leafy vegetables, shellfish, hard water	Builds bones and teeth and maintains bone density and strength; helps prevent osteoporosis in older population; plays a role in regulating heart beat, blood clotting, muscle contraction, and nerve conduction; may help prevent hypertension
Chloride	750 mg***	Table salt, fish, pickled and smoked foods	Maintains normal fluid shifts; balances pH of the blood; forms hydrochloric acid to aid digestion
Magnesium	280 mg (women), 350 mg (men)* 1 cup spinach = 160 mg	Wheat bran, whole grains, raw leafy green vegetables, nuts (especially almonds and cashews), soybeans, bananas, apricots, hard water, spices	Aids in bone growth; aids function of nerves and muscles, including regulation of normal heart rhythm
Phosphorus	800 mg* 1 cup milk = 993 mg 1 serving chicken = 231 mg	Meats, poultry, fish, cheese, egg yolks, dried peas and beans, milk and milk products, soft drinks, nuts; present in almost all foods	Aids bone growth and strengthens teeth; important in energy metabolism
Potassium	2,000 mg** 1 cup raisins = 524 mg 1 banana = 400 mg 1 small potato = 400 mg	Oranges and orange juice, bananas, dried fruits, peanut butter, dried peas and beans, potatoes, coffee, tea, cocoa, yogurt, molasses, meat	Promotes regular heartbeat; active in muscle contraction; regulates transfer of nutrients to cells; controls water balance in body tissues and cells; contributes to regulation of blood pressure
Sodium	500 mg*** 1 frozen pot pie = 1.6 g	All from salt	Helps regulate water balance in body; plays a role in maintaining blood pressure
Chromium	50–200 mcg**	Meat, cheese, whole grains, dried peas and beans, peanuts, brewer's yeast	Important for glucose metabolism; may be a co-factor for insulin
Copper	1.5–3.0 mg**	Shellfish (especially oysters), nuts, beef and pork liver, cocoa powder, chocolate, kidneys, dried beans, raisins, corn oil margarine	Formation of red blood cells; co-factor in absorbing iron into blood cells; assists in production of several enzymes involved in respiration; interacts with zinc
Fluorine (fluoride)	1.5–2.5 mg**	Fluoridated water, foods grown with or cooked in fluoridated water; fish, tea, gelatin	Contributes to solid bone and tooth formation; may help prevent osteoporosis in older people
Iodine	150 mcg*	Primarily from iodized salt, but also seafood, seaweed food products, vegetables grown in iodine-rich areas, vegetable oil	Necessary for normal function of thyroid gland; essential for normal cell function; keeps skin, hair, and nails healthy; prevents goiter
Iron	10 mg (male), 15 mg (female, during child-bearing years) 4 oz calves liver = 12 mg	Liver (especially pork liver), kidneys, red meats, egg yolks, peas, beans, nuts, dried fruits, green leafy vegetables, enriched grain products, blackstrap molasses	Essential to formation of hemoglobin (the oxygen-carrying factor in the blood); part of several enzymes and proteins in the body
Manganese	2–5 mg** 1 cup peanut butter = 2 mg	Nuts, whole grains, vegetables, fruits, instant coffee, tea, cocoa powder, beets, egg yolks	Required for normal bone growth and development, normal reproduction, and cell function
Molybdenum	75–250 mcg**	Peas, beans, cereal grains, organ meats, some dark green vegetables	Important for normal cell function
Selenium	55–70 mcg* 4 oz fish = .038 mg	Fish, shellfish, red meat, egg yolks, chicken, garlic, tuna, tomatoes	Complements vitamin E to fight cell damage by oxygen
Zinc	12–15 mg* 5 oysters = 160 mg 2 slices whole wheat bread = 2 mg	Oysters, crabmeat, beef, liver, eggs, poultry, brewer's yeast, whole-wheat bread	Maintains normal taste and smell acuity, growth, and sexual development; important for fetal growth and wound healing

  * Amount adequate to meet the needs of practically all healthy persons except pregnant or lactating women; established by Food and Nutrition Board of National Academy of Sciences.
  ** No RDA established; estimated safe intake given.
  *** Estimated minimum requirement of healthy persons.

Adapted by permission from the University of California at Berkeley Wellness Letter, Copyright © Health Letter Associates, 1992.

National Institutes of Health 1994 Recommendations for Optimal Calcium Intake

GROUP	OPTIMAL DAILY INTAKE
Children (6–10 years)	800–1200 mg
Teens and young adults (11–24 years)	1200–1500 mg
Men (25–65 years), women (25–50 years), and postmenopausal women on estrogen	1000 mg
Men (65 years), women (65 years), and postmenopausal women not on estrogen	1500 mg
Pregnant and lactating women	1200 mg

Note: The preferred source of calcium is calcium-rich foods such as dairy products, especially low- and non-fat dairy products. Calcium-fortified foods and calcium supplements are other means by which calcium intake can be reached in those who cannot or choose not to eat calcium-rich foods.

Source: NIH Consensus Development Conference Statement on Optimal Calcium Intake, June 6–8, 1994.

TABLE 8.L Calcium intake for males and females in United States, 1988–91.

Male	Average Intake (mg)	% Recommended (RDA)
2–23 mo.	850	130
2–5 y	870	109
6–11 y	1007	121
12–19 y	1211	101
20–39 y	1061	122
40–59 y	842	105
60–79 y	850	106
80+ y	721	90

Female	Average Intake (mg)	% Recommended (RDA)
2–23 mo.	796	123
2–5 y	807	101
6–11 y	867	102
12–19 y	810	68
20–39 y	765	88
40–59 y	670	84
60–79 y	680	85
80+ y	626	78

Source: National Health and Nutrition Examination Survey III, Phase I, 1988–91 as reported in Looker et al., *Calcium Intake in United States.*

Calcium will command even more attention if reports linking increased calcium intake with prevention of colon cancer in high-risk families prove true. Researchers have observed a return to normal of precancerous colon cells after 8 weeks of calcium supplementation in subjects from families with a high incidence of colon cancer. Several large studies now have reported reduced colon cancer risk among high calcium consumers as well.

The average calcium intake for males and females is shown in Table 8.L. As you can see, women thus far have done a poor job of getting the calcium they need. Men basically have done okay. With the current average calcium intake for women being closer to 650 mg or less a day, achieving the new NIH recommendation of 1200 mg ultimately means a significant increase in calories unless a supplement is taken. Because men in general consume more calcium than women, they can achieve even the highest recommended intake by simply drinking one more glass of milk at 90–150 calories, depending on fat content. A woman would need one to four additional glasses of milk depending upon which set of recommendations she would choose to follow. Again, depending on fat content, this could mean an increase of as much as 360–600 calories every day. The literature is quite clear that getting calcium from food is the best and safest way to achieve recommended goals. Nonetheless, because of concerns regarding weight control, supplementation issues are also considered here.

How to get more calcium safely is a controversial issue. As with all the minerals, information to guide you is limited. The best advice for the moment includes the following recommendations and precautions:

1. Try to get more calcium from the foods you eat. Good sources of calcium are listed in Table 8.M. The lactose in milk products enhances absorption of calcium, which makes them good sources. When vitamin D is added to these products, they are even better because vitamin D also increases calcium absorption. Vitamin C does the same, so eating an orange with milk is a good choice. High-fat, as well as high-protein, diets encourage calcium excretion. As such, low-fat or skim dairy products actually offer more calcium than whole milk. Avoid heavy consumption of caffeine. For every 150 mg of caffeine consumed (about one cup of coffee), 5 mg of calcium is lost from the body. Drinking at least one glass of milk a day, however, seems to minimize this impact over time.

2. Take a supplement if you can't or won't get enough calcium from the foods you eat, but don't count on a supplement to replace calcium-rich foods in your diet. Large doses of calcium supplements may inhibit absorption of iron, zinc, manganese, copper, and manganese and, in susceptible individuals, can cause kidney stones, especially calcium nitrate. The calcium in milk and milk products does not seem to cause these problems. Thus, food remains the best source of calcium. If you do decide to take a supplement, make sure it is just that. Some criteria to guide selection of a supplement are:

 a. Of the various supplement forms available, calcium carbonate is the easiest to compound into small tablets. Because it interferes with iron absorption, it is best to take it in between meals or at least not with iron supplements or major food sources of iron. Older people, however, should take it at mealtime, when their stomach acidity is greatest. Whatever your age, taking smaller doses several times a day can increase absorption up to 20%.

 b. Avoid supplements with the words "dolomite," "bone meal," or "oyster shell" on the label. These products may contain lead contaminates. Also, don't use products formulated with aluminum and magnesium hydroxide (for example, the antacid Rolaids). These products actually can increase calcium loss.

 c. The amount of calcium available to you from a tablet is called "elemental calcium" and should be listed on the product label. More calcium can be in a tablet than you can get out of it. For example, a tablet of the antacid TUMS contains 500 mg of calcium, but only 200 mg is elemental calcium.

 d. Vitamin D enhances calcium absorption and is included in some supplement formulations.

Care should be taken not to exceed 5–10 mcg (200–400 I.U.) of vitamin D per day, including what you eat. Excess vitamin D can be toxic.

 e. *Any* supplement that doesn't dissolve in 6 ounces of vinegar within 30 minutes at room temperature (stirred every 5 minutes) probably won't dissolve in your stomach either—at least in time for you to derive any benefit.

Iron

Iron is vitally important to life. It is needed to deliver oxygen to the cells, form muscle, produce antibodies, synthesize collagen, convert beta-carotene to vitamin A, and detoxify drugs in the liver, among other things!

The amount of iron you need each day depends upon how much you lose in urine, feces, perspiration, and desquamation (loss of hair, skin cells, and nails). For children, adolescents, and pregnant women, new tissue growth also creates greater need for iron. For the average adult man, iron loss totals about 1 mg/day. Menstruation increases the average iron loss for women to 1.5 mg/day. Because the body absorbs only about 10% of the iron you eat, the recommended intake is 10 mg/day for men and for postmenopausal women. Menstruating women need at least 15 mg of iron each day.

National nutritional surveys have indicated that about 18% of women 19–64 years of age consume the amount of iron recommended; another 26% consume 70% of the recommended amount; the remaining 56% of women consume less than 70%! Men did a lot better; 88% of the men in this age group ate the recommended amount of iron. The fact that women need more iron than men during these years accounts for some of this difference, but not all. Even after age 65, men still eat more iron than women.

Women have difficulty obtaining needed iron because a diet adequate in most other nutrients provides only 6 mg of iron per 1000 calories. Unless a woman eats at least 2500 calories a day, she likely won't get the iron she needs. An iron supplement may be needed; ferrous sulphate probably is the least expensive and most effective form. Whether you need a supplement is best determined through a blood test and discussion of the results with a physician.

Where to get iron and how to get the most iron out of what you eat are important questions, especially for women. The following information about sources of iron provides some answers.

TABLE 8.11 Calcium content per serving of selected foods.

CALCIUM	DAIRY	FRUITS/VEGETABLES	LEGUMES/NUTS/SEEDS	GRAINS	MEAT/FISH/FOWL
Less than 100 mg	1 egg = 28	1 banana = 7 1 apple = 10 1 baked potato with skin = 20 1 c cooked carrots = 48 1 orange = 54 1 c green beans = 61 1 c sauerkraut = 71 1 c mashed sweet potato = 77	1 tbsp peanut butter = 5 1 oz dry roasted cashews = 13 1 oz peanuts = 24 1 oz sunflower seeds = 33 1 c cooked lentils = 50 1 oz filberts = 53 1 oz almonds = 75 1 c chick peas (garbanzo beans) = 80 1 c pinto beans = 86 1 c navy beans = 95	1 c spaghetti noodles = 14 1 c oatmeal = 14 1 slice whole-wheat bread = 20 1 c brown rice = 23 1 plain bagel = 29 1 slice white bread = 32 1 pancake = 36 1 pita bread = 49 1 buckwheat pancake = 59 1 bran muffin = 60 1 English muffin = 96	2 slices bacon = 2 2.8 oz lean beef roast = 4 2.5 oz pork chop = 4 1 hot dog (10/pkg) = 5 2.5 oz lean sirloin steak = 8 1/2 roast chicken breast = 13 3 oz light meat turkey = 16 3 oz broiled halibut = 14 3 oz water-packed tuna = 17 3 oz baked salmon = 26 3 oz baked clams = 59 3 oz crabmeat = 61 3 oz shrimp = 96
100+ mg	1 c 2% cottage cheese = 155 1 c hard ice cream or ice milk = 176	1 c cooked dandelion greens = 147 1 c cooked chopped kale = 179	1 piece tofu = 108 (2½ × 2¾ 1") 1 c refried beans = 141		3 oz canned salmon with bones = 167
200+ mg	1 oz cheddar cheese = 204 1 oz part skim mozzarella cheese = 207 1 oz provolone = 214 1 oz swiss cheese = 272 1 c whole milk = 291 1 c 2% milk = 297 1 c baked custard = 297	1 c cooked broccoli = 205 1 c cooked chopped turnip greens = 249 1 c cooked spinach = 277			1 c oysters = 226
300+ mg	1 c nonfat (skim) milk = 302 8 oz lowfat fruit-flavored yogurt = 343 8 oz lowfat plain yogurt = 415 8 oz nonfat plain yogurt = 452	1 c cooked rhubarb = 341 1 c cooked chopped collard greens = 357			3 oz canned sardines with bones = 372

c = cup; tbsp = tablespoon; oz = ounce

Food sources of iron. Liver is the only really good source of iron. Pork liver offers the most per serving. Unfortunately, liver also has high levels of cholesterol. Perhaps more important, many Americans don't (won't!) eat liver very often. Other meats, cereals, vegetables, and beans provide most of the iron in American diets. Fruits are rather poor sources, although the pulp of fruit has twice as much iron as fruit juice. On paper, eggs seem to be a good source of iron, but only 2% of the iron in egg can be absorbed. Milk and milk products contain little iron. A nonfood source of iron is iron pots and pans; foods cooked in them can pick up additional iron. The amount of iron in selected, frequently consumed foods is listed in Table 8.N.

Absorption of iron.

1. The iron in animal foods is absorbed better than that in vegetables and grains. Consuming meat with vegetables and grains, however, increases the absorption of iron from these sources two to three times.

2. Consuming a source of vitamin C with sources of iron increases its absorption. This also is true when taking a supplement. You will get more iron from a supplement taken with a glass of orange juice than with water.

3. Small amounts of iron are absorbed more easily. Eating small doses of iron three to four times throughout the day is better than consuming one big dose. The same applies to supplements. Also, you will get about twice the iron from your supplement if you take it with a meal rather than take it before eating.

4. Drinking coffee or tea with a meal can decrease iron absorption 40%–95%. Tannins in tea and polyphenols in coffee are iron-binding substances.

Several recent studies have suggested that some people have too much iron and that this excess might increase the risk of cancer and heart disease. More study of this issue is needed to confirm or negate this allegation. However, for those who wish to be cautious, limit consumption of red meat to the recommended 6 ounces per day and don't take iron supplements unless blood tests indicate your supply

TABLE 8.N Iron content per serving of selected foods.

FOOD	SERVING SIZE	CALORIES	MG IRON
Meat, Fish, Eggs, Poultry, Nuts, and Legumes:			
Egg, fried	1 large	83	0.9
Beef roast, lean	3 oz	165	3.1
Hamburger	3 oz	285	3.2
Chicken breast	3 oz	160	1.3
Tuna in water	3 oz	120	1.6
Peanut butter	2 tbsp	178	0.6
Bacon, lean	3 slices	89	2.8
Beef liver	3 oz	195	7.5
Shrimp	3 oz	100	2.5
Haddock, perch, salmon, etc.	3 oz	160	1.0
Raw clams	3 oz	65	5.2
Oysters (7–8 med.)	4 oz	80	6.0
Tofu (soybean curd)	4 oz	85	2.5
Chick peas	½ cup	145	2.9
Sunflower seeds (dry, hulled)	¼ cup	200	2.5
Pumpkin seeds (dry, hulled)	¼ cup	195	3.9
Peanuts (roasted in oil and salted)	¼ cup	210	.7
Filberts	¼ cup	182	1.0 scant
Cereals:			
Cornflakes	1 cup	88	1.9
Shredded wheat	1 biscuit	83	1.1
Saltines (10 grams)	4 crackers	43	0.5
Rice	½ cup	112	0.9
White bread	1 slice	81	0.6
Whole-wheat bread	1 slice	73	0.5
Dairy Products:			
Whole milk	8 oz	157	0.1
2% fat milk	8 oz	121	0.1
Skim milk	8 oz	90	0.1
Cheddar cheese	1 oz	114	0.2
Fruits:			
Apple	1 med	81	0.4
Banana	1 med	105	0.9
Orange juice, frozen	4 oz	56	0.1
Peach	1 med	37	0.5
Vegetables:			
Corn, canned	4 oz–½ cup	98	0.8
Green beans	4 oz–½ cup	52	0.7
Green peas	4 oz–½ cup	88	1.8
Lettuce (100 grams)	¼ head	13	0.5
Tomatoes	1 med	22	0.5
Potato, baked	1 med	93	0.7

is low. Exercising regularly and donating blood periodically also help to control iron levels.

Salt (Sodium Chloride)

The combination of two minerals, sodium and chlorine, is most commonly known as salt. It is given special attention here because diets high in salt are associated with high blood pressure, and American diets *are* high in salt. As previously noted, about one in four American adults has high blood pressure.

Sodium seems to be the mineral responsible for the connection between salt and high blood pressure, but sodium is not solely to blame for this health problem. As noted earlier, low calcium intake, overweight, smoking, race, age, and family history are also risk factors. To further complicate this picture, not all people who eat salt develop high blood pressure, and reducing salt intake certainly doesn't guarantee a return to normal pressure once high blood pressure has developed.

Although some confusion and controversy surround salt and high blood pressure, one fact has emerged rather clearly: Certain people have a genetic propensity to develop high blood pressure and/or to be sodium-sensitive. For these people, a high-salt diet probably will contribute to high blood pressure in time. An estimated 20% or more of Americans may have this tendency, and African Americans are at even greater risk. Long-term high salt intake also may be an important factor, as almost three of four people over age 65 have problems with high blood pressure. Recent research suggests, however, that the impact of high salt intake may be minimized if adequate amounts of potassium and calcium are consumed.

At this point, no one can predict who can eat salt liberally without concern and who cannot. This is unfortunate because desire for salt seems to be acquired through dietary practices and not by a need for it. The body needs only about 115

mg of sodium/day to regulate the balance of water and dissolved substances outside cells (potassium does this inside cells). To allow for variation in individual need plus exercise and environmental conditions, nutritionists suggest that 500 mg of sodium/day should be adequate. This amounts to about 1.3 g of salt (¼ teaspoon) per day. The average American adult, however, eats 10–20 g of salt/day, between 2 and 4 teaspoons.

Why do Americans like salt so much? The explanation may lie in reports from the Food and Drug Administration that American infants consume about the same amount of salt as adults do, 18 g/day, and that toddlers get even more, about 25 g/day. How do they get so much salt? From adults who prepare foods to their own tastes. Indeed, over two-thirds of our intake of salt comes from processed foods.

Guidelines for Reducing the Salt in Your Diet

1. Add little or no salt to food at the table, and certainly not until after you've tasted it.

2. Cut down on salt used in cooking and baking. First cut the amount in half. As you become accustomed to that, reduce it further.

3. Use sodium-free spices and flavorings in place of salt. Some of these are onion, garlic, curry, ginger, nutmeg, parsley, pepper, sage, thyme, mustard, sesame seeds, and vanilla, walnut, lemon, almond, and peppermint extracts. The American Heart Association can provide a more complete list of these, plus low-sodium recipes.

4. Use fresh meats, vegetables, and fruits as much as possible. Frozen vegetables are next best.

5. Reduce intake of canned soups and vegetables, cold cuts, canned meats, hotdogs, sausage, salted and smoked fish, processed cheese, bouillon cubes, and sauces such as worcestershire, soy, and barbeque.

6. Reduce intake of salty snacks such as potato chips, pretzels, salted nuts, crackers, and popcorn.

7. Look for the word "sodium" on product labels even if it's part of another word (e.g., monosodium glutamate, sodium bicarbonate, sodium propionate, sodium saccharin). Avoid as many of these as you can.

8. Limit your intake of pickled vegetables, which contain a lot of salt.

9. Avoid eating at fast-food restaurants. Many of the usual entrees, including hamburgers and fried chicken, are high in sodium (see Table 8.0).

10. Check with your local water district to find out if the sodium content of your drinking water is higher than 45 parts per million. If it is, buy a filter to attach to your tap; otherwise, simply drinking water could nullify your efforts to reduce sodium in your diet.

The use of processed foods doesn't necessarily mean that parents are giving their children "junk food." It simply means that foods you buy in cans and packages often contain a lot of added salt. For example, fresh peas contain only 2 mg of sodium per 3½-ounce serving, but canned peas contain 236 mg. By comparison, an ounce of Planters Peanuts contains only 132 mg, and a 1-oz bag of Lay's Potato Chips has 191 mg of sodium. Indeed, a 10-oz serving of Campbell's Tomato Soup has a whopping 1050 mg. The sodium content of these and other processed and fresh foods is given in Table 8.O. A more complex list is given in *The Sodium Content of Foods*, published by the U.S. Department of Agriculture.

With processed foods composing 55% of the American diet, the difficulty of reducing an overdeveloped taste for salt should be apparent. Difficult or not, that is exactly what health experts are recommending. They believe that limiting salt intake to 6 g/day, equivalent to 2400 mg of sodium, will help curtail the incidence of high blood pressure.

WATER AND OTHER SOURCES OF LIQUID

"Last, but not least" is certainly an appropriate description for the last nutrient to be discussed. Actually, you need more of this than any of the other nutrients, and without it you probably would die within a week. The magic nutrient is water. It supplies no calories for energy, but it is the medium for *all* essential body functions. As such, it is a solvent, growth promoter, lubricant, temperature regulator, catalyst, and source of trace elements. Indeed, the human body is composed largely of water; the average adult body contains about 40–50 quarts.

The average person loses about 2½ to 3 quarts of water daily in urine, perspiration, feces, and evaporation in the lungs. In hot environments or with heavy exercise, water loss can approach 4 quarts a day. To maintain optimum functioning, this fluid has to be replaced each day.

A guide to estimating the amount of water you need each day is 1 quart or 4 cups for every 1000 calories consumed. For most people, that means drinking between 8 and 16 cups of water every day. Fortunately, you don't actually have to drink this much water, because the food you eat contains water. Fruits and vegetables have an especially high water content, most about 80%. Meats are about 50% water, breads 35%. Water also is created inside the body through various metabolic reactions. In all, these sources probably will provide almost half the water you need; you have to drink the rest. If you have a choice, hard water is better than soft water. Soft water seems to contribute to an increased incidence of high blood pressure and heart disease.

It is generally recommended that you consume a minimum of six to eight glasses of water per day. Some of this can be in the form of other beverages such as milk, which is 87% water, and bottled waters.* Soft drinks also are a source of water, but they are loaded with sugar (only about 10% of the soft drinks sold are "diet"). An estimated 25% of the sugar we eat annually comes from soft drinks. For those needing only extra calories and more water in their diets, soft drinks are a good choice because, in general, the only nutrients they have are calories and water!

Colas, regular or diet, also give you a dose of caffeine fairly equivalent to that in a cup of coffee or tea, depending on how the latter is brewed. The caffeine in a 12-oz cola drink ranges from 40 to 72 mg. A cup of instant tea has about 25 mg of caffeine; brewed tea has twice as much or more. Instant coffee has about 65 mg of caffeine per cup; perked coffee may contain as much as 140 mg, and drip coffee, 155 mg or more.

Caffeine is a stimulant to the heart and central nervous system and a relaxant to the digestive system and kidneys. In small doses, as in one or two cups of coffee, caffeine can enhance the efficiency of the heart and other muscles and increase mental alertness and thought processes. Larger doses, however, can mean trouble. Drinking three to four or more cups of coffee in succession can cause rapid and irregular heart rhythms, shakiness, headache, diarrhea, and excessive urine output. All of these reactions are unpleasant and certainly not conducive to health. The major concern with caffeine, however, is its possible long-term effects. Many studies, primarily of coffee drinkers, have indicated a possible link between caffeine and increased risk of heart disease, cancer, fibrocystic breast disease, and birth defects. To date, research has failed to confirm a caffeine connection to any of these health problems. In a recent major study, however, pregnant women who drank 1½–3 cups of coffee a day had twice the risk of miscarriage and those who drank more than three cups a day had three times the risk.

---

*Mineral water, seltzer, and club soda are especially popular drinks today. The health benefits of these drinks beyond increased water intake have not been established. Some of them do offer extra minerals, but large amounts can be a hazard. Too many minerals can upset the body's natural balance of these substances. People with heart disease or high blood pressure should examine labels closely to see if sodium is one of the minerals present, as in club soda.

TABLE
8.0 Sodium content of selected foods.

FOODS	PORTION	SODIUM (MG)
DAIRY		
Milk	1 cup	120
Chocolate milk	1 cup	150
McDonald's chocolate shake	1	330
Ice cream, hard	1 cup	108
Ice cream, soft	1 cup	153
Cheddar cheese	1 oz	176
Cottage cheese	1 cup	910
Mozzarella cheese	1 oz	106
Swiss cheese	1 oz	74
Swiss, processed	1 oz	388
Homemade chocolate pudding	1 oz	146
Jello chocolate instant pudding	1 cup	880
Yogurt, fruit-flavored	1 cup	133
Egg	1 whole	69
Egg white	1 white	50
FATS		
Butter	1 pat	41
Margarine	1 pat	45
All oils	1 cup	0
French dressing	1 tbsp	188
Low-calorie	1 tbsp	306
Italian dressing	1 tbsp	162
Low-calorie	1 tbsp	136
Thousand Island	1 tbsp	110
Low-calorie	1 tbsp	153
MEATS		
Canned tuna, Del Monte	3 oz	468
Canned shrimp	3 oz	1955
Fresh shrimp	3 oz	180
Salmon, broiled	3 oz	55
Pink salmon, canned	3 oz	443
Halibut, broiled	3 oz	103
Scallops, steamed	3 oz	298
Bacon	2 slices	202
Beef, pot roast	3 oz	46
Chipped beef	2½ oz	3053
Ground beef	3 oz	70
McDonald's Big Mac	1	1510
Burger King Whopper	1	909
Lamb chop	3 oz	47
Ham	3 oz	1009
Pork chop	1 oz	56
Canned lunch meat	1 slice	720
Beef franks	1	504
Bologna	2 slices	578
Kentucky Fried Chicken, original recipe	3 pieces	2285
Broiled chicken	½ or 6 oz	116
Swanson turkey dinner	1	1735
Roast turkey, light	3 oz	54

FOODS	PORTION	SODIUM (MG)
FRUIT		
Apple, large	1	2
Applesauce	1 cup	5
Banana	1	1
Grapefruit	½	0
Cantaloupe	½	24
Honeydew melon	1/10	13
Orange	1	7
Pear	1	1
Strawberries	1 cup	2
GRAINS		
Bagel	1	245
Whole-wheat bread	1 slice	180
Pumpernickel bread	1 slice	277
French bread	1 slice	203
White bread	1 slice	129
Shredded wheat	¾ cup	3
Oatmeal, cooked	1 cup	1
Oatmeal, instant	1 cup	285
Kellogg's Corn Flakes	1 cup	351
Post Raisin Bran	1 cup	370
Pancakes, homemade buckwheat	3	375
Hungry Jack extra light pancakes, 4-inch	3	1150
Rice, cooked without salt	1 cup	0
Instant rice, cooked	1 cup	767
VEGETABLES		
Peas, fresh	½ cup	2
Peas, canned	½ cup	236
Green beans, fresh	1 cup	4
Green beans, canned	1 cup	340
Beets, fresh	½ cup	74
Beets, canned	1 cup	233
Tomatoes, cooked/fresh	1 cup	10
Tomatoes, canned	1 cup	390
Corn, fresh	1 cup	3
Corn, canned	1 cup	572
B & M Brick Oven baked beans	1 cup	810
Potatoes, baked	1	16
Hash brown potatoes, cooked from frozen	1 cup	53
Potato chips	10	133
Sauerkraut	1 cup	1561
MISCELLANEOUS		
Jif peanut butter	2 tbsp	155
Campbell's tomato soup	10 oz	1050
Lipton Cup-A-Soup, vegetable	8 oz	800
Heinz kosher dill pickles	1 large	1137
Nabisco Wheat Thins	16 (1 oz)	240
Planter's peanuts	1 oz	200
Olives, green	10 large	936
Olives, ripe	10 extra large	410
A-1 sauce	1 tbsp	275
Soy sauce	1 tbsp	1029

Until more information is available, the caffeine in several cups of coffee, tea, or soda pop would seem to pose no problem for most people. Pregnant women and people with heartbeat irregularities, however, should check with their physicians about the safety of drinking these beverages. Consumers of caffeine in general might want to consider moderating the amounts they drink in case the possible negative effects of caffeine eventually are confirmed. In all cases, users of caffeinated beverages risk loss of water-soluble vitamins and minerals, especially calcium and magnesium in their urine, because of the diuretic effect of caffeine.

To avoid caffeine, some people have begun drinking decaffeinated coffee and herbal teas. A word of caution is needed in each case. Many decaffeinated coffees contain chemicals derived from the decaffeinating process that some researchers believe may be cancer-causing. Evidence is inconclusive. Coffee decaffeinated by a steam process developed in Switzerland does not contain these chemicals and might be a safer choice for consumers. Water-processed decaffeinated coffee is best if you want to be extra cautious in this matter. A report that decaffeinated coffee increases LDL cholesterol seems to be unjustified and not a good reason for avoiding or giving up "decaf."

Herbal teas have become popular replacement beverages for coffee. Although most of them don't contain caffeine, some do, and in amounts equal to or greater than those in coffee. The product label should indicate this. Besides indicating caffeine content, if any, the label should state the plants used to make the tea. This information is important because many herbal teas come from plants that historically have been used as drugs. Some of these teas actually are poisonous in sufficient quantities. Teas made from sassafras, ginseng, and chamomile are examples. If you want to drink herbal teas, the best advice is to learn first about the plants they are made from and then to drink only dilute preparations.

Alcoholic beverages provide water, too, but they also contain the drug alcohol. Alcohol is a central nervous system depressant. Besides its sedating effect on the brain, it acts as a diuretic. Thus, when you drink alcoholic beverages, you risk loss of water-soluble vitamins and minerals. Heavy use of alcohol also is prominently associated with fatal accidents, liver disease, cancer, cardiovascular disease, gastrointestinal problems, and birth defects.

Technically, alcohol is a nutrient because it provides calories, 7 per gram. Some alcoholic beverages (e.g., wine) contain small amounts of vitamins and minerals but, for the most part, alcohol, like refined sugar, represents empty calories. Because it provides essentially nothing but calories and its presence in the body is not in any way needed, it usually is not considered a nutrient.

On the other hand, limited intake of alcohol—no more than one or two drinks per day—is associated with reduced mortality from CVD, possibly because of increased blood levels of HDL cholesterol. Nevertheless, the many health and psychosocial problems connected with alcohol, plus its addictive qualities, preclude it from being a prescribed approach to CVD. Of course, the potential for birth defects remains even with limited alcohol consumption during pregnancy.

As a beverage or as a nutrient, alcohol offers very little, especially in light of its association with numerous serious health problems. If you are going to consume alcohol, limiting consumption to 1–2 drinks per day is the current recommendation. If weight control is a problem, eliminating the empty calories you get from alcohol would be best. Next best would be no more than one drink per day. Caffeine and alcohol have been considered here as foods and beverages or as components of such. They are discussed further in Chapter 10 as drugs.

THE RDAS AND THE DIETARY GOALS AND GUIDELINES FOR AMERICANS

The primary sources of nutritional recommendations in this chapter are the **Recommended Dietary Allowances (RDAs),** the **U.S. Dietary Goals,** and dietary guidelines issued by prominent public and private health organizations.

The RDAs are established by the Food and Nutrition Board, a committee of the National Academy of Sciences National Research Council (NAS-NRC). They are reviewed and reissued about every 5 years. The board's goal is to recommend a daily intake for each essential nutrient that will be adequate to meet the needs of practically all healthy persons. To accommodate individual variations in need and usage of nutrients, the board's recommendations actually exceed the nutrient requirements for most people. The RDAs for 1989 are listed by sex and age group in Appendix 6.

The U.S. Dietary Goals were issued in 1977 by the Senate Select Committee on Nutrition and Human Needs. They were developed from the recommendations of the nation's foremost nutrition and health experts for reducing the incidence of disability and death from chronic diseases including cardiovascular disease, cancer, and diabetes.

Since that time, dietary goals and guidelines also have been issued by the U. S. Department of Agriculture, the American Heart Association, the American Cancer Society, the Surgeon General of the United States, and the National Research Council. A comparison of these guidelines is offered in Table 8.P. Basically, all these guidelines suggest the following as most important to decreasing the risk for chronic disease:

1. Maintain weight.
2. Increase carbohydrate intake to 55% or more of total calories, but limit refined sugars to 9%–10%.
3. Increase fiber intake.
4. Reduce total fat intake to 30% or less of total calories. Limit saturated fat to 10% or less.
5. Limit cholesterol intake to 300 mg/day or less.
6. Reduce salt intake to 6 g/day or less.
7. Avoid alcohol or limit yourself to 1–2 drinks/day. If pregnant, don't drink at all.
8. Eat a variety of foods, especially lots of fruits, vegetables, and grains.
9. Limit protein intake to recommended levels; do not exceed twice the RDA.

THE 1990 NUTRITION LABELING AND EDUCATION ACT (NLEA)

In November 1990, the **Nutrition Labeling and Education Act (NLEA)** was signed into law, representing the first change in labeling requirements in 20 years and providing consumers with valuable information that did not appear on old labels. In developing regulations for the new law, the Food and Drug Administration has established definitions for terms used to describe food characteristics and new standards for evaluating the nutritional content of food items. All of this was much needed because manufacturers used terms such as "light" to describe weight, color, calories, fat content, or just about any characteristic that might seem attractive, and the previous standards for evaluating food content were based on 1968 RDAs.

Label Requirements

All new labels have to include the following information:

- Common name of the product
- Name and address of manufacturer, packer, or distributor
- Net content in terms of weight, measure, or count

- Ingredient list in descending order by prominence of weight
- Serving size and number of servings per container
- Quantities of specified nutrients and food constituents (called the Nutrition Panel)

In terms of the ingredient list and serving sizes, the FDA set forth some major changes. One major change is the designation of serving size for different food product categories (e.g., cereals). In the past, companies set their own serving size according to their best sales advantage.

Another major change for the new label is the requirement that manufacturers list all ingredients they have used including all additives as well as specific fats and oils. On past labels, manufacturers could simply list oils they might have used in the product (e.g., "soybean oil, coconut oil, or palm oil," without specifying which one).

The Nutrition Panel

As you will note in Figure 8.3, which shows the nutrition panel format, the first information given is serving size and servings per container, followed by the number of total calories and calories from fat per serving. It might have been helpful to many consumers to have the fat content expressed in percent of calories per serving; however, that is not the case. Percent fat can easily be calculated, though, by simply dividing calories from fat by total calories. So the shopper still needs to shop with a calculator in-hand or in-head.

In addition to total calories and calories from fat, the nutrition panel must provide the following quantities in this order:

- Total fat in grams
- Saturated fat in grams
- Cholesterol in milligrams
- Sodium in milligrams
- Total carbohydrate in grams
- Dietary fiber in grams
- Sugar in grams
- Protein in grams
- Vitamin A, vitamin C, calcium, and iron in percent of RDI

The rest of the information on the nutrition panel is based on a new label reference called *Daily Values.* The Daily Values in turn represent two new sets of *dietary standards:* The *Reference Daily Intake* (RDIs) and the *Daily Reference Values* (DRVs). Only the term *Daily Value,* however, appears on the label (in hopes of making label reading less confusing!).

TABLE 8.1 Dietary advice to the public from various government and health groups.

	WEIGHT CONTROL	CARBO-HYDRATE	FIBER	ANIMAL LIPID	VEGETABLE LIPID	TOTAL LIPID	CHOLES-TEROL	SODIUM (NA)	OTHER
American Cancer Society (1989)	Avoid obesity (defined as 40% or more overweight)	55% daily calorie intake Include foods rich in vitamins A and C Include cruciferous vegetables	Increase fiber intake 30 grams fiber per day drink			30% or less daily caloric intake		Avoid salt-cured food or eat occasionally	Drink alcohol in moderation
American Heart Association (1990)	Maintain best body weight	50% or more of calories, emphasizing complex forms		Limit saturated fat to less than 10% of calories	Limit polyunsaturated to less than 10% of calories	Limit total fat to less than 30% of calories	Limit cholesterol to less than 100 mg per 1000 calories Not to exceed 300 mg per day	Limit to 1 gram per 1000 calories Not to exceed 39 grams per day	Limit alcohol to 15% of calories Not more than 50 ml ethanol per day Eat a variety of foods
Dietary Guidelines USDA, HHS (1995)	Balance the food you eat with physical activity Maintain or improve your weight	Choose a diet moderate in sugars	Choose a diet with plenty of grain products, fruits, and vegetables	Choose a diet low in fat and saturated fat		Choose a diet low in fat	Choose a diet low in cholesterol	Choose a diet moderate in salt and sodium	Eat a variety of foods If you drink alcoholic beverages, do so in moderation
Surgeon General's Report, Nutrition & Health (1988)	Achieve and maintain desirable body weight	Increase consumption of whole-grain foods, cereal products, vegetables and fruits	Increase consumption of whole-grain foods, cereal products, vegetables, and fruits	Reduce consumption of fats, especially saturated fat		Reduce consumption of fats		Intake	Alcohol in moderation (no more than two drinks per day)
National Academy of Sciences-National Research Council (1989)		55% calories including five or more servings of fruits and vegetables, and six or more servings of breads, cereals, and legumes		Reduce to less than 10% of calories		Reduce to 30% or less total	Less than 300 mg per day	Total intake of salt = 6 g	No more than 1 oz pure alcohol per day Maintain moderate protein intake Drink fluoridated water Consume RDA for calories

FIGURE
8.3   Using the new food label.

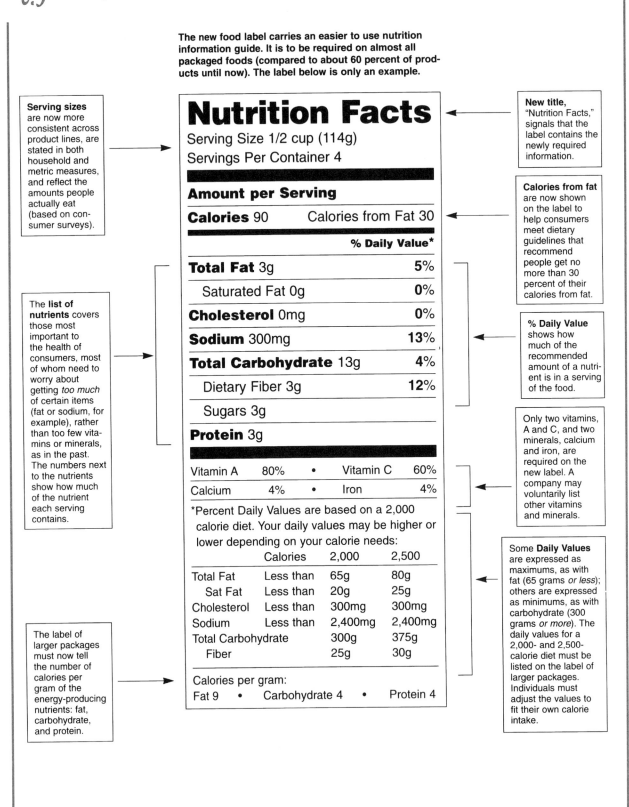

Source: Food and Drug Administration, 1993.

The RDIs actually are the population-adjusted mean of the RDA for protein, vitamins, and minerals. For the interim the new RDIs will be essentially the same as the former USRDA's. New values are being proposed for RDIs of the future. Table 8.Q compares the RDIs currently in use (formerly referred to as USRDA) and the newly proposed RDIs.

The Daily Reference Values (DRVs) actually are based on the U.S. Dietary Goals for total fat, saturated fat, cholesterol, sodium, carbohydrate, fiber, and protein. Listed on the bottom of the nutrition panel are the amounts of these nutrients, in grams and milligrams, that comply with the U.S. Dietary Goals when eating a 2000-calorie diet or a 2500-calorie diet. Specifically, total fat is based on 30% of calories, saturated fat on 10% of calories, carbohydrate on 60% of calories, protein on 10% of calories, and fiber on 11.5% of calories. Sodium content is based on salt intake of 6 grams per day,

and cholesterol on 300 milligrams or less per day.

The percent Daily Values shown on the nutrition panel, then, represent the manufacturers' report to the consumer on the percent of recommended intake for fat, saturated fat, cholesterol, sodium, carbohydrate, and fiber for someone consuming the 2000-calorie diet. The information on the panel regarding the 2500-calorie diet is not used by the manufacturer but is provided for consumers' information only. Furthermore, it is voluntary for the manufacturer to list percent Daily Value for protein.

New Label Definitions

Specific definitions of terms that manufacturers can use have been stipulated. The purpose is to help you know what you are buying, which means, of course, that you have to know the definitions. This is a fairly large challenge, as you can see in

TABLE 8.Q Label reference values (RDIs) current and proposed.*

CURRENT REFERENCE DAILY INTAKES*			PROPOSED REFERENCE DAILY INTAKES*		
Vitamins and Minerals	Units of Measurement	Adults and Children 4 or More Years of Age	Nutrient	Units of Measurement	Adults and Children 4 or More Years of Age
Vitamin A	International Units	5,000	Vitamin A	Retinol equivalents[1]	1,000
Vitamin D	International Units	400	Vitamin C	Milligrams	60
Vitamin E	International Units	30	Calcium	Milligrams	1,200
Vitamin C	Milligrams	60	Iron	Milligrams	15
Folic acid	Milligrams	0.4	Vitamin D	Micrograms[2]	10
Thiamin	Milligrams	1.5	Vitamin E	Alpha-tocopherol equivalents[1]	10
Riboflavin	Milligrams	1.7			
Niacin	Milligrams	20	Vitamin K	Micrograms	80
Vitamin B_6	Milligrams	2.0	Thiamin	Milligrams	1.5
Vitamin B_{12}	Micrograms	6.0	Riboflavin	Milligrams	1.8
Biotin	Milligrams	0.3	Niacin	Niacin equivalents[1]	20
Pantothenic acid	Milligrams	10	Vitamin B_{12}	Micrograms	2
Calcium	Grams	1.0	Phosphorus	Milligrams	1,200
Phosphorus	Grams	1.0	Magnesium	Milligrams	400
Iodine	Micrograms	150	Zinc	Milligrams	15
Iron	Milligrams	18	Iodine	Micrograms	150
Magnesium	Milligrams	400	Selenium	Micrograms	70
Copper	Milligrams	20	Chloride	Milligrams	3,400
Zinc	Milligrams	15			

[1] 1 retinol equivalent = 1 mcg retinol or 6 mcg beta-carotene; 1 alpha-tocopherol equivalent = 1 mg d-alpha-tocopherol (RRR-alpha-tocopherol); 1 niacin equivalent = 1 mg niacin or 60 mg of dietary tryptophan.
[2] As cholecalciferol.
** These label reference values were determined by selecting the highest 1989 RDA value from among those for adults and children 4 or more years of age excluding values for pregnant and lactating females.
* The label reference values currently in use (RDIs) are the same as the USRDAs which were determined by selecting the highest 1968 RDA value from among those for adults and children 4 or more years of age, excluding values for pregnant and lactating women.

FYI 10, which contains some of the commonly used terms, along with their now official definitions. Some study and some practice in shopping will be necessary before these definitions will become thoroughly familiar.

New Label Nuances: Buyer Beware

As with any new law designed to make things better, some things don't get corrected and new problems are created. Such is the case with the Nutrition Labeling and Education Act. The following are nuances in the regulations for the new law that could be misleading. You should be aware of the following:

- The allowable range for serving size is 50%–200% of the designated amount.
- Some designated serving sizes are too small or too large (e.g., the designated serving size for meat is 3 oz, but most people eat more than that in a serving).

- The term "sugars" includes both added and naturally occurring sugars, so foods such as fruit juices and milk will seem high in sugar because they have naturally occurring sugars.
- Fresh meats, poultry, and seafood can be listed as either raw or cooked, and comparing these two forms is nearly impossible.
- 2% fat milk can be labeled "low fat" even though it has 5 grams of fat per serving instead of 3 grams (see definition of low-fat). The only true low-fat milks are skim, nonfat, and 1%.
- Items marked "low-fat" and "low-in-saturated fat" have less fat than items marked "lean" and "extra lean."
- Packaged meals and main dishes labeled "low-fat" or "low sodium" are likely to contain more fat and sodium than you might expect, because of the amount of food in the package or because of more generous labeling definitions for meals than for individual foods. *Read carefully!*

New Definitions for Labeling Terms

Free (synonyms: *without, no, zero*):
Calorie Free: fewer than 5 calories/serving
Sugar Free: less than 0.5 grams/serving
Fat Free: less than 0.5 grams/serving

Low (synonyms: *little, few, low source of*):
Low Calorie: 40 calories or fewer/serving
Low Fat: 3 grams or less/serving
Low Saturated Fat: 1 gram or less/serving
Low Sodium: less than 140 mg/serving
Very Low Sodium: less than 35 mg/serving
Low Cholesterol: less than 20 mg/serving

Lean and Extra Lean (describes meat, poultry, seafood and game):

Lean:	less than 10 grams of fat, less than 4 grams of saturated fat, and less than 95 mg of cholesterol/100 grams or 3½ oz
Extra Lean:	less than 5 grams of fat, less than 2 grams of saturated fat, and less than 95 mg of cholesterol/100 grams or 3½ oz
High:	20% or more of the daily value for a particular nutrient in a serving
Reduced:	contains 25% less of a nutrient or of calories than the regular product
Light:	⅓ fewer calories or ½ the fat or ½ the sodium
More:	contains at least 10% of the Daily Value more than the reference food

THE IMPACT OF GOOD NUTRITION ON HEALTH

The dietary guidelines presented in this chapter leave no doubt that the health experts in the United States believe that what we eat can increase or decrease our risk of developing serious degenerative diseases, especially cardiovascular disease, cancer, and diabetes. In the years to come, researchers will continue to explore and clarify the relationship between nutrition and these conditions, but even today there is no doubt that nutrition does play a critical role.

The same can be said for the role of nutrition in the aging process. As explained in Chapter 3, the physical losses in function that occur with age seem to result primarily from disuse and from cell dysfunction and death. Because cells cannot function properly at any age without an adequate nutrient supply, the importance of good nutrition in maintaining maximum possible function and minimizing premature dysfunction is clear. Though we have only theories to explain what goes wrong with cells to ultimately cause dysfunction after 70–80 plus years, nutrition is a factor in all of these theories. Research indicates that nutrition indeed does have the power to increase or decrease the rapidity of aging.

The impact of nutrition on health extends further than simply minimizing the development of diseases and aging changes. Good nutrition is critical to feeling and doing your best. The importance of adequate nutrients for proper physiological functioning has been noted already; you can't be in top physical condition without it. What you eat also can influence your emotional state. Nutrition has been linked with feelings of depression and, in later life, with symptoms that mimic senility. If health can be described as being able to do the things you want and need to do and feeling that *now* is the best time to be alive, good nutrition is essential to health.

SUMMARY

Variety, quality, and quantity are the key determinants of good nutrition. In terms of quality, your diet needs to contain nutrients the body cannot function properly without and cannot make on its own. The six main categories of these essential nutrients are: protein, carbohydrate, fat, vitamins, minerals, and water. Quantity recommendations are not yet definite for all nutrients, but the U. S. Dietary Goals and the Recommended Dietary Allowances (the RDAs) are the prevailing quantity standards at present.

One of the most critical nutrients is protein, composed of nitrogen-containing components called amino acids. Nine of these amino acids are called essential because the body cannot make them. Any protein containing all nine of these essential amino acids in sufficient quantity for the body to use is called a complete protein; all others are incomplete proteins. All animal products except gelatin provide complete proteins. With the exception of legumes, vegetable proteins are incomplete. By eating certain combinations of vegetables, grains, nuts, and seeds or by eating them with a source of complete protein such as milk, it is possible to get complete protein without actually eating meat. National nutrition studies indicate that the average American overconsumes protein from childhood through old age. Nutrition experts currently advise limiting protein to no more than 10%–15% of total daily calories.

Americans also are eating more fat than the recommended 30% or less of daily calories. The average American consumes about 34% or more of his or her daily calories in fat. About 95% of the fat in the diet is composed basically of three kinds of fatty acids: saturated, monounsaturated, and polyunsaturated. Although most foods actually contain mixtures of all three types, saturated fats predominate in animal products. Diets high in saturated fat increase the risk of cardiovascular disease, whereas diets emphasizing mono- and polyunsaturated fats seem to provide protection from CVD. High-fat diets, regardless of the type of fat, increase the risk of several forms of cancer.

Cholesterol is another type of fat found in the diet of those who consume animal products. Americans eat between 320 and 450 mg of cholesterol a day even though the liver can make all that the body needs and despite the fact that high levels of cholesterol in the blood increase the risk for cardiovascular disease. Reducing cholesterol intake to 300 mg or less is recommended.

All evidence indicates that choosing a low-fat, low-cholesterol diet is advisable for overall good health. This requires an emphasis on vegetables, grains, and fruit, and limited intake of meats such as beef, pork, and lamb, as well as butter and eggs.

The incidence of cardiovascular disease and cancer is lower among people whose diets are high in carbohydrate. Some evidence suggests that the fiber and vitamins and minerals in carbohydrate foods actually may help prevent these problems in addition to supplying the body with essential nutrients. For these reasons, nutrition experts are recommending that Americans increase their carbohydrate intake from the current 46% of daily calories to 55% or more. This recommendation, however, stipulates eating no more than 10% of daily calories in the form of refined sugars. Refined sugars, or simple carbohydrates, contain none of the fiber or vitamins and minerals found in the complex carbohydrates—fruits, vegetables, and grains.

In terms of fuel for body functioning, protein and carbohydrate each provide the body with 4 calories of energy per gram. Fat is more energy-dense, providing 9 calories per gram. Of these three nutrient groups, carbohydrate and fat are the body's preferred fuel sources. If these are in sufficient supply, protein can be "spared" for structural growth and repair, its primary role.

The essential nutrients called vitamins and minerals are substances the body seems to need to grow and to function properly, but they provide no calories for energy. Even with the technological advancements made over the years, much remains unknown about these substances, including how much people actually need for good health. Consequently, controversy prevails regarding the quantities of certain vitamins and minerals that people should consume. Vitamins A, C, and E are prominent examples. It is important to check the validity of claims made for these and other nutrients before consuming large amounts.

Currently 13 vitamins are known to be required by the body and must be consumed. These are the fat-soluble vitamins A, D, E, and K, and the water-soluble B complex (eight total) and C vitamins. The fat-soluble vitamins are carried into the body with the aid of fat in the diet and are stored in fat in the body. Thus, it is not absolutely critical to eat them each day unless the amounts being consumed and in body stores are low compared to recommended intake. In fact, fat-soluble vitamins can accumulate to toxic levels if they are consumed in excess over time. Water-soluble vitamins are not stored in the body to any great extent and thus have to be eaten daily. But even these vitamins, when consumed in very large amounts, can cause undesirable and even harmful side effects.

Twenty-one minerals are known to be essential to body functioning. Calcium, phosphorus, sodium, and potassium are examples of macrominerals, needed in quantities of 100 mg or more per day. Iron, copper, and zinc are examples of microminerals, needed in amounts less than a few mg per day.

Thus far, recommended intake has been established for only 7 of the 21 minerals. Amounts described only as "estimated safe and adequate" have been suggested for seven minerals, and a minimum requirement has been set for two others. This ignorance regarding minerals is potentially dangerous because minerals tend to be toxic at much lower levels than vitamins. Toxicity levels for many minerals have not been clearly established. Because calcium and iron often are lacking in the American diet, and because consumption of sodium and chloride (salt) is close to excessive, specific discussions are provided regarding these minerals.

Because the body daily loses 2½ to 3 quarts of water in urine, perspiration, and feces, and by evaporation in the lungs, this fluid must be replaced every day. This means consuming about a quart of water, or 4 cups for every 1000 calories consumed. Fortunately, food can supply some of this water, leaving 6–8 cups to be consumed in beverage form.

Several governmental agencies and private organizations have proposed nutritional standards and guidelines over the years. Foremost of these have been the Recommended Dietary Allowances (RDAs) and U.S. Dietary Goals. In 1990 the Nutrition Labeling and Education Act (NLEA) required new information to be placed on foodstuffs sold commercially. The Food and Drug Administration was charged with developing definitions to standardize the terms used.

In all, the information provided in this chapter makes one clear statement: Good nutrition is essential for health.

REFERENCES

"Alcohol Alert." 1989. *Tuft's University Diet and Nutrition Letter* 7(March): 1.

Altscul, A., and Grommet, J. 1980. "Sodium Intake and Sodium Sensitivity." *Nutrition Reviews* 38: 393.

American Cancer Society. 1987. *Eating Smart.* New York: ACS.

American Cancer Society. 1988. *Eat Smart with Fruits and Vegetables.* New York: ACS.

"Antioxidants Re-examined." 1994. *Harvard Women's Health Watch* 1(11): 1.

"Baby 'Label' Arrives." 1993. *Nutrition Action Healthletter* 20(March): 7–9.

Barrett-Connor, E., et al. 1993. "Coffee-associated Osteoporosis Offset by Daily Milk Consumption." *Journal of the American Medical Association* 271(4): 280–283.

Bernard, P., et al. 1993. "Content in 70 Brands of Dietary Calcium Supplements." *American Journal of Public Health* 83(8): 1155–1160.

Blot, W. J., J. Y. Li, et al. 1993. "Nutrition Intervention Trials in Linxian, China: Supplementation with Specific Vitamin/Mineral Combinations, Cancer Incidence, and Disease-specific Mortality in the General Population." *Journal of the National Cancer Institute* 85(18): 1483–1492.

Brody, J. 1987. *Jane Brody's Nutrition Book.* New York: Bantam Books.

"Buying Guide: Sugar Substitutes." 1986. *University of California Berkeley, Wellness Letter* 2 (June): 9.

"Caffeine: Grounds for Concern?" 1994. *University of California Berkeley, Wellness Letter* 10(March): 4–6.

"Caffeine Update: The News is Mostly Good." 1988. *University of California Berkeley, Wellness Letter* 4(10): 4–5.

"Calcium: Maximizing Its Benefit." 1994. *Johns Hopkins Medical Letter: Health After 50 6* (Feb.): 4–5.

"Calcium: Vital for Women and Men." 1994. *Consumer Reports On Health* 6(2): 13–15.

"Can Vitamin C Save Your Life?" 1994. *Consumer Reports On Health* 6(3): 25–27.

Connor, S. 1989. "The Cholesterol–Saturated Fat Index for Coronary Prevention: Background, Use, and a Comprehensive Table of Foods." *Journal of the American Dietetic Association* 89: 807–816.

"Daily Dietary Fat and Total Food-energy Intakes—Third National Health and Nutrition Examination Survey, Phase 1." 1994. *Morbidity & Mortality Weekly Report* 43(Feb.): 116–117, 123, 125.

Dinsmoor, R. 1986. "Seeking a Suitable Sweetener." *Diabetes Self-Management*, March–April: 26–28.

"Does Beta-carotene Prevent Cancer—or Cause It?" 1994. *Consumer Reports On Health* 6(8): 85–87.

"Does Salt Raise Your Blood Pressure?" 1994. *Consumer Reports On Health* 6(April): 42–43.

"Don't Be Jittery About Decaf." 1990. *University of California Berkeley, Wellness Letter* 6 (February): 5.

Evans, W., Rosenberg, I. H., and Thompson, J. 1992. *Biomarkers*. New York: Simon & Schuster.

"First, Antioxidants. Now It's Phytochemicals!" 1994. *American Health* 13(July/Aug.): 92, 94.

"Fish Oil Capsules vs. Fish." 1994. *University of California Berkeley, Wellness Letter* 10(June): 4.

Food and Nutrition Board, Committee on Dietary Allowances. 1989. *Recommended Dietary Allowances*, 10th ed. Washington, DC: National Academy of Sciences.

"Free Radicals and Antioxidants: Finding the Key to Heart Disease, Cancer, and the Aging Process." 1991. *University of California Berkeley, Wellness Letter* 8(Oct.): 4–5.

Gey, K. F., et al. 1987. "Plasma Levels of Antioxidant Vitamins in Relation to Ischemic Heart Disease and Cancer." *American Journal of Clinical Nutrition* 45: 1368–1377.

Glomset, J. 1985. "Fish, Fatty Acids, and Human Health." *New England Journal of Medicine* 312: 1253.

Greger, J. L. 1988. "Effect of Variations in Dietary Protein, Phosphorous, Electrolytes and Vitamin D on Calcium and Zinc Metabolism." *Nutrient Interactions*, edited by C. W. Bodwell and J. W. Erdman, Jr. New York: Marcel Dekker.

Grobbee, D., et al. 1990. "Coffee, Caffeine, and CVD in Men." *New England Journal of Medicine* 323: 1026–1031.

Guthrie, H. 1986. *Introductory Nutrition*. St. Louis: C. V. Mosby.

Heaney, R. P., and Recker, R. R. 1986. "Distribution of Calcium Absorption in Middle-Aged Women." *American Journal of Clinical Nutrition* 43: 182–185.

Henry, H., et al. 1985. "Increasing Calcium Intake Lowers Blood Pressure: The Literature Reviewed." *Journal of the American Dietetic Association* 85: 182–185.

Hubbard, J., et al. 1985. "Nathan Pritikin's Heart." *New England Journal of Medicine* 4: 52.

Hui, Y. 1985. *Principles and Issues in Nutrition*. Monterey, CA: Wadsworth.

"Iron: Too Much of a Good Thing?" 1994. *Consumer Reports On Health* July 76–77.

Jenkins, D., et al. 1989. "Nibbling vs. Gorging: Metabolic Advantages of Increased Meal Frequency." *New England Journal of Medicine* 321: 929–934.

Kies, C. 1989. "Copper, Manganese and Zinc: Micronutrients of Macroconcern." *Food and Nutrition News* 61(March/April): 2.

Krombout, D., et al. 1985. "The Inverse Relationship Between Fish Consumption and 20-year Mortality from Coronary Heart Disease." *New England Journal of Medicine* 312: 1205.

Lang, S. 1984. "Beyond Bran." *American Health* 3(3): 64.

Liebman, B. 1990. "The HDL/Triglyceride Trap: An Interview with Wm. Castelli." *Nutrition Action Newsletter* 17: 5–7.

Looker, A. C. et al. June 6–8, 1994. *Calcium Intake in the United States*. Paper presented at the National Institute of Health Consensus Development Conference on Calcium.

McBean, L. D. 1987. "Food Versus Pills Versus Fortified Foods." *Dairy Council Digest* 58 (March–April).

McCarron, D. A., et al. 1987. "The Calcium Paradox of Essential Hypertension." *American Journal of Medicine* 82(supplement): 27–33.

Menkes, M., and Comstock, G. 1984. "Vitamins A and E and Lung Cancer." *American Journal of Epidemiology* 120(3): 342–349.

Mensinki, R. P., and Martin, K. B. 1990. "Effects of Dietary Trans Fatty Acids on High Density and Low Density Lipoprotein Cholesterol Levels in Healthy Subjects." *New England Journal of Medicine* 323: 439–447.

"Might Americans Be Taking in Too Much Iron?" 1993. *Tufts University Diet & Nutrition Letter* 10(11): 3–6.

"Minerals: Facts and Fancy." 1991. *University of California, Berkeley Wellness Letter*.

National Dairy Council. 1989. *Calcium: A Summary of Current Research for the Health Professional*. Rosemont, IL: NDC.

National Osteoporosis Foundation. 1989. *Boning Up on Osteoporosis—A Guide to Prevention and Treatment*. Farmington, MA: NOF.

National Research Council. 1990. *Diet and Health Implications for Reducing Chronic Disease Risk.* Washington, DC: National Academy of Sciences.

Nieman, D. C., Butterworth, D. E., and Nieman, C. N. 1992. *Nutrition* Dubuque, IA: Wm. C. Brown Publishers.

"On the Margarine-Butter Controversy." 1994. *Tufts University Diet & Nutrition Letter* 12(5): 1–2.

Ornish, D. 1990. *Dr. Dean Ornish's Program for Reversing Heart Disease.* New York: Random House.

Ornish, D. 1993. *Eat More, Weigh Less.* New York: HarperCollins.

"Phytochemicals: Plants Against Cancer." 1994. *Nutrition Action Healthletter* 21(3): 1, 9–11.

"Pressing Garlic for Possible Health Benefits." 1994. *Tufts University Diet & Nutrition Letter* 12(7): 3–6.

Public Health Service, Department of Health and Human Services. 1988. *The Surgeon General's Report on Nutrition and Health* (PHS publication #88-50210). Washington, DC: Government Printing Office.

"Pumping Immunity." 1993. *Nutrition Action Healthletter* 20(3): 1, 4–7.

"Salt—Adjusting for Age." 1988. *University of California Berkeley, Wellness Letter* 5(February): 2.

Samet, J. M., et al. 1985. "Lung Cancer Risk and Vitamin A Consumption in New Mexico." *American Review of Respiratory Disorders* 131: 198–202.

Sanborn, C. F. 1990. "Exercise, Calcium and Bone Density." *Sports Science Exchange* 2(24): 271–274.

Schaafasma, G., et al. 1987. "Nutritional Aspects of Osteoporosis." *World Review of Nutrition and Diet* 49: 121–159.

Schiffman, S., et al. 1987. "Aspartame and Susceptibility to Headache." *New England Journal of Medicine* 317: 1181.

Shah, B. G. 1987. "Calcium Supplementation with Antacids." *Journal of American Medical Association* 257: 541.

Siger, F., and Whitney. 1994. *Nutrition: Concepts and Controversies*, 6th ed. Minneapolis: West Publishing.

Smolin, L. A., and Grosvenor, M. B. 1994. *Nutrition: Science and Applications*. New York: Saunders College Publishing.

Spencer, H. 1986. "Minerals and Mineral Interactions in Human Beings." *Journal of American Dietetic Association* 86: 864–867.

Spencer, H., et al. 1988. "Do Protein and Phosphorus Cause Calcium Loss?" *Journal of Nutrition* 118: 657–660.

"The Coffee Connection." 1994. *Harvard Women's Health Watch* 1(8): 2–3.

"The Heart Health-E Vitamin?" 1994. *Nutrition Action Healthletter* 21(Jan./Feb.): 8–10.

"The Salt Shakeout." 1994. *Nutrition Action Healthletter* 21(2): 1, 5–6.

"The Truth About Calcium." 1988. *Consumer Reports* May: 288–291.

"To Take Antioxidant Pills or Not: The Debate Heats Up." 1994. *Tufts University Diet and Nutrition Letter* 123(3): 3–6.

"Tumor Growth Halted with Synthetic Vitamin E." 1993. *American Institute for Cancer Research Newsletter* 41: 9.

U.S. Department of Agriculture, Department of Health and Human Services. 1982. *The Sodium Content of Your Food* (Home & Garden Bulletin #233). Washington, DC: Government Printing Office.

U.S. Department of Health and Human Services. 1989. *Nutrition Monitoring in the U.S.* Washington, DC: Government Printing Office.

U.S. Senate Select Committee on Nutrition and Human Needs. 1977. *Dietary Goals for the United States*, 2d ed. Washington, DC: Government Printing Office.

Valsey-Gehser, M., and Eskin, N. 1987. *Canola Oil Properties and Performance*. Winnipeg, Manitoba: Canola Council.

"Vegetarianism: You Can Get By Without Meat." 1980. *Consumer Reports* 45(June): 357.

"Vitamin C Protects Blood from Radicals." 1989. *Science News* 136(August): 133.

"Vitamins: Facts and Fancy." 1991. *University of California, Berkeley Wellness Letter.*

Weinsier, R. 1985. "Recent Developments in the Etiology and Treatment of Hypertension: Dietary Calcium, Fat, and Magnesium." *American Journal of Clinical Nutrition* 42: 1331–1338.

"We're Still Taking Our Beta Carotene." 1994. *University of California, Berkeley Wellness Letter* 10(10): 1–2.

Whitney, E. N., and Rolfes, S. R. 1993. *Understanding Nutrition.* St. Paul: West Publishing.

Willet, W., and Ascherio, A. 1994. "Trans Fatty Acids: Are the Effects Only Marginal?" *American Journal of Public Health* 84(5): 722–724.

"Wrap-Up: Minerals." 1986. *University of California Berkeley, Wellness Letter* 2(January): 4.

Checking-Up on Eating Well

✓ How well are you eating? Do you really know?

✓ What guidelines can you follow to choose a health-promoting diet for yourself?

✓ How can you shop for and prepare the most nutritious foods?

✓ Should you be taking supplements?

According to the statistics reported in Chapter 8, Americans in general need to change many of their eating habits in order to enjoy optimum vitality and longevity. The problem is that even statistically supported evidence doesn't cause very many people to change their behavior. People all have a tendency to read the evidence, believe it, be concerned about it, and yet not *do* much about it. It's easy to think that these statistics apply only to other people, but only a nutrition "check-up" will indicate whether that's true or not.

You may think that, although your diet could certainly use some improvement, overall it's not that bad. Or you may be rather sure your diet is poor. One way or another, checking-up on your diet—comparing it to the recommendations—is the best way to find out what, if anything, you need to change or improve. The techniques and procedures to help you do this type of dietary analysis are provided in the first part of this chapter. The second part of the chapter offers practical guidelines you can use as needed to implement the recommendations in Chapter 8. Eating patterns, use of supplements, and the selection and preparation of food to help you eat well are addressed.

NUTRITIONAL ASSESSMENT

Determining whether or not you are well-nourished is quite an involved task. A complete nutritional assessment would require in-depth personal history, anthropometric measurements, a physical examination, and biochemical and dietary analyses. The specific data that would be collected under each of these categories are indicated in Tables 9.A and 9.B. The services of trained professionals obviously would be required to analyze all of this material appropriately. The assessment would be both time-consuming and expensive. If you are in nutritional trouble, however, it could be worth it for your quality and quantity of life.

Although diet analysis is just one small part of a thorough nutritional assessment, it does provide an inexpensive, do-it-yourself way of "guestimating" whether you are eating well enough to provide the nutrients you need. If the results suggest that you are significantly

over- or undereating in terms of calories or specific nutrients, you then might seek professional consultation.

Of course, a diet analysis does not indicate if you are properly metabolizing and absorbing the food you eat, so periodic physical examinations and blood tests could be beneficial even if your diet analysis shows no problems. This precaution could be especially important if one or more of the nutritional risk factors or deficiency symptoms listed in Tables 9.A and 9.B apply to you.

Several methods are available today for analyzing your diet. Keeping a food diary of everything you eat for 3–7 days and then comparing the nutrient content of what you actually ate with the recommended dietary allowances and the Dietary Goals for Americans is one of the more accurate methods. Numerous computer programs are available for doing such an analysis; *Food Processor* and *Dine* are two examples. Given your height, weight, sex, age, and activity level, along with the data from your food diary, the computer can calculate your personal RDA and do all the nutrient comparisons in a matter of seconds.

If you do not have access to a computer, you can also do this type of diet analysis by hand using a government publication called *The Nutritive Value of Foods*. A sample page from that publication is shown in Figure 9.1. As you can see, the amounts

TABLE 9.A Nutritional assessment data: Possible causes/indicators of poor nutrition status.

MEDICAL PROBLEMS	DIET PRACTICES/PROBLEMS
Recent major illness/surgery	Very low calorie intake
Over- or underweight	Fad diets
Anorexia/bulimia	Fasting 10 days or more
Diarrhea or vomiting	Dental problems
Heavy smoking	Chewing/swallowing difficulty
Alcoholism	
AIDS	SOCIOECONOMIC CONDITIONS
Cancer	
Radiation or drug therapy	Inadequate income
Cardiovascular disease	Inadequate knowledge
Hyperlipidemia	Inadequate food storage
Hypertension	or preparation
Diabetes	Living/eating alone
Diseases of lung, liver, or kidney	
Neurologic disorders	ANTHROPOMETRIC MEASURES
Depression	
Other	Height
Drug use, regular or long-term	Weight
Legal: Prescription and	Skinfold or other body fat indicator
nonprescription	
Illegal	

Adapted from *Understanding Nutrition*, 6th ed., by E. Whitney and S. Rolfes (Minneapolis: West, 1993).

TABLE
9.B
Nutritional assessment data: Possible laboratory tests and physical indicators of vitamin and mineral deficiency/toxicity.

VITAMIN		SELECTED PHYSICAL SIGNS/SYMPTOMS OF DEFICIENCY (D)/TOXICITY (T) IN ADULTS	LAB TESTS
Vitamin A	(D)	Triangular gray spots on eye; dryness of eyes; night blindness; dry, scaly, "goosebump" skin	Serum vitamin A Serum carotene
	(T)	Joint pain, bleeding, loss of appetite, loss of hair, menstrual cessation, jaundice	
Thiamin (B$_1$)	(D)	Muscle weakness, calf-muscle pain, loss of ankle and knee-jerk reflex, edema in lower limbs	Erythrocyte transketolase
Riboflavin (B$_2$)	(D)	Redness, scaling, and cracking at corners of mouth; magenta-colored tongue; light sensitivity; mental confusion	Erythrocyte glutathione reductase
Niacin (B$_3$) (Nicotinic acid)	(D)	Enlarged, reddened, "smooth" tongue; irritability; bilateral skin irritation on backs of hands, forearms, legs, etc.	Urinary N-methyl-nicotinamide
	(T)	Skin burning, itching, and flushing; nausea and diarrhea	
Pyridoxine (B$_6$)	(D)	Cracking at corners of mouth; enlarged, red tongue; irritation of sweat glands; weakness; nervousness	Serum vitamins Tryptophan load test
	(T)	Nerve damage	
Folacin (Folic acid)	(D)	Cracked and swollen tongue, diarrhea, anemia	Red cell folate
Cobalamin (B$_{12}$)	(D)	Smooth, swollen tongue; numbness in fingers and toes; skin sensitivity; anemia; lemon-yellow color	Serum B$_{12}$ Urinary methyl-malonic acid
Vitamin C	(D)	Bleeding, spongy gums; pinpoint hemorrhages into skin; weakness; poor wound healing	Serum vitamin C Leukocyte vitamin C
	(T)	Cramps, diarrhea, nausea	
Vitamin D	(D)	Bone softening and bending, muscle cramps and twitching	Serum alkaline phosphatase
	(T)	Calcification in soft tissue, loss of appetite, thirst, nervousness	
Vitamin E	(D)	Rare: red blood cell fragility; possible edema and flaky dermatitis	Erythrocyte hemolysis test Plasma tocopherol
	(T)	Not definitely known. Some reports of cramps, diarrhea, possible impaired clotting time, increased blood lipids in women using oral contraceptives, decreased serum thyroid hormone	
MINERAL			
Calcium	(D)	Osteoporosis, uncontrollable muscle contractions, seizures	Serum calcium
Potassium	(D)	Muscle weakness, hypotension, respiratory failure, arrhythmia	Serum potassium
	(T)	Abnormal heart function	
Magnesium	(D)	Uncontrollable muscle contractions, nervousness and tremors, nausea, lethargy, arrhythmias	Serum magnesium
Iron	(D)	Fatigue, weakness, pallor, headache, difficulty breathing upon exertion	Hemoglobin Hematocrit Serum ferritin
Iodine	(T)	Iron deposits in tissues, bronze-colored skin, blackened stools, arrhythmias, infections	Serum protein-bound iodine
	(D)	Goiter, sluggishness, weight gain	
Zinc	(D)	Impaired sense of taste and smell, poor appetite, slow wound healing, infections, impaired growth	Serum zinc Hair-zinc
	(T)	Nausea, exhaustion, anemia, diarrhea	

From *Understanding Nutrition*, 6th ed., by E. Whitney and S. Rolfes, (Minneapolis, MN: West Publishing, 1993); and *Nutrition*, 2nd ed., by D. Niemen (Dubuque, IA: Wm C. Brown, 1992).

FIGURE 9.1

Sample page from *The Nutritive Value of Foods.*

Item No	Foods, approximate measures, units and weight (weight of edible portion only)	Grams	Water Percent	Food energy Calories	Protein Grams	Fat Grams	Fatty Acids Saturated Grams	Monounsaturated Grams	Polyunsaturated Grams	Cholesterol Milligrams	Carbohydrate Grams	Calcium Milligrams	Phosphorus Milligrams	Iron Milligrams	Potassium Milligrams	Sodium Milligrams	Vitamin A value International units	Vitamin A value Retinol equivalents (RE)	Thiamin Milligrams	Riboflavin Milligrams	Niacin Milligrams	Ascorbic acid Milligrams	Item No
Poultry and Poultry Products																							
	Chicken:																						
	Fried, flesh, with skin:[53]																						
	Batter dipped:																						
656	Breast, 1/2 breast (5.6 oz with bones)-- 4.9 oz	140	52	365	35	18	4.9	7.6	4.3	119	13	28	259	1.8	281	385	90	28	0.16	0.20	14.7	0	656
657	Drumstick (3.4 oz with bones)-- 2.5 oz	72	53	195	16	11	3.0	4.6	2.7	62	6	12	106	1.0	134	194	60	19	0.08	0.15	3.7	0	657
	Flour coated:																						
658	Breast, 1/2 breast (4.2 oz with bones)-- 3.5 oz	98	57	220	31	9	2.4	3.4	1.9	87	2	16	228	1.2	254	74	50	15	0.08	0.13	13.5	0	658
659	Drumstick (2.6 oz with bones)-- 1.7 oz	49	57	120	13	7	1.8	2.7	1.6	44	1	6	86	0.7	112	44	40	12	0.04	0.11	3.0	0	659
	Roasted, flesh only:																						
660	Breast, 1/2 breast (4.2 oz with bones and skin)-- 3.0 oz	86	65	140	27	3	0.9	1.1	0.7	73	0	13	196	0.9	220	64	20	5	0.06	0.10	11.8	0	660
661	Drumstick, (2.9 oz with bones and skin)-- 1.6 oz	44	67	75	12	2	0.7	0.8	0.6	41	0	5	81	0.6	108	42	30	8	0.03	0.10	2.7	0	661
662	Stewed, flesh only, light and dark meat, chopped or diced-- 1 cup	140	67	250	38	9	2.6	3.3	2.2	116	0	20	210	1.6	252	98	70	21	0.07	0.23	8.6	0	662
663	Chicken liver, cooked-- 1 liver	20	68	30	5	1	0.4	0.3	0.2	126	Tr	3	62	1.7	28	10	3,270	983	0.03	0.35	0.9	3	663
664	Duck, roasted, flesh only-- 1/2 duck	221	64	445	52	25	9.2	8.2	3.2	197	0	27	449	6.0	557	144	170	51	0.57	1.04	11.3	0	664
	Turkey, roasted, flesh only:																						
	Dark meat, piece, 2-1/2 by																						
665	1-5/8 by 1/4 in-- 4 pieces	85	63	160	24	6	2.1	1.4	1.8	72	0	27	173	2.0	246	67	0	0	0.05	0.21	3.1	0	665
	Light meat, piece, 4 by 2 by																						
666	1/4 in-- 2 pieces	85	66	135	25	3	0.9	0.5	0.7	59	0	16	186	1.1	259	54	0	0	0.05	0.11	5.8	0	666
	Light and dark meat:																						
667	Chopped or diced-- 1 cup	140	65	240	41	7	2.3	1.4	2.0	106	0	35	298	2.5	417	98	0	0	0.09	0.25	7.6	0	667
	Pieces (1 slice white meat, 4 by 2 by 1/4 in and 2 slices dark meat, 2-1/2																						
668	by 1-5/8 by 1/4 in)-- 3 pieces	85	65	145	25	4	1.4	0.9	1.2	65	0	21	181	1.5	253	60	0	0	0.05	0.15	4.6	0	668
	Poultry food products:																						
	Chicken:																						
669	Canned, boneless-- 5 oz	142	69	235	31	11	3.1	4.5	2.5	88	0	20	158	2.2	196	714	170	48	0.02	0.18	9.0	3	669
670	Frankfurter (10 per 1-lb pkg)-- 1 frankfurter	45	58	115	6	9	2.5	3.8	1.8	45	3	43	48	0.9	38	616	60	17	0.03	0.05	1.4	0	670
671	Roll, light (6 slices per 6 oz pkg)-- 2 slices	57	69	90	11	4	1.1	1.7	0.9	28	1	24	89	0.6	129	331	50	14	0.04	0.07	3.0	0	671
	Turkey:																						
672	Gravy and turkey, frozen-- 5-oz package	142	85	95	8	4	1.2	1.4	0.7	26	7	20	115	1.3	87	787	60	18	0.03	0.18	2.6	0	672
673	Ham, cured turkey thigh meat (8 slices per 8-oz pkg)-- 2 slices	57	71	75	11	3	1.0	0.7	0.9	32	Tr	6	108	1.6	184	565	0	0	0.03	0.14	2.0	0	673
674	Loaf, breast meat (8 slices per 6-oz pkg)-- 2 slices	42	72	45	10	1	0.2	0.2	0.1	17	0	3	97	0.2	118	608	0	0	0.02	0.05	3.5	[54]0	674
675	Patties, breaded, battered, fried (2.25 oz)-- 1 patty	64	50	180	9	12	3.0	4.8	3.0	40	10	9	173	1.4	176	512	20	7	0.06	0.12	1.5	0	675
676	Roast, boneless, frozen, seasoned, light and dark meat, cooked-- 3 oz	85	68	130	18	5	1.6	1.0	1.4	45	3	4	207	1.4	253	578	0	0	0.04	0.14	5.3	0	676
Soups, Sauces, and Gravies																							
	Soups:																						
	Canned, condensed:																						
	Prepared with equal volume of milk:																						
677	Clam chowder, New England-- 1 cup	248	85	165	9	7	3.0	2.3	1.1	22	17	186	156	1.5	300	992	160	40	0.07	0.24	1.0	3	677
678	Cream of chicken-- 1 cup	248	85	190	7	11	4.6	4.5	1.6	27	15	181	151	0.7	273	1,047	710	94	0.07	0.26	0.9	1	678
679	Cream of mushroom-- 1 cup	248	85	205	6	14	5.1	3.0	4.6	20	15	179	156	0.6	270	1,076	150	37	0.08	0.28	0.9	2	679
680	Tomato-- 1 cup	248	85	160	6	6	2.9	1.6	1.1	17	22	159	149	1.8	449	932	850	109	0.13	0.25	1.5	68	680

[53] Fried in vegetable shortening.

[54] If sodium ascorbate is added, product contains 11 mg ascorbic acid.

of six vitamins, five minerals, fat, protein, carbohydrates, and calories are given for commonly consumed food; more than 900 foods are listed. If you consume adequate amounts of these key nutrients and a minimum of 1200 calories per day, your diet probably provides all the other vitamins and minerals you need. The Recommended Dietary Allowances for individuals of different ages and gender also are included in the publication, for comparison purposes. As almost every major nutrition textbook includes a copy of this document, obtaining it for yourself can be as easy as a trip to the library or bookstore. You can also locate it in the government section of the library, or you can purchase it directly from the Government Printing Office in Washington, DC.

You also can compare the total calories you consume in a day with your caloric expenditure. This should be of some help in analyzing your present weight control problems and preventing future ones. Instructions for calculating your daily caloric expenditure were given in Chapter 7. It would be best, of course, to calculate your expenditure for the same days you record your food intake. If done carefully, this should provide the most accurate estimate of your caloric expenditure. You can, however, estimate your expenditure using the formula given in Table 9.C or using the values listed in the RDA tables in Appendix 6. The RDA tables for energy expenditure will be your least accurate estimate unless you are exactly the height and weight and activity level (light to moderate) of the reference people in the table.

If you wish to utilize the food diary method, specific instructions and forms that you can use to complete your data collection and analysis are included in Lab 25, Appendix 9. You can use Forms 1 and 2 to record your food intake and energy expenditure. Forms 3–7 will assist you in comparing the nutrient value of your diet with the RDAs and the Dietary Goals for Americans.

Another way to analyze your diet is the *diet recall* method. This method relies on your recall of what you have eaten during a specified time period. To obtain this information you are generally asked to respond to a series of questions about your eating habits—the kinds of foods you eat and the quantities and frequency. This technique can produce an analysis of your diet in less than 30 minutes, but its accuracy depends on your memory and honesty. It can provide a lot of valuable information, but it cannot provide the detail, in terms of vitamins, minerals, and calories, that you can obtain using the food diary technique.

The diet recall instrument presented in Lab 24 was developed by the Lipid Atherosclerosis Nutrition Staff of the Oregon Health Sciences University, Portland, Oregon. Called the Diet Habit Survey Quiz, this instrument is designed to evaluate your current eating habits in comparison with the goals of the New American Diet. The New American Diet was developed by Sonja Connor, R.D., and William Conner, M.D., based on international data regarding diet and disease prevention and, in particular, a five-year family heart study. This study was funded by the National Institutes of Health to determine what desirable dietary changes the general population would be willing and able to adopt.

Results of the family heart study showed that people could make health-enhancing changes in their diet, but not overnight. The book *The New American Diet* contains a description of three phases of dietary modifications leading from the typical American diet toward the Dietary Goals for Americans and even beyond. The dietary behaviors that typify each phase are summarized in Figure 9.2. The behaviors constituting Phase III of the New American Diet actually represent more stringent goals in terms of fat, cholesterol, and salt intake than do the Dietary Goals for Americans. The current American diet, the 1989 Dietary Goals for Americans, and

TABLE 9.C   Estimated daily caloric need.

ACTIVITY LEVEL	CALORIES PER POUND EXPENDED
1. Very sedentary: no activity; confined to house	13
2. Sedentary: typical American with office job/light work	14
3. Moderate: #2 plus weekend recreation	15
4. Very active: complies with American College of Sports Medicine standards of vigorous exercise 3×/wk	16
5. Competitive athlete: vigorous activity	17+

Formula: Weight in pounds × Activity Level Expenditure

Example: 120 lb. female × Sedentary Activity Level
120 lb. × 14 = 1680 calories
Estimated daily caloric need = 1680 calories

Adapted from American Heart Association, Dallas.

FIGURE

9.2   Summary of the three phases of the New American Diet.

THE NEW AMERICAN DIET STEP BY STEP

PHASE I: SUBSTITUTIONS

This is accomplished by:
- avoiding egg yolks, butterfat, lard and organ meats (liver, heart, brains, kidney, gizzards);
- substituting soft margarine for butter;
- substituting vegetable oils and shortening for lard;
- substituting skim milk and skim milk products for whole milk and whole milk products;
- substituting egg whites for whole eggs;
- trimming fat off meat and skin from chicken;
- choosing commercial food products lower in cholesterol and fat (low-fat cheeses, egg substitutes, soy meat substitutes, frozen yogurt, etc.).
- modifying favorite recipes by using less fat or sugar and vegetable oils instead of butter or lard;
- decreasing use of table salt and using lower sodium salt (Lite Salt)

PHASE II: NEW RECIPES

This step involves:
- reducing amounts of meat and cheese eaten and replacing them with chicken and fish;
- eating meat, chicken or fish only once a day;
- cutting down on fat; as spreads, in salads, cooking and baking;

- eating more grains, beans, fruits and vegetables;
- making low-fat, low-cholesterol choices when eating out;
- finding new recipes to replace those that cannot be altered;
- using few products containing salt

PHASE III: A NEW WAY OF EATING

The final phase means:
- eating meat, cheese, poultry, shellfish, and fish as "condiments" to other foods, rather than as main courses;
- eating more beans and grain products as protein sources;
- using no more than 4–7 teaspoons of fat per day as spreads, salad dressings and in cooking and baking;
- drinking 4–6 glasses of water per day;
- keeping extra meat, regular cheese, chocolate, candy, coconut and richer home-baked or commercially prepared food for special occasions (once a month or less);
- enjoying a wide variety of new food and repertoire of totally new and savory recipes;
- decreasing amount of salt used for cooking

From *The New American Diet* by S. Connor and W. Connor (New York: Simon & Schuster, 1986).

the New American Diet are compared in Table 9.D. The Diet Habit Survey, Lab 24, will allow you to see how your own diet compares.

CHOOSING A HEALTH-PROMOTING DIET

Just as diagnosing a disease doesn't cure it, neither does a dietary analysis automatically improve one's diet. In the first instance, a prescription of some sort is generally given in hopes of restoring health. Prescriptions also have been written to help people select foods that optimize healthy functioning and minimize risk of disease. The Food Guide Pyramid

and the National Research Council's 1989 *Diet and Health* recommendations are two of these. If you are one of the few people whose diet analysis indicated you are eating well in all categories of comparison, congratulations! The information in the rest of this chapter will simply help you refine your already good nutritional habits. If your diet did not meet recommendations, the following dietary "prescriptions" could make a significant difference in your well-being now and in the future.

Food Guide Pyramid

In 1992 the U.S. Department of Agriculture introduced the Food Guide Pyramid as the new guide for Americans to use in selecting foods to meet their nutrient requirements as well as the Dietary Goals for Americans (discussed later in this chapter). The Food Guide Pyramid replaces the Basic Four Food Groups, which had been the guide in use since 1956. As shown in Figure 9.3, the Food Guide Pyramid divides foods into five major categories and recommends a range of servings in each category. The five major categories are (1) bread, cereal, rice, and pasta; (2) vegetables; (3) fruits; (4) milk, yogurt, and cheese; and (5) meat, poultry, fish, dry beans, eggs, and nuts. There actually is a sixth group, fats, oils, and sweets, but rather than a serving recommendation, it has a "Use Sparingly" caution.

The pyramid shape is meant to reflect the number of servings to be eaten each day from each of these categories to meet nutrient requirements. The Bread, Cereal, Rice, & Pasta group is at the base of the Food Guide Pyramid, with 6–11 servings recommended. The Vegetable and the Fruit groups share the next level, with 3–5 and 2–4 servings recommended, respectively. The Milk, Yogurt, & Cheese group and the Meat, Poultry, Fish, Dry Beans, Eggs, & Nuts group are next to the top of the pyramid and, thus, have the smallest recommended number of servings at 2–3 for each group. The Fats, Oils, & Sweets group at the top of the pyramid are not recommended in any amounts except "sparingly" because they provide

TABLE

9.0   Comparison of the current American diet, Dietary Goals for Americans, and New American Diet, Phase III.

	CURRENT AMERICAN DIET	DIETARY GOALS FOR AMERICANS, 1989	NEW AMERICAN DIET (PHASE III)
Fat, percent (%) of total calories	34+	<30	20
Saturated fat (% of total calories)	12+	<10	5
Monounsaturated fat (% of total calories)	15	10+	8
Polyunsaturated fat (% of total calories)	7	10	7
Protein (% of total calories)	16	10–15	15
Carbohydrate (% of total calories)	46	55+	65
Cholesterol (mg/day)	320–450	<300	<100
Salt (grams/day)	10–20	<6	<6

From *Prescription for Lower Chronic Disease Risk: Less Fat and More Fruits, Vegetables and Complex Carbohydrates*, by the National Research Council (Washington, DC: National Research Council, 1989); *Surgeon General's Report on Nutrition and Health*, by the Department of Health and Human Services (DHHS Publication #PHS 88–50210) (Washington, DC: Government Printing Office, 1988); *The New American Diet*, by S. Connor and W. Connor (New York: Simon & Schuster, 1986) and *Morbidity & Mortality Weekly Report* 43, Feb. 25, 1994.

so many calories but few of the required nutrients. Examples of what constitutes a serving for each of the five food groups are included in Figure 9.3.

If you "eat the pyramid" each day in terms of number of servings, you could do very well in terms of getting the nutrients you need. Depending upon the foods you select from each category, you also could end up eating too many calories, too much fat, and too much salt. Although the narrative that accompanies the Food Guide Pyramid does suggest foods to "select" and foods that should be "limited," just looking at the pyramid itself suggests that all that is required is a certain number of servings per food group. The term "limit" isn't specific or directive, given the wide range of eating habits people have, and not everyone will even read the narrative.

Another potential problem in making healthful food selections lurks in the Meat, Poultry, Fish, Dry Beans, Eggs, & Nuts group. The fat content of even lean meat is much greater than dry beans, for example, and nuts are much higher in fat than fish. These foods also have a fiber difference. By lumping protein sources together, the Food Guide Pyramid suggests that two to three "lean" hamburgers per day would be just fine for protein. Although that is true for protein, the total fat and saturated fat content of even one "lean" hamburger would not make it an advisable selection every day let alone *several* hamburgers per day!

To address some of the problems with the Food Guide Pyramid, the Center for Science in the Public Interest (CSPI) has developed a modification of its own. CSPI's Healthy Eating Pyramid* has three different panels: an Anytime panel, a Sometimes panel, and a Seldom panel, including recommended foods and serving sizes (see Figure 9.4). The Anytime panel suggests foods in each food group that are low in fat and saturated fat and have no other major drawbacks such as being high in salt or sodium. "Anytime" means that these are good choices every day and even several times a day, according to the number of servings recommended.

The Sometimes panel suggests foods that have moderate amounts of fat or saturated fat, or that are high in unsaturated fats, sodium, cholesterol, or added sugar. Foods made from white flour or white rice are also on this panel. "Sometimes" means to choose no more than two or three of these foods per day or, if more, then extra-small servings.

Most of the foods on the Seldom panel are high in fat and saturated fat; some have moderate amounts of fat but are high in sodium, cholesterol, or added sugars. "Seldom" means small portions *and* no more than two or three times per week.

In addition to the specific recommendations regarding food choices, CSPI's Healthy Eating Pyramid categorizes the low-fat, high-fiber dry beans with its vegetable group. The number of

---

*You can get a three-dimensional model of the Healthy Eating Pyramid by writing to CSPI-Pyramid, Suite 300, 1875 Connecticut Ave, NW, Washington, DC 20009. A two-dimensional model was published in the December 1992 issue of CSPI's *Nutrition Action Health Letter,* an excellent monthly publication with the latest and "hottest" nutrition news and analysis of issues and foods.

FIGURE
9.3
Food Guide Pyramid: A guide to daily food choices.

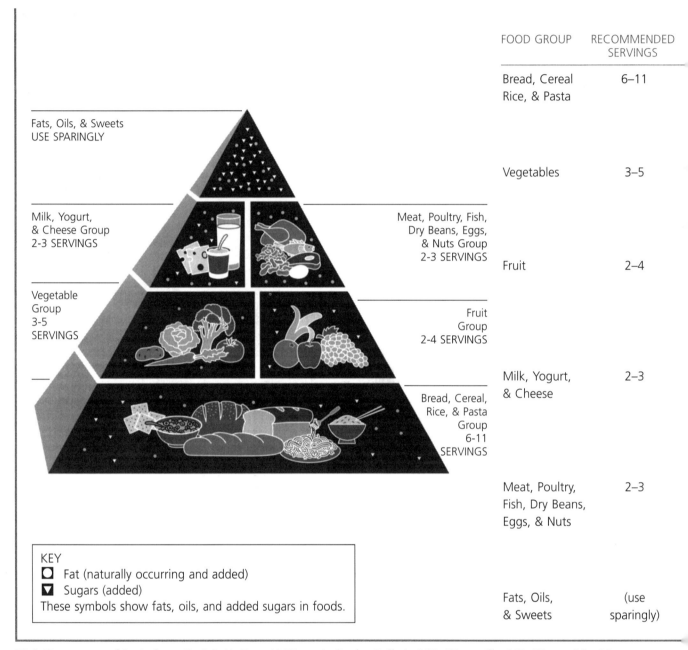

FOOD GROUP	RECOMMENDED SERVINGS
Bread, Cereal Rice, & Pasta	6–11
Vegetables	3–5
Fruit	2–4
Milk, Yogurt, & Cheese	2–3
Meat, Poultry, Fish, Dry Beans, Eggs, & Nuts	2–3
Fats, Oils, & Sweets	(use sparingly)

Fats, Oils, & Sweets
USE SPARINGLY

Milk, Yogurt,
& Cheese Group
2-3 SERVINGS

Meat, Poultry, Fish,
Dry Beans, Eggs,
& Nuts Group
2-3 SERVINGS

Vegetable
Group
3-5
SERVINGS

Fruit
Group
2-4 SERVINGS

Bread, Cereal,
Rice, & Pasta
Group
6-11
SERVINGS

KEY
▢ Fat (naturally occurring and added)
▼ Sugars (added)
These symbols show fats, oils, and added sugars in foods.

U. S. Department of Agriculture, *Food Guide Pyramid* (Home & Garden Bulletin 252) (Hyattsville, MD: Human Nutrition Information Service, 1992).

servings for the Vegetable and Beans group is increased by one, for a total of 4–6 servings, and the number of servings for the Fish, Poultry, Meat, Nuts, & Eggs group is reduced by one, for a total of 1–2 servings.

Another feature of CSPI's Healthy Eating Pyramid is the Mixed Food category, which lists frequently consumed food combinations such as sandwiches, burritos, pizza, salads, and so forth.

The popularity of these foods makes this extra category extremely valuable in trying to make healthy food choices.

The serving sizes for CSPI's Healthy Eating Pyramid also are somewhat different from those listed by the USDA for the Food Guide Pyramid. CSPI has chosen slightly larger serving sizes, which are more reflective of the amounts most people perceive as a serving. For example, two

SERVING EXAMPLES FOR THE FOOD GROUPS OF THE FOOD GUIDE PYRAMID

SIZE EXAMPLES	SELECTION RECOMMENDATIONS
1/2 cup cooked cereal 1 oz dry cereal 1 slice bread 2 cookies 1/2 medium doughnut	Choose whole-grain breads, cereals, and grains such as whole-wheat or rye bread, oatmeal, and brown rice. Use high-fat, high-sugar baked goods such as cakes, cookies, and pastries in moderation. Limit fats and sugars added as spreads, sauces, or toppings.
1/2 cup cooked or raw chopped vegetables 1 cup raw leafy vegetables 3/4 cup vegetable juice 10 French fries	Eat a variety of vegetables, including dark-green leafy vegetables such as spinach and broccoli, deep-yellow vegetables such as carrots, sweet potatoes, and corn, legumes such as kidney beans, and other vegetables such as green beans and tomatoes. Cook by steaming or baking. Avoid frying, and limit high-fat spreads or dressings.
1 medium apple, banana, or orange 1/2 cup chopped, cooked, or canned fruit 3/4 cup fruit juice 1/4 cup dried fruit	Choose fresh fruit, frozen without sugar, dried, or fruit canned in water or juice. If canned in heavy syrup, rinse with water before eating. Eat whole fruits more often than juices; they are higher in fiber. Regularly eat citrus fruits, melons, or berries rich in vitamin C. Only 100% fruit juice should be counted as fruit.
1 cup milk or yogurt 1½ oz natural cheese 2 oz process cheese 2 cups cottage cheese 1½ cups ice cream 1 cup frozen yogurt	Use skim or low-fat milk for healthy people over 2 years of age. Choose low-fat and nonfat yogurt, "part skim" and low-fat cheeses, and lower-fat frozen desserts such as ice milk and frozen yogurt. Limit high-fat cheeses and ice cream.
2-3 oz cooked lean meat, fish, or poultry 2–3 eggs 4–6 tablespoons peanut butter 1½ cups cooked dry beans 1 cup nuts	Select lean meat, poultry without skin, fish, and dry beans often. Trim fat, and cook by broiling, roasting, grilling, or boiling rather than frying. Limit egg yolks, which are high in cholesterol, and nuts and seeds, which are high in fat. Be aware of serving size; 3 oz of meat is the size of an average hamburger.
Butter, mayonnaise, salad dressing, cream cheese, sour cream, jam, jelly	These are high in energy and low in micronutrients. Substitute low-fat dressings and spreads.

slices of bread (on a sandwich, for example) are considered a serving by CSPI, compared to one slice for the USDA.

More help with food selections from the major food categories of meats, fruits, vegetables, cereals, grains, and beans can be found in Appendix 7, CSPI's Eating Smart Shopping Guide. For the frequent or even occasional fast-food consumer, nutrient analyses as provided by Kentucky Fried Chicken, McDonalds, Burger King, Taco Bell, Wendy's, Pizza Hut, Baskin Robbins, and TCBY are found in Appendix 8.

Whichever pyramid model you find most useful, "eating the pyramid way" should lead you in the right direction in terms of getting the nutrients you need. With careful food selections, you also should be able to achieve the dietary goals and guidelines for Americans discussed next.

FIGURE
9.4   Healthy Eating Pyramid.

ANYTIME PYRAMID

Catsup
Olives
Mustard
Mayonnaise, *fat-free*
Salad dressing, *fat-free*
FATS, SWEETS, & CONDIMENTS

Buttermilk
Cheese, *fat-free*
Cottage cheese, *fat-free or low-fat*
Milk, *skim or 1% fat*
Plain yogurt, *non-fat*
DAIRY FOODS
(2 to 3 servings a day)

Seafood, *all*
Pork tenderloin
Tuna, *in water*
Chicken breast or drumstick, *no skin*
Egg white or substitute
Beef top or eye of round, *Select*
Turkey, except wing, *no skin*
FISH, POULTRY, MEAT, NUTS, & EGGS
(1 to 2 servings a day)
(Trimmed; baked or roasted.)

Vegetables, *fresh, frozen, or canned*
Vegetable juice, *no-salt or light*
Beans (eg., Black, Garbanzo, Pink, Pinto, Great northern, Kidney)
Split peas, Lentils, Black-eyed peas
VEGETABLES & BEANS
(4 to 6 servings a day)

Fruit, *fresh, frozen, dried, or canned with juice*
Fruit juice
FRUITS
(2 to 4 servings a day)

ANYTIME

Bread, English muffins, Rolls, Bagels, *whole wheat or whole grain*
Breakfast cereals, *cold, whole grain, low-sugar* (eg., bran flakes, Cheerios, Grape-Nuts, Life, Nutri-Grain, shredded wheat, Total, Weetabix, Wheaties)
Breakfast cereals, *hot, whole grain, low-sugar* (e.g., oatmeal, Wheatena)

Bulgur
Corn tortillas
Crackers, *whole grain, low-fat* (e.g., crispbread, Triscuits)
Pasta
Popcorn, *air-popped*
Rice, brown
Pretzels, *whole grain, unsalted;* Tortilla chips, *no-oil*

BREAD, CEREAL, RICE, PASTA, & BAKED GOODS *(6 to 11 servings a day)*

Bean burrito
Cheeseless pizza
Grilled chicken sandwich
Pork & beans

Garden salad w/chicken chunks & light dressing

Canned soup, *low-sodium*
Spaghetti w/tomato sauce

Vegetable pita sandwich
Stir-fried vegetables & rice w/chicken or seafood
Turkey *(fresh-cooked)* sandwich

MIXED FOODS

SOMETIMES PYRAMID

Jelly
Sugar
Oils, Mayo.
Salad dressing
Salt, Soy sauce
Margarine, *diet, tub*
FATS, SWEETS, & CONDIMENTS

Milk, *2% fat*
Sherbet
Ice milk
Ice cream, *non-fat*
Frozen yogurt, *all*
Cottage cheese, *4% fat*
Fruit yogurt, *non-fat or low-fat*
Cheese, Cream cheese, Sour cream, *light*
DAIRY FOODS

Turkey roll
Turkey, *w/skin*
Tuna, *in oil*
Chicken nuggets
Nuts, Peanut butter
Pork loin (except blade)
Beef round or sirloin steak
Chicken breast or drumstick, *w/skin;* thigh, *no skin*
FISH, POULTRY, MEAT, NUTS, & EGGS
(Trimmed; baked or roasted.)

Avocado
Cole slaw

French fries
Guacamole
Hash browns
Potato chips
Corn chips
Potato salad

V8 juice
Tomato juice, *(canned)*
Soybeans
Tofu

Cranberry sauce, *canned*
Fruit, *canned in syrup*
Fruit "drinks," "blends," "cocktails," or "beverages"

VEGETABLES & BEANS

SOMETIMES

FRUITS

Angelfood cake
Fig bars
Pancakes, Waffles
Oatmeal raisin cookies
Gingersnaps
Molasses cookies
Pretzels

Rice, white
Packaged rice mixes
Tortilla chips, *light*
Bread, English muffins, Rolls, Bagels (eg., multi-grain, oatmeal, rye, pumpernickel, white)

Biscuits
Croissants
Cakes, Cookies, Granola bars, *fat-free*
Breakfast cereals, *refined* (e.g., corn flakes, Rice Krispies)

Crackers, *refined* (e.g., saltines, oyster)
Crackers, *not low-fat* (e.g., cheese, Ritz)
Breakfast cereals, *heavily sweetened* (e.g., Cap'n Crunch, Frosted Flakes)

BREAD, CEREAL, RICE, PASTA, & BAKED GOODS

Baked potato w/cheese
Beef or chicken burrito
Canned or dried soup
Cheese pizza

Chef salad w/light dressing
Chicken taco
Hummus w/pita

Lasagna w/meat
McLean Deluxe
Macaroni & cheese

Peanut butter & jelly sandwich
Roast beef sandwich
Spaghetti w/meatballs
Tuna or chicken salad sandwich

MIXED FOODS

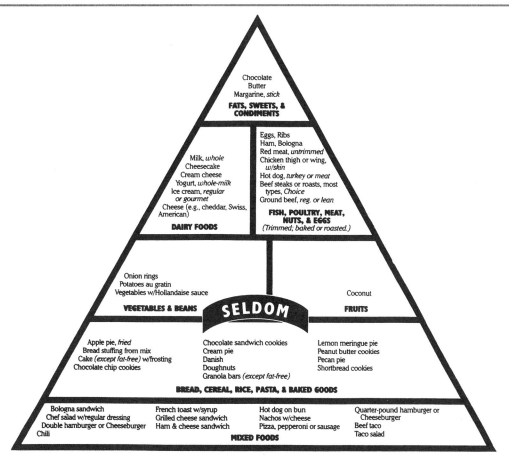

SERVING SIZES

Mixed Foods

7 oz (about 2 slices) pizza
1 cup soup, cooked spaghetti, or chili

Bread, Cereal, Rice, Pasta, & Baked Goods

2 slices bread
½ cup dense cereals (like granola)
1 cup other cooked cereal or pasta
¾ cup cooked rice
2 waffles
3 pancakes
1/20 cake
1 oz (2 to 3) cookies
⅛ pie
½ oz (about 4) crackers
1 oz (about 14) chips

Vegetables & Beans

1 cup lettuce
½ cup cooked vegetables or beans

Fruit

1 medium fruit

½ cup canned fruit
1 cup juice

Dairy Foods

1 cup milk, yogurt, or ice cream
1 oz cheese
½ cup cottage cheese

Fish, Poultry, Meat, Nuts, & Eggs

4 oz cooked meat, poultry, or seafood
1½ oz shrimp
3 oz tuna
2 oz (two slices) luncheon meat
1 hot dog
1 egg
2 tbsp peanut butter
¼ cup nuts

Fats, Sweets, & Condiments

1 tbsp margarine, butter, or oil
1 tbsp catsup, mayonnaise, soy sauce, or jelly
1 tsp mustard
2 tbsp salad dressing

Dietary Goals and Guidelines

After the U.S. Dietary Goals were issued in 1977, with the hopes of reducing the incidence of chronic disease, the U.S. Department of Agriculture in 1980 developed a list of basic dietary recommendations to guide people in reaching these goals. The recommendations, called the Dietary Guidelines for Americans, have been revised to reflect the National Research Council's 1989 report, *Diet and Health*. This report updates the original U.S. Dietary Goals and now represents the most current and comprehensive scientific analysis of the health risks and benefits of various dietary practices. The 1995 Dietary Guidelines for Americans are as follows:

- Eat a variety of foods.
- Balance the food you eat with physical activity.
- Maintain or improve your weight.
- Choose a diet with plenty of grain products, fruits, and vegetables.
- Choose a diet low in fat, saturated fat, and cholesterol.
- Choose a diet moderate in sugars.
- Choose a diet moderate in salt and sodium.
- If you drink alcoholic beverages, do so in moderation.

These guidelines are a very general summary of the specific dietary goals recommended in *Diet and Health*. These dietary goals for Americans are:

1. Minimize:
   a. Total fat intake to 30% or less of total calories
   b. Saturated fat intake to 10% or less of total calories
   c. Cholesterol intake to 300 mg or less per day
      (1) Substitute fish, skinless poultry or lean meats, and low-fat dairy products
      (2) Limit fried foods, oils and fats, egg yolks, and other fatty foods
2. Consume 55% or more of total calories in carbohydrate, including:
   a. Five or more servings of fruits and vegetables, especially green and yellow vegetables and citrus fruit
   b. Six or more servings of breads, cereals (especially whole grains), and legumes
3. Eat sufficient protein to meet the RDA (0.8 grams per kilogram of body weight) but not more than twice that amount, or 1.6 grams. For the average-weight woman and man, 5 and 7 ounces of meat or fish respectively at 8 grams of protein per ounce would meet the RDA.

4. Don't drink alcohol at all if pregnant. Otherwise, if you wish to drink, limit consumption to two cans of beer, two small glasses of wine, or two average cocktails per day.
5. Minimize salt intake to 6 grams or less, about 1 teaspoon, per day.
6. Maintain weight by balancing calorie intake with activity level.
7. Ensure sufficient calcium intake by consuming two to four servings of non-fat (preferably, or low-fat) milk products. Children 2 years of age or younger should consume whole milk products.
8. Drink fluoridated water, if at all possible, to protect teeth and bones (or otherwise maintain recommended fluoride intake).
9. Don't take vitamin and mineral supplements in excess of 100% of the RDA unless recommended by a health professional.

An easy way to follow most of these guidelines is simply to choose most of the foods you eat from the Anytime panel of CSPI's Healthy Eating Pyramid. More specific suggestions for adding starch and fiber to the diet and avoiding too much fat, cholesterol, sugar, alcohol, and salt were presented in Chapter 8. Combining these suggestions with the recommended food selections from the Healthy Eating Pyramid produces a diet plan that provides the RDAs you need and minimizes your risk of major chronic diseases. This plan emphasizes fruits, vegetables, and grains, accompanied by smaller amounts of lean meats and dairy products, and very limited quantities of high-fat foods such as gravies, baked goods, dressings, and alcohol.

GETTING THE MOST FROM YOUR FOOD

Deciding what foods are best to eat is only part of your diet planning job. How often you eat, what you buy at the store, and how you prepare it all influence the nutrients you get from food. The following information may help you with these choices.

Three Meals or More

If you usually eat very little food until after 5:00 P.M., you may not be as well-nourished as your diet analysis indicates. The body simply doesn't handle large amounts of nutrients very well. For example, you may recall that the absorption rate for iron is low when a large amount is supplied all at once and is much higher when only small amounts are available. Therefore, the recommendation is to eat small amounts of iron throughout the day. This recommendation also applies to consuming sources of complete protein.

Small, frequent meals are recommended, too, as a means of controlling weight and body fat. In essence, the body makes best use of food in small amounts, a minimum of three times per day, or preferably four to six. Eating in relation to your activity patterns also seems to help the body use food better. If you are more active during the day, that's when to eat most of your food. "Breakfast like a king, lunch like a prince, and dinner like a pauper" seems to be the best advice, though most people do not eat this way. If you can move slightly in that direction, you will be doing a better job of eating to enhance yourself.

Health-Wise Shopping

Getting the most for your money is every consumer's goal. This is easier said than done. When you walk into a supermarket, you are faced with 8,000 to 10,000 items from which to choose. Some general guidelines are offered here to help you make the most nutritious selections.

1. Read labels. Ingredients are listed in descending order according to their weight in the product. Decide if the first several ingredients are what you want to get from that product. If not, don't buy it, or check another brand. It might have more of what you want. To review label definitions in current use, refer to Chapter 8.

2. When buying cereals, breads, and other grain products, choose those that list "whole grain" as the first ingredient, rather than refined or bleached ingredients. You will get more vitamins and minerals. For the same reason, choose "enriched" over "unenriched," "stoneground" grain over any other form, and brown rice over white.

3. Choose fresh fruits and vegetables over canned. Frozen is the next best choice, and perhaps your best choice if you can't shop often. Fresh produce can lose significant amounts of vitamins if stored in the refrigerator several days. To minimize losses, refrigerate produce in moisture-proof bags, or at least in the vegetable crisper section. When buying fresh produce, select the fruits and vegetables that are darkest in their natural color. Dark greens and deep yellows, oranges, and reds offer the most vitamin A (beta-carotenes).

4. Buy fresh meats if you can, but frozen meats, fish, and poultry offer similar nutrient content *if* they have been wrapped well.

Cooking It Right for You

How food is cooked also has a significant effect on nutrients you get. The concern here is largely with loss of water-soluble vitamins, but increasing nutrient content is also a possibility. For example, frying food markedly increases its caloric content. Using iron pots and pans will add some iron to the foods you prepare in them. To minimize loss of water-soluble vitamins in cooking:

1. Minimize exposure of foods to water; the B and C vitamins dissolve in it.
   a. Don't soak vegetables to wash or store them.
   b. Use as little water as possible in cooking, and cook for the shortest time possible. Microwave cooking may increase retention of nutrients.
   c. If cooking time is prolonged, as in braising or stewing meat, use the broth in some way (e.g., for soup or in dressing).
   d. Cook vegetables whole if possible. The more you cut them up, the greater the vitamin loss.

2. Use the best cooking methods for preserving vitamins—pressure cooking, steaming, boiling, poaching, and stewing.
   a. Although significant vitamin loss occurs with the last three of these, because of the water exposure, using the broths recaptures the vitamins.
   b. Microwave cooking, oven broiling, roasting, and frying do less damage to vitamins than braising or stewing (if you can't or won't reuse the broth), but frying so significantly adds fat and calories to the diet that it can't be recommended.
   c. Charcoal broiling or barbecuing is believed to add carcinogens to foods through the smoke and flames. Wrapping foods in foil or placing them in a pan to protect them from the smoke and flames can eliminate this problem but also may reduce desired flavors. A compromise is to raise the grill higher above the flames or coals and cook foods more slowly.

3. Do not overcook meats; this causes loss of the B vitamin thiamin (unless the broth is eaten) and can decrease the availability of certain amino acids.

4. Prepare salads as close as possible to the time they'll be eaten. This will preserve vitamin C.

DECIDING ABOUT SUPPLEMENTS

At this point you may be thinking, "This is too much to bother with! I'll just take a supplement to make sure I'm getting what I need." Although you might need a supplement, you should not assume that supplements can be substitutes for food. The first problem is a practical one: No supplement on the market contains all the nutrients you need. That creates the problem of trying to buy some or all of the nutrients you need individually and then combining them in the appropriate amounts so you're not getting too much of one or too little of another. Too much of one nutrient might interfere with absorption or utilization of another. Too little of another nutrient might make it worthless, or render another nutrient unusable, and so on! This description is meant to sound confusing and complex because that's the situation regarding supplements today. Not even the experts can tell you how to use supplements in place of a good diet, because the information simply isn't available. Anyone who claims such knowledge is deliberately or unintentionally misrepresenting the state of the art in nutrition.

Experimentation is ongoing, not only in regard to what we need to function but also in terms of possibly curing disease. In some research the effects of megadoses of vitamins and minerals (10 or more times the known or assumed requirement) are being examined, but no hard evidence is available from which to derive safe recommendations at this time. In fact, these studies generally are indicating that all vitamins and minerals can be toxic in large enough doses. Anyone who chooses to take such large amounts sporadically or on a regular basis is taking a risk.

The truth is that relatively little information exists about how much of the different nutrients the body needs, what combinations promote the greatest utilization of what is consumed, and exactly when the body needs what. Clearly, however, all the nutrients the body requires are present in foods. It also is known which foods contain a lot of nutrients and which contain only a few. This is the knowledge base behind the recommendation to eat a variety of high-quality foods in moderation throughout the day. With the help of diet-planning guides such as the Food Guide Pyramid and the Healthy Eating Pyramid, eating becomes far easier than relying on supplements, and certainly a more pleasurable way to try to meet nutritional needs. Thus, the important points regarding supplements are:

1. To obtain the necessary vitamins and minerals, there is no adequate replacement for food.

2. The word *supplement* means "added to," not "substituted for."

Some people may need to supplement nutrients in their diets as discussed in Chapter 8. Also, a detailed list of conditions that might cause a person to require supplementation was given in Table 9.A. The more common of these conditions are summarized in FYI 1, accompanied by suggestions as

FYI

Situations in Which Supplements Are Useful

The following are common conditions in which vitamin supplements—or increased consumption of vitamin-rich foods—are valuable.

1. *Pregnancy and breast-feeding* increase a woman's vitamin requirements. A multiformula tablet with iron meets these needs. All women of child-bearing age need extra iron, whether from foods or supplements.

2. *Oral contraceptives* lower bloodstream vitamin levels by disrupting the body's ability to utilize B vitamins (particularly niacin and B_6). Some physicians recommend a B-complex tablet to counter this.

3. *Smoking* depletes vitamin C supplies by as much as 30%, which can be harmful, depending upon dietary habits. A small supplement (100 mg) will be enough to compensate.

4. *Dieting* reduces overall vitamin intake, at times dangerously, and this is especially true for the fad diets and very low calorie diets. Unless the diet is balanced nutritionally (an example is Weight Watchers), multivitamin tablets are needed.

5. *Alcohol* can disrupt diet. Multitablets (especially those high in B-complex vitamins, which absorb alcohol) may prevent serious physical damage.

6. *Caffeine*, taken in large quantities from coffee, tea, or cola drinks, causes the body to flush out water-soluble vitamins more rapidly. Small daily supplements of the B-complex and C vitamins will replenish supplies.

7. *Vegetarians* who eat no animal products at all need a supplement of vitamin B_{12}.

8. Older people whose diets are limited in quantity or quality need supplementation.

to the vitamins or minerals probably needed. If you find yourself described in this list, you may need a supplement of vitamins or minerals, or both. Your safest action would be to take a supplement that provides no more than the recommended amount of the nutrient(s) you need. If you think more than that would be better, take some time to find out what is known about the effects of large amounts of that vitamin or mineral before using yourself as a guinea pig. Some reliable sources to consult are listed in FYI 5 in Chapter 8. Also read some of the references provided at the end of Chapter 8 regarding vitamin and mineral studies.

The seriousness of some of the conditions listed in Tables 9.A and FYI 1 warrants additional comment. Excessive drinking, anorexia/bulimia, extreme fad diets (such as liquid protein formulas), and very low calorie diets or fasting are more than just nutritional problems. They are potentially life threatening. A vitamin/mineral supplement may help offset some of the negative effects of nutritional problems such as these, but it won't solve the problem. The most important action to take if you are trying to cope with one or more of these problems is to *seek professional help*. Alcoholics Anonymous, eating disorders groups, Overeaters Anonymous, and Weight Watchers are some good starting points. The people involved with these groups have all struggled with similar problems and can provide support, information, and direction in locating additional sources of help as needed.

SUMMARY

Nutritional studies indicate that the average American needs to change some eating habits to enjoy optimum vitality and longevity. Unfortunately, most people don't know if they are eating better or worse or the same as the "average" person. You can, however, determine how well you are eating by comparing your diet to nutritional recommendations.

The Food Guide Pyramid and the Healthy Eating Pyramid are recommended guides for selecting foods that provide the required nutrients while helping you avoid excessive fat, cholesterol, sugar, alcohol, and salt. Getting the most from the food you select can depend upon when you eat it and your shopping and cooking skills. Eating smaller meals, three times or more a day, allows the body to make the best use of food. Eating in relation to your activity pattern is also helpful in this regard. Shopping skills that promote a healthier diet include careful reading of labels, buying whole-grain products, and choosing fresh vegetables, fruits, and meats whenever possible.

CHOICES IN ACTION

Now it's time to check up on your eating behavior. Lab 24, "Diet Habit Survey," gives you an opportunity to compare your eating habits with those of the average American, and then with the goals recommended in the New American Diet as well as the 1989 U.S. Dietary Goals for Americans. Or, keep a food diary for a day—or better yet, a week. Lab 25, "Nutritional Assessment," helps you calculate your caloric intake and expenditure for a 24-hour period; the percent of protein, fat, and carbohydrate calories you consume; and your nutrient components relative to the RDA.

If you want to do a quick check-up on some of your favorite foods or meals in terms of their potential to promote fatty deposits on blood vessels, use Form 6 from the Nutritional Assessment Lab (Lab 25). Using this form, you can calculate the Cholesterol–Saturated Fat Index (CSI) for any individual food or meals.

How you cook food can influence its nutrient content significantly. Frying markedly increases the caloric content of any food. Prolonged cooking in water generally causes major losses of B and C vitamins. Recommended cooking techniques include pressure cooking, steaming, boiling, poaching, and stewing. The last three of these do cause significant vitamin losses, but these can be regained if the broth is used, as in a soup.

Regarding vitamin and mineral supplementation, *there is no adequate replacement for food to obtain all the vitamins and minerals you need.* Among the people who may need to supplement nutrients in their diet are those who consume very low calorie diets, drink excessive amounts of alcohol, have been ill for a long time, and take oral contraceptives. The safest choice is a supplement that provides no more than the recommended amount of the needed nutrient(s).

Probably the two most important dietary practices that Americans need to work on are: (a) eating small amounts of food more often, and (b) avoiding fatty foods.

REFERENCES

Andresky, J. 1985. *Vitamins in Nutrition and Health.* Englewood, CO: Morton Publishing.

Brody, J. 1987. *Jane Brody's Nutrition Book.* New York: Bantam.

Center for Science in the Public Interest. *CSPI Healthy Eating Pyramid: An Eater's Guide.* 1992. Washington, DC: CSPI.

Connor, S. 1989. "The Cholesterol–Saturated Fat Index for Coronary Prevention: Background, Use, and a Comprehensive Table of Foods." *Journal of the American Dietetic Association* 89: 807–816.

Connor, S., and Connor, W. 1986. *The New American Diet.* New York: Simon & Schuster.

"CSPI Healthy Eating Pyramid." 1992. *Nutrition Action Healthletter* 19: 8–9.

Dennison, D. 1994. *DINE Healthy* [computer program]. West Amherst, NY: DineSystems.

"Don't Send Nutrients Down the Drain." 1991. *University of California Berkeley, Wellness Letter* 7: 7.

"Daily Dietary Fat and Total Food-Energy Intakes— Third National Health and Nutrition Examination Survey, Phase 1." 1994. *Morbidity & Mortality Weekly Report* 43: 116–117, 123, 125.

Food and Nutrition Board, Committee on Dietary Allowances. 1989. *Recommended Dietary Allowances,* 10th edition. Washington, DC: National Academy of Science.

Gettz, E., and Geltoy, R. 1994. *The Food Processor version 6* [computer program]. Salem, OR: ESHA Research.

Guthrie, H. 1986. *Introductory Nutrition.* St. Louis: C. V. Mosby.

Hui, Y. 1985. *Principles and Issues in Nutrition.* Belmont, CA: Wadsworth.

Hunter, B. 1985. "Risky Cooking Practices: Don't Get Burned." *Consumer's Research* 68(May): 29.

National Research Council. 1989. *Prescription for Lower Chronic Disease Risk: Less Fat and More Fruits, Vegetables and Complex Carbohydrates.* Washington, DC: Government Printing Office.

National Research Council. 1990. *Diet and Health Implications for Reducing Chronic Disease Risk.* Washington, DC: National Academy of Sciences.

Nieman, D. C., Butterworth, D. E., and Nieman, C. N. 1992. *Nutrition.* Dubuque, IA: Wm. C. Brown Publishers.

Rinzler, C. 1985. "The Chemistry of Cooking." *American Health* 4(December): 42.

Siger, F., and Whitney, E. N. 1994. *Nutrition: Concepts and Controversies,* 6th edition. Minneapolis: West Publishing.

Simko, M., et al. 1984. *Nutrition Assessment.* Rockville, MD: Aspen Systems.

Smolin, L. A., and Grosvenor, M. B. 1994. *Nutrition: Science and Applications.* New York: Saunders College Publishing.

Solomons, N., and Allen, L. 1983. "Functional Assessment of Nutritional Status: Principles, Practice and Potential." *Nutrition Reviews* 41: 33.

Surgeon General's Report on Nutrition and Health. 1988. (DHHS Pub. No. PHS 88-50210). Washington, DC: Government Printing Office.

"The ABC's of Taking Supplements." 1985. *Tufts University Diet and Nutrition Letter* 3(May): 7.

"The ABC's of Taking Vitamins." 1981. *Consumer's Digest* 20(July-August).

"The Dietary Guidelines Become More User Friendly." 1991. *Tufts University Diet and Nutrition Letter* 8(January): 3.

U. S. Department of Agriculture. 1992. *Food Guide Pyramid.* (Home & Garden Bulletin 252). Hyattsville, MD: Human Nutrition Information Services.

U. S. Department of Agriculture, Department of Health and Human Services. 1970. *Calories and Weight: U.S.D.A. Pocket Guide* (Home and Garden Bulletin #153). Washington, DC: Government Printing Office.

U.S. Department of Agriculture, Department of Health and Human Services. 1981. *Nutritive Value of Foods* (Home and Garden Bulletin #72). Washington, DC: Government Printing Office.

U.S. Department of Agriculture, Department of Health and Human Services. 1995. *Dietary Guidelines for Americans*, 3rd edition (Home and Garden Bulletin #232). Washington, DC: Government Printing Office.

U.S. Senate, Select Committee on Nutrition and Human Needs. 1977. *Dietary Goals for the United States*, 2d edition. Washington, DC: Government Printing Office.

Whitney, E. N., and Rolfes, S. R. 1993. *Understanding Nutrition*. St. Paul: West Publishing.

Williams, M. 1992. *Nutrition for Fitness and Sport*, 3d edition. Dubuque, IA: Wm. C. Brown Publishers.

"Wrap-up: Minerals." 1986. *University of California Berkeley, Wellness Letter* 2(January): 4.

10

Choosing to Protect Yourself:

STDs, Drugs, and Violence

✔ Can you protect yourself from STDs and still have an active social life?

✔ How can you tell whether or not someone you're dating has an STD?

✔ How can you avoid becoming a victim of drug abuse?

✔ Are you an easy target for crime?

✔ Do you know how to protect yourself when you're in danger of assault?

This above all: to thine own self be true,
And it must follow, as the night the day,
Thou canst not then be false to any man.

William Shakespeare, Hamlet,
(Act 1, Sc.3, 78–80)

Choosing to protect yourself in life gives you the best chance of attaining what you can be. It allows you to "be there" for those who love you. And, by your example, you may help others to choose to protect themselves.

Protecting yourself from sexually transmitted diseases (STDs), substance abuse, and violence requires both offensive and defensive strategies. There are at least four basic protective strategies or actions:

1. *Learn as much as possible about STDs, about the drugs you take and/or might be exposed to, and about violence, especially when you might be most vulnerable.* Learn which behaviors place you at risk and which behaviors protect you.

2. *Be honest with yourself about your weaknesses.* Under what circumstances might you allow yourself to be vulnerable to a risky situation? Could you imagine yourself getting talked into drinking even when you know you're going to be driving? Would you have unprotected sex with someone you have met recently and are feeling passionately attracted to if he or she didn't request using a condom? Would you have unprotected sex with someone you are in love with, or do drugs with someone you trust? Make a list of all the situations in which you think you might take a chance.

3. *Once you know your possible weak points, plan in advance how you will handle yourself* should you face one of these moments. What will you say? What will you do to protect yourself rather than place yourself at risk? Make a list for yourself of the behaviors, situations, environments, personal policies, or goals you could use to help you through your weak moments.

4. *A key part of behavior planning is to talk about your concerns with people you trust and care about.* Discussing self-protection with your sexual partner or a friend might help both of you. At the least, talking up front and in advance about how you want to be in a given situation takes off some of the pressure to give

in during a potentially weak moment. You will have announced your intentions, and people will know what to expect or not expect from you. Likewise, the more you talk about your intentions—your personal policies for self-protection—the more confidence you will gain in yourself to do what you say you will do.

This chapter offers information about STDs, potentially abusive substances, and violence—how you become a victim and how you can protect yourself.

SEXUALLY TRANSMITTED DISEASES

Sexually transmitted diseases (STDs) are diseases transmitted primarily by sexual contact, meaning by direct person-to-person contact of warm, moist body surfaces and by exposure to body fluids, specifically, blood, semen, vaginal secretions, and breast milk. The most prominent STDs are chlamydia, gonorrhea, genital warts, genital herpes, hepatitis, syphilis, and HIV disease. These are major concerns because of their alarmingly high incidence, long-term consequences, and/or potential threat to life itself. The annual number of new cases of these STDs in the United States is shown in Figure 10.1.

Sexually transmitted diseases have been around for a long time. Descriptions of what are thought

FIGURE 10.1

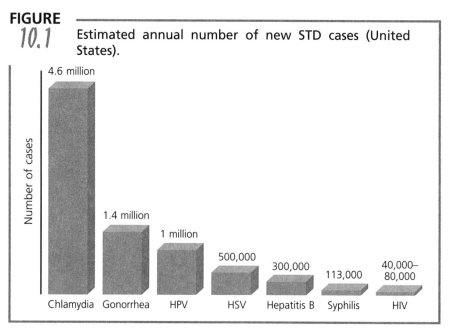

Estimated annual number of new STD cases (United States).

Surgeon General's Report on HIV Infection & AIDS June 1993, p. 1
Donovan, P., Testing Positive: STD & Public Health Response, AGI, NY. 1993, pp. 10–17 (Division of STD/HIV Prevention. Annual Report, 1994. Centers for Disease Control & Prevention. Atlanta: 1995.)

to be gonorrhea and syphilis are found in the Old Testament of the Bible (Leviticus 21:18, Numbers 31:2–23, and Deuteronomy 28:27–29). Ancient Greek physicians gave the name herpes (meaning "to creep") to the STD that resulted in sores that seemed to creep over the body surface. STDs used to be called venereal diseases or social diseases, although one seldom hears that terminology any more, because STDs are contracted primarily through social relationships that culminate in sexual behavior and/or by sharing needles/syringes when using drugs.

Approximately 12 million new cases of STDs occur in the United States each year, as shown by age group in Figure 10.2. Two-thirds of these new cases occur among people under 25 years of age. Three million of these occur among teenagers aged 13–19, that is, about one in every eight teens. As many as 56 million or more Americans (1 in 5) are thought to have a long-term or life-long viral infection such as genital herpes or genital warts. As of mid-1995, more than 300,000 Americans had died since 1980 from HIV infection that developed into AIDS. For people 25–44 years of age, AIDS is now the leading cause of death.

Why are STDs still with us, and in such big numbers? Throughout the centuries many factors have deterred efforts to minimize or eliminate transmission of these diseases. The risk factors discussed below are important to examine because they suggest how you can protect yourself.

Risk Factors for STDs

1. *Sex.* First and foremost, as the label STD implies, these diseases are transmitted primarily by sexual interactions. Obviously, abstaining from sex would eliminate risk of some STDs and severely curtail the risk of others. Next to abstinence, sex between uninfected partners in a long-term monogamous relationship affords the least risk of STDs. Those who have sex under any other circumstances are at greater risk, and the risk increases as the frequency of sex and the number of partners increases.

2. *Ignorance and "silent" infections.* Not all sexually active people know about STDs or how to protect themselves. And even if they do know about STDs, they may not know they are infected and do not think protective measures are necessary. For example, a person can carry HIV, the AIDS virus, for 6 months before testing positive. Symptoms may not appear for years. During this time, however, anyone who has sex with this person may become infected.

3. *Multiple sex partners.* Having many sex partners magnifies the possibility of spreading STDs, as each new sexual liaison actually represents sexual interactions with all of the other sex partners each person has been with. This means that if you and a partner had sex last night, and last year both of you had sex with three other people, and for the last seven years all of those people had sex with three other people each year, then you were actually exposed to 4,908 other people last night.

4. *Early-onset sexual activity.* The earlier sexual behavior begins in a person's life, the more likely the person will have multiple partners, and therefore the more likely the person will contract an STD. Of females in the United States aged 15–19 in 1971, 36% reported having had intercourse. The percentage was 47% in 1982 and 53% in 1988. Of males 17–19 years of age in the United States, 66% reported being sexually active in 1979; the percentage was 76% in 1988.

5. *Feeling invulnerable—the "not me" syndrome.* Feelings of invulnerability cloud judgment. "It can't/won't happen to me—at least, not this time!" and "she (he) is too nice to have an STD" are both common ways of thinking that invite people to forego protective behavior, to take a chance. What is abundantly clear about STDs is that NO ONE IS INVULNERABLE, regardless of age, race, economic group, religion, or any other factor.

6. *Substance abuse.* Substance use and abuse lessen

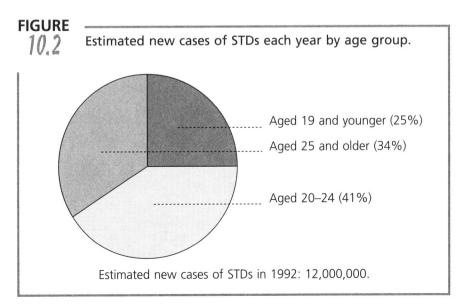

FIGURE 10.2 Estimated new cases of STDs each year by age group.

Aged 19 and younger (25%)

Aged 25 and older (34%)

Aged 20–24 (41%)

Estimated new cases of STDs in 1992: 12,000,000.

Source: Centers for Disease Control and Prevention, *Division of STD/HIV Prevention, 1994 Annual Report*, Atlanta, 1995.

precautionary behavior. It encourages taking a chance. And, if equipment is shared by injection drug users, substance abuse can be directly responsible for transmitting some types of STDs, such as HIV and syphilis.

7. *Social mores and pressures.* Social mores associate STDs with illicit sex and immoral behavior. As a consequence, a person who has an STD may feel embarrassed or fear rejection by a potential sex partner should he or she admit the infection and/or suggest protective measures.

8. *Failure to use protection against STDs.* In 1988, only 20% of sexually active women 15–44 years of age said their sexual partner used a condom. In 1991 only 27% of sexually active men aged 20–39 reported using a condom within a 4-week period. In 1993, only 8% of people who had more than one sexual partner during the previous year reported using a condom consistently. Given that the condom is one of the few disease–protection devices available for those who choose to be sexually active, the implications of these statistics should be obvious. The estimated risk of acquiring selected STDs during a single act of unprotected intercourse is shown in Figure 10.3. As you can see, women are more at risk than men are in some cases.

The risk factors for STDs help suggest those behaviors that provide the most protection from STDs in general. A brief look at these choices is provided in FYIs 1 and 2. However, each STD has its own peculiarities, and for any one disease, there may be additional things you could do to protect yourself. Individual STDs are discussed in the next section.

Most Prevalent STDs

Chlamydia

An estimated 3 to 10 million people contract chlamydia each year, making it the most common sexually transmitted disease in America. This infection is especially prominent in women.

Transmission. The tiny chlamydia bacterium usually is transmitted via vaginal intercourse.

Symptoms. In 70% of cases, no early symptoms are apparent. Symptoms may take weeks or months to appear. Symptoms in males include painful, burning, and difficult urination, as well as a thin urethral discharge. Female symptoms, when they occur, also include painful, burning urination, as well as a yellowish vaginal discharge, lower abdominal pain, and bleeding between periods.

Consequences. If untreated, chlamydia infections can lead to pelvic inflammatory disease (PID), a severe infection of female pelvic organs.

FIGURE The risk of contracting an STD in one act of unprotected intercourse with an infected partner.

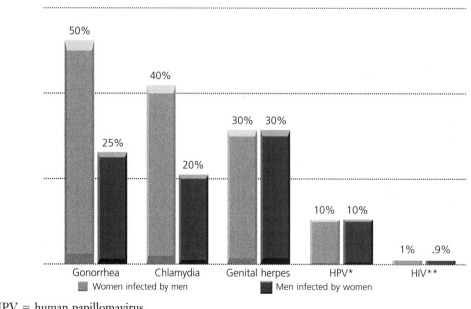

*HPV = human papillomavirus.
**HIV = human immunodeficiency virus.

Source: *Preventing Pregnancy, Protecting Health; A New Look at Birth Control Choices in the United States*, by S. Harlap, K. Kost, and J. D. Forrest (New York: AGI, 1991), p. 43.

General Protective Behaviors

1. *Sexual abstinence.* The chances of exposure to an STD are extremely small for people who are not sexually active, unless they inject drugs or are the unborn baby of an infected mother. *Abstinence is your safest behavior choice.*

2. *Limited number of sexual partners.* The number of sexual partners can be limited in the following ways:

   - *Establish a personal policy of "no sex" until each of you has been tested and examined for STDs.* Remember signs and symptoms of STDs aren't always evident even to the infected person. This means no sex for at least 6 months to allow for the HIV test to be highly accurate. This policy automatically eliminates one-night stands for sex only or sex with a person who is only casually interested in you. ("No sex" does not preclude all forms of intimacy, just those that involve penetration of any body opening and/or exposure to blood, semen, and vaginal fluids.)

   - *Get in and stay in a monogamous relationship with an uninfected person.* Monogamous means only one person for the long term, not a few weeks or months. Monogamous applies to both people in the relationship. "Uninfected" means you have followed the policy suggested in number one. There is no other way to know with any degree of certainty whether someone has an STD.

   - *Be honest and open in communicating with your partner.* Communication that is open and honest starts at the beginning of a relationship and builds trust. In this case, the trust is for a monogamous relationship or the courage and compassion to admit otherwise.

Because untreated gonorrhea also leads to PID, a brief description of PID is presented in the discussion of the consequences of gonorrhea. PID can result in blockage of the fallopian tubes and sterility for women; 75% of all fallopian tube blockages test positive for chlamydia. Although men do not get PID, the chlamydia bacterium can infect and cause scar tissue blockage of the vas deferens, which can result in sterility.

If women become infected with chlamydia during pregnancy, spontaneous abortion and stillbirth are possible. Further, about 182,000 infants become infected during the birth process each year.

Diagnosis and treatment. Because chlamydia and gonorrhea share the symptoms of painful, burning urination and vaginal or urethral discharges, the only way to determine specifically that chlamydia is the cause of the infection is to culture the bacteria from swabbings of the infected areas.

Seven days of antibiotic treatment kills chlamydia. Both sexual partners (or multiple partners) must be treated simultaneously. Otherwise the infection will just be passed back and forth. A follow-up examination should occur one week after the antibiotic treatment to determine that the drug has been successful. There can be no sexual intercourse until the treatment has been found to be successful.

Gonorrhea

Approximately one-half million cases of gonorrhea are reported each year. This number may be closer to 1 million, as not all cases are reported. The incidence of gonorrhea has been increasing gradually since the late 1950s.

Transmission. The gonococcal bacterium thrives in warm, moist places such as the mucous membranes of the mouth, throat, rectum, cervix, and urinary tract. Consequently, genital, oral–genital, and anal–genital contact are the modes of transmission. When exposed to cold or dryness, the bacterium dies within a few seconds, making the toilet seat and the doorknob possible, but extremely unlikely, as modes of transmission.

Symptoms. Men may have symptoms within 2 days to a week after infection. The main symptom is burning urination with urethral discharge. After 2 to 3 weeks, painful urination tends to decrease and the bacterium travels on to infect the prostate and testicles. About 10% of men have no symptoms and, therefore, remain silent carriers. For women, the most common early symptom is no symptom. About 80% of women have no sign of infection until their male partner discovers his infection. If gonorrhea is found early in a woman, it usually is during a routine gynecological screening.

Always Use Protection

Aside from abstinence, condoms in combination with spermicide provide the best overall protection—provided you know how to use them. Condoms do not make any sexual encounter *safe;* they just make it *safer* or less likely for transmission of STDs.

To have a condom with you means nothing. To know how to use a condom and to use one every time you have sex is to protect yourself. The following suggestions are offered for using condoms. The first seven apply to both the male and the new female condom.

1. Always have more than one condom with you.
2. Use condoms made only from latex or polyurethane (those made from animal membrane do not prevent HIV transmission).
3. Avoid exposing the condom to heat of any kind (such as in your back pocket, glove box, or sunlit shelf); heat damages condoms.
4. Always check the expiration date before using a condom.
5. Never open the package with your teeth or fingernails; you might tear the condom.
6. Never use a condom twice.
7. Practice before you need to use one. Get an ample supply, go home, and practice until you can open the package and put the condom in the vagina or on the penis in the dark, correctly and quickly.

FOR MALE CONDOMS:

1. Use only water-based lubricants such as K–Y jelly or Astroglide; anything with oil in it will cause a latex condom to break within minutes (if a lubricant doesn't wash off your hands easily with plain water, leaving no greasy feeling, it has oil in it). A note to women: Some yeast infection medications contain oil.
2. Condoms with a receptacle tip allow the most room for ejaculated semen. If using a condom without a receptacle tip, leave 1/2 inch of condom loose at the tip of the penis.
3. Put the condom on the penis as soon as it is erect, and hold the condom in place after climax so it doesn't slip off. Withdraw the penis from the vagina, mouth, or anus before the erection subsides.

FOR FEMALE CONDOMS:

1. Insert the condom into the vagina (this can be done up to eight hours before sex, but it probably is better to do it within an hour or two before).
2. Remove the condom after sex and before standing.
3. Do not use in combination with the male condom.
4. Use a lot of lubricant between the condom and the penis.

When symptoms do appear in women, they are likely to be unusual vaginal discharge or bleeding, painful urination, fever, painful intercourse, and pelvic pain. The latter three symptoms suggest that the infection has progressed to the cervix and fallopian tubes.

Consequences. Sterility becomes a possibility if the gonorrhea is untreated. These bacteria also can get into the bloodstream and infect the membranes lining the heart and the joints.

If untreated, gonorrhea, like chlamydia, can lead to pelvic inflammatory disease (PID)—any severe and extensive bacterial infection of female pelvic organs. Approximately 10–15% of women who have one episode of PID are left sterile; of those who have three episodes of PID, 50–75% become sterile.

Chlamydia and gonorrhea are the two leading causes of PID, accounting for 90% of the incidence; this is about 11% of all women of reproductive age. Symptoms of PID vary considerably.

Typical symptoms of PID caused by gonorrhea are sudden severe pelvic pain, fever, shaking chills, and heavy vaginal discharge or bleeding.

Diagnosis and treatment. Accurate diagnosis requires culturing the gonococcal bacterium from infected tissues. The treatment is a one-week regimen of antibiotics. A follow-up examination one week after treatment is essential because some strains of the gonococcal bacterium have become resistant to some antibiotics. Sexual partners must be treated at the same time, regardless of whether they have symptoms. Sexual intercourse must cease until the treatment has been declared successful.

Human Papilloma Virus (HPV) (Genital Warts)

Human papilloma virus infection, more commonly known as genital or venereal warts, is thought to be the most common viral STD in the United States, infecting some 20–40 million Americans. An estimated 10% of the sexually active population has the virus, and at least a million new cases occur each year.

Transmission. HPV is extremely contagious. Direct contact of any sort, sexual or nonsexual, can spread this virus from one person to another. Infected individuals can even spread the virus to various areas of their own body by touch. In addition to visible warts, HPV can cause inconspicuous or invisible lesions on the vulva, vaginal wall, and penis. Even when these lesions are not visible, they can produce and shed viral particles that are easily transmissible.

Symptoms. Genital warts usually begin to appear 1 to 8 months after infection. At first these warts look like small, round elevations on the skin, which grow in size and number, often blending together into a cauliflower-like growth. Genital warts can appear on the buttocks, anus, inner thighs, vagina, vulva, cervix, and penis.

Consequences. Of the fifty types of this virus, some are implicated in cervical cancer. HPV has been found in about 90% of the cervical cancers tested. HPV also may be involved in cancers of the vagina, vulva, and penis. It is important to note, however, that most cases of genital warts are *not* caused by the HPV types linked to cancer.

Treatment. Physicians can remove visible warts by cauterization, freezing, laser, and surgery. There is no way to deal with invisible lesions or to eliminate the virus from the body without the possibility of recurrences. And there is no vaccine for HPV. Consequently, the pool of infected persons continues to increase.

Genital Herpes Virus Infection

Prior to HIV/AIDS, genital herpes probably was the most feared sexually transmitted disease. The infection is lifelong, with recurrent episodes, and there is no cure. At least 30 million Americans have contracted the herpes virus, and a half-million more become infected each year.

Two types are of concern here, herpes simplex virus type I (HSV-1) and herpes simplex virus type 2 (HSV-2). Approximately 85% of upper-body infections, such as cold sores and fever blisters, are caused by HSV-1 and approximately 85% of genital infections are caused by HSV-2. However, each of these virus types can attack both oral and genital tissues.

Transmission. Typically, HSV-1 and HSV-2 cause sores to develop on the body surface or internally. Any contact with them risks infection. Genital-to-genital contact or genital–to–mouth contact is the usual mode. The virus also can be transferred by touching open sores with hands or towels

and then touching other body parts. Transmission can occur when sores aren't present, but the risk is considerably higher when sores are present.

The virus is capable of crossing the placenta and infecting the fetus of a pregnant woman. This is most likely if the virus is acquired early in pregnancy. The result can be miscarriage or, if the baby is born, mental retardation or defective sight or hearing.

Symptoms. One or more sores appear 2–12 days after contact with an infected person. The most common sites of genital infection for women are the labia and, less commonly, the vagina. The most common sites for men are on the penis and within the urethra. Sores can appear on the inner thighs and buttocks of either sex.

The first sign of a developing sore is a tingling, itching, or burning sensation at the site. Within hours, small red marks appear, and within a few more hours red-rimmed, fluid-filled blisters form. Over the next 2–10 days, the blisters break and "weep," and scabs form. Formation of the scab indicates the healing process has begun. A first attack could take 4 weeks to heal completely; usually after that, healing is complete within 2 weeks. During this initial outbreak other symptoms may be swollen lymph nodes, fever, and aching muscles.

Healing of the sores does not mean the virus is gone. The virus remains alive but dormant in the nerve tissue around the site of the sore and can be reactivated, usually by stress, hormonal changes, certain foods, and mechanical irritation such as tight clothes.

If a mother has sores present when giving birth, the baby's risk of becoming infected is very high. As the baby has no immunity and the virus is attracted to nerve tissue, the baby's brain is often attacked, leading to mental retardation. If the virus gets into the baby's eyes, the danger of partial or complete loss of sight is high. Consequently, if herpes is known or suspected in the mother, Cesarean birth may be required for the baby's safety.

Diagnosis and treatment. A physician must culture cells from a sore within 3 days of its appearance to tell if the herpes simplex virus is present and which type it might be. If a person has been infected with herpes simplex virus for some time, a blood test will show antibodies indicating whether a sore is a herpes infection.

There is no vaccine for herpes infections at this time, although there is promise of one. If and when a vaccine is developed, it will not be able to protect those who are already infected, of course. The drug most often prescribed to treat genital herpes infections is Acyclovir. It shortens or decreases the frequency of outbreaks.

Viral Hepatitis

Viral hepatitis is a mild to very serious infection of the liver. Actually, three forms are caused by three distinctive viruses: hepatitis A, hepatitis B, and hepatitis C. The estimated incidence per year for hepatitis A is 130,000, for hepatitis B, 300,000, and hepatitis C, 150,000.

Transmission. All three types of viral hepatitis are highly contagious and can be transmitted sexually and nonsexually. The fecal matter and all body fluids from an infected person, including saliva, tears, sweat, blood, urine, vaginal secretions, and semen, contain the hepatitis virus. Thus, the virus is transmitted easily by any intimate sexual contact that exposes mucous membranes (in the mouth, vagina, urethral opening, and anus) to infected fluids. Probably two-thirds of hepatitis B infections result from sexual transmission.

Other modes of transmission include drinking or eating food or water contaminated with body fluids or feces from an infected person who did not wash before preparing foods; sharing needles for drug injections or for piercings or tattoos; sharing toothbrushes, razors, and manicure equipment; and changing soiled diapers or linens from an infected person and not thoroughly washing hands afterwards. Transmission by blood transfusion is now rare because of careful testing.

An infected person is able to transmit the virus as much as 4–6 weeks before experiencing any symptoms. Furthermore, more than half of those infected with hepatitis B and C may never develop symptoms, and approximately 10% may become carriers of the virus. None of these people may know they are infectious, so they would have no motivation to try to protect others from the virus they carry.

Symptoms. For all three types of this virus, early symptoms of infection are flu-like, including low-grade fever, fatigue, headache, loss of appetite, nausea, and abdominal pain. Later symptoms of jaundice (yellow skin and eyes) and darkened urine indicate liver involvement. People who have chronic or long-term infections and carriers are at high risk of developing liver cancer and cirrhosis.

A person infected with hepatitis A usually experiences only the early symptoms, beginning 2–6 weeks after exposure. Full recovery is typical within 3 weeks, after which time the person is no longer infectious.

Symptoms of infection with hepatitis B and C appear more gradually, 1–6 months after exposure, *IF* at all. Three of four people infected with hepatitis C and about half of those with hepatitis B do not experience any of the flu-like symptoms, even though they are contagious.

Consequences. Hepatitis B and C viruses both may stay in the body for a lifetime, so their hosts always are infectious and vulnerable to long-term liver problems. Half of those infected with hepatitis C and 10% of those with hepatitis B develop cirrhosis or cancer of the liver or some other serious liver disease.

Diagnosis and treatment. Blood tests are used to detect hepatitis and carriers of each type. Unfortunately, no drug is available yet as a cure. Treatment consists of rest, good nutrition, and avoiding alcohol and other drugs (birth control or estrogen replacement) that put a strain on the liver until liver function returns to normal.

A vaccine is available for hepatitis B. It is recommended highly if you are at high risk of being exposed to hepatitis B. This includes health-care workers, anyone living with or having sex with an infected person, anyone who has multiple sex partners, regular recipients of blood products, IV drug users, and travelers to areas of the world where hepatitis B is widespread. Also, all babies born to women with hepatitis B should be vaccinated at birth.

In 1995 the FDA approved a new vaccine called Havrix, for hepatitis A. Havrix should provide long-term protection. It is recommended for those at high risk for contracting hepatitis A, such as international travelers, soldiers stationed in developing countries, and health-care workers.

Syphilis

Rates of reported cases of syphilis have doubled in the United States since 1984. About 113,000 new cases are reported each year. *Chemically dependent female prostitutes have been a major source of syphilis in recent years.* Of the STDs, syphilis is especially serious because it always gets into the bloodstream and becomes a systemwide problem.

Transmission. A spiral-shaped bacterium called a spirochete is the cause of syphilis. It dies within a few seconds of exposure to air. Thus, sexual intercourse, kissing, or intimate body contact is required for transmission. Syphilis is contagious, however, only when external sores are present (during the first two stages). Sores may be visible, such as on the penis, or hidden inside the rectum or vagina. The infected person might not be aware that he or she is contagious with syphilis because the sores are not painful.

Any woman who has syphilis or becomes infected during pregnancy can pass the disease to the developing fetus. Successful early treatment of the infected mother-to-be should ensure the child's safety. Without treatment, the pregnancy is likely to result in miscarriage, stillbirth, or birth defects.

Signs and symptoms. Unless it is treated and cured, syphilis progresses through four stages, ultimately causing permanent damage.

1. *Primary syphilis.* Spirochetes multiply and migrate throughout the body for 10–90 days before the first symptom, called a chancre, appears at the exact spot where it entered the body. Any contact with the chancre is most likely to transmit syphilis. Usually the chancre is on or near the sex organs, but it can be on the lip, tongue, finger, or any other part of the body. Very often it is within the vagina, where it won't be noticed, as it is painless. With or without treatment the chancre disappears spontaneously in 3–6 weeks. Not until this point will blood tests for syphilis become positive.

2. *Secondary syphilis.* One to 6 months after the chancre disappears, other symptoms begin to appear. The most common symptom is a rash that does not itch. It may cover the entire body but most commonly develops on the palms of the hands or soles of the feet. Also moist sores filled with spirochetes may develop around the sex organs or in the mouth, making any kind of sexual or intimate behavior—certainly sexual intercourse or even kissing—extremely risky. The infected person also may have a sore throat, headache, fever, joint pain, and patchy hair loss. Secondary syphilis lasts from several days to several months and then, with or without treatment, disappears.

3. *Latent syphilis.* This stage begins when the rash and symptoms of secondary syphilis disappear. It lasts from a few months to a lifetime, the latter being the case for most people. Now the disease is no longer contagious by contact. It still can be transmitted, however, from a pregnant woman to her fetus.

During latent syphilis no external sign of disease is present. Only a blood test can show that a person is infected. During this period, however, the spirochete is progressively invading brain, spinal cord, and heart/blood vessel tissues. When the damage to these organs is sufficient to cause symptoms, the late stage of syphilis begins.

4. *Late or tertiary syphilis.* The late stage of syphilis usually appears 10–20 years after initial exposure. It is characterized by permanent damage to vital organs. Brain damage, spinal cord damage, heart disease, and blindness are the most common problems.

Human Immunodeficiency Virus (HIV) Disease

An estimated 1–1.5 million Americans are infected with HIV, about one in every 250 Americans. This is actually a small number compared to the 30–40 million Americans infected with the genital herpes virus or the genital warts virus. Nonetheless, HIV disease has become the STD of greatest concern today because of the high mortality rate associated with AIDS—the final stage of HIV disease—and because of the alarming rate at which HIV infection is spreading.

Of the 1,119 Americans diagnosed with AIDS in 1982, 119 were still living in 1993. More than 300,000 Americans have died of AIDS as of late 1995. Most of these deaths are in the 15–44 age group.

Transmission. Once the human immunodeficiency virus has entered the body, it lives and multiplies primarily in the white blood cells of its human host specifically in the immunity-producing cells called T lymphocytes. Within a few days to a week, the newly infected person is capable of passing the virus to someone else. The individual is then infectious throughout the entire course of the disease.

The virus can survive only in a moist environment. Any body fluid containing enough white blood cells can transfer the virus to another person. These body fluids are, in order of greatest virus content, blood (including menstrual blood), semen (including "pre-ejaculate"), vaginal secretions, and breast milk. Unless blood is present in sweat, tears, saliva, vomit and/or urine, these fluids do not carry enough virus to transfer the virus successfully to another person.

The virus in blood, semen, vaginal fluids, and breast milk can infect another person only if it can gain entry into that person's body via a break in the skin or exposure to mucous membrane that lines the mouth, eyes, nose, vagina, rectum, and urethra. The virus can pass through intact mucous membrane; no break, cut, or tear in the tissue is necessary. Breaks, tears, or sores in the mucous membrane, however, increase the likelihood of transmission.

The following *do not* transmit HIV:

- insects
- pools and hot tubs
- toilet seats
- door knobs
- drinking fountains
- phones
- shaking hands
- kissing and hugging
- working or living with an infected person
- using objects or eating food handled by an infected person
- giving blood

Only three modes of transmission satisfy all the conditions HIV needs to survive and to penetrate the body:

1. sexual contact
2. parenteral contact (via the bloodstream)
3. perinatal contact (to unborn child).

1. *During sexual contact,* mucous tissues usually are exposed to semen, vaginal secretions, and possibly some blood. For men the small urethral opening at the end of the penis offers a point of entry for the virus, and the urethra is lined with mucosal tissue for the virus to penetrate. For women, the entire vaginal cavity is lined with mucous tissue, providing a large area for the virus to penetrate. Thus, females are more susceptible to HIV infection via vaginal intercourse with an infected partner than are males.

Anal intercourse provides the same conditions plus the additional opportunity for the virus to enter the body through tears in rectal tissue, which is thinner and not as expandable as vaginal tissue. *Oral sex,* in which infected semen, vaginal secretions, or blood gets into the mouth, also provides a large mucous area for HIV to penetrate.

Whether the sexual liaison is heterosexual or homosexual is irrelevant as long as these opportunities for transmission arise during sexual contact and one of the sexual partners is infected. Worldwide, approximately 70% of AIDS cases have been the result of heterosexual transmission. In the United States, HIV first appeared in the homosexual population. Injection drug users were next in number, and then heterosexuals. The current trend is toward a greater increase in heterosexual transmission. As shown in Figure 10.4, reported AIDS cases from heterosexual transmission doubled for both men and women between 1989 and 1992. The greater increase in incidence in the United States is in heterosexual women.

The sexual behaviors of kissing, hugging, and masturbation, even mutual masturbation, will not result in infection as long as no blood, semen, or vaginal fluids are exposed to mucous tissue or breaks in the skin. (A quick dip of the hands in some lemon juice or vinegar will tell you quickly if you have any skin breaks there!)

2. *Parenteral contact* refers to direct exposure of the bloodstream to infected fluids. Injection drug use with shared equipment, especially needles and syringes, is by far the major mode of transmission in this category. If injection drug users were to use new needles and equipment to inject themselves every time they used a drug, HIV infection would not be transmitted by injecting drugs. Needles used for tattooing, piercing, electrolysis, acupuncture, and for injecting steroids, insulin, or any other substances also can transfer HIV if they are reused or not properly sterilized after use on an infected person. Again, exclusive use of new needles for each new client eliminates this problem.

Other opportunities for direct infection of the blood include surgical procedures and blood transfusions, personal injuries, and first-aid procedures. Receiving a transfusion of infected blood today is highly unlikely, as donated blood units are tested rigorously and donors are tightly screened. The American Red Cross estimates the chances of receiving an HIV-contaminated unit of blood in the United States at 1 in 250,000 units. However, the chance of contaminated units may be higher in parts of the country where HIV infection rates are higher. Donating autologously (for yourself) is the safest way of dealing with blood transfusions.

Providing first aid to anyone who is bleeding could certainly provide opportunity for infection. You can protect yourself using surgical gloves and a pocket mask with a one-way valve for CPR, which

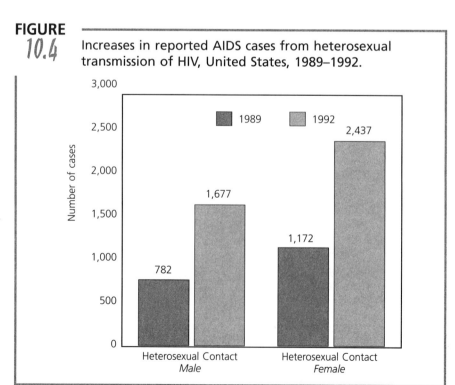

FIGURE 10.4 Increases in reported AIDS cases from heterosexual transmission of HIV, United States, 1989–1992.

Source: *Surgeon General's Report,* 1992.

you can obtain from the Red Cross. This provides protection from direct blood contact at wound sites and at the mouth.

3. *Perinatal contact* refers to exposure of the unborn child of an infected woman to her blood during pregnancy, birth, or breast-feeding. The fetus and mother share the same blood supply constantly for 9 months, yet only one in four of these babies becomes infected. Of those infected, about 20% die before 18 months of age. In recent studies the incidence of infected babies born to infected mothers was markedly reduced when the mother took the drug AZT during the last 6 months of pregnancy. More research is needed to confirm this approach. Currently there is no other way to protect the unborn infant. Infected mothers have to forego breast-feeding, of course.

Symptoms and diagnosis. The human immunodeficiency virus attacks the immune system, eventually rendering its human host incapable of fighting off any sort of infection. This process is described here in four stages (some experts use 6 stages).

Only the fourth and last stage of HIV disease has the diagnostic features of AIDS, acquired immunodeficiency syndrome. In 1993 the Centers for Disease Control and Prevention in Atlanta refined the definition of AIDS as follows: (a) testing positive for HIV and having one of 26 "opportunistic infections" or cancers, or (b) testing positive for HIV and having fewer than 200 T4 lymphocytes per cubic milliliter (800–1600 T4 cells is the normal range).

Testing positive for HIV means detecting antibodies to HIV in the blood. Two blood tests are commonly used: the ELISA (enzyme-linked Immuno Sorbant Assay) and the Western Blot test.

The earliest point at which an infected person might have developed enough antibodies for detection is about 3 weeks, but few newly infected people test positive at this time. By 24 weeks, or 6 months, after infection, 99% of infected people will test positive. A very small number may not test positive for a year or more after infection. In essence, people who engage in any sexual behavior that might expose them to HIV cannot say for certain that they are not infected until testing negative 24 weeks after exposure to HIV. Yet, during this 6-month period, if they are infected, they can infect others. Neither can they say for

sure that they are infected until they test positive for HIV. Some people become infected with just one exposure to HIV; others do not.

The symptoms, testing and infectious status, and duration of four stages of HIV disease are as follows:

Stage 1: Initial infection
Symptoms: flu-like, but this goes away
Test: probably negative, which may be inaccurate
Infectious: probably within several days to a week
Duration: days/weeks

Stage 2: HIV-infected but asymptomatic
Symptoms: none
Test: highly accurate 24 weeks after exposure
Infectious: yes
Duration: months/years

Stage 3: HIV-infected and symptomatic
Symptoms: any or all of the general indicators of poor health, including but not limited to weight loss, fever, sweats, yeast infections, swollen glands, nausea
Test: accurate
Infectious: Yes
Duration: months/years

Stage 4: AIDS
Symptoms: those related to any of 26+ specific diseases (e.g., Kaposi's sarcoma, pneumocystis carenii pneumonia, TB, AIDS dementia) plus any of the generalized symptoms listed in Stage 3.
Test: accurate
Infectious: yes
Duration: varies, eventually fatal

STD Hotlines

For more information on STDs in general or for answers to specific questions, call your local health department, STD/AIDS unit, or the following hotlines:

Toll-free: National STD Hotline 1-800-227-8922
(8 A.M. – 11 P.M. EST M–F)

Toll-free: National AIDS Hotline 1-800-342-AIDS (2437)
(open 24 hours)

Herpes Resource Center Hotline 1-919-361-8488
(9 A.M. – 7 P.M. EST M–F)

Treatment. Currently, HIV disease has no cure or preventive vaccine or any promise of a vaccine in the near future. Almost all people who became infected 10–15 years ago have progressed to stage 3 or 4 by now or have died. A few people are surviving HIV infection with no clear explanation for their fortitude.

Several drugs seem to be able to delay the progress of HIV disease. Azidothymidine (AZT) and Dideoxyinosine (DDI) are two drugs that have been used for some time. Unfortunately, their side-effects have been greater than the benefits for some people. Over time, users of these drugs also may become resistant to their effects.

Currently the best prescription for anyone infected with HIV is to take care of and nurture his or her health and strength through good nutrition, exercise, sufficient rest, and stress management. Insufficient as this prescription might seem, especially to an infected person, it has a double impact, one for the virus and one for the person. It promotes the greatest physiological strength to battle HIV, and it also provides the greatest capacity for living life to the fullest each day, doing the things one wants to do and feeling positive about oneself. In essence, it is a prescription for quality living even with HIV.

SUBSTANCE USE AND ABUSE

Protecting yourself from the consequences of substance abuse, your own or someone else's, is the focus of this section. As with sexual behaviors that transmit STDs, drug use and abuse are complicated by people's desire for personal enjoyment, physical satisfaction, psychological relief, ego support, peer approval, social rituals, economic gain, political advantage, and power. To deal with these issues, you should know something about the substances themselves—what they do for and to a person.

WHY DO PEOPLE USE DRUGS?

Throughout history, people have used drugs and become dependent on them. During this century, however, drug use and abuse have reached epidemic proportions. No one reason can be offered as an explanation. Theories that seek to explain drug-using behavior center on the *predisposition* certain people may have to certain drugs, be it

genetically determined (such as metabolism), or problems in psychological development derived from childhood, or a way to cope with stress. Whatever the reason, researchers have found that each type of drug produces a specific psychological state, or an altered reality, and that chronic users choose a specific drug because of the state it induces.

From the first experience of an altered state, the person may or may not seek that experience again. If the reason is "just to see what it's like," the person's motivation is experimental or curiosity. If the altered state is sought repeatedly, the motivation changes. It may be for perceived pleasure, to escape from a world that seems stressful, or to satisfy physical and psychological addictions. Compulsive users find that virtually every aspect of their lives revolves around obtaining, maintaining, and using the drug. These individuals, described as being drug-dependent, are controlled physically, psychologically, and socially by their drug habit. Their willingness to exploit others, including those who love them the most, to obtain drugs is a vivid reminder of how completely dependent users can become. Between the one-time user whose motivation is curiosity and the daily abuser is a continuum that can be described in terms of motivation and frequency of use (Figure 10.5).

Drug rehabilitation research has documented lack of self-identity as a deep-seated cause of drug abuse. In contrast, people who are comfortable with themselves are less inclined to try to alter their self-perception through drugs. Many rehabilitation programs are aimed specifically at the formation of a positive identity. Another psychological problem—call it alienation, estrangement, or indifference—is manifested in the individual's withdrawal into a lonely, hopeless inner world.

Drugs, Violence, and Crime

Anyone listening to the news in the 1990s knows all too well that drug use often is linked to violence

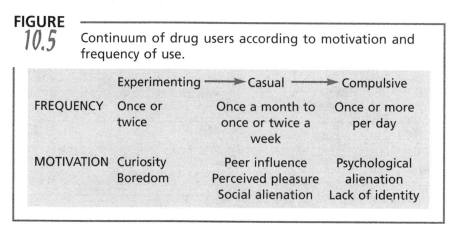

FIGURE 10.5 Continuum of drug users according to motivation and frequency of use.

	Experimenting ⟶	Casual ⟶	Compulsive
FREQUENCY	Once or twice	Once a month to once or twice a week	Once or more per day
MOTIVATION	Curiosity Boredom	Peer influence Perceived pleasure Social alienation	Psychological alienation Lack of identity

and crime. Legal drugs such as alcohol and illegal drugs such as cocaine, amphetamines, and PCP affect a person's physiological function, cognitive ability, and mood. These effects increase the likelihood that users will act violently. In addition, to obtain money to buy drugs, drug users may commit violent or other illegal acts. The connection between drug use, robbery, prostitution, embezzlement, and drug dealing is well documented.

The use and abuse patterns of some of the more widely used legal and illegal drugs are discussed next, weighing the benefits and risks of using these drugs. From the discussion, you can determine ways to protect yourself from becoming a victim of drug abuse.

Alcohol

The human organism does not require alcohol, yet throughout history alcohol has been an integral part of life in most parts of the world. Political leaders celebrate important agreements with a toast. Glasses are raised to toast the bride and groom or the New Year. Elaborate establishments are built to provide places to gather and consume alcohol. The average household contains some form of alcoholic beverage. In the United States, a temporary prohibition of alcohol from 1920 to 1933 produced the largest episode of civil disobedience in the country's history.

Alcohol is not consumed only when one feels deviant or defiant. It is not used only to mask stress, insecurity, or depression or to give a person courage. It is a cultural adjunct. To some extent and for some people, alcohol consumption is pleasant and pleasurable. For many others, though, especially people with emotional problems and those who overindulge, alcohol presents a problem—a self-inflicted, individual problem for which society as a whole pays a great price.

The Societal Costs of Alcohol

More than half of the adult U.S. population drinks alcohol. Many people do so without any problems. More than 18 million Americans, however, are believed to have significant problems associated with alcohol. They contribute significantly to the staggering $80 billion loss to the U.S. economy each year in the form of lost production and medical costs. Of the 50,000 deaths each year from motor vehicle accidents, about half are alcohol-related. Cirrhosis of the liver remains the fourth leading cause of death for middle-aged men and fifth for women. The percentage of homicides and suicides committed under the influence of alcohol is difficult to assess but is believed to be considerable. A greater awareness by pregnant women of the effects of alcohol on the fetus shows promise in reducing the incidence of fetal alcohol syndrome.

With the possible exception of the teenage drinking problem, which has worsened, the number of drinkers and the severity of their problem, as well as deaths attributed to alcohol, have remained fairly constant over the last decade. Unfortunately, little progress has been made in understanding the factors that cause alcoholism. Similarly, little progress has been made in alcohol treatment techniques, and little new information has been uncovered on how alcohol affects the human organism.

The alcohol contained in alcoholic beverages is ethyl alcohol, or ethanol. Because of its chemical structure, ethanol has the power to depress the action of the central nervous system, and its depressant actions brings about most of the commonly observed drinking behaviors. The first observable effects of ethanol are those controlled by the higher centers of the brain, located primarily in the frontal area. For some unknown reason, one's

Avoid Overindulging in Alcohol

To avoid slipping past a pleasurable social interaction into intoxication:

- The party atmosphere should be relaxing, and whatever can be done to make everyone mix should be done. One reason people drink too much at social gatherings is that they cannot seem to get conversations going.

- The volume of music should be low enough to allow people to socialize. Again, when you cannot talk, you drink more.

- Food should be served. It not only slows down the absorption of alcohol but also satisfies some oral needs to supplant the continual sipping of drinks. Good food also takes some of the spotlight off alcohol. Foods that have some protein content are best: for example, cheese and crackers, Swedish meatballs, hard-boiled eggs, cheese fondue, pizza, and bite-sized cold cuts.

- Activities should be going on, with some effort to get everyone involved. Dancing, games, sports, and good conversation quickly become the focus, and drinks can just add to the enjoyment.

Source: *On Drink*, by Kingsley Amis (New York: Harcourt, Brace, Jovanovich, 1973).

learned social inhibitions are the first to be affected. Possibly this part of the brain controls complex behaviors; millions of nerve cells are required to "think," and even small amounts of alcohol may interfere with this process. Research shows that alcohol may impede the brain's capacity to switch from one source of information to another. In addition, alcohol impairs motor functioning.

Research shows that alcohol causes some people to become more aggressive in certain circumstances but not in others. This may be related more to personality than to the situation. For example, when male social drinkers drink in competitive group situations, their interpersonal aggression increases. Research also is linking alcohol to a large percentage of domestic violence episodes.

Drinking and Driving

Alcohol is involved in about half of all highway deaths. About 22,000 people a year (400 a week)

FIGURE 10.6 — Factors that contribute to alcoholism.

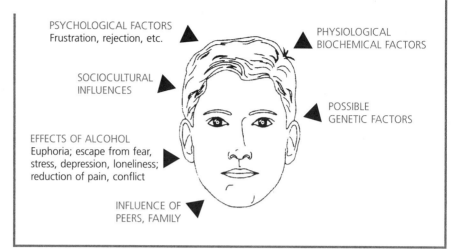

- PSYCHOLOGICAL FACTORS Frustration, rejection, etc.
- PHYSIOLOGICAL BIOCHEMICAL FACTORS
- SOCIOCULTURAL INFLUENCES
- POSSIBLE GENETIC FACTORS
- EFFECTS OF ALCOHOL Euphoria; escape from fear, stress, depression, loneliness; reduction of pain, conflict
- INFLUENCE OF PEERS, FAMILY

die because some people choose to drive while intoxicated. About half of those killed each year are *not* the ones who had been drinking. If it were not for drinking drivers, six in 10 young adults killed in automobile accidents would still be alive.

As many as 60% of all alcohol-related accidents are single-vehicle crashes, which usually involve running off the road or running into something. Yet few people think their driving is affected seriously by alcohol. A study of eight professional race drivers who doubted that their

---

A C T I V I T Y

PRESCRIPTION FOR HEALTH

You can protect yourself from alcohol abuse in several ways. *Best Advice:* Don't drink at all. Alcohol has few, if any, health benefits. *Second Best:* Drink in moderation. Don't glorify alcohol or your ability to consume it. Learn to recognize the signs of overdrinking and use these as a signal to slow down. Common signs are loud talking, slurred speech, walking unsteadily, dropping things or spilling drinks, perspiring, and turning red or pale in the face.

Don't drink and drive. Carpool, select a designated driver who will not drink, call a friend, take a taxi, hitch a ride, or stay the night. And don't let your friends drive if they've been drinking. Stay in control. Learn how to keep track of your blood alcohol level by knowing your weight, the amount of alcohol you've consumed, and your drinking time. Keep yourself busy with interesting and active pursuits. Avoid friends who do little else besides drink for their recreation.

If you find yourself. . .

- drinking, even in moderation, every day

- finding that your drunken exploits are all you have to talk about
- missing your early classes because of hangovers
- getting drunk regularly
- drinking to dull the hurt of loneliness and to counteract frequent depression
- driving after drinking
- needing to brag constantly about your ability to drink. . .

you should seriously consider cutting down on how much and how often you drink, for you are developing an addictive behavior pattern. If cutting down is difficult for you to do alone, seek help. NOW.

Talk to your doctor or a counselor about the possibility that you are drinking too much. Be honest. If you aren't comfortable in doing this, look up the telephone number for Alcoholics Anonymous (AA) and call. Ask how you can tell if you are drinking too much and if AA can assist you in finding help.

performances would be affected yielded the following results:

- 7 mistakes while sober
- 22 mistakes when impaired
- 42 mistakes when intoxicated

Alcohol-Related Medical Problems

Well-documented alcohol-related medical problems include:

Alcoholism
Cancer
Cardiovascular disorders
Cirrhosis
Endocrine disorders
Fetal alcohol syndrome
Gastrointestinal disorders
Neurological impairment

Space does not allow in-depth coverage of each of these conditions. Suffice it to say, the $80 billion spent annually in the United States on the social, legal, and medical costs of dealing with these problems, on top of the incalculable human suffering they cause, is sobering. Figure 10.6 summarizes the possible causative factors in the development of alcoholism.

Tobacco

Following alcohol, the nicotine present in tobacco is the second most widely used drug in the United States. Approximately 55 million Americans smoke daily. Nicotine meets the established scientific criteria for being classified as a dependency-producing drug. It causes physiological dependence in both animal and human experiments. Under experimental conditions, when habitual use is discontinued, nicotine withdrawal symptoms ensue, including EEG (brainwave) changes, measurably impaired intellectual and psychomotor performance, irritability, aggressiveness, anxiety, insomnia, and fatigue. These symptoms sometimes can be relieved by chewing nicotine-containing gum. Tobacco use, like use of other abused drugs, often is peer-initiated. Social support for tobacco use allows for tolerance and habitual patterns to develop with repeated use.

Smoking Tobacco

Nicotine is not only an addictive drug, but also a deadly drug. More than 485,000 Americans die prematurely from tobacco-related illness. Cigarette smoking is now recognized as the largest single preventable cause of premature death and disability

in our society. Projections by the American Cancer Society and the Veterans Administration reported differences of between 7 and 9 years in life expectancy between continuing smokers and non-smokers. Other studies indicate that men who have smoked cigarettes throughout their lives will die nearly 18 years earlier than men who never started. A 30-year-old man who smokes will reduce his life expectancy on average by about one-fourth.

Cigarette smoking annually causes:

- 147,000 deaths from cancer
- 240,000 deaths from diseases of the circulatory system
- 61,000 non-cancer deaths from diseases of the respiratory system
- 14,000 deaths from diseases of the digestive system
- 4,000 infant deaths resulting from mothers smoking
- 4,000 deaths as a result of fires and accidents
- nearly 15,000 deaths from ill-defined and miscellaneous diseases

Add to that the deaths caused by smoking pipes and cigars, passively inhaling environmental tobacco smoke, and chewing and snuffing tobacco, and the total U.S. death toll from tobacco may be more than a half million—more than a fourth of all deaths from all causes. Since 1979 the number of smokers has dropped slightly. In a breakdown by age groups, 22% of youth and 40% of adults are regular smokers. By age 12, one of five youngsters smokes. One alarming increase in smoking patterns is that of girls; the smoking pattern of high school girls now approximates that of high school boys.

Smokeless Tobacco

There has been a resurgence in the use of all forms of smokeless tobacco in the United States, with sales increasing about 11% each year since 1974, and resulting in an estimated 22 million users. Several forms of tobacco are either chewed or sniffed. Snuff is a finely ground tobacco sold in circular cans. Users commonly place a pinch of snuff between the lip and gum; it also is placed on the back of the hand and sniffed through the nose. Another form of smokeless tobacco, chewing tobacco, is loose-leafed and sold in a pouch. It also is placed between the lip and gum for a time and then spit out. Another type is the plug that is sold in brick form, from which the user cuts or bites off a piece. Using smokeless tobacco results in blood levels of nicotine approximating those after cigarette smoking, and preliminary evidence indicates

ACTIVITY

WHY DO YOU SMOKE?

The Horn–Waingrow Smoking Motives Questionnaire addresses most schools of thought on motivations for smoking by assessing six factors: sensory-motor stimulation, nervous system stimulation, pleasure, reduction of tension, habit, and addiction. Addiction is the strongest motivation and sensory-motor stimulation the weakest.

Based on the motives for smoking, at least four different types of smokers have been identified. If you are a smoker, which type are you? If you are not a smoker, you may use this information to understand the smoking behavior of a friend or relative. If you smoke, the knowledge of why you smoke may help motivate you to quit.

1. Do you smoke more in times of crisis? Have you quit smoking several times but lapsed back into smoking during stressful times? Is the cigarette a sedative, reducing feelings of fear, anger, and nervousness? If so, you can be classified as a *negative-effect smoker,* one who smokes a cigarette as a crutch in times of crisis or as a sedative to relieve feelings such as nervousness, anger, shame, and disgust. This kind of need fulfillment offers tremendous reinforcement, and smoking becomes a pleasurable experience.

2. Do you find yourself lighting one cigarette before the other is completely out? Does the absence of a cigarette make you feel uncomfortable? Do you constantly feel a strong desire to smoke? If so, chances are that you are an *addictive smoker,* one who uses cigarettes to satisfy needs or to solve problems, one who feels more normal with a cigarette than without one.

3. Do you really like to smoke and enjoy the taste of smoke? Does smoking relax you? Does it add enjoyment after a meal? Do you get pleasure from manipulating the cigarette, blowing smoke rings? Do you think you look older and more sophisticated when you smoke? If so, you probably are a *positive-effect smoker,* often called a pleasure smoker.

4. If you are running out of cigarettes constantly, you likely underestimate the amount you smoke. You're a chain smoker, but the habit is so automatic that the cigarette is out of the pack and into your mouth almost without conscious thought. You may find that cigarettes don't taste particularly good, but you seem to have one lit at all times. Often you light up only to find one lit in the ashtray. If this behavior describes your smoking pattern, you have a smoking habit. You are a *habitual smoker.*

Source: Daniel H. Horn, National Clearinghouse for Smoking and Health, Health and Human Services.

that smokeless tobacco use also leads to nicotine dependency.

With the use of smokeless tobacco, increases in heart rate and blood pressure have been observed in 3 to 5 minutes. It has the potential for causing cancer of the oral cavity, pharynx, larynx, and esophagus. Smokeless tobacco also can produce harmful effects on the soft and hard tissues of the mouth, causing bad breath, discolored teeth, receding gums, and periodontal destruction. Smokeless tobacco can contribute to cardiovascular disease in the same way as smoked tobacco, and its use is discouraged especially by individuals who have high blood pressure.

The relationship of smoking to stress has been investigated frequently. Smokers consistently score higher than nonsmokers on nearly all anxiety measures. In addition, smokers often are seen as especially sensitive to stress because, as a group, they lack coping resources and resort to smoking in an attempt to cope. Subjective distress is one of the most frequently reported triggers for smoking. Highly anxious smokers likewise have been found to have lower expectations of being able to produce desired outcomes, which translates into lower self-

confidence. Although failure to meet internal expectations is difficult to measure, it often results in low self-esteem, which has been observed more in smoking than in nonsmoking teenagers. Because failure tends to result in diverting efforts from assigned tasks, no wonder teenage smokers seem to fail more in school than nonsmokers do.

Passive Smoking

Smoking cigarettes in public is a strongly disputed issue centering on individual rights: the rights of the smoker to smoke versus the rights of the nonsmoker to breathe air unpolluted by smoke. At least 1,200 different toxic chemicals have been identified as products of tobacco smoke. Smoke is a mixture of hot air and gases that suspend small particles called tars in cigarette smoke. Many of the particles contain **carcinogens,** substances that are known to cause cancer. One such chemical, benzopyrene, is among the most potent carcinogens known. Also contained in the particulate matter are chemicals called phenols, which are thought to speed up or activate dormant cancer cells.

Scientific studies show clearly that nonsmokers in the presence of smokers are affected by the

A C T I V I T Y

GIVING UP THE HABIT

Tobacco use may produce both psychological and physical dependence. Smoking is one of the more difficult dependencies to end, perhaps because smoking was acceptable for so long and smokers developed the dependency early and continued it for decades. Smoking cessation treatment results in short-term success rates as high as 70%, but these rates decrease significantly to an average of between 6% and 15% a year later.

There are more than 30 million former smokers in the United States and another 30 million people who have tried to quit but failed. The reasons some people succeed and others fail are not well understood, but many researchers believe that success is a result of a combination of personal motivation and an effective plan of action. Successful smoking cessation programs tend to include the following core elements.

Motivation or commitment. Motivation is all-important and can be increased through:

1. Education about the harmful effects of smoking
2. Knowledge of psychological patterns of smokers
3. Examination of the motivation and commitment to becoming a nonsmoker

Breaking the habit. Whatever the underlying psychological reason compelling an individual to smoke, a habit has developed and a habit must be broken. Smokers seldom are aware of how much they do smoke, so an initial record-keeping phase, in which the smoker records all the cigarettes smoked, is deemed necessary. A tapering-off process toward a targeted quitting date in 3 to 6 weeks is characteristic of most successful programs as are behavior modification techniques associated with the buying, carrying, or handling of the cigarette.

A healthy lifestyle. A third component of an effective program often is not included in smoking cessation programs, and this oversight undoubtedly contributes to the high failure rates. This phase focuses on psychological needs that smoking traditionally has satisfied. The goal is to extinguish these needs and develop lifestyle skills that will help the nonsmoker remain a nonsmoker. The basic components are:

1. *Relaxation and stress-management skills.* Nearly every smoker uses cigarettes to control one or more of the following factors:
   - excess anxiety
   - low self-esteem
   - excess anger
   - depression
   - stressful lifestyle
   - inability to relax

2. *Diet.* Many smokers are nervous eaters who have substituted smoking for eating. Often, when smoking stops, eating and weight gain problems emerge. This creates fear in weight-conscious smokers. Close attention to diet and weight-management counseling are essential to the success of most smoking cessation programs.

3. *Exercise.* Exercise not only is integral to a healthy lifestyle but also may be essential to smoking cessation programs because it:
   - Builds confidence and self-esteem
   - Reduces anxiety and excess stress
   - Burns calories
   - Is antiethical to the physical deterioration caused by smoking

All these activities tend to help smokers in their efforts to kick the habit.

After support. Most people who quit smoking and then start again do so within a few weeks of quitting. Recidivism can be reduced through *relapse training.* Two important factors are related to relapse:

1. The need to smoke is still present. Even though smokers have changed their overt smoking behavior, they either did not eliminate the triggers, or cues, to smoke or they did not establish a new behavior as a substitute for smoking when the triggers arise.

2. The all-or-nothing attitude of some smokers makes them feel like total failures if they have one or two cigarettes after they have "quit." This undermines their self-image and sets in motion a vicious cycle that further increases their motivation to smoke.

Source: *Changing Health Behavior* by D. Girdano and D. Dusek (Scottsdale, AZ: Gorsuch Scarisbrick, Publishers, 1988), pp. 215–238.

smoke, especially young children who live in a household of smokers. Smoking one cigarette releases into the air surrounding the smoker approximately 70 milligrams of particulates and 25 milligrams of carbon monoxide. The level of carbon monoxide in smoke-filled rooms often reaches 80 parts per million. The Environmental Protection Agency considers this amount hazardous, exceeding the limits set for occupational exposure. Smoke-filled automobiles and smoke-filled rooms often are in violation of pure air quality standards. To make matters worse, because the sidestream temperatures are cooler and some constituents of the smoke are not oxidized completely, the sidestream smoke may be more potent than the smoke inhaled by the smoker.

Increased knowledge of the hazards of smoking in general and the studies of sidestream smoke, combined with increased sensitivity for air-pollution problems and the movement toward individual rights, has led to pressure against smoking in public. Smoking on airplanes and in many municipal buildings and public places has been severely limited or banned. Most hotels, motels, eating establishments, and other privately owned enterprises now give the customer a choice of a nonsmoking room or section.

Protecting Yourself

To protect yourself from being or becoming a victim of tobacco use, especially smoking, you can choose to take one of the following actions, depending on your situation.

1. *Individuals who use tobacco and would like some help in quitting.* If you are going to join a program, research it to see if it has the components mentioned in this text, and make sure you are convinced you can be successful. If you are going it alone, at least get some guidance from the numerous private, government, and association program materials.

2. *Individuals who do not use tobacco and would like to be protected from those who do* (breathing sidestream smoke). The most obvious self-protection activity is to manipulate your environment so as not to be around individuals using tobacco. Practice assertiveness. Ask that individuals not smoke in your presence, and back it up with action by leaving if they continue. Do not support businesses that don't offer nonsmoking accommodations. Finally, decline friends' invitations to join them in using tobacco.

3. *Individuals, especially teenagers and young adults, who might be susceptible to developing a habit of use.* For guidelines, refer to the suggestions at the end of the section on drug use in general.

Marijuana

Marijuana is derived from the flowers and the top leaves of the female *Cannabis sativa* plant, a weed of the hemp family. The plant produces resin, a sticky yellow substance, as a protective shield against the elements. Marijuana plants grown in hotter, sunnier climates produce more resin to protect themselves from the sun's heat. The resin contains the active drug ingredient tetrahydrocannabinol (THC). Cannabis has a number of strains, the strength of each depending on the amount of active THC it contains. In the United States the weakest, and most widely used, preparation is derived from the tops of uncultivated flower shoots and is called "pot," "grass," "weed," and other names. The strongest is made from the resin and is called hashish. In the Western world, cannabis usually is smoked, and in this form it is considered more potent than when taken orally in drinks or food.

The most verified effect of marijuana on humans is a temporary increase in heart rate related to the amount taken. With the smoking or ingestion of marijuana, the eyes redden because of vasodilation of blood vessels. Research continues to confirm early findings that marijuana use decreases hand steadiness and increases body sway while standing erect. When experiments demand uncomplicated responses to a simple stimulus, marijuana has little effect on reaction time, but when the task is complex, performance is impeded. The subjects of experiments also are affected adversely by marijuana when they are asked to detect and respond to peripheral light cues in their visual field. These effects may hinder driving and other machine-operating skills. Simulator studies show that marijuana intoxication impairs driving skills. Also, glare recovery time (after driving into headlights at night, for example) is longer in marijuana-intoxicated drivers.

Research concerning the health hazards of cannabis continues. Street samples of marijuana have continued to become more potent, now averaging more than 4% compared to less than 1% a decade ago. Evidence that marijuana reduces the body's immune response seems conclusive. Marijuana use is associated with greater use of other drugs, with less participation in conventional activities, with a history of psychiatric hospitalization, with lower self-perceived psychological well-being, and with more involvement in other socially deviant activities. A study of marijuana use by adolescents found that it is used as a means of escaping from problems and relieving stress and that it reinforces the individual's unwillingness to face problems. From the time of early popularization of marijuana, users have reported negative experiences ranging from mild anxiety to acute panic, and an acute brain syndrome including disorientation, confusion, and impaired memory.

Chronic marijuana use is likely related to a lack of motivation in many young and older users alike. Which came first, the amotivation or the smoking of marijuana? According to the National Institute of Drug Abuse, the motivational effects are related highly to use and normal motivation may return when the person ceases using the drug. More than half of the high school seniors in the study who quit using marijuana said they did so because of "loss of energy or ambition," and about 40% of the daily users thought it interfered with their ability to think and contributed to their loss of interest in other activities.

Regarding the often-reported medicinal effects of marijuana, the conclusions are mixed. It has been recommended for hundreds of problems, including insomnia, pain, anxiety, and tension, and used as such sporadically throughout history. Research regarding the medical effects of THC on some maladies has been positive, and special approval for experimentation and prescription has aided individuals with glaucoma and asthma, those who have nausea and vomiting from cancer therapy, and those with epileptic seizures.

Stimulants

Drugs that stimulate the central nervous system have been in use for centuries. Natives of the high Andes chewed on coca leaves to help them contend with a harsh high-altitude existence, and coffee beans and tobacco have long been used for their stimulatory qualities. Suspecting that synthetic substances could produce an adrenaline-stimulating effect, researchers discovered amphetamines in the 1920s. Because of the intense response by the nervous system to the various stimulants, these drugs came to be abused. Reactions include elevation of mood, loss of appetite, alertness, wakefulness, and attentiveness. The stimulants include cocaine, amphetamines, and caffeine, among others.

The mechanism of action of the stimulants appears to be that of mimicking the action of the central nervous system, probably by increasing the release of one or both of the neurotransmitters dopamine and norepinephrine. This occurs in specific brain areas such as the cortex, which is responsible for thinking and judgment and the reticular activating system, which is responsible for our wakefulness and alertness. The site of amphetamine action in this part of the brain explains behavioral reactions such as the elevation of mood and loss of hunger. These combined reactions of alertness, wakefulness, and attentiveness are characteristics of the stress reaction, or the "fight-or-flight" syndrome. The following physiological reactions occur:

1. Constriction of blood vessels
2. Increased heart rate and strength of myocardial contractions
3. Rise in blood pressure
4. Dilation of the bronchi
5. Relaxation of intestinal muscle
6. Mydriasis (dilation of the pupil)
7. Increased blood sugar levels
8. Shorter blood coagulation time
9. Increased muscle tension
10. Stimulation of the adrenal glands

Cocaine

Cocaine is a powerful central nervous system stimulant derived from the leaves of the coca shrub native to South America. Coca plant leaves are made into cocaine paste, which in turn is converted into cocaine base and then into cocaine hydrochloride. Cocaine comes in three basic forms: the rock form, the flake form (considered by connoisseurs to be a delicacy), and the most common "street coke," the powder form, which usually is diluted. Cocaine almost always is cut (mixed) with synthetics such as Procaine, Benzocaine, and speed.

In its pure form, cocaine is a white crystalline powder that looks like sugar (hence the nickname "snow"). It is sniffed (snorted) in powder form, liquefied and injected, or made into "freebase" and smoked. Smoking freebase produces a shorter and more intense "high" because the drug enters the blood more rapidly than through the mouth or nose. Cocaine that can be smoked now is readily available on the illicit market as "crack." Because crack is easy to produce and thus is available at lowered cost, the dangers of increasing use and the likelihood of becoming cocaine-dependent are magnified.

Cocaine is a powerful drug, capable of altering the psychophysiological state of the user significantly. A lethal dose is approximately 1.2 grams for most individuals if the entire amount is taken orally at one time. Early publications regarded cocaine as nonaddictive; physical dependency and withdrawal were believed not to occur. Today these views are being reassessed. The effects of chronic use are becoming more apparent. Experts in the field now consider tolerance and withdrawal as definite entities in chronic cocaine use.

In addition to possible physical dependence, cocaine induces a high level of psychic dependence and often results in a destructive type of drug abuse. As the effects wear off, feelings of depression and fatigue often set in. Headache, discomfort, and depression often lead to a strong desire to get high again. Understanding the desire for continued use is not difficult. If a strong psychological drive motivates frequent and heavy use, the user goes into the second stage, called *cocaine dysphoria*, experiencing apathy, nervousness, insomnia, and weight loss from anorexia.

If the second stage is unabated over several months, the user likely will go into a third stage, the psychotic state, almost indistinguishable from acute paranoid schizophrenia. Hallucinations, hypomanic behavior (compulsive repetitive behavior), and delusional paranoia characterize this stage.

The purity of "street" cocaine increased markedly—from 29% to 73% pure—between 1982 and 1984. Illicit cocaine now is not only significantly purer, but also is much less expensive than a decade ago. Treatment centers specializing in cocaine dependence are springing up throughout the country, but to date no unique mode of treatment for cocaine abusers has been developed. All of the programs stress the need for total abstinence, learning to manage impulsive drug-using behavior, and developing insight into the destructive role of the drug in the user's life. Three of four cocaine users interviewed who called the 800–COCAINE help line reported a loss of control over their use; two-thirds were unable to stop despite repeated attempts. Nine in ten users interviewed in the 800–COCAINE sample reported serious emotional and physical consequences of use.

Drug-related emergency room visits, deaths from overdose, and serious clinical problems show a higher rate of increase for cocaine than for any other abused drug. The increase in cocaine use in the past few years has been accompanied by a dramatic increase in cocaine-related hospital emergency room visits, verifying the increase in hardcore abuse.

Amphetamines

Amphetamines have been used as stimulant drugs for a number of years. One of the first uses of Benzedrine was as a vasoconstrictor for nasal passageways—the Benzedrine Inhaler was introduced in 1932. Later this inhaler was removed from the market because of its frequent abuse.

Further research led to development of an amphetamine closely related to Benzedrine, called Dexedrine, and led to the discovery of methylamphetamine ("speed"). Of the three, Dexedrine probably is used the most medically because, even though its stimulatory effects on the central nervous system are greater than those of the other two, if has fewer side-effects. This is one of the main reasons Dexedrine is the amphetamine used most frequently in diet pills.

Subjective effects of amphetamines include a feeling of euphoria, a sense of well-being, reduced appetite, talkativeness, hyperactivity, and a feeling of heightened mental and physical power. A single dose (5 to 15 milligrams) of amphetamine can produce these symptoms. Administering the drug in emergencies, when a person must stay awake and alert over a longer than usual time, has been found useful. If wakefulness is longer than 1½ to 2 days, irritability, anxiety, and other undesirable effects likely will develop.

Therapeutic or medical use of the amphetamines is decreasing, as many authorities believe these drugs are no longer needed. Therapeutic use of amphetamines still is accepted in treating symptoms of narcolepsy (a sleep disorder) and hyperkinetic behavior in children with organic brain damage. Some medical professionals are no longer using these drugs to treat obesity, because of their long-term ineffectiveness and because other nonamphetamine stimulants may work to suppress appetite in the short-term.

Because the use of amphetamines is of questionable value, taking these drugs may be considered misuse. The misuse of amphetamines generally revolves around:

1. Weight control
2. Better physical performance
3. Better mental performance, alertness, or relief from general lassitude.

One abuse pattern often seen is that of taking low-dose oral amphetamines compulsively on a daily basis in a desperate attempt to maintain a stimulated pace of life, to reinforce chemically an outgoing personality, to keep the mood elevated, and to hold back the inevitable depression that sets in as the body rebounds from the chronic stimulation. The pattern usually entails taking uppers in the morning and afternoon and downers such as alcohol and barbiturates at night. To reduce some of the nervous side-effects of amphetamine stimulation, many commercial brands add sedatives, usually barbiturates, to the amphetamines, producing an unintentional barbiturate dependence.

Another pattern of amphetamine abuse lies in the intravenous use of high-dose methamphetamines. As tolerance develops, users progress from doses of around 10 to 40 milligrams several times a day to many times that amount. Much has been written on the aggressiveness and violence associated with the "speed scene." Violence is especially likely to break out when all available speed has been used. The fatigued and irritated user then goes out in search of more speed or a safe place to crash (to come down off the drug). Both situations can easily trigger hostility. Some regions of the country are experiencing an epidemic use of "crystal meth" or "ice," a highly potent form of methamphetamine, and its ever-present violent subculture.

Caffeine

Coffee drinking in America is an extension of the European custom brought to this country centuries ago. In Europe, coffee houses were the common meeting places for conversation, political argument, and camaraderie. Coffee drinking continues to be a custom that gives one an excuse to sit down to converse or take a "time out." The coffee break became a national institution partly because of the need for a rest from work but also because of the stimulation this beverage offers. The chemical caffeine belongs to the xanthine group of drugs. Xanthines are powerful amphetamine-like stimulants that can increase metabolism and create a highly awake and active state. They also trigger release of the stress hormones, which are capable of increasing heart rate, blood pressure, and oxygen demands on the heart, among other effects.

Coffee is the most frequently consumed source of caffeine in America. Other caffeine sources are tea, chocolate, cola and soft drinks, anti-sleep preparations, and other over-the-counter drugs such as appetite suppressants and analgesics.

People who drink more than one or two cups of coffee every day develop some tolerance, physical dependence, and most likely some psychological dependence on the coffee habit. Individuals who drink more than two cups of coffee a day often believe they cannot get started in the morning without their coffee and drink it continually throughout the day to keep going. Withdrawal from caffeine occurs when those who have become tolerant to it abruptly discontinue its use. Symptoms of withdrawal include headache, irritability, lethargy, mood changes, sleep disturbance, and mild physiological arousal.

Many consider caffeine consumption of more than 250 milligrams per day to be excessive, as it can have adverse effects on the body. (The average brewed 6-ounce cup of coffee contains about 110 milligrams of caffeine, as well as other xanthines: theobromine and theophyllin.) Overconsumption of caffeine can result in:

- restlessness
- nervousness
- excitement
- insomnia
- flushed face
- diarrhea
- muscle twitching
- rambling flow of thought and speech
- cardiac arrhythmia (irregular heartbeat)
- periods of inexhaustibility
- psychomotor agitation
- gastrointestinal complaints

Caffeine also may stimulate secretion of the digestive enzyme pepsin within the stomach. In an empty stomach this enzyme, combined with the natural oils in coffee, can irritate the stomach lining—a reason why those who already have ulcers should cut out caffeine products. Medical uses of caffeine include treatment for drowsiness and fatigue and treatment for migraine and other vascular headaches.

Sedative Hypnotics

As the dangers of sedative hypnotics—barbiturates and nonbarbiturates—have become apparent, their medical use as antianxiety and antitension drugs is declining. These drugs have been found to create tolerance (and cross-tolerance to other depressant drugs) and psychic and physical dependence. Withdrawal after chronic abuse is more traumatic than that caused by any other drug, mainly because of the life-threatening convulsions that accompany withdrawal. The tranquilizers that have largely replaced the barbiturates unfortunately have been found to pose potential dangers identical to the earlier sedative hypnotics: tolerance, dependence, and overdose, primarily. Illicit use of sedative hypnotics has increased dramatically. Policy-makers of federal drug abuse organizations have called for a reevaluation of barbiturate use. Some of the problems seen with these drugs are the following.

1. Barbiturates are used more frequently than any other drug as a means of suicide.
2. Accidental death occurs from otherwise less-than-lethal levels of barbiturates when they are used in conjunction with alcohol.
3. Barbiturates have been abused consistently since their arrival on the market. Their abuse has been linked with violent behavior and with accidents from motor clumsiness.
4. Withdrawal from barbiturate dependence poses serious medical considerations, as it is life-endangering to the user.

Opiates

The family of opiates derives from opium extracts of the parent plant *Papaver somniferum.* Processing produces crude heroin, which is dried and crushed to form white heroin, the injectable drug seen in the United States. It resembles talc or flour in consistency and may have a heroin content of 95% or more before it is adulterated.

The heroin user's preferred form of administration is intravenous because of the immediate rush. Other forms of administration are snorting (sniffing), intramuscular injection (skin-popping or joy-popping), and smoking. Heroin and the other opiates exert their effects by depressing the central nervous system. This depressant action works to relieve pain and, in large doses, to induce sleep. Overdose causes death because of the drug's depressant action on the respiratory center in the brain.

Heroin produces immediate effects: a flush of euphoria, an elevation of mood, and a feeling of peace, contentment, and safety. This is why heroin has such addictive potential.

Common physical effects of the opiates are:

- respiratory slow-down
- constipation
- constriction of pupils of eye
- hypotension
- suppressed sex drive
- release of histamine

Contrary to common belief, high-dose users of the opiates can function quite adequately. Aside from the danger of unsterile needles and other factors inherent in the lifestyle of the heroin user, the addict does not deteriorate physically as much from chronic use as other drugs such as alcohol. Nevertheless, diseases such as hepatitis, septicemia, and endocarditis accompany the use of unsterile needles, and abscesses are common among heroin addicts. Another cause of death in heroin addicts is cardiovascular collapse because of allergic reaction to the injected substance.

According to one school of thought, three major factors create heroin dependence: life situation, personality, and pharmacology of the drug. It often is said that people start to use drugs for one reason but often continue using them for very different reasons. This is particularly true in the case of heroin users. This is because opiates can create a personality complete with specific drives, needs, and values that may be entirely different from those the individual has when not addicted. Research has added credence to this long-held hypothesis.

The number of heroin-dependent persons seems to have stabilized in the last few years. Estimates are approximately one-half million users in the United States. Although the abuse of heroin and other narcotics remains a significant public health problem, the ills associated with opiate abuse continue to be more social than medical. Thievery and prostitution are the most common consequences of having a habit that is both expensive and debilitating and that precludes useful employment. About 80,000 opiate-dependent individuals are in treatment at any given time in the United States. Some centers advocate drug programs such as methadone maintenance, and some advocate drug-free therapeutic communities.

Hallucinogens/Psychedelics

Among the natural hallucinogens are nutmeg, certain morning glory seeds, and jimson weed. The prototype of "manufactured" hallucinogens—which have basically the same effects on the body—is lysergic acid diethylamide-24, better known as LSD. For many years LSD was ingested in the form of a sugar cube containing a drop of LSD. Today it appears more often as a tablet or soaked into heavy blotter paper, from which it is placed under the tongue or licked off. It begins to affect the brain in about 40 minutes to an hour or more, and the effects continue about 12 hours.

One of its first visual manifestations is that of ever-changing colors and shapes of objects and the appearance of rainbow-like halos around lights. The senses are further affected with possible synesthesia (a crossing of sense responses such as hearing colors and seeing sounds). The person may be entranced by the deepness of colors, the beauty of a single object, the pureness of sound. While LSD enhances visual and auditory perception, it is detrimental to other senses. Time and space perceptions are lost, and because of its stimulatory nature, LSD permits many extra stimuli to enter thought processes. Sounds and sights may flash on and off, tripping thought processes that have been long forgotten.

An acute psychological danger with this drug is that ego boundaries may disappear. For example, the floor may seem to become part of the body, and stepping on the floor may evoke bodily pain. The ego may be inflated to heights beyond compare (pure omnipotence) or to extreme lows, where suicide may seem to be the only way out. Thinking loses its logic. Users may become fixated on illogical "truths" that occur to them during an LSD experience.

A well-publicized chronic reaction to LSD is the flashback, although not everyone who takes LSD experiences this phenomenon. It seems to occur most often in cases in which the user has had a bad experience. Feelings of paranoia, unreality, and estrangement often accompany the flashback, along with distorted visual perceptions and prickly or tingling sensations creeping over the body.

Other abused hallucinogens include mescaline, the psilocybin mushroom, and PCP. The latter has replaced LSD as the most abused hallucinogen overall. The effects of PCP mimic schizophrenic thinking, and PCP ingestion is a leading cause of psychiatric admission. The illegal manufacture of PCP is lucrative and relatively easy because its chemical components are widely available commercially and impossible to control. Although PCP use seems to be decreasing overall, its use in some populations such as high school seniors has increased.

Designer Drugs

An emerging problem in the drug abuse arena is that of analogs of drugs of abuse. These are synthetic compounds created by underground chemists and designed to mimic psychoactive drugs. The chemists change the molecular structure of a drug, which also may change its potency, length of action, euphoric effects, and toxicity. These drugs became illegal since passage of the Anti-Drug Abuse Act of 1986, but they are difficult to control. MDMA, which is a synthetic hallucinogen billed as Ecstasy and a heroin substitute called China White, likely will add to the incidence of drug-taking in this category.

These analogs have been dubbed "designer" drugs in the media, which may create an impression that they somehow are special or desirable. They often contain contaminants, however, and can have serious adverse side-effects. Counting exactly how many people have overdosed on these drugs and how many fatalities can be attributed to them—or even the extent of their use and availability—is impossible. The evidence, however, is ample to generate concern among public health officials, especially as the use of cocaine decreases and the use of hallucinogens increases.

Protecting Yourself from Drug Abuse

Protecting yourself from drug abuse once again focuses on the choices individuals have concerning their personal situation:

1. *Individuals who use drugs and would like help in quitting.* Help is available and usually is free, offered by government-funded medical groups. College students can contact their health or counseling center. Outside the university, help often is drug-specific. Sometimes a telephone call to an anonymous hotline is a first step. For many years, self-help groups such as Al-Anon, Alateen, and Adult Children of Alcoholics (ACOA) have existed for the families and friends of alcoholics. These groups, which have no dues or fees, also can help families of drug abusers.

Support groups patterned after those serving the families of alcoholics have been formed specifically for families of drug abusers. Nar-Anon is for people whose lives have been affected by a drug abuser. Families Anonymous focuses on the families of drug abusers, as well

as those concerned about runaways and delinquents. COCANON family groups are for people whose lives have been affected by a friend's or family member's cocaine habit. These groups are organized into local chapters, usually listed in the phone book. They exist to help the families of drug users rather than to address the needs of the users themselves. In the groups, members share experiences and common concerns and work to understand better how the drug abuse problem affects them. The anonymity of all participants is protected and respected.

2. *Individuals who do not use drugs and would like to be protected from those who do.* The most obvious self-protection activity is to manipulate your environment so as not to be around individuals using drugs. Exposure to drugs usually leads to social or legal problems and often to violence. Practice assertiveness. Ask that individuals not use drugs in your presence. Back it up with action, and leave if they continue. Finally, be prepared mentally to decline friends' invitations to join them in using drugs.

3. *Individuals, especially teenagers and young adults, who might be susceptible to developing a drug habit.* To help influence this decision, education strategies combine social influence and personal and social skills training. These approaches supply factual information about drugs, what they can do and

Drug Abuse Resources

Local chapters of the following groups usually can be found in the phone book. National headquarters numbers and addresses are given below. They can provide local referrals and other information. The alcohol-related groups also offer support for families of someone addicted to cocaine.

NATIONAL HOTLINES

National Institute on Drug Abuse: 800-662-HELP
Cocaine help line: 800-COCAINE

OTHER RESOURCES

COCANON Family Groups, P.O. Box 64742-66, Los Angeles, CA 90064; 213-859-2206
Families Anonymous, P.O. Box 528, Van Nuys, CA 91408; 818-989-7841
Nar-Anon Family Group Headquarters, World Service Office, P.O. Box 2562, Palos Verdes, CA 92704; 213-547-5800
Adult Children of Alcoholics, Central Service Board, P.O. Box 3216, Torrance, CA 90505; 213-534-1815
Al-Anon/Alateen, Family Group Headquarters, 1372 Broadway, 7th floor, New York, NY 10018-0862; 212-302-7240

cannot do. This information is supplemented by analyses of motivations and need fulfillment associated with drug use. Surveys provide students with feedback concerning drug use by their peers, correcting the misperception that everybody does it. Skill development is designed to make students aware of social pressures to use drugs and to teach specific skills (e.g., refusal skills) with which to resist these pressures. Drug education provides the stimulus for students to clarify their values with regard to health, risk-taking behavior, and drugs so rational decision-making processes can be developed.

Personal Safety from Crime and Violence

Although most of us feel safe in our daily lives, crime and violence are a fact of life today, so learning how to protect ourselves is necessary. First, we should be aware of situations that may lead to violence or crime and avoid them. Much criminal activity is rooted in the drug scene, from the smuggling and sale of illicit drugs by dealers, to the stealing of money and goods by users to buy drugs, to accidents, altercations, rapes, and murders by people who are under the influence of drugs. Another source of crime is the dysfunctional family, in which violence is endemic. Police officers often consider domestic violence calls to be the most potentially dangerous to their own safety. Some people become victims of crime because they hold an attitude of "it won't happen to me." This prevents people from taking precautionary or preventive measures. Accepting that crime can happen to you is the first step to self-protection. Beyond that, you must deliberately take steps to learn and apply self-protection measures. Protecting yourself translates into learning about crime—who's doing it and how and where you might be most at risk. Protecting yourself means becoming skilled in self-protection. Just as you try to eat healthfully and to exercise for fitness, you can learn and apply measures to protect yourself from violent crime. FYI 6 sets forth six principles of self-protection. (Note: Weapons will not be discussed here, but if you decide upon a weapon, be sure to get training on how to use it, how to take care of it and how to safeguard it from the hands of children.)

Steps to Self-Protection

Think of self-protection as a line of defense beginning with (a) prevention, moving then to (b) avoidance, then to (c) assertiveness, and, ultimately, if the first three don't prevail, to (d) physical self-defense. In the first line of defense the idea is to prevent the opportunity for crime to occur. This doesn't mean that crime can't and won't occur if you take preventive measures. It relies on probabilities; it will be less likely to occur.

Prevention

Prevention requires taking precautions regularly in advance of any problems. This discourages crime and criminals. Prevention involves all aspects of your life, from how you carry yourself and present yourself, to protecting your home and yourself at home, to protecting yourself on the street, on buses, on trains, in taxis, at the bank or cash machine, while driving, at work, at restaurants, and so forth.

How you carry yourself really refers to how others see you. Do they get an image of a victim or a nonvictim? You want to project an image of confidence, of being in charge, of being alert to your surroundings. Do you walk with determination, or do you seem to apologize for the space you take up on the sidewalk? Do you make eye contact with the people you encounter, or do you look at the sidewalk and study your shoes? Do you have your shoulders up and back and your head up, or do you have rounded shoulders and a head-down look? In essence, you may be able to prevent attack just by exuding a commanding and alert presence.

Protecting your home requires that you be aware when coming and going from your residence. Install a peephole in your exterior doors so you know who is there without opening the door and do not let any stranger into your home, even if the person says it is an emergency. Without opening the door, offer to telephone for the help needed. Outside lighting is another priority; consider a motion-sensor light. Own a dog. Install electronic alarms. Possibly one of the most important prevention measures for home safety is to install deadbolt locks on all exterior doors. To fortify the lock, add a reinforced strike plate that is attached with three-inch screws.

Protecting yourself on the street involves minimizing opportunities for crime. For example, instead of carrying a purse, wear a fanny pack, which is harder to rip off than a loosely held purse. If you must carry a purse, wear it under a coat or strapped diagonally across your chest with the flap turned toward your body. Carry pepper spray (check on the legality in your state first) so it can be seen. Buy pepper spray that has 1–2 million heat units. Personal alarms work well also; of course, they must be carried so they can be engaged easily.

Principles of Self-Protection

Most people are not prepared for violent attack. They don't know what to do. For normally nonviolent people to protect themselves in threatening situations, they have to adopt an attitude of power and apply six basic principles.

1. *Be alert.* You can learn to be alert. Being alert means being aware of your surroundings. Make a habit of anticipating what and who might be a threat to your safety. As you are out and about, practice asking yourself on-the-spot questions. How many people did I just pass? What kind and color of car just went by? Know what and who is behind you, and pay special attention to anything "out of place" such as someone from the gas company asking for permission to enter your house or noticing in your rear-view mirror that the same car has been behind you for an unusually long time. *Alertness gives you warning.*

2. *Be decisive.* You can accentuate decisiveness. Play "what if" games with yourself. What if someone seems to be following you while you are walking down the street. What can you do? The first thing is to be sure this individual is actually following you. Cross the street, and go in the opposite direction. If the person is still there, you can be sure he or she is following you. Now what can you do? Go inside a convenience store or get into a group of people and stay with them. The bottom line is to make a decision about what you are going to do and do it. Don't hesitate or deviate. Don't ponder the decision. Make a decision and commit to it. *Decisiveness gives you a course to pursue.*

3. *Be aggressive.* Let the assailant worry about his or her life. Don't hold back. Strike so the assailant is incapable of further action. Strike the eyes, nose, throat, or groin. Knee the groin rather than kick the shin, stomp on the foot, or slap at the head (the latter blows would not hurt the assailant much but certainly could enrage him/her). *Debilitate the assailant.* If you initially can't imagine doing this, imagine doing it for a loved one (a child, a mate) and, with practice, ultimately for yourself. How can you cultivate this kind of a response? Think of the greatest indignation you can imagine happening to you or to a loved one, and get angry. Anger allows us to block out our own imminent peril and concentrate on destroying the "bad person." *Aggressiveness allows you to carry out your plan with all the power you've got!*

4. *Be fast.* Be quick. Retaliate instantly. Don't hesitate. A delayed reaction by the victim is all the assailant needs to take control of the situation. Most criminals have the least control over victims in the first crucial seconds of an attack. While you wait for the "perfect time to make your move," the assailant is getting more and more control. *An immediate defense minimizes the control the assailant has over you!*

5. *Be cool.* This means maintaining self-control. Keep your concentration under pressure. Participating in sports is a good way to train this component. *Staying focused circumvents distraction.*

6. *Be a surprise.* By doing what your attacker least suspects—fighting back—you throw the assailant off balance. The unexpected is disconcerting, which means the assailant becomes less in charge of the situation. The criminal does not expect a victim to fight back. In rape cases, victims who fight back have been found to suffer less psychological trauma than those who don't, and the incidence of injury seems to be similar regardless of strategy used—fighting or nonresistance.

Trust your instincts. If you think someone is following you, or the only person you see on the street ahead of you is acting suspiciously, your instincts are alerting you to possible danger. Pay attention to those signals, and take a different action than you had planned. If a stranger asks for directions, don't let him or her get too close. Don't let any stranger take your hand—ever. Don't enter unfamiliar areas that you cannot observe first: Make a wide swing around corners, stay wide from alleys, and the like. Use window glass of stores to check your rear visibility. Walking or jogging with a dog on the streets keeps an assailant off-guard; he or she doesn't know if the dog is attack-trained.

To protect yourself when using public transportation, carry exact change so you don't have to pull out your wallet to pay your fare. On a bus, sit up front near the driver, and pick an aisle seat versus an inside seat. On a subway, pick a well-lit car with a lot of people. As you enter a taxi state the company and the license number and in a non-threatening way, let him/her know you'll remember the number. You might state "those are the exact numbers I play in the lottery!"

Be especially careful at the bank. This is a prime hangout for muggers. Be alert to people loitering outside the bank (in cars, on foot) as well as inside the bank. If you find reason to be "on guard" go to another bank. It takes only seconds for someone to put an ice pick into your tire when they see you getting a cash withdrawal. They simply follow you from the bank until your tire goes flat and then offer you help (which is relieving you of your money.) Be as private as possible at the teller window. Complete your transaction with your back blocking observers' view. Before leaving the teller window, put cash immediately into your wallet or purse or inside a jacket pocket.

Using automatic teller machines is more hazardous than most transactions because you normally aren't surrounded by other people. Avoid ATMs late at night, particularly if they are isolated. A potential mugger on a bicycle a block away can be where you are in seconds.

Car safety involves looking in the back seat before getting in the car and also looking *under* the car, as assailants have been known to lie in wait under a car. You are particularly vulnerable when loading groceries or children into the car. Your back is to the world, and you are focused on what you are doing. If the parking lot is mostly deserted, ask for customer service with groceries. Don't leave items where they are visible to potential thieves. Put your purse on the floor, under your knees.

If you think you're being followed, drive to the nearest police station. If you don't know where the police station is, drive to an all-night store or gas station and ask someone to call for help. Keep the car doors locked and windows rolled down only enough for ventilation but not enough for someone to gain access. Carry a cellular phone so help is just a phone call away. If someone threatens you and tries to get you out of your car, put it in gear and drive off. At work and at restaurants, avoid isolated restrooms, particularly those located near an outside exit. Go with someone if this is the case. Parking structures and surface lots pose considerable risks. Go with someone to your car, and then drive that person to his or her car. Don't flash money. And don't place yourself in isolated situations with people you don't know well.

Avoidance

After you've taken all the preventive measures possible, and still find yourself in a potentially bad situation, the second line of defense is avoidance. If you're walking down the street and see what looks like a potential for trouble, cross the street and walk down the other side, or go around the block and come back up to your course, but on the other side of the problem.

If you come home and find your door open or other tipoffs that someone unexpected has been in your home, leave immediately and call police.

Likewise, if you are in the house and hear unexpected noises outside that alert your "sixth sense," call police and go to a safe area in the house. If someone is on the verge of getting in, you need to get out and go for help.

If a car bumps your car, particularly in an isolated location, stay in your car with doors locked and windows rolled up. Exchange information through the window glass or indicate that you want to drive to a gas station or store (where there are people). Getting out of the car to exchange insurance information and look over the damage is a compelling temptation that you must resist. Many cases of "bumper rape" and car jackings have happened within this context. As soon as you get out of your car, you are at the assailant's mercy.

If someone grabs you by the sweater, coat, or shirt, slip out of the garment and run while yelling for help. Preferably yell "fire, fire, fire," as people are more likely to respond to fire, which is a known danger.

Assertiveness

If you need help, yell about what is going on— "purse snatch," "rape," "car jacking"—to gain public attention and let people know what is happening. Many safety experts recommend yelling "fire" to attract attention and public involvement. "Fire" implies that it might be *their* house, *their* car, which is hard to ignore.

Use the loudest "karate-like" yell you can muster, rather than yelling "help" repeatedly. The karate-like yell is disconcerting to attackers and empowers the victim.

Physical assertiveness may be called for in combination with verbal assertiveness. In combination, it might be played out this way: "I said no. Leave me alone!" and cross the street while looking over your shoulder directly at the individual to show that you're on guard. If someone struggles with you for your purse, throw the purse in one direction and run the other direction, all the time yelling "purse snatch." Or if you are held up on the street, pull a money clip out of your pocket or purse, throw it one way and run the other, yelling "fire."

Self-Defense

The last line of defense is self-defense. It is last because it carries the most risk. All the strategies that go before pose little risk. If you have carried out the three previous steps and still find yourself in jeopardy, you must decide to *resist* (use self-defense skills for protection) or to go along with the assailant's promises and hope that, by doing nothing, the assailant will spare you. Usually, the first words out of a criminal's mouth are "Do what I tell you and you won't get hurt." That command makes victims easier to control and, therefore, easier to violate.

Conventional wisdom has purported that if you resist (particularly women), the assailant is more likely to harm you. New evidence, however, indicates that if you resist, you actually stand a better chance of escaping. One study of women who were attacked showed that, of those who resisted, 39% avoided further injury, 37% escaped, and 22% scared off the attacker. Other studies show that, of women who have been assaulted, nearly 75% who did something to protect themselves—fight, run, talk, yell—escaped or reduced injury.

The idea of self-defense is to *incapacitate or debilitate* the assailant so you can escape from harm. As noted earlier, when you kick or scrape a shin, or stomp down on an instep of the foot, all you do is make the assailant angry, which escalates the attack. Self-defense experts advocate attacking the eyes, nose, larynx, groin, and knees. Blows to these areas incapacitate the assailant and terminate the assault. You should deliver multiple blows, with all the force you can muster.

Everyone should be trained in self-defense skills. It is one more step in staying in control of yourself. Among the many organizations offering instruction are YMCAs, YWCAs, colleges and universities, some public schools, police crime-prevention programs, and martial arts centers. Most large cities have private programs. Model Mugging is one such program.

Police cannot be everywhere, and you are not always accompanied by a friend or "protector." Therefore, being prepared to protect yourself is essential. J. J. Bittenbinder, a police detective who travels the country lecturing on self-protection, sums up his overall advice in the following four points:

1. Be a tough target—be the one the criminal doesn't choose, whether that be you, your house, or your car.

2. Deny privacy—don't ever let someone take you to a secondary crime scene (e.g., being forced into an assailant's car, taken to the storage room at work).

3. Attract attention—yell "fire," throw a rock through someone's house window to get attention, run into a crowded restaurant for help, set off your personal alarm.

4. Do something—take some kind of action. Use your chemical spray, strike at the vulnerable body parts, run while screaming "fire."

Let's look next at some of the "crimes of our times," how they usually happen, and what we can do to prevent them.

Date and Acquaintance Rape

The National Victim Center (NVC) defines rape, date rape, and acquaintance rape as follows. *Rape* involves the use of force, or threat of force, with penis penetration of a victim's vagina, mouth, or rectum. *Date rape* is a sexual assault by an individual with whom the victim has a "dating relationship and the sexual assault occurs in the context of this relationship. *Acquaintance rape* is a sexual assault by an individual known to the victim.

The NVC states that almost four of five rapes are committed by attackers who know their victims. This is consistent with data from the *Ms.* Project on Campus Sexual Assault, funded by the National Institute of Mental Health, which found that more than 84% of those raped knew their attacker and that 57% of the rapes occurred on dates. Acquaintance rape is the predominant rape crime today.

The NVC and the Crime Victims Research and Treatment Center (CVRTC) released a report in 1992 entitled, *Rape in America: A Report to the Nation*, which stated that 683,000 American women are raped each year; in essence, this is one in every eight adult women. The *Ms.* Project on Campus Sexual Assault surveyed 6,000 students from 32 college campuses, with males and females equally represented. The study found that one in four college women had been victims of rape or attempted rape and that one in 12 of these college men admitted committing acts that fit the definition of rape or attempted rape.

Perpetrators of acquaintance rape (including date rape) tend to have some characteristics in common. They:

- become intimate or personal too soon (someone hitting on you when you barely know him)
- have negative attitudes about women (you might notice his making degrading comments about other women in your presence)
- are controlling, i.e., tells you what to wear, where you will go, what you can say, which friends you can see, etc.
- drink excessively, gets drunk frequently and tries to push drinks on you
- are intrusive, i.e., unwanted touches, jokes etc.
- accepts violence as a way of life, enjoys violent movies, is abusive to animals, etc.

You are now aware of characteristics of those who rape. This knowledge permits you to be selective

Rape Prevention Guidelines

To prevent acquaintance or date rape:*

1. Be clear about what you want; make sure your body language is reinforcing what you are saying.
2. Don't fall for, "If you loved me you would."
3. Minimize drinking and avoid drugs, and avoid socializing with people who take drugs.
4. Set sexual limits for yourself, and communicate those limits clearly to your date.
5. Don't do things you don't want to do just to be polite. Be assertive by clearly expressing what you want and what you don't want.
6. Listen to your feelings, trust your feelings, and act as a result of your feelings.
7. Protest loudly and clearly if things get out of hand.
8. Avoid isolated settings.
9. Contribute financially to the date so neither "owes" anything to the other except "thank you" for a nice time."
10. Double-date, or meet your date at the event (e.g., movie theater, game) until you feel totally comfortable with that person.

---

* These guidelines are applicable to men seeking to avoid unwanted intimacy as well.

---

about individuals with whom you choose to be. If, despite your best judgment, you still find yourself in a situation that jeopardizes your safety, then there are additional guidelines offered in FYI 7 to prevent the situation from escalating to rape.

If, despite your best efforts to be selective and preventive, you still find yourself in an escalating rape situation, your decision now is whether to resist or submit. That decision should be made in light of the following three questions:

1. *What is your location?* 3 P.M. in the parking lot of a shopping mall is different from 3 A.M. in that same parking lot. In the first case, if you yell, someone could hear you. In the second case, there is someplace to run for help.

2. *What is your personality?* The success of resistance depends largely on the victim's ability to apply it. Do you tend to be passive/dependent or independent/assertive? The former does not lend itself (without training) to being resistive in a crisis situation. The latter personality does lend itself to resistance in threatening situations.

3. *What is the perpetrator's motivation?* Physical resistance will discourage one type of rapist but excite another. Test the person by first talking back, yelling for help to see what the reaction to

your action is. If the perpetrator acts startled—keep up the action. If the perpetrator becomes violent, back off momentarily and rethink an opportunity for escape.

Answers to these three questions provide the information needed to know whether to resist or submit. No one answer applies universally.

Sometimes, victims don't tell anyone. One major reason they don't tell is because they assume the "shame and blame" for what happened. It's unfortunate that there is shame, but there is no room for self-blame. The victim is *not* to blame; the person committing the rape (whether an acquaintance, a friend, or someone unknown) is to blame.

Victims tend to bear their burdens alone. Years later, the trauma can be released by a reminder of the rape, and the tragedy that occurred years ago plays out as if it happened just yesterday. The best action for a victim of acquaintance rape or date rape is to report it immediately by calling 911, insist on a rape advocate being present during the report (reporting doesn't mean you have to prosecute), talk about it with close friends, and get counseling. It's best to deal with the trauma right away.

Spousal Abuse

The term "spousal abuse" refers to actions one partner takes to intimidate, control, or harm the other in the context of an intimate relationship. The abuse may be emotional, psychological, or physical; the relationship may exist within or outside of legal marriage; and it can be heterosexual or homosexual. Females are more likely than males to be victims of violence by intimates. Annually, 572,000 women are victimized by someone with whom they are intimate, compared to approximately 49,000 men. More than half of all female homicide victims in the United States are killed by an intimate male partner. Therefore, we will use the female gender to denote the victim and the male gender for the abuser, bearing in mind that the information is applicable to abusers of both genders.

It is estimated that 2–4 million women are victims of abuse each year, with more than 1 million women seeking medical care for abuse-related injuries. One out of every four women in this country will suffer some kind of violence at the hands of an intimate and very few will tell anyone. Spousal abuse happens in one of every four homes in America. A woman is more likely to be injured, raped, or killed by her male partner than by any other type of assailant.

Violence toward family members is passed from generation to generation. Abusers and abusive people alike tend to come from abusive families. Once people are victimized by physical violence in their own home, their risk of being victimized again is high. An apology and affection follows the abuse, followed eventually by another abusive episode, and so the cycle continues.

Among typical characteristics of abusers, they:

- lack communication and negotiation skills
- are extremely jealous
- have a friendly personality when out in public but are explosive at home
- dislike women; treat them as objects
- blame wife/girlfriend for things that go wrong in their lives
- are guarded and manipulative
- are demanding, even if the partner is ill
- "allow" the wife/girlfriend to go out in public only in their presence
- take total control of the finances

Abusers slowly and deliberately weave a web that isolates the partner. Because they control the finances, they control the partner's behavior.

"An ounce of prevention is worth a pound of cure" is an adage that fits like a glove in this situation. The first place to stop abuse is before it starts. The best way is to truly get to know the person with whom you are planning to spend your life, as well as the family. Do you detect any signs of abuse? If you do, get out before you get in too deep.

If you are in an abusive situation, call a hotline or shelter for information and help. If you are an abuser, or see yourself as having the above characteristics, get help. You need to understand why you are the way you are and how to get out of this web. Individual counseling followed by couple counseling offers an alternative.

Sexual Harassment

Sexual harassment has existed in the workplace since women first began to work outside the home and is historically documented back to the colonial times. In occupational settings, 42% of women and 15% of men experience sexual harassment. It theoretically has been illegal since passage of the Civil Rights Act of 1964. The legal definition for sexual harassment was issued by the U.S. Equal Employment Opportunity Commission (EEOC) in 1980. This definition includes two classes of harassing behavior: (a) attempts to extort sexual cooperation by subtle or explicit threat of job-related consequences, and (b) verbal or physical conduct that is unwelcome or offensive.

Men experience sexual harassment, but to a much lesser extent than women. In two studies, both in college settings, 11% and 9% of men reported sexual harassment. These data are in contrast to a review of studies on college women which estimated somewhere between 20–30% had been victims of sexual harassment. In a study of 133 medical trainees' in internal medicine, 73% of the women and 22% of the men had been sexually harassed during their training. Rates tend to be higher for graduate students than for undergraduate, which in turn are higher than those for high school students.

In a study of sexual harassment at a state college in Pennsylvania, both men and women reported having experienced sexist comments, physical advances, and explicit sexual propositions. Most of the harassment reported came from male faculty members, and generally from just one faculty member, as opposed to many faculty members.

In general, perpetrators tend to be co-workers or peers rather than people in positions of authority. One well-recognized study (U.S. Merit Systems Protection Board) found 40% of harassers to be superiors. Perpetrators are more likely to be male. In another study, 96% of harassers were men in female cases and 55% were men in cases of male victims.

Several authors have attempted to construct a hierarchy of sexually harassing behaviors, ranging from mild to severe. Mild forms of harassment can be remarks of a sexual nature, repeated requests for a date, whistles, and staring. More serious are sexual propositions and unwanted physical contact of a nonsexual nature. The most severe forms are sexual propositions linked to job enhancement or job threat, unwanted physical conduct of a sexual nature, and sexual assault.

Sexual harassment, like the crimes of acquaintance rape and domestic violence, is able to flourish because victims don't fight back and tend not to report it. As a victim, you may choose to submit to the harassment, ignore the behavior, avoid the perpetrator, confront the perpetrator, change a job or class, report the behavior to a superior or a grievance committee, or seek legal assistance. The dynamics are much the same as in other abuse situations.

Stalking

The National Victim Center defines stalking as "the willful, malicious and repeated following or harassing of another person." As of 1993, all 50 states and the District of Columbia have some form of anti-stalking law.

More than 200,000 cases of stalking occur in the United States each year. Of these cases, half involve threats of violence. Women are disproportionately the victims of stalking.

The stalker can be a friend, lover, worker, or neighbor, but in most cases the stalker is an ex-spouse or ex-lover. Stalkers mix up the emotions of love, anger, rage, and retribution. They ultimately demand total commitment from their victims. They mentally terrorize their victims. Their behaviors range from driving by the victim's home repeatedly, to appearing on the doorstep, ringing the doorbell at 3 A.M., to following the victim everywhere, day or night.

Victims of stalkers many times end up changing their lives drastically. Changes can be as innocuous as screening telephone calls or as extreme as leaving behind family, friends, and careers to take on a new identity in a different location.

Some protective tips are:

- If you spot suspicious behavior early, put an end to the relationship at once. Suspicious behaviors describe someone who gets abusive or irrationally upset when you say "no" to something this person wants, snoops into your personal life behind your back, and shows up at places uninvited.
- Reject the stalker. Be explicit in your communication (e.g., "I'm not interested in you now and I'm positive I never will be").
- Don't try to talk, reason, or negotiate with the stalker; refuse to be flattered or reactive.
- Cut off all contact. When you don't respond, the stalker will get the message.
- Tell friends, family, employer about the stalker.
- Contact the telephone company to inquire about any services that might be helpful (e.g., caller ID, documentation of telephone calls made to your number).
- Document everything (phone messages, letters; keep a notebook stating as many *details* as possible, with emphasis on threats; take pictures; use a video recorder).
- Educate yourself about the crime of stalking; acquire a copy of your state's stalking law from the District Attorney's office.
- With documentation, call the police; report each incident directly after it has occurred; obtain a copy of the report and number.
- Consider a civil injunction or temporary protective order.
- Have a plan (keep important phone numbers with you at all times; have a suitcase of "essentials" in the trunk of your car; keep extra money on hand regularly; keep the gas tank full).
- If you have to relocate, don't leave a "paper trail" (pick up and hand-carry copies of medical records, children's school records; obtain a post office box; arrange for a trusted friend or relative to forward mail; don't leave forwarding addresses).

Car Prowls

Car prowls usually happen at scenic sites when people park and hike a distance to view a scenic/historical site. These crimes occur during the nicer weather months, as early as April and as late as October or November. Robbers punch out a window, door, or trunk lock to quickly steal anything left in the car: radio, credit cards, wallets, cellular phone, checkbooks. Deputy Fred Hill of the Oregon Police says a car prowl can be done in 7 seconds, and the thief usually walks away with $200 per car.

Some preventive tips are:

- Leave valuables at home, if possible.
- Don't count on your valuables being safe if you leave them in the trunk or under the seat.
- Don't park in an isolated area.
- Hike and sight-see in the morning; car prowls are more prevalent in the afternoon.
- Look around before you leave your car. Do you see people sitting in parked cars for a long time? Do they seem out of place?
- Carry your purse, camera, and similar valuables with you.
- If you have a choice of cars, take one with a local plate (maybe a rental car) for your scenic drive. Out-of-state vehicles are particularly vulnerable because the thieves know the owners are not going to return to prosecute them.

Carjacking

Carjacking is a type of robbery that involves theft or attempted theft of a motor vehicle by force or threat of force. There were 25,000 carjackings in the United States in 1992. Based on National Crime Victimization Survey data from 1992, the offender succeeded in stealing the car in 52% of the carjackings. According to this same report, men are more likely victims of carjackings than women, Blacks than Whites, and people younger than 35. Most carjacking victims escaped without injury. Carjackers usually have a weapon, most often a handgun. The FBI estimates that a carjacking can take as little as 15 seconds. In one variation, the "bump-and-run," thieves in one car pull up behind a car and bump it. When the driver gets out to inspect the damage, the thieves demand the car.

About two-thirds of carjackings occur after dark, most commonly on the street or in a parking lot or public garage. Carjackings are more likely to occur in a city than in suburbia or rural areas.

Some preventive/protective tips are as follows:

Parking:

- Don't park in dark, isolated areas.
- Before getting out of your car in a parking lot, look around to spot anyone or anything suspicious. If so, stay in your car or drive away.
- As you approach your car, look around and under your car before getting in; make sure your keys are in your hand.
- If a potential carjacker approaches you, make a scene if people are within earshot.
- No matter what, don't get back into the car with the carjacker. Even if he/she has a gun, run.

While driving:

- Be aware of and alert to your surroundings at all times.
- Keep your car doors locked and windows rolled up; use the air conditioner for ventilation.
- If you are stopped at a traffic signal and someone tries to get in your car, run the light.
- Don't let yourself get blocked in at intersections.
- Don't pick up hitchhikers.
- Don't stop to help someone in distress. If you have a cell phone, call 911, or stop and call as soon as you can get to a phone.
- Stay away from rest stops; if you must use one, park up front where other people are around.
- Know where you are going.
- Tell someone where you are going and when he or she should hear from you.
- Drive in the center lane on highways to reduce your chances of being a "bump-and-run" victim.
- Make sure your car is in good operating condition.

- Drive with passengers whenever you can.
- Have a cell phone with you.

Home Burglary

The Uniform Crime Report (UCR) of the FBI defines burglary as the unlawful entry of a structure to commit a felony or theft. The FBI estimates that in 1993, a burglary occurred in the United States every 11 seconds. Burglars sometimes end up raping or committing other types of personal assault regardless of their original intent.

Two of every three burglaries are residential, and 67% involve forcible entry. Burglaries are equally likely to occur during the day as during the night. The average loss for residential burglary was $1,185. More residential burglaries took place between July and December than January through June. Most burglaries occur in urban settings, fewer in suburbia, and even fewer in rural areas.

Most burglars are opportunists; they look for the easy mark. Burglars are looking for cash and small, easy-to-carry things they can turn into cash. Make your home a tough target through the following measures.

Outside:

- Install good outside lighting.
- Keep trees next to the house trimmed (no branches from ground to 8 feet); they can provide easy access to adjacent windows.
- Keep shrubs pruned to a height that doesn't allow someone to hide behind them.
- Don't have high fences; they give burglars privacy in which to do their work leisurely.

Leaving for vacation:

- Check your home to make sure windows and doors are locked.
- Activate your alarm.
- Leave blinds and curtains as usual.
- Ask a neighbor to watch your house; stop mail and newspaper deliveries; put timers on your lights so they come on in various rooms at various times; arrange to have someone mow and water the lawn and plants.
- Disconnect the garage door opener so a thief can't take off with your car, or drill a hole through the track and attach a heavy-duty padlock.

Doors/windows/locks:

- Exterior doors should be solid wood (1¾ inches) or metal; install a peephole; more than

1/8 inch between door and door jam allows for a crowbar; be sure door hinges are on the inside.

- Locks should be 40 inches from any glass on doors; use at least two locks on each exterior door; use deadbolt locks with at least a 1-inch bolt that inserts into a reinforced strike plate that has been installed with three-inch screws.
- Sliding glass doors should have a metal Charley bar or a lock that slides a pin through the two doors.
- Windows should have folding gates easy to open from inside for second story windows (not recommended for lower story because of fire), or a pin to slide through upper and lower window frames.
- Have the locks rekeyed when you move into a home new to you.

Alarm:

- Consider installing an alarm system, preferably hooked up to central monitoring.

Family behavior patterns:

- Don't open your door to strangers.
- Keep exterior doors locked at all times.
- Always check to see that windows and doors are locked before leaving home.

- Don't leave children younger than 12 home alone.
- Instruct family members how to handle phone calls in general, and specifically when no one else is home.
- Keep electronic equipment out of sight from windows and doors.
- Keep a dog or put a large dog bowl with water outside your door; post "beware of dog" signs on your property.

If you come home to a house in disarray or suspicious-looking:

- Don't go in. Go to a neighbor's home. Call 911.

Don't advertise:

- Don't post wedding or funeral notices in the paper. Some burglars watch for these notices and strike during the service.
- If you do have to post the above notices, have someone stay at home while you are gone.
- Don't leave your garage door up with no car in the garage. An empty garage is an invitation to burglars.

Neighborhood watch:

- Watch out for each other informally; formally, form neighborhood watch groups or patrols.

CHOICES IN ACTION

Take this opportunity to honestly evaluate your risk of HIV infection or of contracting any other STD by completing Lab 26, "STDs: Reducing Your Risk," and Lab 27, "HIV Risk Checklist." If you drink alcohol, smoke, or use any other kind of drug, Labs 28 and 29 ("Alcohol Quiz," and "Why Do You Smoke?") can be used to evaluate your knowledge, motivations, and responses to these drugs and may reveal some insights and directions for minimizing or managing the impact of these drugs on your life. Use Lab 31 "Check Out Your House or Apartment," to analyze the safety and security of the place you live. Discuss with family and/or friends the best ways to respond to the potential dangers described in Lab 32, "Potentially Threatening Situations: What Could You Do?".

REFERENCES

"AIDS: Have We Turned the Corner?" 1993. *University of California Berkeley, Wellness Letter* 9: 1–2.

Alan Guttmacher Institute. 1993. *Facts in Brief: Sexually Transmitted Diseases (STD's) in the United States.* Washington DC: AGI.

Alan Guttmacher Institute. 1994. *Sex of America's Teenagers.* Washington, DC: AGI.

American College Health Association. 1990. *The ABC's of Viral Hepatitis.* Baltimore: ACHA.

American Medical Association Council on Scientific Affairs. 1981. "Marijuana: Its Health Hazards and Therapeutic Potentials." *Journal of the American Medical Association* 246(16): 1823–1827.

Amis, Kingsley. 1973. *On Drink.* New York: Harcourt Brace Jovanovich.

Baker, N. L. 1989. *Sexual Harassment and Job Satisfaction in Traditional and Nontraditional Industrial Occupations.* Unpublished doctoral dissertation. Los Angeles: California School of Professional Psychology.

Bart, P. 1985. *Stopping Rape.* Pergamon Press.

Billings, A. G., and Moos, R. H. 1983. "Social-Environmental Factors Among Light and Heavy Cigarette Smokers: A Controlled Comparison with Non-Smokers." *Addictive Behaviors* 8: 381–391.

Bittenbinder, J. J. 1992. *Street Smarts: How to Avoid Being a Victim.* Schaumburg, IL: Video Publishing House.

Byer, C. O., and Shainberg, L. W. 1994. "Sexually Transmitted Diseases." In *Dimensions of Human Sexuality* (pp. 155–188). Dubuque, IA: WCB Brown & Benchmark Publishers.

"Can You Bank on the Blood Supply?" 1993. *University of California Berkeley, Wellness Letter* 9: 6–7.

Cease Fire. September 1994. Healing the Planet III: A Symposium & Workshop. Los Angeles, CA: UCLA Extension.

Centers for Disease Control and Prevention. 1985. *Chlamydia Trachomatis Infections: Policy Guidelines for Prevention and Control.* Atlanta: CDC.

Centers for Disease Control and Prevention. 1988. *Smoking and Health: A National Status Report.* Rockville, MD: U.S. Department of Health and Human Services.

Centers for Disease Control and Prevention. 1993. *Division of STD/HIV Prevention Annual Report, 1992.* Atlanta: CDC.

Centers for Disease Control and Prevention. 1993. "Facts About Adolescents and HIV/AIDS."

HIV/AIDS Prevention. Atlanta: U.S. Department of Health and Human Services.

Centers for Disease Control and Prevention. 1994. *Division of STD/HIV Prevention Annual Report, 1993.* Atlanta: CDC.

Centers for Disease Control and Prevention. 1994. *Monthly Vital Statistics Report.* Hyattsville, MD: U.S. Department of Health and Human Services.

Centers for Disease Control and Prevention. 1994. *Quarterly Update: AIDS in the United States.* Atlanta: Centers for Disease Control.

Centers for Disease Control and Prevention. 1994. *Sexually Transmitted Disease Surveillance Report, 1993.* Atlanta: U. S. Department of Health and Human Services.

Centers for Disease Control and Prevention. 1995. *Division of STD/HIV Prevention Annual Report, 1994.* Atlanta: CDC.

Centers for Disease Control and Prevention. 1995. *HIV/AIDS Surveillance Report, 1994.* Atlanta: U.S. Department of Health and Human Services.

Centers for Disease Control and Prevention. 1995. *Sexually Transmitted Disease Surveillance Report, 1994.* Atlanta: U. S. Department of Health and Human Services.

Charney, D. A., and Russell, R. C. 1994. "An Overview of Sexual Harassment." *American Journal of Psychiatry* 151(1): 10–17.

Cheraskin, E., and Ringsdorf Jr., W. M. 1978. *Psychodietetics.* New York: Bantam Books.

Cleary, J. S., Schmieler, C. R., Parascenzo, L. C., and Amrosio, N. 1994. "Sexual Harassment of College Students: Implications for Campus Health Promotion." *Journal of American College of Health* 43(1): 3–10.

Cooper, J. 1989. *Principles of Personal Defense.* Boulder, CO: Paladin Press.

Council on Scientific Affairs, American Medical Association. 1992. "Violence Against Women: Relevance for Medical Practitioners." *Journal of the American Medical Association* 267: 3184–3189.

Cutright, M. J. March 1991. "Teen Dating in the '90's." *Redbook* pp. 18, 20, 23.

Danks, H. September 13, 1994. "Carjackers Terrorize Woman for 12 Hours. *The Oregonian* p. B8.

Dolan, C. J. Feb./Mar. 1994. "Young Women: Whether a Date or Stranger-Rape Is Rape." *Women's Self Defense* p. 70–73.

Donovan, P. 1993. *Testing Positive: Sexually Transmitted Disease and the Public Health Response.* New York: Alan Guttmacher Institute.

Drugs, Crime, and the Justice System 1992: A National Report from the Bureau of Justice Statistics. 1992. Washington, DC: U.S. Government Printing Office.

Dusek, D., and Girdano, D. *Drugs: A Factual Account.* New York: McGraw-Hill.

Fackelmann, K. 1992. "Herpes, HIV, and the High Risk of Sex." *Science News* 141: 68.

Facts in Brief: Sexually Transmitted Diseases (STDs) in the United States. 1993. Washington, DC: Alan Guttmacher Institute.

Fitzgerald, L. F. 1992. *Sexual Harassment in Higher Education: Concepts and Issues.* Washington, DC: National Education Association.

Fitzgerald, L. F. 1993. Sexual Harassment. *American Psychologist* 48(10): 1070–1076.

Gerstein, D. R., and Lewin, L. S. 1990. "Special Report: Treating Drug Problems." *New England Journal of Medicine.*

Girdano, D., and Dusek, D. 1988. *Changing Health Behavior.* Scottsdale, AZ: Gorsuch Scarisbrick, Publishers.

Glantz, M. D., editor. 1984. *Correlates and Consequences of Marijuana Use.* Washington, DC: U.S. Department of Health and Human Services.

Glover, E. D., et al. "Smokeless Tobacco Research: An Interdisciplinary Approach." *Health Values* 8(3): 21–25.

Gorman, C. 1992. "Invisible AIDS." *Time Magazine* (Aug. 3): 30–37.

Greden, J. F. 1981. "Caffeinism and Caffeine Withdrawal." In J. H. Lowinson and P. Ruiz, (eds.), *Substance Abuse: Clinical Problems and Perspectives*, pp. 167–184. Baltimore: Williams and Wilkins.

Greenleaf, V. D. May/June 1990. "Women and Cocaine." *New Realities* p. 21–27.

Griffith, H. W. 1988. *Complete Guide to Prescription and Non-Prescription Drugs.* Los Angeles: Body Press.

Harlap, S., Kost, K., and Forrest, J. D. 1991. *Preventing Pregnancy, Protecting Health: A New Look at Birth Control Choices in the United States.* New York: Alan Guttmacher Institute.

Hazelwood, R. R., and Harpold, J. A. June 1986. Rape: The Danger of Providing Confrontational Advice. *FBI Law Enforcement Bulletin* pp. 1–5.

Herrnstein, R. J. 1990. "Addictions and Other Pathological Choices." *American Psychology* 45(3): 356.

Hollister, L. 1983. "Cannabis: Finally a Therapeutic Agent?" *Drug and Alcohol Dependence* 11: 135–145.

Holloway, M. March 1991. "Trends in Pharmacology: Rx for Addiction." *Scientific American* pp. 95–103.

Isaac, N. E., Cochran, D., Brown, M. E., and Adams, A. L. 1994. "Men who Batter." *Archives of Family Medicine* pp. 3, 50–54.

Johnson, A. E., Nahmias, A. J., Magder, L. S., Lee, F. K., Brooks, C. A., and Snowden, C. B. 1989. Distribution of Genital Herpes (HSV-2) in the U.S.: A Seropidemiological National Survey Using a New Type-Specific Antibody Assay. *New England Journal of Medicine* 321: 1–12.

Komaromy, J., Bindman, A. B., Haber, R. J., and Sande, M. A. 1993. Sexual Harassment in Medical Training. *New England Journal of Medicine* 328: 322-326.

Kost, K., and Forrest, J. D. 1992. "American Women's Sexual Behavior and Exposure to Risk of Sexually Transmitted Diseases." *Family Planning Perspectives* 24: 244–254.

Leigh, B., Temple, M. D., and Tracki, K. 1993. "The Sexual Behavior of U.S. Adults: Results from National Survey." *American Journal of Public Health* 83(10): 1400–1408.

Loy, P. H., and Stewart, L. P. 1984. "The Extent and Effects of Sexual Harassment on Working Women." *Sociological Focus* 17(1): 31–43.

McCarthy, N. June 5, 1994. "Columbia Gorge Car Clouters Get a Fast Start." *The Oregonian.*

McConnell, H. February 1991. "Many Marijuana Users Need Help." *The Journal of the Addiction Research Foundation*; p. 34.

Monteverde, G. August 1994. Interview with AIDS Educator, Multnomah County Health Department. Portland, Oregon.

Mulroy, D. Feb/March 1994. Travel Advisory: Carjacking, Drive-by Shootings, What Next? *Women's Self Defense* pp. 12–13.

National Highway Traffic Safety Administration. 1989. *Drunk Driving Facts.* Washington, DC: U.S. Department of Transportation.

National Institute of Drug Abuse. 1984. *Student Drug Use in America.* Washington, DC: U.S. Government Printing Office.

National Institute of Drug Abuse. 1990. "NIDA Monitors Hawaiian 'Ice' Epidemic." *NIDA Notes* 5(2): 22. Washington, DC: U.S. Government Printing Office.

National Victim Center. 1992. *At a Glance: Acquaintance Rape* (Tech. Rep. Vol. 1. No.1). Arlington, VA: National Victim Center.

_____ 1994. *Stalking* (Tech. Rep. Vol 1. No. 63). Arlington, VA: National Victim Center.

_____ 1994. *Stalking and the Law* (Tech. Rep. Vol. 1. No. 43). Arlington, VA: National Victim Center.

National Victim Center in Conjunction with Crime Victim Research and Treatment Center at the Medical University of South Carolina. 1992. *Rape in American: A Report to the Nation.* National Victim Center.

Nelson, M. B. August 1993. "Women Fight Back." *Shape* pp. 83–85.

Ninth Report to the U.S. Congress. 1982. *Marijuana and Health.* Washington, DC: U.S. Department of Health and Human Services.

Office of Justice Programs. 1994. *Carjacking* (NCJ - 147002). Washington, DC: U.S. Department of Justice.

_____. 1994. *Domestic Violence: Violence Between Intimates* (NCJ - 149259). Washington, DC: U.S. Department of Justice.

Perrine, S. November 1990. "Crime-Proof Your Home." *Parents* pp. 74–77

Puente, M. July 21, 1992. "Legislators Tackling the Terror of Stalking." *USA Today* p. 9.

Quigley, P. 1989. *Armed and Female.* New York: E. P. Dutton, c/o Viking Penguin Inc.

Razzi, E. November 1993. Burglarproof Your Home. *Kiplinger's Personal Finance Magazine* pp. 71–76.

Rose, J. E., Srijati, A., and Murray, M. E. 1983. "Cigarette Smoking During Anxiety-provoking and Monotonous Tasks." *Addictive Behaviors* 8(4): 353–359.

Schwartz, R. H., Luxenberg, M. G., and Hoffmann, N. G. "'Crack' Use by American Middleclass Adolescent Polydrug Abusers." *Journal of Pediatrics* 118(1): 150–155.

Scully, D., and Marolla, J. 1993. "Riding the Bull at Gilley's: Convicted Rapists Describe the Rewards of Rape." In P. Bart and E. G. Moran (Eds.), *Violence Against Women* pp. 26–46. Newbury Park, CA: Sage Publications.

Sonenstein, F. L., Pleck, J. H., and Ku, L. C. 1989. "Sexual Activity, Condom Use and AIDS Awareness Among Adolescent Males." *Family Planning Perspectives* 21: 152–158.

Sonenstein, F. L., Pleck, J. H., and Ku, L. C. 1991. "Levels of Sexual Activity Among Adolescent Males in the United States." *Family Planning Perspectives* 23: 162–167.

Staff. January 1994. "Get Street Smart!" *Prevention* pp. 69–74, 127.

Stephens, J. Feb./Mar. 1994 "10 Inexpensive But Vital Ways to Protect Your Home from Criminals." *Women's Self Defense* pp. 26–29.

Stets, J. E., and Straus, M. A. 1990. "Gender Differences in Reporting Marital Violence and Its Medical and Psychological Consequences." In M. A. Straus & R. J. Gelles (eds.), *Physical Violence in American Families: Risk Factors and Adaptations to Violence in 8,145 Families* pp. 151–165. New Brunswick, NJ: Transaction Publishers.

Stine, G. 1993. *Acquired Immune Deficiency Syndrome.* Englewood Cliffs, NJ: Prentice Hall.

Strong, S. February/March 1994. "Last Word." *Women's Self Defense* p. 82.

Surgeon General's Report to the American Public on HIV Infection and AIDS. 1993. Washington, DC: Government Printing Office.

Terpstra, D. E., & Baker, D. E. 1987. "A Hierarchy of Sexual Harassment." *Journal of Psychology* 121: 599–605.

Thompson, W. June 12, 1994. "Every 30 Minutes a Car Is Stolen in Portland, and Every 19 Seconds in the U.S." *The Oregonian.*

Tortora, G., et al. 1992. *Microbiology,* 4th ed. Menlo Park, CA: Benjamin-Cummings.

U.S. Surgeon General. *Reducing the Health Consequences of Smoking, Years of Progress—A Report of the Surgeon General.* Rockville, MD: Office of Smoking and Health.

Walter, H. J., Vaughan, R. D., Gladis, M. M., et al. April 1992. "Factors Associated with AIDS Risk Behaviors Among High School Students in an AIDS Epicenter." *American Journal of Public Health* 82: 528–532.

Warshaw, R. (1988). *I Never Called It Rape.* New York: Harper & Row, Publishers.

Washington, A. E., and Katz, P. 1991. "Cost of and Payment Source for Pelvic Inflammatory Disease." *Journal of the American Medical Association* 266(18): 2565–2569.

Weddington, W. W., et al. "Changes in Mood, Craving, and Sleep During Short-Term Abstinence Reported by Male Cocaine Addicts." *Archives of General Psychiatry* 47: 861–868.

Williams, S. G., Hudson, A., and Redd, C. 1982. "Cigarette Smoking, Manifest Anxiety and Somatic Symptoms." *Addictive Behaviors* 7(4): 427–428.

Wilson, J., and Shook, J. A. 1994. "Counseling." *Women's Self Defense* 58: 60, 61.

Youngwood, C., and Hoyt, C. April 1993. "Rape: How to Protect Yourself. *McCall's* pp. 108–116.

Understanding Stress

✔ What is stress?

✔ What causes stress in your life?

✔ What is the relationship between stress and illness?

✔ Is stress always harmful?

✔ Is the environment or your personality the more important cause of stress?

To be optimally healthy, we must possess the ability to live in harmony with our environment, meeting its demands while minimizing the detrimental effects of excess stress. The topic of stress involves attention to manifestations of stress in the body, the effects of stress on health, and the common causes of stress. These issues are addressed in this chapter.

BASIC DEFINITIONS

Stress refers to the body's reaction to outside pressures; it is manifested in the build-up of pressure, the strain of muscles tensing, and psychophysiological (mind and body) arousal that can fatigue the body systems to the point of malfunction and disease. A **stressor** is any condition or event that causes a stress response; it may be physical, social, or psychological—even imaginary.

Stress management involves understanding the stress response, recognizing the stressors, developing stress reduction skills, and incorporating these regularly into your lifestyle. Stress management is the topic of Chapter 12.

The difficulty in managing stress is that it permeates every aspect of life. Physically, the body responds to stress in a variety of ways. The physical effects of stress are influenced by behavior, which in turn is determined by factors such as psychological make-up, emotions, personality, social learning, and habituation. Philosophical and spiritual influences, in the form of commitments and joy in living, also play a role in stress and the stress response.

PHYSICAL STRESS

Physical stress means strain, pressure, or force on a system. In the context of the human organism, it describes the body's reaction to the environment through the build-up of internal pressure and the strain of muscles tensing for action. In the final analysis, stress is physical. Physical pressure, if prolonged, is what can fatigue or damage the body to the point at which it affects health adversely.

Stress evokes a natural physical defense mechanism that has allowed human beings to survive. Without it we would not survive even the relatively tame world most of us live in today. Stress is a physical response that protects our physical lives. We need stress and do not want to—nor can we—eradicate our stress response. The goal is to manage stress by diminishing excess stress in our lives, the stress that is detrimental. Imagine a cave-dweller holding a club dripping with blood in his hand, and a slain sabertooth tiger in the background. Your imaginary X-ray vision allows you to view inside the man's stomach, which reveals a peaceful scene representative of a calm state. Now picture modern man or woman in a business suit, clenched jaw, squinting eyes, furrowed forehead, shaking a fist at the boss in the background. Your ability to see inside the stomach shows a raging inferno, indicative of emotional turmoil. The significance of an appropriate versus an inappropriate stress response becomes clear.

Walter B. Cannon defines stress as the "fight-or-flight syndrome." He notes that when one becomes stressed, proper use of that stress is either to fight off the threat or to run from it. In either case the body prepares itself through a myriad of physiological mechanisms, and the mechanisms endowed to modern humans are the same as those used by our cave-dwelling ancestors. Cave-dwellers were able to handle, or dissipate, their stress more appropriately because, when aroused by fear for their life, they battled with the tiger to kill or be killed. Or they chose to run and escape with their life. Either option resulted in the use and dissolution of internal stress build-up. In our modern society, in contrast, our options for dissipating stress usually do not include a physical response. In our imagined scene, the threat is the boss. We cannot hit the boss with a club or shout angrily at him or her. We cannot run from the threat, and in many cases we cannot even talk about our grievances. Nonetheless, the stress response has been activated. Pressure builds up. The muscles strain to strike out or to hold back our natural response. Externally, nothing happens. Internally, the body is a raging inferno of stress and tension.

Stress Is:

POSITIVE

- When it forces us to adapt, thus increasing our coping skills
- When it increases our awareness of problem areas

NEGATIVE

- When it exceeds our ability to cope, fatigues our systems, and results in behavioral or physical problems

The stress response of modern humans often is inappropriate to both the situation and its level of intensity. Although physical stressors still exist, often the stressors of modern society are primarily ego or social-related. In addition, these stressors may continue for a long time. When a stressor is ego-related or involves a social situation, it cannot be solved by a physical response. The stress response to the boss, one of marked tension in the body, is inappropriate for the degree of threat involved; it also is inappropriate in intensity, which refers to the magnitude and duration of the stress. Intense stress is necessary at times and usually is not detrimental to health unless it is repeated too often. After an intense response, the elevated physiological parameters usually drop to normal within 24 to 48 hours. Examples of stressors that might stimulate such an intense response include a strenuous bout of exercise, a physical attack, an automobile accident or near miss, and a medical procedure involving harsh drugs or surgery. The stress goes up during the event, comes down afterward, and then is gone. The opposite end of the stress continuum is characterized by a low level of anxiety that persists, but at such a low degree that the body tolerates it.

Stressors occur daily. They are part of life. When the body tolerates the stress and when performance is good, the stress is deemed positive, healthy, and challenging. Hans Selye, one of the pioneers of the modern study of stress, terms this **eustress,** positive, action-enhancing stress. It is what gives the athlete the competitive edge and the public speaker the enthusiasm to project optimally.

Eustress helps us overcome lethargy. Selye uses the term **distress** to denote negative, debilitating, or harmful stress. Distress indicates that the situation is beyond one's coping capacity and performance will suffer. It produces overreaction, confusion, poor concentration, performance and test anxiety, and usually results in below-par performance. Prolonged distress moves the organism into the health danger zone.

Optimal stress is a point between eustress and distress at which performance should be its best. At this point the stress is intense enough to motivate and prepare one physically to perform optimally, yet not intense enough to cause the body to overreact, become confused, or sustain harmful effects. Figure 11.1 illustrates this concept.

An optimal level of stress is the point at which stress increases health and performance. Distress or overload begins when stress continues to increase and performance begins to suffer. At this point, though the effect may be difficult to recognize, health also begins to suffer. One of the primary goals of this chapter is to increase your awareness of what stress is and how it affects you. The best way to find your optimal stress level and to recognize and prevent debilitating distress is to develop the ability to recognize the signs and symptoms of distress and then reduce them. Although that sounds simple enough, it isn't. The human organism characteristically becomes accustomed to its level of arousal, which, after a time, becomes the body's normal state. People become "immune" to their stress arousal if it lasts a few weeks or so. The body's sensitivity to stress arousal

FIGURE 11.1 Stress and performance: The point of optimal performance.

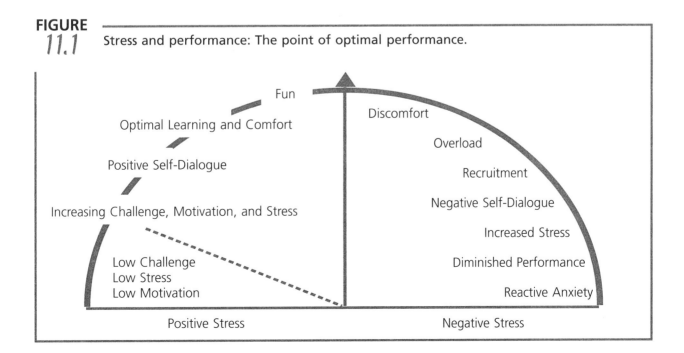

becomes dulled. Lack of awareness, however, does not mean the effects of stress arousal are any less of a problem.

The solution is to increase your sensitivity to the signs of distress. Stress is a phenomenon unique to each individual. The final product, stress arousal, is unique to you. That uniqueness lies in the specific stress symptoms you manifest. Researchers in the field of psychophysiology have identified hundreds of physiological and behavioral effects of excessive stress arousal. The ones you experience represent your unique pattern of response.

To begin developing an awareness of your own signs and symptoms of distress, a checklist is provided in the accompanying activity. Some of the potential signs of arousal are listed in three major categories: musculoskeletal, visceral, and mood/disposition. When some of these signs or symptoms are present, this usually means you have gone beyond the optional point of stress arousal and continued arousal will be detrimental to your performance and health.

STRESS RESPONSE

The signs and symptoms of stress arousal occur when a physiological system of the body becomes stimulated excessively. The normal functioning of that system has been altered, and if the condition persists for an extended time, damage may result. Prolonged overactivation of an organ system can fatigue that system eventually and result in temporary or permanent pathological change or disease. In addition, prolonged stimulation may lower resistance to disease.

After exposing laboratory animals to various stressors, Hans Selye observed the detrimental effects of stress arousal. He was among the first to recognize the relationship between stress and disease, and he formulated a model that helped to illustrate the body's response to stress. This model, which has become known as the **general adaptation syndrome (GAS),** has three stages: the alarm reaction, the stage of resistance, and the stage of exhaustion.

1. In the *alarm stage* the body shows generalized stress arousal. No specific organ system is affected, although most, and in some cases all, of the body systems reveal measurable changes.

2. The *resistance phase* is marked by channeling the arousal into one or several organ systems. Some researchers describe this process as *adaptation to stress.* The human body, which is programmed to survive, seems to channel the arousal into less sensitive systems, such as the muscular system, thereby reducing the immediate danger to the body. In contrast, stress arousal in some parts of the nervous or cardiovascular systems can become life-threatening in a short time. Selye realized that the adaptation process can contribute to development of stress-related illness. "Disease by adaptation" forms the basis of the modern concept of the psychosomatic disease. The specific organ or system to which stress arousal has been channeled ultimately may fatigue and malfunction. Chronic resistance eventually may diminish the ability of that system to function, and disease will result. Your responses to the activity may indicate the systems in your body that adapt to stress arousal and may become weakened.

3. Because the resistance or adaptive process is limited, *exhaustion* eventually may set in. The exhaustion of a weakened system may force another system to become involved in the resistance phase, or the entire body may exhaust its ability to control the arousal and collapse. Usually the body can resist stress arousal for a long time. In the process of resisting, however, systems deteriorate. The cardiovascular system is particularly vulnerable. Chronic heart disease and hypertension, among other conditions, can indicate exhaustion and result in death. Alternatively, alleviation of the stress may result in *resolution.*

F*Y*I

General Adaptation Syndrome

1. Alarm phase
   - Complex physiological response
   - Initiated by presence of stressors
   - Triggers release of adrenalin, muscle tension, increased heart rate and blood pressure

2. Resistance phase
   - Body mobilizes to combat stressor

3. Exhaustion phase
   - Resources become depleted
   - Resistance breaks down
   - Disease or death may result

A C T I V I T Y

STRESS CHECKLIST

Check (✓) any symptoms you experience on a somewhat regular basis. Depending upon the symptoms present, you may have moved beyond the optimal point of stress arousal.

MUSCULOSKELETAL SIGNS

✓ stiffness in neck

✓ trembling or shaking fingers and hands

✓ twitching muscles (specific muscle _eye muscles (around eye)_)

_____ difficulty standing still or sitting quietly

✓ stuttering or stammering speech

✓ frequent headaches (location on head _around eyes_)

_____ tense muscles (specific muscles _____)

_____ quivering voice

✓ nervous mannerisms (e.g., biting nails, pulling hair, tapping feet)

_____ other _____

VISCERAL SIGNS

_____ heart pounding

_____ lightheaded or faint

✓ cold chills

_____ cold hands

_____ cold feet

✓ dry mouth

_____ profuse sweating (location _____)

✓ upset stomach

✓ sinking feeling in stomach

✓ frequent digestive disturbance

_____ moist or sweaty palms

_____ flushed or hot face

_____ other _____

MOOD AND DISPOSITION

_____ preoccupied

_____ frequent insomnia

✓ feeling uneasy or uncomfortable

_____ nervous or shaky

✓ feeling confused

_____ forgetful

_____ feeling insecure

_____ overexcited

_____ feeling angry

_____ irritated

_____ worried, anxious

✓ exhausted

_____ other _____

RESPONSE SYSTEMS

Each of the system responses discussed here is a natural response necessary for the fight-or-flight response. When taken to excess, and especially when prolonged, the responses become debilitating. Although the central mechanisms for arousal are basically the same for all individuals, each person reacts to prolonged stress arousal differently. Why some individuals respond to their stressors by developing ulcers and others by developing high blood pressure has been questioned since the inception of theories about the relationship between mind and body in the development of disease. Franz Alexander, one of the early pioneers in psychosomatic medicine, proposed that emotional conflicts can affect specific internal organs. More recently, Bernie Siegel concluded that individuals suffering from psychosomatic disease develop sensitive organs in the body and these organs become fatigued from the overactivity.

In a complex hypothesis, these researchers explain that if an individual is often angry, for example, the body stimulates the muscles, organs, and hormones necessary to fight or defend themselves. These organs eventually fatigue from the overactivity, become weakened, and perhaps become diseased. Ernest Rossi and Milton Erickson proposed that stressed people cope in any way possible to alleviate the original stressful situation. The individual usually becomes accustomed to that response to stress, so the body continues to react in this newly learned way to stressful situations. As mentioned previously, the organ or system that is responding to prolonged stress arousal eventually breaks down from exhaustion. The specific ways in which long-term stress affects various systems are discussed next. These include the nervous, muscular, gastrointestinal, cardiovascular, skin, and immune systems.

Nervous System

The nervous system is the initiator of the complex and complete stress response, and it also is a response organ because stress increases neural excitability. A small amount of stress produces just enough arousal to get people "up," excited, motivated to do what they have to do. Too much stress makes people jittery or nervous and often results in difficulty concentrating and making decisions. Performance anxiety, inability to make decisions, and emotions such as fear and anger can cause further physiological stress. A vicious cycle develops when physiological arousal of the nervous system incites increased anxiety and increased hostility, which in turn cause even greater nervous system arousal.

Stressful events, situations, or experiences produce this generalized stress arousal. Once the stressor is appraised, the arousal response begins. Appraisal or awareness of the stressor begins in the lower centers of the brain nearest the spinal cord. Depending on the appraisal of the stressor, appropriate body systems are asked to help solve the stressful problem. Upon resolution of the problem or disappearance of the stressor, the system attempts to get the body back to normal. By responding to a stressor, the body learns a response that may continue increasing the readiness to respond, so the central nervous system becomes hyperactive.

Apart from the more measurable physical responses of the brain to stress are psychological or mood responses. During rest and relaxation the psychological nature of the brain is said to be in **homeostasis,** meaning that the subjective moods of the individual are in harmony, promoting a healthful relationship between mind and body. During the stress response, in contrast, psychological mechanisms of the mind are thrown into turmoil. A "mood disturbance" is one frequent characteristic of the stress reaction. Stress commonly evokes feelings of confusion, fear, and extreme emotional sensitivity, as well as feelings of being threatened.

Muscular System

The system that most people associate with the effects of stress is the muscular system. The body has two muscular systems: the voluntary and the involuntary. The **voluntary muscle system** is the one that allows us to move our muscles. Again, a slight increase in tension helps to improve performance because it gets our muscles ready to act. Excessive muscle tension, however, causes a variety of muscular problems, such as tension headaches, a widespread complaint in our society today. Tension headaches seem to be caused by increased muscle tension in the neck muscles, the muscles around the head, and especially the muscles of the upper back (the trapezius muscles). These muscles are involved in what is called the "defense posture." When people are threatened, they prepare themselves for battle, which causes them to tense up in readiness. Chronic readiness usually is not noticed until that tension causes a great deal of pain. Chronic tension headaches and chronic muscle spasms are common responses of the voluntary muscle system to stress.

The involuntary muscle system deals mainly with the internal body organs. Changes in the tonus and mobility of the gastrointestinal system, for example, may cause many difficulties such as difficulty swallowing, diarrhea, constipation, and spastic colon.

Gastrointestinal System

The gastrointestinal system consists of the esophagus, stomach, small and large intestines, and rectum. In the stomach, stress reactions cause an increase in hydrochloric acid and a decrease in the protective mucus that lines the stomach and the small intestine. The mucus layer normally protects these areas from peptic enzymes and hydrochloric acid. Harold Wolf was one of the first individuals to study gastric response to stress, using a now-famous research subject named Tom. Through a natural hole in Tom's stomach, researchers were able to see that when Tom became aroused (especially when he was angered), blood filled the tissues in the lining of his stomach, the lining became frail, and at times hemorrhaging even occurred. It was easy to deduce that ulceration could occur as a result. Researchers also measured increases in the production of hydrochloric acid during times of stress.

Stress also causes changes in metabolic activity. For example, an overall mobilization of protein occurs. This causes various difficulties. For example, if the stress reaction lasts a long time, antibody production decreases. If the situation is prolonged, the individual may become more susceptible to viral and bacterial illnesses. Another aspect of protein mobilization is *muscle wasting*. The flight-or-fight response is an *immediate* reaction designed to save the individual's life *right now*. The body is not worried about what is going to happen later; it has to live through the stress event now. Therefore, available proteins are used to produce enzymes for metabolic activity, and few go into the production of muscle. Over time, this protein allocation causes overall muscle wasting.

Fat metabolism during the stress response also increases. This is simply a mechanism for getting usable energy into the body cells. During a stress situation, glucose (which normally is available to all body cells) is shunted into the central nervous system. This is because the central nervous system can burn only glucose, and fat must be mobilized so the cells have something to burn. Because modern people rarely use physical movement as a response to stress, this output of fat is not needed, and the fat circulates in the system until finally it is reabsorbed into storage tissue. Evidence shows that this circulating fat may be deposited along arterial walls and thus contribute to the development of atherosclerosis.

Cardiovascular System

In the cardiovascular system, stress brings about an overall increase in activity. If you are going to run away or fight, you are going to need more blood, especially in the muscles. To accommodate this need, the heart rate increases. Individuals who are anxious or who have a high level of chronic stress tend to have a faster heart rate, even at rest. In addition, stroke volume and cardiac output are greater; more blood is being pumped out of the heart with each beat. At the same time, to get more blood to the muscles vasoconstriction increases blood pressure and eventually may be responsible for causing vascular headaches, worsening atherosclerosis, and aggravating conditions such as Raynaud's disease and Berger's disease.

The heart, through its nervous connections with the brain, is capable of anticipating physiological and metabolic demands by increasing heart action before it actually is required. As we've seen before, however, anticipation of such a demand often increases activity but then the brain thwarts the final action. Thus, the response of the cardiovascular system is to no avail. Many psychological states increase cardiovascular activity when no action actually is required. A new or unusual experience frequently elevates the heart rate, as do fear, anger, anxiety, and most situations that threaten the ego.

Another cardiovascular problem related to stress is consistently elevated blood pressure, or hypertension. Because the primary work of the heart is to overcome the pressure in the arteries to which the blood must flow, increasing blood pressure greatly increases the work of the heart and contributes to cardiovascular problems. A chronically stressed person often has a chronically overworked heart.

Skin System

To think of the skin as a separate system capable of responding to stress arousal may seem unusual; nevertheless, its complex function and intricate nervous control make it a sensitive response system, and its accessibility makes it a convenient window into the body. Each of the millions of cells that make up the skin system contains chemicals of an electrical nature. As the body expresses itself, the chemical activity of the skin cells changes, producing different patterns of electrical activity that can be measured on the skin's surface. Although it is sometimes difficult to interpret, police authorities use it in lie detector tests, and health professionals use it to help understand a person's emotions, motivations, and problem-solving techniques.

Temperature is another basic response system of the skin. Small blood vessels under the skin change in response to emotion. During tense, anxious periods, they shut down and allow less blood to pass, causing the skin temperature to become lower and the skin to appear pale. At other times the blood vessels open and allow the skin to flush with blood, raising the skin temperature. With this type of response pattern, prolonged emotional responses can change the activity of the skin long enough to result in malfunction and disease.

Immune System

Based on extensive medical experience, physicians and researchers recognize that thoughts, emotions, attitudes, and beliefs have a great deal of bearing on health, disease, and the ability to recover from illness. The link between emotions and disease is through the immune system.

The immune system may become compromised in stress-related illness in three basic ways: (a) underactivity, (b) hyperactivity, and (c) misguided impulses. These three types of dysfunctions are typified, respectively, by cancer, asthma, and rheumatoid arthritis. Underactivity, or depression of the immune system, occurs in response to stress-induced release of adrenal cortex hormones. Researchers have found that even slight suppression of the immune system greatly increases susceptibility to bacteria and viruses. The hyperactive immune response seen in asthma involves irritation of the mucous lining of the airways in the lungs. When the lining is irritated, the resulting hyperimmune response can cause symptoms ranging from mild discomfort to respiratory failure. *Autoimmune diseases* are the result of a misguided immune system that attacks its own tissues as well as those of invading bacteria and viruses. Autoimmune disorders caused by breakdowns in communication within the nervous, endocrine, and immune systems often are associated with immune deficiency syndromes, injuries, aging, and malignancies.

With prolonged stress arousal, any or all of the biochemicals, organs, and systems involved will be affected until fatigue occurs. When fatigue of the immune system begins, infections, common colds, and slight skin conditions appear. As the fatigue continues, the conditions grow worse and more serious illnesses begin to set in. When the immune response to disease elements is diminished to 50%–60%, the body may respond with persistent and repeated infections requiring antibiotics; summer colds; serious skin disease or inflammation; and chronic respiratory system conditions such as bronchitis, asthma, or tuberculosis. Immune system fatigue diminishes the body's capability to resist all invading viruses, bacteria, and toxins.

Other Responses

Several other minor physiological responses occur during stress arousal. One is increased sodium (salt) retention, which can feed back and aggravate the increase in blood pressure. Another is increased sweating of the underarms, palms of the hands, and soles of the feet. If these areas are constantly wet, it may be a sign that you are responding to a situation with anxiety or stress.

CAUSES OF STRESS: STRESSORS

Why does a person become stressed? What are the causes? How does personality influence stress arousal? The answers to these questions are different for each person. The causes of stress are unique. Even though stress has a dozen common causes, each person's response is different, depending upon the stressors and how they interact with the individual's personality and are affected by his or her lifestyle. The amount of stress is determined by lifestyle situations, especially relationships inside and outside of work. Basic personality and the physical environment are other critical variables. Table 11.1 outlines the factors that make up these general categories of stressors.

TABLE 11.1 Major classification of stressors.

CLASS	STRESSOR
Lifestyle	Adaptation
	Overload
	Frustration
	Deprivation
Personality	Self-concept
	Time-urgency
	Anger and hostility
	Need for control
	Anxiety and anxious-reactivity
Environment	Biological rhythms
	Nutrition
	Overcrowding
	Noise
	Pollution
	Toxic wastes
	Drugs

Lifestyle

Lifestyle, how one lives in the sociocultural environment, often is mentioned as the most important determinant of stress. Lifestyle encompasses the events of our lives, as well as our daily work and play activities. Lifestyle includes what we eat or otherwise ingest and factors of our physical environment including the noise, the hurry, and the pressure we encounter every day. Lifestyle also incorporates people with whom we interact, and human interaction possibly is the most potent stressor of all. Even people we don't know can be significant stressors in our lives. For example, we all have had our stress aroused by politicians or editorialists with views that offend us. Four categories of lifestyle factors that influence the stress response are adaptation, overload, frustration, and deprivation. These are discussed below in more detail.

Adaptation

The stress response exists to help us adapt to change. Consequently, the more change we experience in our lives, the more stress we have. Major events and abrupt changes in our lives can throw us off balance and upset our natural equilibrium or homeostasis. To survive, we must adapt to these events and changes, and **adaptation** consumes energy as the body fights to restore balance. Some events require major adaptation; others require only minor adjustments. More than two decades ago researchers Thomas Holmes and Richard Rahe compiled a list of life events, both positive and negative, that required individuals to change their lives or adapt to some degree. The result of their efforts was the Social Readjustment Rating Scale, a simple paper-and-pencil test that assigns a numerical value to life events based on the severity or degree of the change involved. A high score on this test was found to be correlated positively with subsequent illness rates in those individuals, making this test an important tool for studying adaptive stress.

Based on this work, similar scales have been developed that validate this precept for specific populations. Although most studies do show that individuals with more severe life-change events have more stress and more illness, many people who experience the same life events do not have ill effects. This is because of differences in coping abilities, the influence of individual perception of the life event, past experience, susceptibility, and other factors.

The self-scoring Stressor Self-Test included in this chapter was designed to give you an indication of the aspects of your lifestyle that may be causing you stress. We have broken the test into several sections, and as you complete each part, remember that it is an educational tool designed to promote awareness. It in no way substitutes for the diagnostic procedures physicians and psychologists use. Any concerns about your physical or mental health should be directed to a qualified health professional. The Stressor Test, Part 1, a variation of the Social Readjustment Rating Scale, will give you an indication of the events in your life that require your adaptive energy.

Higher scores indicate an increased vulnerability to stress because of a drain of adaptive energy, but you must take into consideration that the importance of life events lies not so much in whether the change is positive or negative, a major life event or a minor one, as on your perception of the significance of the event to your life. The significance and impact of these life events also depend on your coping ability and your support systems.

Overload

Your body has the ability to respond to stress, and as it does so, it becomes conditioned to be increasingly sensitive to stress. When your life becomes overloaded, your stress response system eventually becomes overresponsive and overstressed. **Overload** is defined as a state in which the demands of life exceed one's capacity to meet them. The term *overstimulation* often is used synonymously with overload. Most of us occasionally feel that the pressures of life are building up faster than our ability to deal with them, or that there simply are not enough hours in the day or days in the week to accomplish what has to be done. This is overload. As a result of overload, you might become tired and irritable, get more colds or other illness symptoms, begin to feel fatigued and less sociable, and become less and less enthusiastic about life. The Stressor Test, Part 2 is presented as a self-check of overload factors in your life.

Overload can come from many aspects of your life. The most prevalent source of stress resulting from overload in most people's lives is their work, which can include school. Work stress has several common causes. One of these is called *quantitative overload*, which means that an individual tries to do too many things at one time, tries to meet too many deadlines, and tries to be in too many places at the same time. Another cause of work stress is *qualitative overload*, which occurs when individuals find themselves in situations where the work is beyond their ability, such as after a promotion or during training for a new task. Qualitative overload has become more prevalent in this age of computers and high technology. Individuals who have

A C T I V I T Y

THE STRESSOR TEST, PART 1:
ADAPTATION

Below is a list of some common life events usually perceived as stressful. Check the ones you have experienced in the last 12 months.

Major change in work or school:

_✓_ increase in hours per week

_____ increase in responsibility

_____ increase in authority

_____ decrease in pay 25% or more

_____ increase or decrease in autonomy

_✓_ work shift change (long-term)

_____ loss of job or suspension from school

_✓_ problems with superiors

_____ change of job or school

_____ change of school major

Total number of checks x 2 = _6_

Major change in interpersonal relationships:

_✓_ marriage

_____ divorce or break-up of long-term relationship

_____ serious problems with partner (e.g., infidelity, arguments)

_____ serious restriction of social life

_✓_ major disagreements with family

Total number of checks x 4 = _8_

Major change in lifestyle:

_____ change of residence more than 100 miles away

_____ incurrence of a large debt

_____ problems with the law

_____ death of a close friend or family member

_____ serious illness of a close friend or family member

Total number of checks x 4 = _0_

Major change in health status:

_____ injury or illness resulting in loss of time at work or school

_____ problems with drugs or alcohol

_____ unwanted pregnancy (male or female partner)

_____ premature end of a pregnancy

_____ birth of a child

Total number of checks x 4 = _0_

Add the sum of the four sections to arrive at a score for this test.

TOTAL SCORE _14_

A score between

0–20	= low risk in adaptation
20–40	= low to moderate risk
40–60	= moderate to high risk
60+	= high risk

been doing the same job for many years suddenly may find that their job has changed and evolved beyond their present ability level. Time pressures, deadlines, decision making, and performance anxiety also are stress producers. Performance anxiety can be especially stressful to those who, in their jobs, are responsible for other people's lives and well-being, or for large sums of money.

If your work is being a student, you may experience similar forms of overload. Our society's demand for higher education has created a highly competitive academic environment reaching back into the primary grades. Students are pressured to do well academically to ensure admission to college. College students then must compete for honor status to be considered for graduate or professional schools. Test anxiety is a major problem in college, and academic overload can lead to poor self-concept and emotional disturbances, and to students dropping out of school.

In addition to work, other areas in our lives contribute to overload. For instance, we may experience *urban overload*, which arises from having too many people in too small a space. Cities generate overload stimulation in the forms of stress-producing noise, pollution, crowding, and competition for everything from parking places to restaurant tables. One must move faster just to keep pace in an environment of unfamiliar, seemingly uncaring, faces. Even your home may be a source of overload; for some people, crowding, noise, lack of privacy, cooking, cleaning, and repair work make leaving the house to go to work the most pleasant part of the day.

Frustration

Closely related to overload is the stress engendered by **frustration** at being blocked from doing what we want to do. We may have the feeling that with all those people getting in the way, we are being kept from accomplishing the goals we set for ourselves. Our work and our personal lives have the potential to cause us great frustration, whether from time restraints, competition, disappointed expectations, or other factors. Some common aspects of work that may result in job-related frustration are:

1. *Job ambiguity:* not knowing exactly what the job entails, or not knowing what is expected of you or how you will be evaluated.

2. *Role conflicts:* having to play a role that does not fit your beliefs or values.

3. *Bureaucracy:* dealing with complex rules, excessive paperwork, stifled creativity, poor communication, or some combination thereof.

4. *Discrimination and prejudice:* having to submit to biases that have the potential to stifle anything from day-to-day activities to long-range opportunities and dreams.

5. *Socioeconomic opportunities:* experiencing the power-lessness and hopelessness of the disadvantaged, and perhaps being held back from playing a meaningful role in life.

The Stressor Test, Part 3 is a self-measure of your frustration level.

Deprivation

Deprivational stressors, the opposite of overload, may be just as stressful. **Deprivational stress is the boredom engendered from living a lifestyle or working at a job that is not demanding or challenging. Deprivation is not always related to performing highly repetitive tasks. It also may exist when an individual is not active enough over a long period. Too much passive entertainment (such as television viewing), overindulgence in antisocial or antimotivational alcohol or drugs, too much time alone, and being out of work are all examples of deprivation. Research on loneliness, lack of activity, and lack of purpose indicates that these factors are associated with diminished self-esteem, decreased social stimulation, and spiritual disintegration. All of these social indicators of excessive stress arousal have been associated with increased susceptibility to illness and accidents. The Stressor Test, Part 4 helps you measure your level of deprivation.

Personal Beliefs and Behaviors

We can change our environment and reduce the stimulation we receive from change, overload, and frustration. If the required changes involve other people, though, they may be difficult to make. It is more efficient to change oneself, reducing stress by modifying stressful personality traits. Thus, personal beliefs and behaviors are perhaps the most important variable in the classification of stressors

---

A C T I V I T Y

THE STRESSOR TEST, PART 2: OVERLOAD

Choose the most appropriate answer for each of the following statements and place the letter of your response in the space to the left of the statement.

_____ 1. I find myself with not enough time to do the activities I really enjoy.
(a) almost always (b) often (c) seldom (d) almost never

_____ 2. I feel people expect too much from me.
(a) almost always (b) often (c) seldom (d) almost never

_____ 3. I feel less competent than I think I should.
(a) almost always (b) often (c) seldom (d) almost never

_____ 4. I find myself getting anxious about my work or school.
(a) almost always (b) often (c) seldom (d) almost never

_____ 5. I feel that I have too much responsibility.
(a) almost always (b) often (c) seldom (d) almost never

_____ 6. I have difficulty falling asleep because I have too much on my mind.
(a) almost always (b) often (c) seldom (d) almost never

_____ 7. I feel, when I make a mistake, it is because of being rushed.
(a) almost always (b) often (c) seldom (d) almost never

Scoring: a = 4, b = 3, c = 2, d = 1

TOTAL SCORE _____

7–13 = low vulnerability to stress from overload
14–20 = moderate vulnerability
21–28 = high vulnerability

---

presented earlier. Stress-prone personal characteristics, attitudes, and values interact with our environment. Certain personality characteristics may cause us to be more susceptible to stress; thus may make us more or less prone to stress caused by environment and lifestyle. We can hold down stress by manipulating the environment to try to eliminate or avoid most major stressors, but in our modern, fast-paced society, to completely eliminate stressors would be next to impossible. Therefore, the most efficient path usually is to develop low-stress personality characteristics. Aspects of personality that influence response to stress include: self-concept, time urgency, anger and hostility, the need for control, and anxiety and anxious-reactivity.

Self-Concept

Self-concept also is called self-perception and self-regard. Individuals all have an opinion of themselves, and that opinion is based on a great many factors, experiences, and self-evaluations. The causes and effects of low self-concept are too complex to discuss in detail here. Actually, we are faced with a "chicken and egg" problem because low self-esteem is both the cause and the reinforced result of problems in social interactions. This problem is cyclical. People tend to like other people who are outgoing, assertive, creative, and interesting, and who can make decisions about what they want and how to achieve it. We like these qualities in ourselves also.

Low self-esteem usually prevents people from asserting themselves, from getting their ideas heard, and so on. Low self-esteem leads to poor performance and, subsequently, to reinforcement of the problem. Frustration, anxiety, and hostility—psychological manifestations of stress—often result. A person who recognizes him- or herself in this description may feel helpless to escape the cycle but should realize that help is available and that the cycle can be broken. Counseling is an important first step. Recognizing the stress-inducing aspects of this problem and seeking to reduce the stress are important. The Stressor Test, Part 5 is presented to indicate your self-concept.

Time-Urgency, Anger, Hostility, and the Need for Control

Our society's race against the clock is a major source of stress. Virtually every organization imposes some form of time pressure over those within that organization, whether it is a business, a family, or a classroom. Stressful as organizational time restraints can be, our internal clocks cause the most significant stress arousal, especially for those who have a time-urgency personality trait. These individuals tend to have a heightened sense of time and almost always are worried about how long some thing is going to

A C T I V I T Y

THE STRESSOR TEST, PART 3: FRUSTRATION

Choose the most appropriate answer for each of the following statements and place the letter of your response in the space to the left of the statement.

_____ 1. I feel stifled or held back in my personal life or at work.
(a) almost always (b) often (c) seldom (d) almost never

_____ 2. I find myself upset because things have not gone according to my plan.
(a) almost always (b) often (c) seldom (d) almost never

_____ 3. I find myself frustrated.
(a) almost always (b) often (c) seldom (d) almost never

_____ 4. I feel that I am in a rut.
(a) almost always (b) often (c) seldom (d) almost never

_____ 5. I perceive myself as lost, or in the wrong job or school.
(a) almost always (b) often (c) seldom (d) almost never

_____ 6. I feel as though I'm a victim of discrimination.
(a) almost always (b) often (c) seldom (d) almost never

_____ 7. I feel like pushing people or things out of my way.
(a) almost always (b) often (c) seldom (d) almost never

Scoring: a = 4, b = 3, c = 2, d = 1

TOTAL SCORE _____

   7–13 = *low vulnerability to stress from frustration*
   14–20 = *moderate vulnerability*
   21–28 = *high vulnerability*

A C T I V I T Y

THE STRESSOR TEST, PART 4: DEPRIVATION

Choose the most appropriate answer for each of the following statements and place the letter of your response in the space to the left of the statement.

_____ 1. I find myself bored.
(a) almost always (b) often (c) seldom (d) almost never

_____ 2. I feel that my life or work is not stimulating enough.
(a) almost always (b) often (c) seldom (d) almost never

_____ 3. I find myself becoming restless.
(a) almost always (b) often (c) seldom (d) almost never

_____ 4. I wish my life were more exciting.
(a) almost always (b) often (c) seldom (d) almost never

_____ 5. I find myself daydreaming.
(a) almost always (b) often (c) seldom (d) almost never

_____ 6. I find myself with nothing to do.
(a) almost always (b) often (c) seldom (d) almost never

_____ 7. I feel overqualified to be doing what I'm doing.
(a) almost always (b) often (c) seldom (d) almost never

Scoring: a = 4, b = 3, c = 2, d = 1

TOTAL SCORE _____

   7–13 = *low vulnerability to stress from deprivation*
   14–20 = *moderate vulnerability*
   21–28 = *high vulnerability*

take. The time-urgency personality trait has been studied extensively as part of the famous cardiovascular **Type A personality** construct originally formulated by Friedman and Rosenman. Type A individuals tend to be impatient, driven by an excessive time and task orientation, and more often prone to excessive feelings of anger and hostility.

As problematic as the time-urgency trait is, the behavior and personality traits of anger and hostility are what have been shown to be the most lethal stress producers. These personality characteristics are the most significant characteristics of the Type A pattern in relation to developing cardiovascular disease. The precipitating factor behind hostility seems to be cynical mistrust. The tendency to always draw hostile conclusions about people and events results in a chronic defensive posture and attack strategy that activates the body's nervous and hormonal response systems, especially the cardiovascular system. It is as though the body were saying, "If we are going to be constantly angry and defensive, we might as well just stay that way and avoid all these ups and downs."

Thus far, research has not explained sufficiently how and why a person develops Type A characteristics, although our society clearly is time-conscious and competitive and does reward hard work and achievement. Nevertheless, one can work hard and be successful without being excessively hard-driving, competitive, and controlling.

Dr. David Glass has argued that the core of the Type A behavior pattern is the need for control. The competitiveness, time-urgency, hostility, and low tolerance for frustration in these individuals all may be seen as expressions of a need to overcontrol themselves and their environment. In an attempt to test Glass's hypothesis, other researchers also found that Type A individuals have an exaggerated need to control their lives.

The noted psychologist Albert Bandura stated, "It is mainly perceived inefficiency in coping with potentially aversive events that makes them fearsome. To the extent to which one can prevent, terminate, or lessen the severity of aversive events, there is little reason to fear them." Thus, it can be

ACTIVITY

THE STRESSOR TEST, PART 5: SELF-CONCEPT

Choose the most appropriate answer for each of the following statements and place the letter of your response in the space to the left of the statement.

_____ 1. I feel I don't have much going for me.
  (a) almost always (b) often (c) seldom (d) almost never

_____ 2. I'm uncomfortable around members of the opposite sex.
  (a) almost always (b) often (c) seldom (d) almost never

_____ 3. I'm uncomfortable around my superiors.
  (a) almost always (b) often (c) seldom (d) almost never

_____ 4. Whenever something goes wrong, I blame myself.
  (a) almost always (b) often (c) seldom (d) almost never

_____ 5. I shun new endeavors because of fear of failure.
  (a) almost always (b) often (c) seldom (d) almost never

_____ 6. I have a strong need for recognition and approval.
  (a) almost always (b) often (c) seldom (d) almost never

_____ 7. I boast about myself.
  (a) almost always (b) often (c) seldom (d) almost never

Scoring: a = 4, b = 3, c = 2, d = 1

TOTAL SCORE _____

7–13 = low vulnerability to stress from self-concept
14–20 = moderate vulnerability
21–28 = high vulnerability

argued that the most powerful stressor of all is the real or imagined loss of control. What may contribute to all of the psychosocial and personality stressors examined here is a real or imagined loss of control over one's life.

In his now classic text, *Psychological Stress and Coping Processes*, Dr. Richard Lazarus theorized that the greater the degree to which a person perceives himself or herself to be in control of a situation, the less severe the stress reaction will be. Geer and colleagues showed that just the expectation of control over stressors can be effective in reducing stress. In their studies, one group of students was deceived into believing that their reaction times to shock could reduce the frequency of the shocks they would receive. The experimenters then reduced the number of shocks for all subjects, regardless of their reaction times. The group of subjects that were told they were, indeed, controlling the reduction experienced a decrease in their level of distress, measured by skin conductance. A similar group of subjects who received an equal number of shocks, yet were told they had no control over them, experienced an increased stress response. Thus, anything that adds to the feeling of self-control is likely to reduce the severity of the stress reaction.

Many notable researchers offer considerable evidence that a real or imagined sense of control over self or environment is a powerful stress-reducing mechanism. Fisher compiled perhaps the most impressive array of evidence indicating that a sense of control may be the single most powerful stress management tool one can mobilize. Control also is central to the **hardiness** concept, a psychological behavior pattern characterized by good control, commitment, and challenge. Hardy people are healthier, experience less stress, and recover from illness faster.

Part 6 of the Stressor Test addresses time-urgency, anger and hostility, and the need for control.

Anxiety and Anxious-Reactivity

Anxiety is a well-documented *reaction* to stress, and being anxiety-prone is also a *cause* of excessive stress. Some individuals exhibit an extreme anxiety reaction to stress, persisting long after the stressor has been eliminated. In these individuals the body's reaction to stress *becomes* the stress. They do not seem to possess the feedback dampening mechanisms normally used to cope with stress anxiety. The body seems to become so conditioned to react with anxiety that, with the slightest amount of stress, the body immediately assumes the maximum anxiety response, which then is prolonged.

Speilberger has offered a complete explanation of anxiety. His definition of the anxiety reaction, also called *state anxiety*, is a response to a stimulus that is perceived as threatening. The way we perceive a threat is unique to each of us. Fears are not always grounded in logic, nor can logic alone explain them away or diminish the stress response.

Anxiety and fear produce similar responses in the body and in many ways are the opposite of anger. Anger fills the body with blood and excessive pressure, as if to prepare us for the fight. The anxiety reaction is one of fear, of diminished blood to organs, lowered internal pressure, and a sense of hiding or being frozen in position, hoping not to be seen by the threat. The anger response is to

A C T I V I T Y

THE STRESSOR TEST, PART 6: TIME URGENCY, ANGER AND HOSTILITY, NEED FOR CONTROL

Choose the most appropriate answer for each of the following statements and place the letter of your response in the space to the left of the statement.

_____ 1. I catch myself rushing without a need to do so.
    (a) almost always (b) often (c) seldom (d) almost never

_____ 2. I hate to wait.
    (a) almost always (b) often (c) seldom (d) almost never

_____ 3. I try to make my activities competitive.
    (a) almost always (b) often (c) seldom (d) almost never

_____ 4. I feel guilty when I'm not being productive.
    (a) almost always (b) often (c) seldom (d) almost never

_____ 5. I tend to lose my temper or get irritable.
    (a) almost always (b) often (c) seldom (d) almost never

_____ 6. When frustrated, I feel like hitting something.
    (a) almost always (b) often (c) seldom (d) almost never

_____ 7. I seem to eat and walk faster than most people.
    (a) almost always (b) often (c) seldom (d) almost never

Scoring: a = 4, b = 3, c = 2, d = 1

TOTAL SCORE _____

    7–13 = low vulnerability to stress from time-urgency, anger and hostility, and need for control
    14–20 = moderate vulnerability
    21–28 = high vulnerability

strike back, whereas the fear response is to hide. The body prepares for both. **Anxiety** has been described as *chronic fear*, and anxious-reactivity as the body becoming increasingly stressed when sensing the fear arousal. For example, the anxious response may produce an awareness of hands trembling, heart pounding, or stomach gurgling. This "awareness," whether conscious or subconscious, feeds the anxious stress response, so the stress response becomes more severe. One of the most important stress reduction techniques is to lessen the body's tendency to be overly sensitive to stress arousal. The relaxation techniques presented in Chapter 12 are designed for this purpose. Here, the Stressor Test, Part 7 allows a quick self-check of anxiety and anxious reactivity.

Emotions

An **emotion** is an energy complex made up of ideas, beliefs, attitudes, and opinions, as well as past experiences, postures, and actions. Emotions are basic to the way we think, act, make decisions, and what we believe to be true. Our emotions are basic motivators. They guard our basic needs, and they enrich and intensify our lives. Emotional responses learned early in life are reactions to basic needs and external stimuli. As we grow older, we also learn to create emotional patterns from our thoughts until they become fairly habitual. Because we are taught directly or indirectly not to show all of our emotions, however, we develop negative self-talk that becomes part of our emotional patterns. If we do not like the way an emotion feels or aren't allowed to express it, we can block it out of our consciousness altogether.

Through our ability to relive stressful situations, we learn how to scare ourselves to death, worry ourselves until we are distraught, and catastrophize even the most harmless situation. By the same token, we can retrieve pleasure, joy, laughter, and happiness by thinking about times when we felt those emotions. The Stressor Test, Part 8 helps to assess your emotions.

ACTIVITY

THE STRESSOR TEST, PART 7: ANXIETY AND ANXIOUS-REACTIVITY

Choose the most appropriate answer for each of the following statements and place the letter of your response in the space to the left of the statement.

___ 1. I tend to imagine the worst things happening in any situation.
(a) almost always (b) often (c) seldom (d) almost never

___ 2. I re-live instances or situations again and again in my mind.
(a) almost always (b) often (c) seldom (d) almost never

___ 3. I feel my stomach sinking or my heart pounding.
(a) almost always (b) often (c) seldom (d) almost never

___ 4. I have trouble falling asleep at night.
(a) almost always (b) often (c) seldom (d) almost never

___ 5. I have difficulty speaking or notice my hands and fingers trembling.
(a) almost always (b) often (c) seldom (d) almost never

___ 6. I am tense.
(a) almost always (b) often (c) seldom (d) almost never

___ 7. I feel as though difficulties are piling up.
(a) almost always (b) often (c) seldom (d) almost never

Scoring: a = 4, b = 3, c = 2, d = 1

TOTAL SCORE _____

7–13 = low vulnerability to stress from anxiety and anxious-reactivity
14–20 = moderate vulnerability
21–28 = high vulnerability

Emotional Energy

Emotional energy carries messages that we have named fear, anger, and so on. Take a moment to gasp as though surprised or frightened. The body instantaneously braces itself. Muscles contract, the lungs and heart modify their action, and if taken further, this experiment can cause all systems involved in this emotion to alter their functions. Through nerve stimulation, the muscles tense, the heart beats faster and harder, respiration quickens and deepens, and the pupils of the eyes dilate. Glands are stimulated to modify their secretions. The adrenals begin dumping out hormones to help answer the emergency signals. The emergency signal demands attention. It may signal joy or humor, or it may portend danger. Also, it may be rooted in the external world or within a thought pattern that has little external base. The response to the emergency signal is the emotional reaction pattern, or as we first identified it in this book, it is the stress response.

If the emotion is positive, tension builds and then is released, as a shout or laughter perhaps.

When the emotion is negative, tension builds up and tends to be stored. Usually during this time, negative self-talk increases the tension. Emotional messages do not dissipate until they are delivered.

Emotional "Stuffing"

As children grow into adolescence, they learn that loud laughter and silly giggling are not acceptable in public. They are rewarded for not crying, reprimanded for displaying anger, and chided for being afraid. They are asked not to show that they have been emotionally hurt, to be selective about whom they should love, and to contain their exuberance. They have to "stuff" their emotions. It is no wonder that most adults engage in negative self-talk when they get angry, are hurt or fearful, or even want to shriek with pleasure.

John Bradshaw points out that dysfunctional families deny their children the right to feel or to talk about feelings. This keeps children from being in touch with what they are feeling. First, they are shamed out of expressing any feelings, and second, they aren't allowed to talk about their feelings. In some families children are allowed to express only negative emotions, such as guilt.

Everyone denies emotions to some extent. When a person gets angry and says, "I'm really silly to get mad," the emotion is not honored. But it happens anyway, and it is stored in the body with all the other anger that has been denied and not released. Release of an emotion is necessary before the body can go back to a relaxed state or back into balance. Most of us know the effectiveness of a good laugh or cry as a release to make us feel better.

Breaking Unhealthy Emotional Habits

As noted, honoring our emotions, releasing them, and going about our business is healthy. Because most negative emotional responses are habitual patterns to perceived dangers, we can learn to break those habits rather than suffer the physiological consequences of an unwarranted emergency signal. One way to do this is by relaxing.

A time-honored, efficient, and effective way to relax in any situation is to do deep, **diaphragmatic breathing,** in which air is taken to the deepest lobes of the lungs. Another way to break old negative emotional response patterns is to act on them as soon as you notice that you are thinking negative thoughts or saying negative things to yourself. At that time, tell yourself, "Stop it!" Then, after noting your negative thinking pattern, replace it with relaxation or positive thoughts, or just focus on and enjoy what you are doing and experiencing at the present time.

We can experience the patterns, honor them, and learn to release the tension that otherwise can lead to poor health. *If the emotional energy is not released, disease or behavioral symptoms will result.* The Stressor Test, Part 8 is a self-test of your emotions. Intervention exercises specific to anger and fear are presented in Chapter 12. Some general relaxation training is always helpful, especially meditation and visualization, in which you scan the

body, focusing on the feelings that may be attached to any stress point in the body.

Environmental Stressors

The concept of environmental stress stems from the relationship the human organism has with its environment. This type of stress is influenced only somewhat by an individual's personality or thought process, but a definite relationship exists between one's behavior and the stress *imposed* by the environment. The four general classes of environmental stimuli that can contribute to distress are: biological rhythms, what we eat, the environment itself (overcrowding, noise, air and water pollution, toxic wastes), and drugs. Drugs are covered in Chapter 10, so only the first three classes of environmental stressors will be covered here.

Biological Rhythms

Time always has been recognized as one of our greatest stressors. Although most people associate time-induced stress with society's deadlines and

---

A C T I V I T Y

THE STRESSOR TEST, PART 8: EMOTIONS

Choose the most appropriate answer for each of the following statements and place the letter of your response in the space to the left of the statement.

1. In situations I find difficult to handle, I get angry.
   (a) almost always (b) often (c) seldom (d) never
2. It is difficult for me to say no to other people.
   (a) almost always (b) often (c) seldom (d) never
3. I am depressed.
   (a) almost always (b) often (c) seldom (d) never
4. When I am unhappy, I just have to wait until something good happens to me to change my mood.
   (a) almost always (b) often (c) seldom (d) never
5. When I am angry at someone, I generally keep it to myself.
   (a) almost always (b) often (c) seldom (d) never
6. When I find myself angry I do not know why.
   (a) almost always (b) often (c) seldom (d) never
7. It is difficult for me to laugh at myself.
   (a) almost always (b) often (c) seldom (d) never

Scoring: a = 4, b = 3, c = 2, d = 1

TOTAL SCORE _____

    7–13 = low vulnerability to stress from emotions
   14–20 = moderate vulnerability
   21–28 = high vulnerability

time restrictions, other aspects of time also influence our lives. The natural world runs on time: solar or light time, lunar time, seasonal time, and so on. The human body also runs on time: temperature time, metabolic time, energy time, and hormonal time, to mention just a few. Social, cultural, technological humans have arrogantly ignored their **biological rhythms** for the sake of convenience and conformity. We try to synchronize work and recreation schedules with what is socially and economically efficient. We utilize artificial light, and we speed through time zones. All of these things and more act to change *the body's natural tempo*. As a result, we are out of synchrony with our bodies, and this leads to undue irritability, emotional instability, and increased susceptibility to illness.

What We Eat

Especially during stressful times, high levels of certain vitamins are needed to maintain proper functioning of the nervous and endocrine systems. These are vitamin C and the vitamins of the B complex, particularly vitamins B_1 (thiamin), B_2 (riboflavin), niacin, B_5 (pantothenic acid), B_6 (pyridoxine hydrochloride), and choline. The B-complex vitamins are especially important in the stress response because deficiencies of vitamins B_1, B_5, and B_6 can lead to anxiety reactions, depression, and insomnia. Chapter 8 covers nutrition in depth.

Another type of environmental stressor is food additives and pesticides. *Food additives* are used to improve the texture, flavor, quality, and attractiveness of foods. Little concrete evidence has accumulated on the long-term effects of additives, although headlines and newscasts often warn consumers about the potential hazards of some additives. A rule of thumb is that any artificial chemical on food is unnatural and not good for the body; however, what constitutes an unsafe amount most likely will be debated for years.

Pesticides are unlike additives in that they were created to poison living things. Pesticides are designed to attack a specific pest and then disappear so that no residue remains in food to harm the consumer. In reality, pesticide use seldom can be so well controlled, and there is reason for concern that hazardous pesticide residue might drift onto other crops, pollute the water, contaminate the soil, and accumulate in the tissue of animals and people. Average consumers can assume that their produce contains pesticides unless it is marketed specifically as "organic," and can sidestep some possible dangers by washing the food and rinsing thoroughly.

The conscious manipulation of nutritional behavior to control stress may be referred to as nutritional engineering, which includes making the diet adequate and varied. A well-rounded diet helps avoid overconsumption of any one constituent and strengthens the body's defenses against many stress-induced and stress-related diseases. When used as one of the stress-reducing strategies, it can prove to be a powerful addition to the holistic program for stress management, discussed in Chapter 12.

Environment Itself

The effect of the environment on health depends on (a) the degree of stress, and (b) the condition of the body. The immune system is the system that ultimately protects the body. The healthier the person is, the stronger are his or her defenses against overstimulation from the environment. The impact of environment also is determined by the amount of, and duration of exposure to, the stress-producing element. The body usually can handle stressors one, or even a few, at a time. Multiple stressors can act synergistically so that small doses of several stressors overwork the immune system and create a negative environmental impact. Most environmental problems can be attributed to the world's burgeoning population and increased industrialization.

Overcrowding. Overcrowding (or overpopulation) is a psychosocial and environmental factor contributing to stress. Almost all the environmental stressors discussed here are related in some way to overcrowding. Experiments with animals have revealed that crowding produces excessive stress-hormone secretion, excessive adrenaline secretion, atrophy of the thymus gland (which involves the immune system), atrophy of secondary sexual characteristics, and elevated blood pressure. "There is abundant evidence that among animals, at least, crowded living conditions and their immediate consequences . . . impose a stress that can lead to abnormal behavior, reproductive failure, sickness and even death. Human beings feel the impact of increased population as overstimulation from lack of space, more noise, more cars, more toxins, more crime, increased pollution and more intense competition."

Crowding is not solely a function of space and people but also of an individual's perception or feeling of being crowded. Three people may constitute a crowd in one situation (e.g., a tiny elevator or office), and 33 might not be a crowd in a different situation (e.g., a big party or sporting event). In any event, if you perceive yourself as being crowded or inhibited by the presence of others, overcrowding exists and is a psychosocial stressor for you.

Studies of crowding in penal institutions have revealed that inmates confined to cells with many other prisoners have higher blood pressure in general than do prisoners in less crowded cells. Highly crowded cells create an atmosphere of insecurity and depersonalization, which is more frustrating and inhibitive than less crowded cells.

Social psychologist Stanley Milgram developed the concept of overload to explain the impersonal attitude often observed in urban dwellers. He viewed the large urban center as a vast collection of potential stressors—mass media, mass transportation, vast technological innovations, intense interpersonal stimulation, a deadline-oriented society, and excessive and diverse responsibilities. These all combine in the city to form an aggregation of potential stressors. He suggested that the lack of interpersonal concern is actually a coping mechanism by which city dwellers deal with the bombardment of excessive social stimuli (overload) prevalent in most large cities. Therefore, impersonality is a defense mechanism that protects urbanites' psychological well-being by shielding them from all but the most necessary environmental demands placed on them.

Noise. The study of noise as a stressor is somewhat complex. Noise impacts us both psychosocially and biologically, and it can produce a stress response in one or more of the following ways:

1. By causing physiological reaction through stimulation of the sympathetic nervous system
2. By being annoying and subjectively displeasing
3. By disrupting ongoing activities

As item 2 indicates, noise can act as a stressor in a strictly psychological way (apart from any physical impact). This occurs when noise is perceived as unwanted or somehow inappropriate. This reaction, and the accompanying stress response, depends upon the specific situation. For example, a conversation at a distance of 3 feet generates only about 60 decibels (dB), far below the pain threshold; but if you are trying to study for a final exam, this conversation could become stressful. What may be music to you may be noise to someone else. Regardless of a person's adaptive characteristics, noise in excessive quantity or quality is distressful.

Environmental pollution. The four most significant manmade pollutants in the air are:

1. *Carbon monoxide* comes from fuel burned for transportation and for energy in homes, as wastes from manufacturing, and from solid wastes being burned for disposal.
2. *Photochemical oxidants* arise from other contaminants in the air when sunlight strikes them. Photochemical smog pollution irritates the body's sensitive, exposed tissues—eyes, mucous membranes of the nose and throat, and lungs.
3. *Nitrogen dioxide* occurs during high-temperature fuel-burning and can cause lung disease and lowered resistance to infection.
4. *Sulphur dioxide and suspended particles* arise primarily from the burning of coal, oil, and other industrial products. Together with high concentrations of suspended particulate matter, sulphur oxides are major components of smog and can affect health seriously by taxing the immune system and causing respiratory disease.

Thermal pollution is another form of air pollution found in urban areas that have a minimum of trees, soil, and standing water, and where the reflecting surfaces of pavements and buildings concentrate the heat. Thermal pollution adds to the stress people in crowded environments face. Heating and cooling of homes, driving cars, and energy-consuming industrial processes, especially without adequate safeguards for industrial wastes, are the primary causes of thermal pollution.

An increasingly serious environmental stressor is *water pollution*, which affects animals living in water directly and, eventually, human beings. When chemicals such as nitrates and phosphates (usually from sewage or fertilizer) are released into lakes and ponds, microorganisms in the water use them as nutrients. Nitrates and phosphates support the growth of large quantities of algae, which fill the body of water with dead plant material. Certain bacteria thrive on this dead matter, break it down and, in the process of consumption, use up the water's oxygen. This process, called **eutrophication,** eventually results in the death of waterways and all life forms in the water, including fish. A more insidious form of water pollution is direct dumping of human and industrial toxic waste into water used for human consumption. More than half of the water systems in the United States have been judged as substandard.

The pollution link between water and soil has become a subject of concern. Traditional thinking was that the land would filter or absorb pollutants and surrounding water would be safe from *land pollutants.* That was when contaminants deposited in the ground were nontoxic, mostly biological waste products. People and animals always have excreted solid wastes onto the earth. Bacteria break down waste material and return its constituents to the soil. Plants then use those compounds as fertilizers. The plants either die or are eaten and are themselves recycled. As long as human wastes were not dumped in huge quantities, the system worked. But the current human waste removal system is a waterborne system, and in most large cities purifying the water is becoming more difficult and expensive. Small towns are not exempt either, as many town wells now are being polluted by overburdened septic systems.

Modern society's most serious pollution problem is *toxic waste*, mostly industrial waste products. Of the more than 70,000 chemicals commercially used in the United States, only a few have been tested for their health effects. Two major toxic waste categories are heavy metals and halogenated compounds. Halogenated compounds, or PCBs, are used as insulating material. PCBs are a practically indestructible toxin that appears eventually in the food supply and can impair the immune system. Exposure may result in liver disease, cancer, acne, hair loss, eye damage, or reproductive abnormalities.

Another toxic waste with well-documented genetic danger is *radioactive waste*, mostly from nuclear power plants. The danger from nuclear accidents is ever present, as human beings are capable of making human errors. Even without accidents, an immense amount of dangerous radioactive waste will not decay for 10,000 years, and it currently is accumulating faster than there are places to dispose of it.

The Stressor Test, Part 9 gives you the chance to check your own environmental stressors.

Drugs

Although coffee is not usually considered a drug, it is discussed under this heading because it contains a sympathomimetic agent, caffeine. Sympathomimetic agents are chemical substances that mimic the sympathetic stress response. Many foods contain these sympathomimetic substances naturally, and consumption of these foods triggers a response in the body proportional to the amount

consumed and one's individual susceptibility to the chemical. Coffee is the most common of these sympathomimetic stressors, as it contains caffeine, a chemical that belongs to the xanthine group of drugs. Xanthines are powerful amphetamine-like stimulants that increase the metabolism rate and create a highly awake and active state. They also trigger the release of stress hormones, which are capable of increasing heart rate, blood pressure, and oxygen demands upon the heart. Extreme or prolonged stress hormone secretion can even initiate myocardial necrosis, or destruction of heart tissue.

The effects of nicotine as they relate to stress are almost identical to those of caffeine. Tobacco contains nicotine and, like caffeine, nicotine is a sympathomimetic chemical. As such, it is capable of all the adverse reactions of the sympathetic nervous system noted earlier. Thus, nicotine can trigger a stress response. Nicotine stimulates the adrenals, releasing hormones that elicit the stress

A C T I V I T Y

THE STRESSOR TEST, PART 9: ENVIRONMENT

Choose the most appropriate answer for each of the following statements and place the letter of your response in the space to the left of the statement.

1. I play music at a level that makes conversation difficult.
(a) almost always (b) often (c) seldom (d) never
2. The noise level in my work environment makes conversation difficult.
(a) almost always (b) often (c) seldom (d) never
3. I drink at least _____ cups of coffee or tea per day (excluding herbal tea).
(a) 7 or more (b) 5–6 (c) 3–4 (d) 2 or fewer
4. I smoke tobacco.
(a) more than 2 packs/day (b) 1–2 packs (c) less than 1 pack (d) never
5. I am exposed to the sidestream smoke of others around me:
(a) more than 4 hrs/day (b) 2–4 hrs/day (c) less than 2 hrs/day (d) not at all
6. I run, walk, or ride my bike on city streets crowded with motor traffic.
(a) almost always (b) often (c) seldom (d) never
7. I drink _____ alcoholic beverages per week.
(a) 7 or more (b) 5–6 (c) 3–4 (d) 2 or fewer

Scoring: a = 4, b = 3, c = 2, d = 1

TOTAL SCORE _____

7–13 = low vulnerability to stress from the environment
14–20 = moderate vulnerability
21–28 = high vulnerability

response of accelerated heart rate, blood pressure, respiration rate, and release of fatty acids and glucose into the blood, among other body reactions. Both caffeine and nicotine contribute to one's vulnerability to stress and thus are not recommended for consumption in any amount, but the use of tobacco is considerably more dangerous to overall health.

People take other chemical substances, including alcohol, for various reasons. A common motivation is to get "high" or experience an altered state of consciousness, often in an attempt to reduce the excess stress of coping with life. Competent coping is defined as remaining in control and optimally healthy while meeting the demands of life. Incompetent coping is the inability to meet demands, or sacrificing health or control in the coping attempt. In the incompetent coping situation the individual requires unhealthy physical or psychological help to cope.

Drugs have the ability to alter present reality. Drugs are taken to help *do* something one feels incapable of doing or to *be* something a person is not. When people are comfortable with "who they are" (known as self-acceptance), they are better able to accept their performance as it is without the performance negatively impacting the way they feel about themselves. Individuals who master most of life's tasks will feel good about themselves and less inclined to alter their true perception of themselves.

Altered States

Altered states can be induced through activities such as meditation, daydreaming, or drug-taking. To induce these states by mind direction rather than drug use is healthier. Currently, many popular techniques are offered to induce a self-transcendent, altered state of consciousness through mind direction or control. Yoga, medication, muscular relaxation, autogenic training, and biofeedback are a few examples. They are active and creative, requiring and promoting self-control and self-discipline.

SUMMARY

The stress response is a natural physical response that accelerates the body's defenses when threatened. In prehistoric times, before egos, bosses, traffic, and time deadlines, threats were physical and sporadic. Now the threats that may trigger a stress response are social and psychological.

The primary stressors for modern humans are lifestyle factors including adaptation to change, overload, frustration, and deprivation; personality factors such as self-concept, time urgency, hostility, anger, need for control, and anxiety; environmental factors such as pollution, noise, biological rhythms, nutrition, and overcrowding. Each of us responds to the presence of these stressors in a different way, determined by our lifestyle, experience, coping ability, and perception of the event or stressor. If coping abilities are not adequate and the stress response lasts too long, the body's defenses can fatigue, organ systems can deteriorate and physical illness can result.

Now that you have an awareness of what causes stress, the techniques presented in Chapter 12 can be used to manage stress.

CHOICES IN ACTION

If you haven't done so already, take a few moments to complete the nine Stressor Tests in this chapter. Knowing the primary sources of stress in your life should help you focus your stress management efforts. Lab 33, "Stress Response Analysis," helps you outline the stress you may have in your life.

REFERENCES

Achterberg, J. 1985. *Imagery and Healing.* Boston: Shambhala.

Achterberg, J., and Lawlis, G. 1984. *Imagery and Disease.* Champaign, IL: Institute for Personality and Ability Testing.

Alexander, F. 1965. *Psychosomatic Medicine.* New York: Norton.

Bandura, A. 1982. "Self-Efficacy Mechanism in Human Agency." *American Psychologist* pp. 122–147.

Borysenko, J. 1994. *Minding the Body, Mending the Mind.* Reading, MA: Addison-Wesley.

Bowers, K., and Kelly, P. 1949. "Stress, Disease, Psychotherapy, and Hypnosis." *Journal of Abnormal Psychology* 88(5): 490–505.

Bradshaw, J. 1992. *Homecoming.* New York: Bantam.

Dembroski, T., MacDougall, J., and Musante, L. 1984. "Desirability of Control Versus Locus of Control." *Health Psychology* 3: 12–26.

Fisher, S. 1984. *Stress and Perception of Control.* Hillsdale, NJ: Erlbaum.

Friedman, M., and Roserman, R. 1974. *Type A Behavior and Your Heart.* New York: Alfred Knopf.

Girdano, D. A., Everly, G. S., and Dusek, D. 1996. *Controlling Stress and Tension: A Holistic Approach*, 5th edition. Englewood Cliffs, NJ: Prentice Hall.

Glass, D. C. 1977. *Behavior Patterns, Stress, and Coronary-Prone Behavior.* Hillsdale, NJ: Erlbaum.

Greer, J. H., Davison, G., and Gatchal, R. 1970. "Reduction of Stress in Humans Through Nonveridical Perceived Control of Aversive Stimulation." *Journal of Personality and Social Psychology* 16: 731–738.

Holmes, T. S., and Rahe, R. H. 1968. "The Social Readjustment Rating Scale." *Journal of Psychosomatic Research* 213: 213–218.

Kobasa, S. C. 1979. "Stressful Life Events, Personality and Health." *Journal of Personality and Social Psychology* 37: 1–11.

Lazarus, R. S. 1966. *Psychological Stress and Coping Process.* New York: McGraw-Hill.

Lynch, J. J. 1966. *The Broken Heart: The Medical Consequences of Loneliness.* New York: McGraw-Hill.

Milgram, S. "The Experience of Living in Cities." *Science* 165: 1461–1468.

Muramoto, N. September 1988. "Natural Immunity: Insights on Diet and AIDS." *East West Journal* p. 50.

Rossi, E. 1994. *The Psychobiology of Mind-Body Healing.* New York: Norton.

Selye, H. 1956. *The Stress of Life.* New York: McGraw Hill.

Selye, H. 1974. *Stress Without Distress.* New York: Signet.

Siegel, B. S. 1995. *Love, Medicine and Miracles.* New York: Harper & Row.

Speilberger, C. D. 1972. *Anxiety: Current Trends in Theory and Research*, Vol. 1. New York: Academic Press.

Wolf, S., and Wolff, H. G. 1947. *Human Gastric Function*, 2d edition. New York: Oxford University Press.

Managing Stress

✓ How can your stress response be changed?

✓ How can you modify a stressful environment?

✓ How can you change lifestyle patterns that may contribute to stress?

✓ Is it possible to change beliefs or life philosophies that contribute to stress?

The skills of stress management are not difficult to learn. Provided you are motivated, the means are within your grasp. The components of a stress management program can be ordered into three steps:

1. Quiet the external environment to reduce the stressors in your life.
2. Quiet your internal environment to reduce stimulation of the nervous system.
3. Condition your mind to reduce stress-inducing thoughts.

A large part of stress reduction entails learning how to truly relax. Several relaxation techniques are presented to conclude the chapter.

QUIETING THE EXTERNAL ENVIRONMENT

The following activities are designed to quiet the external environment and, by so doing, reduce the stressors in your life (discussed in Chapter 11). These activities should increase your awareness of life events and then be used to restructure your environment, thought patterns, and behavior.

ACTIVITY
To Combat Adaptive Stress

Adaptive stress occurs when we must adjust to events and changes in our lives. To combat it:

1. Establish daily routines at home, work, school: a regular eating and physical activity program; set sleeping patterns; rest and relaxation times and places. You might establish certain hours of the week as a "mental health getaway." Make sure this is a time when you engage in truly relaxing behavior. A vacation in which you travel usually is not free from adaptive stress, so vacations don't count as mental health days unless they are truly relaxing to you.
2. Plan for change. Adopting the belief that change is a constant in life can prepare you emotionally and psychologically for change. When it comes, it is expected. Some changes are positive, such as meeting a new friend or beginning a new hobby or relationship. Others are negative, such as an unexpected death. Regardless of the nature of changes, all are reminders that change occurs constantly. A helpful exercise is to write a specific plan of

action for change. To do this, follow these steps:
   a. Get a clear mental picture of the present situation that is causing the stress in your life. Write or draw it on a piece of paper.
   b. Get a good picture of the situation as you would like it to be, making sure it is a picture you can achieve on your own. Once a realistic picture is clear in your mind, write or draw it on paper.
   c. Prepare a detailed, sequential plan to get from your present situation to your ideal situation.
3. Use time management techniques to carry out your plan:
   a. Define the ideal outcome so it is crystal clear in your mind.
   b. List the main subtasks in sequential order—what must be done first, second, and so on.
   c. Under each subtask, identify what resources (people and materials) you will need; what skills (new and old) you should have; what proof you will insist upon to know that each subtask is complete; what may block your action at each subtask; and how to get around those blocks.
   d. Identify activities that must be ongoing through the period of change.

ACTIVITY
To Relieve Frustration

To relieve frustration, it must be expressed in some way that brings insight. The following suggestions may be helpful.

1. Express your frustration by talking with someone else or by writing your thoughts down on paper.
2. Find new alternatives to the frustrated goal.
3. Keep a journal of frustrating experiences.
4. Examine personal beliefs that may be producing frustration.
   a. Ask yourself, "What would a person have to believe to become frustrated in such a situation?" Examine some possible answers to your question. The objective is to listen to your answers as you would if a friend were talking. How realistic are you to believe what you believe, and how is that thinking holding you back? The statements below are examples of personal beliefs that might cause you to feel frustration.
      ▪ I must not change my beliefs, attitudes, or actions, because they have gotten me this far in life.

- I will be seen as an inferior person unless I do well and win the approval of others.
- I cannot exist without sincere and constant love and approval from everyone in my life.
- I must be able to do at least one thing with complete competence.
- Justice, fairness, and equality must prevail or life is unbearable.
- I must not experience or show negative emotions because they make me perform poorly and others don't like them.
- I should get what I want, when I want it, regardless of what others think or do.
- Others must not criticize me unjustly.
- Others will treat me the way I think I should be treated.

b. After identifying the belief upon which the frustration is based, turn the belief around so it becomes positive. Make a positive statement. An example for the statement, "Others must not criticize me unjustly" might be: "Others may criticize me unjustly, but that's because they're generally critical people who don't know how to relate in any other way. It's their problem, not mine. I did a good job."

that your feelings of overload are being brought on by a person, negotiate with that person to reduce the load or the deadline. Learn to say what you want and how you feel. For example:

- When you feel that someone is imposing more work or responsibility on you than you think is appropriate at the time, tell the person that the timing is inappropriate.
- If you do not wish to do a task, say "no."
- Ask for help from those around you. Sit down and look at your load objectively in relation to others around you.

4. Determine your optimal stress level (the point at which stress increases health and performance).

5. If you are working under a deadline (the most obvious form of time overload), control much of this stress by effective time management. When the task seems too formidable, use the model for time management in FYI 1 to set priorities and schedule tasks into a workable, efficient order.

Break down a large task into its smallest workable parts, and treat each as a separate task with its own deadlines and requirements. As each small task is finished, add it to the others until the large task is completed. As an

ACTIVITY
To Alleviate Overload

You suffer from overload when faced with excessive demands to the point at which your stress response is aroused. Overload is a function of four major factors:

1. Time pressures
2. Excessive responsibility or accountability
3. Lack of support
4. Excessive expectations of yourself and by others

Consider the following techniques for alleviating the stress of overload.

1. Practice time management and set priorities.
2. Keep a journal of events that are overwhelming.
3. Avoid overcommitments. Learn to say "no." Learn to negotiate. If you perceive

FYI

A Model for Time Management

Time management involves matching the best combination of time demands with your supply of available time. The following steps provide a means of achieving that goal.

TIME DEMANDS

1. List all of the tasks that have to be completed within the given time interval. (For example, on Monday consider what things have to be done during the coming week.)
2. Estimate how much time will be needed to complete *each* task.
3. Go back and increase each of the time estimates in step 2 by 10% to 15%. This will provide some cushion for error or for unexpected problems.

TIME SUPPLY

4. Look at your calendar for the week. Identify the blocks of time available *each* day for completing the necessary tasks.
5. Match the tasks with the available time blocks in such a way as to make use of available time most constructively.
6. Many times you will find that there simply is not enough time available to complete all of the tasks. Therefore, you must *prioritize* the tasks. List the tasks in order of their importance so the most important tasks will be completed. If extra time is available, go on to other, less important tasks.

example, consider a 50-page report or term paper. Writing 50 pages may seem to be a formidable task. When the paper is reduced to its parts, however, each part may be only 5 pages, a much more manageable task.

6. Delegate responsibility. Learn to ask for support.
7. Examine your personal beliefs regarding expectations of yourself and others.
   a. What you expect from others is a good reflection of what you expect from yourself. If others cannot please you with their performance, you probably cannot please yourself with your performance. Some of the negative beliefs that may arise here are:
      - Work is not done until it is done perfectly.
      - I always must perform at 90% effectiveness, creativity, and intellectual excellence or I will be considered sloppy.
      - Others cannot do the job as well as I can.
      - If you want it done right, you have to do it yourself.
      - The world has no room for a person who performs at less than maximum effort all the time.
   b. After identifying the belief upon which the frustration is based, turn the belief around so it becomes positive. Make a positive statement for each belief. An example for the statement, "Work is not done until it is done perfectly" might be: "Perfect is relative to each person in each situation. If I always try to do my best work within the constraints of the situation, I'll be satisfied."

ACTIVITY
To Counteract Deprivation

Deprivation can be particularly frustrating because it is difficult to conceive solutions and inertia sets in. The following ideas have worked for people who are frustrated by deprivation.

1. Keep a journal of your feelings. Writing down feelings about loneliness, boredom, or lack of involvement helps alleviate deprivational stress in two ways:
   a. It is an active process that also may include creativity.
   b. Expressing negative emotions helps to release them.
2. Plan activities. YMCAs offer activities for small fees. Also available are spas and health clubs,

although these are usually more expensive. Most colleges have a physical education department and campus recreation. Collect catalogs or call these establishments to compile a list of possible activities. Choose one or two that you always have wanted to do. Join a social group. Obtain information on support groups, single-parent groups, play-reading groups and so forth. Your community may have a formal listing of social support groups available in the area. If you have a special interest but no established group exists, start a group by placing a notice in your apartment building or dorm, or run an advertisement in the local paper.

3. Learn to ask for human contact. This requires learning assertiveness skills (discussed under suggestions for gaining self-esteem).
4. Examine beliefs that keep you isolated or bored. What would a person have to believe to remain unhappily in that situation? Possible negative beliefs are:
   - I don't deserve the company of fun and interesting people.
   - I can't disclose who I am to others or they won't like me.
   - People will only hurt me and take advantage of me.
   - It takes too much effort to make friends.
   - I'm perfectly happy being by myself.

ACTIVITY
To Control Environmental Stress

Environmental stressors are those external to yourself. You will be surprised to find how many you can avoid or control.

1. Practice assertiveness skills when someone is invading your space with their noise. Limit your exposure to noisemakers and consider using earphones to listen to music to avoid invading the space of others.
2. Regulate your diet as discussed earlier, and avoid stimulants.
3. Try to live and travel in accordance with your natural rhythms. When you are tired, rest. Fatigue promotes incompetent coping.
4. Minimize exposure to pollutants that reduce immune system efficiency.

ACTIVITY
To Enhance Poor Self-Esteem

Everyone can work toward a more positive self-concept. Low self-esteem is a result of negative beliefs about oneself, negative self-talk, which fuels the negative beliefs, and the way life experiences are perceived. Enhancing the self-concept requires breaking the negative spiral. The following techniques present a number of levels of possible change.

1. List your resources. On paper, write all the resources you have in your life. You are alive and have attained a certain number of years. What do you have going for you that has helped you get to where you are now? In listing resources, include:

   a. Physical, material resources such as income, clothing, housing, money

   b. Social support resources such as family, friends, teachers, counselors

   c. Internal resources such as empathy, tenacity, sense of humor, honesty, good friend to others, and so on

   Once you have listed as many items as possible in each category, write each resource on a 3" × 5" card and place a new card on the top of the deck each day. Upon reading the daily resource, repeat several times to yourself or aloud that you possess this quality or resource. Merely reading the words on a card is not enough to enhance how you feel about yourself; you also must internalize the resource and accompany it with a positive feeling.

2. Make affirmations. **Affirmations** are statements confirming that you already have what you envision having. They are written in the first person, present tense. They are positive statements accompanied with positive feelings.

   a. Clearly get in mind what you want. For example: "I want to weigh 140 pounds."

   b. See yourself clearly in the situation, having obtained what you want (as in item a). If you cannot see yourself having completely attained your goal, drop back to a point where you can see yourself. Work forward from there.

   c. Experience the good feeling of having accomplished what you want.

   d. Make a meaningful statement regarding the accomplishment of getting what you want:

   It's easy for me to _____.

   I enjoy having _____.

   I'm becoming more and more _____.

   These statements should focus on the characteristic or quality you want ("I enjoy being self-confident"), not the ability to get there (e.g., "I can become self-confident"). They should be as specific as possible; an affirmation of "I'm losing weight easily and quickly" can be stated more specifically, "I'm reaching my goal of 140 pounds easily and quickly." Inserting action words such as "easily" and "quickly" creates movement from the present situation to the affirmed situation. Words that trigger feelings also are helpful (e.g., joyously, excitedly, lovingly).

   e. Write affirmations for all aspects of your life—physical, social, emotional, spiritual, occupational, intellectual—so you will have a well-rounded life.

   f. Say your affirmations at least once a day, but preferably two, three, or more times throughout the day. Times typically committed to affirmations are upon rising and before going to sleep. Other likely times are when waiting for appointments, while driving, or scheduled times at work, home, or school.

3. Use positive self-talk. Negative self-talk perpetuates negative feelings about yourself and also continues to affirm negative self-beliefs.

   a. Monitor yourself for one day and write down all the words and phrases you say to yourself that are negative. Enlist the help of others around you by having them identify statements they hear you say about yourself.

   b. For each negative phrase you have identified over the period of a day, write a positive follow-up. For example, a negative phrase might be: "You big dummy." Follow it with, ". . . but I like you anyway."

   c. After this exercise, each time you hear yourself saying something negative about yourself, add something positive.

   d. After mastering c (above), each time you begin to say something negative about yourself, substitute a positive statement; don't even bother to say the negative statement.

4. Give and accept compliments.

   a. Practice giving compliments to others, and study how others accept them. Do they just say, "Thank you," or do they add a statement of humility? Make your compliments sincere by commenting on something you really like. Begin with your friends, then expand to others in your work or study space, sales clerks, service people, and so on.

   b. Begin to accept compliments by responding with a smile and a "thank you." Make no follow-up statement unless it is a positive confirmation of the compliment (e.g., "Thank you; I really like it, too").

5. Become more assertive.

   a. Verbal assertiveness means saying what you like or dislike about someone or something without being degrading. It is getting what you want, but not at the expense of someone else's self-esteem. Some people confuse assertiveness with aggressiveness. Aggressive communication is demanding, bossy, patronizing, or demeaning, insisting that someone obey your wishes. It is an act of verbal pushing and shoving, with no consideration for the other person's self-esteem. When the other person does not comply or agree, the aggressor insists that he or she is "dumb" or "stupid" or "crazy" for not agreeing. When people respond to a situation aggressively they should expect counteraggression, alienation, and defensiveness from the other person. Communication is virtually blocked, and all who are involved come away from the situation feeling anxious, angry, and misunderstood.

b. At the opposite end of the scale from aggression is nonassertive or passive behavior. Many have learned from childhood to be passive placaters who do not ask for what they want. Their mode of operation is to manipulate. They sit back wishing that someone would notice their needs and fulfill them; or they set up subtle and roundabout ways of getting what they want. Manipulators use guilt and blame to get others to do what they want. They control others with "shoulds, oughts, and ifs." Nonassertiveness is related highly to low self-concept.

c. In becoming more assertive, know your rights to:
- Say no and not feel guilty.
- Change your mind.
- Take your time in planning your answer or action.
- Ask for instructions or directions.
- Demand respect.
- Do less than you possibly can.
- Ask for what you want.
- Experience and express your feelings.
- Feel good about yourself, no matter what.

Assertiveness training involves operationalizing these rights.

6. Examine your negative beliefs. As discussed in some of the other categories, negative beliefs are the basis for negative feelings and behaviors. What are the core self-concept beliefs upon which you conduct your life? Some possible beliefs that may stem from early childhood are:
- I'm an unlovable person.
- I do things so poorly that nobody could like me.

- No matter how hard I try, things always turn out badly.
- Nobody likes me, so why should I try?
- I'm unworthy of others' love and attention.

When you treat yourself in an unloving way or behave in a way that deprecates yourself, ask, "What must a person believe to behave in such a self-deprecating way?" Then turn the belief around to a positive statement, and repeat it whenever you notice you are being unkind to yourself.

The beliefs that are the basis of your relationship with yourself also are the foundation for your beliefs about other people. This knowledge can be used to your advantage by changing your attitudes toward others to become more accepting, compassionate, and loving. As you release judgment toward others, you may release judgment toward yourself. A simple affirmation about others, such as "People do the best they can with what they have at any given time," allows one to let others be where they are without having to judge their actions. A statement like this doesn't mean others cannot grow and learn other ways of doing things; it merely says they are doing the best they can. That affirmation can be extended to the self in stressful times: "I'm doing the best I can with what I have right now."

ACTIVITY
To Counteract Time-Urgency, Anger, and Hostility

Changing harmful Type A traits that have built up over time will require a lot of effort and will take time, but it is possible. The following suggestions have been applied successfully.

1. Use time management. Review the time management process described under "overload."

2. Set goals and alternative goals to avoid rushing into tasks without having adequately planned for them.

3. Practice concentration. Try concentrating completely on one task, finishing it, and then going on to the next.

a. Read material that makes you concentrate—something with difficult concepts rather than simple ones.

b. When working on one plan and another pops into your mind, say "Stop it," and go back to the original plan.

c. Practice meditation, detailed visualization, progressive muscle relaxation, or other relaxation training techniques (discussed later in the chapter) in which you must focus on one thing at a time.

d. If a good idea about something else pops up in the middle of the project, jot it down and go back immediately to the original project.

4. Practice thought-stopping. Reduce negative self-talk using the techniques presented in the "self-concept" category, above, and in item 3, on concentration.

5. Practice anger management.

   a. Keep an anger diary for one week. On a 3" × 5" index card for each incident, jot down what precipitated the anger; how you re-acted; how you felt before, during, and after the anger incident; what you expected from others in the situation; why you think others acted the way they did; your self-talk before, during, and after the incident; and how long the self-talk lasted.

   b. Write a list of coping self-talk statements. Under the headings (1) Before the incident, (2) When physiologically aroused, (3) During the encounter, and (4) After the encounter, write four or five statements each that you can use to help you stay calm during that time.

   c. Use a relaxation technique that works for you (discussed later in the chapter) and, while relaxed, go over in your mind the inci-dent you have chosen. As you play through it, insert an appropriate positive coping state-ment at the four points outlined in b. Review the incident using the coping statements.

   d. When you can re-live this incident with no feelings of anger, choose the next least stress-ful situation from your diary, and repeat the procedure, using your positive coping self-statements.

   e. When you can re-live old incidents without anger, transfer the technique to future poten-tial anger situations in your life.

6. Examine your ego involvement. You know the ego is involved when you ask yourself, "What will someone else think of me if I fail? . . . if I don't do what they want?. . . if the project I'm completing isn't on time?" Ego involvement often is based upon rewards from the system or from one specific person rather than completing the job for the internal reward of a job well done.

7. Examine your beliefs regarding anger, expecta-tions, and perfection. An underlying cause of anger is not getting what we expect, so reducing the incidence of anger involves examining our beliefs about expectations. Typical expectations are based upon beliefs such as:

   ▪ I know how to do it best and quickest.

   ▪ If it's not done my way, it's done wrong.

   ▪ If you can't do it quickly and well, get out of the way.

   ▪ If I do everything "by the book," I'll be rewarded and live happily ever after.

   ▪ If I hurry, I'll get everything done.

After an episode of anger, review your thoughts and behavior. What must you believe to think and behave that way? Upon identifying an irrational or negative belief behind the anger, change it to a positive one such as, "People each have their own way of doing things that are right for them."

ACTIVITY
To Deal with Anxiety

Several techniques have been developed to deal specifically with excess anxiety. Among them are the following.

1. Try **thought-stopping.** This is a technique whereby the stressed person intentionally breaks the anxiety cycle by abruptly leaving the obses-sional thoughts.

   You may be thinking about a situation, such as being worried about not completing an assignment, and jump ahead in your mind to a confrontation. You make your excuse to your professor, he gives his response, and so on. This story will probably never play itself out for a mil-lion reasons. Just *stop* yourself. Return to the here and now. Remember the body does not know the difference between real and imagined stress. A fearful person spends (wastes) a lot of time in these types of unnecessary and stress-inducing daydreams.

2. Write a "fear history." The anxious reactor is typified by fear. To learn more about yourself and how you respond in an anxious manner to stressful situations, write your history of fear. As a child, how did you react when you were fright-ened? How did your parents react when they were fearful? Did you seem to learn the fear reaction from a specific incident?

   Choose an anxious situation from your childhood, and identify the basis of that anxiety. It may have been a realistic reaction for you as a child, but is it still a realistic response now that you are an adult and have more knowledge and experience?

3. Take action. Fear constricts. The opposite of constriction is expansion or movement. When anxiety strikes, make an immediate plan of action so you change the old patterned response to fear. An example is the person lying in bed

who hears a noise outside the window. An anxious reactor may become terrified and paralyzed in bed. Making this situation nonstressful calls for getting up immediately, turning on the lights, and looking for the source of the noise. If the source is found not to be harmful, laughter and a pleasant "good night" to the source can end the incident. If the source is not found, an affirmation of "there's nothing here to be afraid of" can end the incident. If the source is found to be harmful, taking action to correct the situation is the best path to follow.

4. Give away fear.

   a. Write a lengthy, scary letter to yourself about your fear. Make it as fearful as possible. Catastrophize; think of the worst possible situation. Put it away for a day.

   b. Come back the next day and make the letter even worse than it was. Follow the fearful feelings as deeply as you can. Again put it away for a day.

   c. Come back the third day with a red pen or pencil and begin identifying the parts of your letter that have no rational basis.

   d. After identifying which parts of your fear may be rational and which parts are not, release all the unrealistic, unfounded fear that you have put into the letter by burning it in a ceremonial manner.

   e. Take action regarding the fear that is real.

5. Examine your beliefs regarding fear. What are your beliefs about what others can do to you? About your own strength and ability to maintain your security? What is the basis of your beliefs? Change the beliefs to positive statements, and begin to affirm that you are always safe and secure. Nothing can harm you.

ACTIVITY
To Gain Control

Feeling that one has no control over one's life is a root cause of mental/emotional distress. The following may be helpful in gaining a sense of more control.

1. Keep a journal. Whenever you are frustrated at not being able to control all the things and people around you, or you feel that parts of your life are out of control, write your experiences in a journal. Expressing your feeling about the situation in itself will help alleviate stress.

2. Do a calming breathing exercise. When your body is in a state of stress arousal, you are likely to interpret the symptoms as a sign that you are losing control. One way you might begin to

exert more control over your environment is to regain control over your body first. (This exercise is presented in the discussion of Breathing Exercises later in the chapter.)

3. Conduct a reality check. With the reality check, as adapted from Kriegel and Kriegel, when life seems out of control, take the following steps:

   a. Measure in numbers the difficulty of the situation. Get specific. If you cannot assess the difficulty in a number, give it quantitative ratings on a scale of 1 to 10. This causes the mind to think rationally instead of in terms of feelings.

   b. Rate your ability to solve the problem. Have you ever done this or something like it before? How did you do? What resources do you have that helped in the past? What new resources have you developed since that time that would help in this situation?

   c. Examine the consequences. What is the worst thing that could happen? What is the real likelihood (probability) of that actually happening? Rate this on a scale of 1 to 10.

   d. Release the irrational. Develop an action plan for the rational.

4. Let go of judgments. Acknowledge the right of each person to perform in his or her personal manner without judgment from others. If you can internalize the idea that you are the only one responsible for your life, you must extend that to others around you. One person cannot make others do what they do not wish to do. Moreover, one individual does not have the right to manipulate the lives of others. The simple technique here is to say to yourself whenever you begin to judge others, "They're doing the best they can for themselves at this time."

5. Examine your beliefs regarding the need to control others. The less we trust ourselves, the more we try to control others. As in the other discussions regarding beliefs in this chapter, people with a need to control the people and events around them must look at the irrational or negative belief system that is driving them. Some possibilities may be:

   ▪ Everything will fall apart if I don't keep control.

   ▪ The only way people will need me is if I'm in control.

   ▪ No one who is not as bright or as talented as I am has the right to be in control.

   ▪ If I don't control others, they will try to control me.

   ▪ Power is control.

Turn negative or irrational beliefs into positive beliefs and continue to affirm these beliefs by using them as the basis for noncontrolling behavior.

QUIETING YOUR INTERNAL ENVIRONMENT

Generalized relaxation training can be used as a basic intervention technique itself or be used to quiet the body and the mind in preparation for other, more specific interventions. Physically, the body responds to emotions in a variety of ways. Incoming information received by the brain alerts the *subconscious* appraisal pathway. This pathway prepares the body for any potential physical action that might be needed. The *overt* action or outward responses are conscious and occur only after the brain processes and evaluates the situation. Thus, the stress response (physical arousal) can be elicited by conscious, voluntary action or by subconscious, involuntary (autonomic) activation that keeps the body in a state of readiness. The constant state of readiness to respond with the fight-or-flight reaction when such a response is unwarranted is called *emotional reactivity*. If the body remains in this state a long time, the organ systems become fatigued and may malfunction.

Stress and tension responses, anxiety, and illness are a few indicators of the inner workings of the mind and body. Relaxation training can help reduce emotional reactivity. Relaxation training promotes voluntary and autonomic control over some central nervous system activities associated with arousal and promotes a quiet sense of control that eventually influences attitudes, perception, and behavior. Relaxation training fosters interaction with your inner self, and you learn by feeling (visceral learning) that your thinking influences your body processes and your body processes influence your thoughts. You come to know your feelings and emotions as part of your immediate thinking experience. When you have learned to stay in the present, to direct your focus on what is happening right now, and spend less time in needless worry and fantasy, you become more peaceful. Emotional responses become good end points upon which to concentrate healing efforts.

Throughout the day, each new stressful situation leaves a residual amount of tension in the body, the accumulation of which results in an inability to dissipate all the residual tension. The longer you practice relaxation exercises, the more you dissipate your residual tension and increase your general state of relaxation. Gradually, the relaxed state becomes a stable part of your personality. Relaxation activities are designed to quiet your internal environment and reduce stimulation of the nervous system. In addition,

they can reduce sensory stimulation, produce a relaxation response, and then condition that response. The benefits of relaxation activities include:

1. Decreasing body stimulation
2. Producing a calming or relaxation response
3. Conditioning the relaxation response
4. Learning to focus your concentration on one thing at a time
5. Helping separate what is real from what is not real in your life
6. Quieting the internal chatter produced by feeling guilty about the past or worrying about the future

Some representative techniques are discussed in the following pages. These are:

breathing exercises
muscle relaxation, including yoga
visual imagery
biofeedback
physical exercise
meditation

Breathing Exercises

A physiological relationship seems to exist between the brain centers that control respiration and the centers that control general nervousness or reactivity. From the ancient yogis to recent researchers, one basic recommendation for calming the body has been to use a breathing technique involving **diaphragmatic breathing.** A stressed person breathes differently than a relaxed person. The breathing of a person who is stressed is shallow and rapid, whereas a person who is relaxed breathes deeply, as though from the abdomen. In diaphragmatic breathing you actually can feel the abdomen move in and out when you breathe. Simply sitting down for a few minutes several times a day and controlling your breathing teaches your body to respond in a relaxing manner. If you breathe like a relaxed person, you will *be* more relaxed, at least for a short time.

During the course of an average day, many of us find ourselves in anxiety-producing situations. The heart rate increases. The stomach may become upset. Thoughts may race uncontrollably through the mind. During these episodes, we require fast-acting relief from our stressful reactions. The brief exercise described next has been effective in reducing most of the stress reaction we get during acute exposure to stressors. It is a quick way to calm down in the face of a stressful situation. The basic mechanism for stress reduction in this exercise involves deep breathing.

Step 1. Assume a comfortable position. Rest your left hand (palm down) over your navel. Now place your right hand so it rests comfortably on your left. Your eyes should remain open.

Step 2. Imagine a hollow bottle or pouch inside your body, beneath your hands. Begin to inhale. As you do, imagine that the air is entering through your nose and descending to fill that internal pouch. Your hands will rise as you fill the pouch of air. As you continue to inhale, imagine the pouch being filled to the top with air. Your rib cage and upper chest will continue the rise that began at your navel. Make the total length of your inhalation 3 seconds for the first week or so, then lengthen the inhalations to 4 or 5 seconds.

Step 3. Hold your breath. Keep the air inside the pouch. Repeat to yourself, "My body is calm."

Step 4. Slowly begin to exhale, to empty the pouch. As you do, repeat to yourself, "My body is quiet." As you exhale, you will feel your chest and then abdomen fall.

Repeat this four-step exercise four or five times in succession. If you begin to feel lightheaded, stop at that point. If lightheadedness remains a problem, consider shortening the length of the inhalation or decreasing the total number of repetitions of this exercise, or both.

Practice this exercise 5 to 10 times a day. Make it a habit in the morning, afternoon, and evening, as well as during stressful situations. After a week or two of practice, you may want to omit Step 1, the purpose of which is to teach the technique only. Because this form of relaxation is a skill, it must be practiced. Regular, consistent practice will lead to a calmer and more relaxed attitude—a sort of anti-stress attitude—and when you do have stressful moments, they will be far less severe.

Another exercise to promote relaxation and increase your power of concentration is *breath counting*. You may do this sitting or lying down. As before, you will use quiet, normal, diaphragmatic breathing. Concentrate on your breathing. As you breathe in, think "in." Let the air out and think "out." Think, "In . . . out . . . in . . . out." As you breathe out, count each breath. Count the consecutive breaths without missing a count. If you happen to miss one, start over. When you get to 10, start at 1 again. Do this 10 times as you sit quietly. Concentrate, anticipate the breath, and block all other thoughts from your mind.

Muscle Relaxation, Including Hatha Yoga

Most experts in the area of relaxation believe that reducing excess muscle tension not only reduces total body tension and anxiety directly but also helps eliminate the psychological forerunner of the muscle tension indirectly. We know that a person cannot relax the mind or concentrate fully if the brain is being bombarded by muscle tension impulses. Whether reducing muscle tension is an end in itself or a means to an end, it is an essential step in relaxation. Much of the harmful, stress-producing muscle tension is extremely subtle and difficult to detect. If you are thinking defensive thoughts, you start to assume a defensive posture. To think of an action and not have your muscles prepare for the potential action is next to impossible. A tense individual who is defensive and who is imagining action constantly creates a situation in which the body becomes efficient at being tense and adapts by maintaining a chronic state of muscle tension.

If the condition is permitted to exist for an extended time, it may produce or exaggerate a wide variety of physical disorders. A few of the more common of these are tension headaches, muscle cramps and spasms (such as writer's cramp), limitation of range of movement and flexibility, susceptibility to muscle injuries such as tears and sprains, insomnia, and a wide variety of gastrointestinal maladies (constipation, diarrhea, colitis), kidney problems, and dysmenorrhea (irregular menstrual periods). The muscular system is involved in every body process and in every expression of emotion.

Neuromuscular relaxation training trains both the muscles and the nervous system components that control muscle activity. The objective is to reduce the tension in the muscles. Because the muscles make up such a large portion of body mass, muscle relaxation leads to a significant reduction in total body tension as well. Literally hundreds of relaxation techniques have been devised, and almost every relaxation program includes some form of muscular relaxation. The basic objective is to teach the individual to relax the muscles at will by first developing a thinking-feeling awareness of what being relaxed feels like. If you are able to differentiate tension and relaxation, control over tension will follow easily. To accomplish this, you must learn to center on the task or problem and control the mind's tendency to wander aimlessly in daydreams.

Strength, flexibility, and reduction of muscle tension are the rewards of hatha yoga, the most popular type of yoga in the Western world. Hatha yoga uses body positions and exercises to promote physical and mental harmony. It also is used as a technique to quiet the body in preparation for quiet mental states. Most yoga practice starts with hatha yoga because it is said to provide the body with the health and endurance needed to learn more advanced forms of yoga. Positive results can be derived from yoga, especially if the exercises are chosen for specific groups of people with specific outcomes in mind.

A C T I V I T Y

RELAXATION TECHNIQUES

RELAXING MUSCLE GROUPS

A. Head
1. Wrinkle your forehead.
2. Squint your eyes tightly.
3. Open your mouth wide.
4. Push your tongue against the roof of your mouth.
5. Clench your jaw tightly.
6. Repeat all of group A in fairly rapid succession.
7. Relax for 5 minutes and periodically say, "Relax and let go."

B. Neck
1. Push your head back into a pillow.
2. Bring your head forward to touch your chest.
3. Roll your head sideways to your right shoulder.
4. Roll your head sideways to your left shoulder.
5. Repeat all of group B in fairly rapid succession.
6. Relax for 5 minutes and periodically say, "Relax and let go."

C. Shoulders
1. Shrug your shoulders up as if to touch your ears.
2. Shrug your right shoulder up as if to touch your ear.
3. Shrug your left shoulder up as if to touch your ear.
4. Repeat all of group C in fairly rapid succession.
5. Relax for 5 minutes and periodically say, "Relax and let go."

D. Arms and hands
1. Hold your arms out and make a fist with each hand.
2. One side at a time: Push your hands down onto a surface.
3. One side at a time: Make a fist, bend your arm at the elbow, tighten up your arm while holding the fist.
4. Repeat all of group D in fairly rapid succession.
5. Relax for 5 minutes and periodically say, "Relax and let go."

E. Chest, lungs, and back
1. Take a deep breath.
2. Tighten your chest muscles.
3. Arch your back.
4. Repeat all of group E in fairly rapid succession.
5. Relax for 5 minutes and periodically say, "Relax and let go."

F. Stomach
1. Tighten your stomach area.
2. Push your stomach area out.
3. Pull your stomach area in.
4. Repeat all of group F in fairly rapid succession.
5. Relax for 5 minutes and periodically say, "Relax and let go."

G. Hips, legs, and feet
1. Tighten your hips.
2. Lying down, push your heels into the floor.
3. Tighten your leg muscles below the knee.
4. Curl your toes under as if to touch the bottom of your feet.
5. Repeat all of group G in fairly rapid succession.
6. Relax for 5 minutes and periodically say, "Relax and let go."

VISUAL IMAGERY

The visual imagery technique involves using *self-directed mental images of relaxed states.* This simple method centers on conditioned patterns of responses that become associated with specific thoughts. Recall a moment when you allowed your mind to run away, and imagine the worst-case scenario of a potentially threatening event. You may have been worried about not completing a term paper or losing your job, or perhaps you were having problems with a friend or mate. Your muscles feel tense, you have a sinking feeling in your stomach, and the hair may rise on the back of your neck. This represents a conditioned physiological response to that memory. The opposite effect also can be generated, producing an equally dramatic but very different physiological response. Imagining yourself in your favorite relaxation spot, perhaps sitting on a quiet beach with the sun warming your body or fishing in your favorite stream, elicits a relaxation response.

Used as a technique for general relaxation, visual imagery centers on memory recall of relaxing places, events, and experiences in your life. It is a method in which you talk to your body and tell it to relax. A good, quick technique is the relaxation-recall exercise as follows:

Step 1. In a quiet room and in a comfortable chair, assume a restful position. Create a quiet, passive attitude in your mind. Take four deep breaths, feeling both your ribcage and your stomach expand. Make each one deeper than the one before. Hold the first inhalation 4 seconds, the second one 5 seconds, the third one 6 seconds, and the fourth one 7 seconds. Pull the tension from all parts of your body into your lungs and exhale it with each expiration. Feel more relaxed with each breath.

Step 2. Count backward from 10 to zero. Breathe naturally, and with each exhalation, count one number and feel more relaxed as you approach zero. With each count you descend a relaxation stairway and become more deeply relaxed until you are totally relaxed at zero.

Step 3. In your memory go to a favorite relaxation place. Stay there 5 minutes. Vividly recall the feelings of that place and time that were relaxing.

Step 4. Bring your attention back to yourself. Count from zero to 10. Energize your body. Feel the energy, vitality, and health flow through your system. Feel alert and eager to resume your activities. Open your eyes.

Muscle relaxation exercises can be used for general relaxation or for specific control over a single muscle group. The general relaxation exercises include larger sections of the body musculature or the entire body. Exercises that relieve muscle tension most effectively are the ones that contract the muscles fully and then allow full relaxation. The basic technique is:

1. Tense each muscle group separately.
2. As you apply tension, take a deep breath.
3. Hold the tension about 5 seconds.
4. Release the tension slowly as you breathe out while saying silently, "Relax and let go."
5. Relax 30 seconds and repeat to yourself silently, "Relax and let go."
6. Practice this sequence with each muscle group.

Techniques for exercising specific muscle groups are given in the "Relaxation Techniques" activity.

To get your money's worth from vacations and special moments, use them in your visualizations. Emotions and illness are related to your thoughts, so if you replace negative thoughts with positive ones, you can reduce the emotional risk factors related to illness.

Biofeedback

The underlying principle of **biofeedback** is awareness of body function, which is the first and most important criteria for changing stress-causing behavior. In a biofeedback session small electrodes may be attached to the muscle you wish to relax. Electrical impulses from the muscle are transferred through a wire to an instrument that emits a beep for every impulse. The greater the frequency of beeps, the more tense the muscle. Therefore, a person can learn to sense even the most minute change in muscle tension.

Using a similar procedure, one can become attuned to changes in skin temperature, which demonstrate blood flow changes to a specific region of the body. As you can tell, biofeedback magnifies subtle body changes, making them more noticeable. After only a few training sessions, a person usually can learn to feel the changes without the instrument.

Biofeedback can be used as an educational tool that provides information about behavior or performance in much the same way as a bathroom scale gives information about the success of weight gain or reduction efforts. If we learn to feel, our bodies will tell us a lot about their functioning. Likewise, monitoring brainwaves can tell us much about states of consciousness and information processing, which can aid in the voluntary control of consciousness. The possibilities are as numerous as the body systems that can be measured.

In another sense, biofeedback is much more than just a self-monitoring system. It can be used to promote self-exploration, self-awareness, and self-control. Relaxation and tranquillity condition the tone of the nervous system to be less reactive, and gradually you begin to change behavior by becoming a more tranquil person. This process disciplines the mind to reduce the constant internal "chatter," allowing for better concentration in solving problems and often leading to insights and creativity. What started out as an exercise in relaxation quickly turns into a development of self-awareness and self-control.

Physical Exercise

As discussed in Chapter 11, the fight-or-flight response to stress has helped ensure human survival. In fact, no amount of relaxation training can diminish the intensity of this innate reflex. Stress is physical, intended to make possible a physical response to both physical and symbolic threats. Once the stimulation of the event penetrates the psychological defenses, the body prepares for action. The increased hormonal secretion, energy supply, and cardiovascular activity associated with the fight-or-flight response also signify a state of stress, a state of extreme readiness to act as soon as the voluntary control centers of the brain decide what action to take.

Usually the threat is not physical. It holds only symbolic significance. Our lives are not in danger, only our egos. Physical action is not warranted and must be subdued, but for the body organs it is too late. What took only minutes to start will take hours to undo. The stress products are flowing through the body and will activate various organs until these byproducts are reabsorbed into storage or used by the body gradually. While this gradual process is taking place, the body organs suffer.

One solution is to use the physical stress arousal for its intended purpose: physical movement. The increased energy intended for fight or flight can be used instead to run or swim or ride a bike. In this way one can accelerate dissipation of the stress products, and if the activity is vigorous enough, it can cause the body to rebound after exercise into a state of deep relaxation.

Although we often assume recreation is relaxation, they are not necessarily the same. In fact, for most people they usually are not the same because recreation can be stressful, especially if it is competitive. Even though the stress of exercise usually is absorbed by the exercise, the stress of competition often sets in motion thoughts and feelings that linger. These thoughts may even become the stimulus for prolonged emotional arousal with the rehash of missed points, social embarrassment, and self-doubt. Ideally then, exercise to reduce stress should be devoid of ego involvement. Though strenuous, it should be a time of peace and of the harmonious interaction of mind and body. In that sense, it may be the most natural of stress reduction techniques.

Hans Selye is one of many sage advisors who has said that you cannot be stressed and laugh at the same time. If we turn that around and assume that if you are laughing and having fun, you cannot be stressed, we also can assume that having fun and playing are good stress-reduction techniques. That sounds simple enough, but recreation isn't always what it seems. We go on vacations, belong to clubs, play tennis, handball, and golf. We spend a lot of time pursuing recreation. But recreation and relaxing play can be vastly different.

Play is the spontaneous expression of our naturalness and the guru of the right brain. Playfulness denotes spontaneity, self-confidence, joy, being attuned to life, the ability to be focused and immersed or to be in flow, forgetting time and responsibilities; it is the ability to obtain pleasure, to be silly, and to see and experience the less serious side of life. In contrast, imposed structure and organized games frequently block play. Whenever we are told how to play, whom to play with, and how long to play, our naturally playful responses are blocked. Structure implies right and wrong ways of doing things, which heightens the possibility of making mistakes and makes work out of play.

Meditation

Descended from ancient yoga and Zen Buddhism, modern meditative practices represent a mixture of philosophies and techniques. Regardless of their ancestry, all the meditative techniques have two common goals: a quiet body and a quiet mind. A primary goal of meditation is to reduce the surface chatter of the mind. Reduced surface chatter means reduced anxiety. This in turn reduces general arousal, and the mind can achieve the peace and quiet natural to an ego- or self-transcendent state of consciousness.

Meditation reduces the activity of most physical systems and at the same time enables the meditator to be in complete control over emotions, feelings, and memories. Although meditation involves a passive state of mind, it is an active process

that takes thought, preparation, and practice. It is a skill that teaches us to let go of the past, let go of the future, and just "be." Meditation disciplines the mind to tune out the tensions and pressures from others and from ourselves. It tunes us in to our own centeredness, the very basis of our physical, mental, emotional, and spiritual health.

The art of meditation is the ability to attain a relaxed, passive state of concentration while maintaining alertness and control. In the meditative state one is aware of subtle thoughts, energy, and creative intelligence. The meditator is left with a feeling of creativity and accomplishment.

You can form the habit of meditating more easily if you write it into your daily schedule. For this reason, in the early learning stages, you may want to meditate at the same time each day. Try to avoid meditating on a full stomach or when you are very sleepy. If these are the only times you have,

A C T I V I T Y
CONCENTRATION EXERCISES

The following activities will help in the concentration portion of your meditation.

1. Count each exhale while doing deep yogic (diaphragmatic, or very deep) breathing, as explained earlier. Count up to 20 and back down to zero. If you lose count, start again, concentrating only on the breath, not on your ability to count. It doesn't matter if you lose count. Merely begin again.

2. Repeat a word, an idea, or a phrase that depicts peace, beauty, or a spiritual ideal for you. "Om"—a Sanskrit word meaning "one" or "I am one, we are one"—is the universal mantra. More than just spoken, it is chanted softly aloud on each exhalation ("aaaaaaooooooommmmm") at your own pitch and tonality. Group meditation using "Om" as the collective mantra is soothing.

3. Use a visual focus, rather than sound. A candle flame, a picture that produces serenity for you, or a mandala* may be a good eyes-open focus. Whatever visual you use, be sure it does not offer your brain's left hemisphere food for thought, or it will be busy analyzing, planning, evaluating. The circle with a dot in the center, the equilateral triangle with the tip at the top, and the square have been used for centuries as aids to meditation. Some meditators use visual imagery (eyes closed) as their concentrative focus.

*A mandala is a simple geometric pattern used for meditation because the left hemisphere of the brain tires quickly of the simple pattern while the rest of your mind continues to focus on it.

however, meditating is better than passing it up. Sitting in a comfortable chair with arms or in a cross-legged position rather than reclining keeps the spine straight and helps keep you awake. If you'd rather recline during meditation, bend your arm at the elbow with your hand straight up in the air. If you fall asleep, your forearm will fall and awaken you.

During the free-fall period of meditation (step 4 below), when you are open to whatever comes into your mind, you may feel dizzy or nauseous because of the energy flow. Holding the index finger to the thumb may help shut down some of that energy flow.

The process of meditation entails the following steps:

1. Quiet your external environment. Put the telephone ringer to the "off" position. Play some soft classical or other soothing instrumental music (use earphones if you want).

2. Sit with your spine straight, hands folded on your lap, take some deep breaths, and relax your muscles.

3. Spend 10–30 minutes in a concentrative exercise to clear the mind (some examples are given next). Still the active left hemisphere of the brain, and direct your energy.

4. Open your palms and spend 10 minutes in "neutral," a period of not controlling or focusing your thoughts. Flow with whatever you may feel. Stay calm and relaxed with interest. Touch whatever comes to you and let it go.

5. Wiggle around and let the energy flow throughout your body.

6. Get up and go on with your other activities.

PRESCRIPTION FOR STRESS MANAGEMENT

The exercises outlined in this chapter can be learned easily and, when perfected, represent a solid beginning to managing stress. An excellent review of techniques can be found in the book *Principles and Practices of Stress Management.* Now, to get started:

1. Reread Chapter 11 for a better understanding of what stress is and how it can harm your health, decrease your performance, and reduce your happiness.

2. Make a list of your stress-related symptoms, both physical and emotional.

3. Go back to your stress profiles (in Chapter 11) and identify the stressors to which you seem most vulnerable.

4. Plan a program to reduce your stressors and eradicate your negative stress-related symptoms. This will involve:

   a. Establishing desired outcomes. Be specific (for example, deciding to stop biting your fingernails).

   b. Calling upon specific stress-reduction techniques, such as those introduced here.

   c. Matching techniques to your specific needs.

   d. Developing a plan of action complete with practice schedules.

   e. Writing a contract with yourself to include evidence of, and rewards for, success.

5. Carry out the program, including monitoring for progress, changing any program that is not working, evaluating success, and rewarding yourself.

SUMMARY

Three basic steps are required in a stress management program:

1. Quieting the external environment by eliminating or reducing external stressors.

2. Quieting the internal environment (mind "chatter") to reduce stimulation of the nervous system.

3. Conditioning the mind to eliminate thoughts that are stressful.

Specific techniques for reducing externally caused frustration include keeping a journal, changing behavior patterns that invite stress, working on self-concept (including assertiveness training), stopping negative beliefs, and setting positive goals, among others.

Among the tools for quieting the internal environment and quieting the mind are breathing exercises, muscle relaxation exercises, visual imagery, biofeedback, physical exercise, and meditation. The connection between mind and body is clear. Therefore, managing stress requires activities that apply physical and mental/emotional tenets in tandem.

CHOICES IN ACTION

If you have completed Lab 33 (associated with Chapter 11), you have determined the people or types of events that are stressful for you. Lab 34, "Planning a Stress Management Program," helps you determine ways you can cope with your stress.

REFERENCES

Budzynski, T. H., and Peffer, K. 1980. "Biofeed-back Training." In *Handbook on Stress and Anxiety*, edited by I. L. Kutash and L. B. Schlesinger. San Francisco: Jossey Bass.

Carrington, P. 1984. "Modern Forms of Meditation." In *Principles and Practice of Stress Management*, edited by R. Woolfolk and P. M. Lehrer. New York: Guilford Press.

Everly, G. S., and Girdano, D. A. 1980. *The Stress Mess Solution*. Englewood Cliffs, NJ: Prentice Hall.

Gawain, S. 1986. *Living in the Light*. Mill Valley, CA: Whatever Publishing.

Girdano, D. A. 1981. *Better Late Than Never: How to Avoid a Midlife Fitness Crisis*. Englewood Cliffs, NJ: Prentice Hall.

Girdano, D. A., and Dusek, D. 1988. *Changing Health Behavior*. Scottsdale, AZ: Gorsuch Scarisbrick.

Girdano, D. A., Everly, G. S., and Dusek, D. 1996. *Controlling Stress and Tension: A Holistic Approach*, 5th edition. Englewood Cliffs, NJ: Prentice Hall.

Kriegel, R., and Kriegel, M. 1984. *The C Zone: Peak Performance Under Pressure*. New York: Doubleday.

Lehrer, P. M., Woolfolk, R., Rooney, A., McCann, B., and Carrington, P. 1983. "Progressive Relaxation and Meditation: A Study of Psycho-Physiological and Therapeutic Differences Between the Two Techniques." *Behavior Research and Therapy* 21.

Mobily, K. 1982. "Using Physical Activity and Recreation to Cope with Stress and Anxiety: A Review." *American Corrective Therapy Journal* May-June.

Selye, H. 1974. *Stress Without Distress* New York: Signet.

Stoya, J. 1983. "Guidelines for Cultivating General Relaxation: Biofeedback and Autogenic Training Combined." In *Biofeedback: Principles and Practice for Clinicians*, edited by J. V. Basmajian. Baltimore: Williams and Wilkins.

Woolfolk, R., and Lehrer, P. M. 1993. *Principles and Practice of Stress Management*. New York: Guilford Press.

Woolfolk, R. L., Lehrer, R., McCann, B., and Rooney, A. 1982. "The Effects of Progressive Relaxation and Meditation on Cognitive and Somatic Manifestations of Daily Stress." *Behavior Research and Therapy* 20.

Your Self—
Your Choice

✔ Are you experiencing "quality living"?

✔ How healthy are you in each aspect of your life?

✔ How much effort are you making to become all you can be?

✔ What are your goals for each dimension of your life, and what must you do to reach them?

✔ What can you do now to get started?

13

This chapter is for you to write. It is about you: How you are right now, how you would like to be, and what you can do to start becoming the person you want to be. In Chapters 1 and 3 you learned what comprises and what jeopardizes quality living. In Chapter 2 you learned about a process that can help you decide how you want to be and determine how to pursue your goal. In Chapters 4–12 you actually began that process by learning about behaviors that contribute to high-level functioning in all dimensions of life, and you learned how to engage in these behaviors safely and effectively.

To *really* evaluate your status regarding quality living, however, you need to bring all of your knowledge and assessment data together in one "big picture." The forms and exercises in this chapter will help you accomplish this. (Labs 35–39 offer duplicate copies of the forms, for your convenience.)

ASSESSING YOUR CURRENT FUNCTIONAL STATUS

In Lab 1, you had the opportunity to estimate your functional status. Now you have more information on which to base your assessment. Use Form 13.1, the Functional Status Worksheet, to assess your current functional level in each dimension of life. This worksheet provides a checklist of criteria that reflect healthy functioning in each dimension of life, as defined in Chapter 1. For your convenience, the definitions are restated here:

Physical health: The ability to carry out daily tasks with energy remaining for unforeseen circumstances; biological integrity.
Emotional health: The ability to control emotions and express them appropriately and comfortably.
Social health: The ability to interact well with people and the environment; having satisfying interpersonal relationships.
Mental health: The ability to learn, including intellectual capabilities.
Spiritual health: The belief in some unifying force such as nature, scientific laws, or a godlike entity.

ASSESSING YOUR CURRENT EFFORTS

Because *how* you are living your life and your goals, plans, and progress—what you are "becoming"—are also part of experiencing quality living, your "big picture" is not complete until you have indicated your *efforts* to develop your capacities in each dimension of life. Begin by reviewing the lifestyle circle described in Chapter 1 and the personal lifestyle circle you developed for yourself in Lab 2.

Your new lifestyle circle will help you determine how balanced your efforts currently are to develop each dimension of your life—to live a *wellness lifestyle*. It will help you identify those dimensions of your life in which a greater effort might result in higher levels of functioning and more satisfaction in living. Or your lifestyle circle might show that you *are* doing the best you can, even though your functional status might not reflect it because of illness or some other type of limitation, *or* simply because of the delay that sometimes exists between efforts and results, such as when you try to lose weight, lower blood cholesterol levels, or increase fitness.

Use Form 13.2, the Lifestyle Worksheet, to determine your current effort level or lifestyle. FYI 1 provides examples of efforts that comprise a wellness lifestyle.

List the efforts you have made during the last week to develop your capacity in each dimension of life. After completing your "effort list" for each dimension, use a scale of 0 to 10 to rate the intensity of your efforts, with 0 representing no effort and 10 representing your best effort. Use these numbers to shade in the lifestyle circle in Form 13.2. (You may find it helpful to refer back to Figure 1.5 in Chapter 1, which gives examples of lifestyle circles.)

EVALUATING YOUR CURRENT FUNCTIONAL STATUS AND EFFORTS

After completing the Functional Status Worksheet and your Lifestyle Circle, evaluate what your assessments indicate. Does your personal worksheet describe you as functioning in each dimension at a level with which you are satisfied? Is your health status where you would like it to be? Does your lifestyle circle indicate that you are operating at as high a level of effort as you're able to? Are your efforts balanced among the dimensions?

If your answer is "yes" to all of these questions, you are to be congratulated; you undoubtedly are experiencing a high level of quality living. Many if not most of us, however, are not satisfied with our status in one or more areas. We know we could expend more effort at developing ourselves. Nonetheless, we would like to be somehow magically transformed and not have to struggle through the changes that would enable us to improve our functional status. Unfortunately, there is no magic.

FORM
13.1 Functional Status Worksheet.

Directions: This checklist is designed to assist you in assessing your functional status in each of the five dimensions of life. Criteria to consider in determining your status are offered for each dimension, and extra lines are provided for you to add your own criteria, if desired. Circle the number that best describes your current level of functioning for each criterion listed, using the following scale:

0 = Don't know   1 = Low level of functioning   2 = Average functioning
3 = Above-average functioning   4 = High level of functioning

For example, if your muscular strength/endurance is above average, circle the 3 for that category. If your cholesterol level is well within safe limits, circle the 4 for that category (if you have a dangerously high cholesterol level, you would circle 1, indicating a low level of functional status for that category).

Dimension	Criteria to Consider	Current Functional Status				
		Don't Know	Low	Average	Above-Average	High
PHYSICAL	Overall fitness level	0	1	2	3	4
	Cardiorespiratory fitness	0	1	2	3	4
	Muscular strength/endurance	0	1	2	3	4
	Body composition (% fat)	0	1	2	3	4
	Body chemistry profile:					
	Total cholesterol	0	1	2	3	4
	HDL	0	1	2	3	4
	LDL	0	1	2	3	4
	Glucose level	0	1	2	3	4
	Iron intake	0	1	2	3	4
	Heart function:					
	Heart rate	0	1	2	3	4
	Blood pressure	0	1	2	3	4
	Daily rest/relaxation	0	1	2	3	4
	Energy level	0	1	2	3	4
	Recommended nutritional intake:					
	Cholesterol	0	1	2	3	4
	Complex carbohydrates	0	1	2	3	4
	Protein	0	1	2	3	4
	Sodium	0	1	2	3	4
	Calcium	0	1	2	3	4
	Total fat	0	1	2	3	4
	Saturated	0	1	2	3	4
	Unsaturated	0	1	2	3	4
	Fiber	0	1	2	3	4
	Other criteria (specify)					
	_____	0	1	2	3	4
	_____	0	1	2	3	4
EMOTIONAL	Self-esteem:	0	1	2	3	4
	Positive self-talk	0	1	2	3	4
	Self-confidence	0	1	2	3	4
	Self-image	0	1	2	3	4
	Body image	0	1	2	3	4
	Honest expression of emotions	0	1	2	3	4
	Appropriate expression of feelings/desires	0	1	2	3	4
	Other criteria (specify)					
	_____	0	1	2	3	4
	_____	0	1	2	3	4

(continued)

FORM
13.1 Continued.

Dimension	Criteria to Consider	Current Functional Status				
		Don't Know	Low	Average	Above-Average	High
SOCIAL	Stress level	0	1	2	3	4
	Interpersonal relationships:					
	Comfort level with others	0	1	2	3	4
	Number of close friends	0	1	2	3	4
	Satisfying intimate relationships	0	1	2	3	4
	Enjoy interactions with other people	0	1	2	3	4
	Engage in a variety of activities	0	1	2	3	4
	Other criteria (specify)					
	_____	0	1	2	3	4
	_____	0	1	2	3	4
MENTAL	Informed/aware regarding:					
	World events	0	1	2	3	4
	National events	0	1	2	3	4
	Local events	0	1	2	3	4
	Technical information for job	0	1	2	3	4
	Personal growth issues	0	1	2	3	4
	Intellectual abilities:					
	Quick to learn	0	1	2	3	4
	Perceptive	0	1	2	3	4
	Analytical	0	1	2	3	4
	Performance:					
	Quality	0	1	2	3	4
	Productivity	0	1	2	3	4
	Creativity	0	1	2	3	4
	GPA or job evaluations	0	1	2	3	4
	Other criteria (specify)					
	_____	0	1	2	3	4
	_____	0	1	2	3	4
SPIRITUAL	Personal life philosophy:					
	Well-defined ideas about					
	meaning/purpose of life/death	0	1	2	3	4
	Feel at peace with self/life	0	1	2	3	4
	Positive outlook on life	0	1	2	3	4
	Strong identity with self/values	0	1	2	3	4
	Other criteria (specify)					
	_____	0	1	2	3	4
	_____	0	1	2	3	4

(continued)

FORM
13.1   Continued.

CONCLUSION

Tally the number of "Don't Know's," "Low's," & "Avg-High" function ratings you gave yourself in each dimension of your life.

DIMENSION TALLIES	TOTAL # OF ITEMS RATED	DON'T KNOW (#) OF 0's	LOW (#) OF 1's	AVE-HIGH (#) OF 2's, 3's & 4's
Physical	_____	_____	_____	_____
Emotional	_____	_____	_____	_____
Social	_____	_____	_____	_____
Mental	_____	_____	_____	_____
Spiritual	_____	_____	_____	_____

What conclusions can you make regarding your current functional capacity in each dimension?

Physical _____

_____

_____

_____

Emotional _____

_____

_____

_____

Social _____

_____

_____

_____

Mental _____

_____

_____

_____

Spiritual _____

_____

_____

_____

FORM

13.2 **Lifestyle Worksheet.**

1. List your efforts (deliberate choices) during the last week to develop your capabilities in each dimension of your life:

   Physical   *Emotional*   *Social*   *Mental*   *Spiritual*

2. Level of Effort

   Estimate your overall level of effort in each dimension using a scale of 0 (no effort) to 10 (best effort).

   _____   _____   _____   _____   _____

   Physical   *Emotional*   *Social*   *Mental*   *Spiritual*

3. Using the numbers from #2, shade in your effort levels on the Lifestyle Circle. This will allow you to actually *see* how you are living now. (Figure 1.5 in Chapter 1 shows examples of shaded lifestyle circles.)

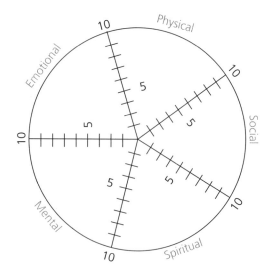

Examples of Efforts Comprising a Wellness Lifestyle

PHYSICAL DIMENSION

Efforts to be physically fit:
- Regular aerobic exercise
- Regular strength and flexibility exercise
- Adequate rest
- Maintaining appropriate weight and lean body mass

Efforts to eat well:
- Low-fat/high-carbohydrate diet/high fiber
- Variety of nutritious foods
- Meeting RDA standards
- Following U.S. Dietary Goals

Efforts to protect self from physical hazards:
- Avoiding ingestion, abuse of, and exposure to harmful substances including cigarette smoke, pollution, drugs, radiation.
- Observing safety precautions such as wearing seat belts, not drinking and driving, wearing appropriate clothing for the weather, keeping any equipment in good repair.

EMOTIONAL DIMENSION

Efforts to promote/maintain self-esteem:
- Acknowledging your personal qualities and accomplishments
- Establishing reasonable expectations of self (stress management)
- Seeking companionship with people who care for and about you
- Expressing feelings honestly

Efforts to control and express emotions appropriately:
- Being assertive but not aggressive
- Listening as well as telling
- Expressing desire without demanding
- Loving without possessing

SOCIAL DIMENSION

Efforts to manage stress:
- Saying "no" if already overburdened
- Planning time for self
- Delegating responsibilities
- Making a daily plan
- Developing interests and engaging in a variety of activities

Efforts to establish satisfying interpersonal relationships:
- Acknowledging and respecting the concerns and feelings of others
- Caring about and helping others
- Identifying others you enjoy doing things with
- Taking time to learn/care about another on an intimate basis

MENTAL DIMENSION

Efforts to expand knowledge/awareness:
- Reading/listening to news and talking with others about local, national, and world concerns
- Reading and taking classes/seminars to gain technical information for job or personal growth and life management skills

Efforts to be self-reliant and productive:
- Using skills and knowledge to be creative and perform capably on job and in personal life

SPIRITUAL DIMENSION

Efforts to develop personal philosophy:
- Reading, talking with others, taking classes regarding established approaches to life philosophy, as from science, religion, philosophy
- Trying out various philosophical/religious options
- Identifying personal beliefs and feelings about life

There are only small steps, which, if arranged appropriately so they fit into a meaningful sequence, can lead to larger steps and eventually to large and permanent changes. Nothing is static. Everything is in process. You are who you are now only at this moment, and you can choose in the next moment to launch yourself in a new direction.

DECIDING HOW YOU WANT TO BE

The next step is to *decide* whether your current functional status and effort levels are where you want them to be. Using Form 13.3, the Long-

Term Goal Worksheet, record the goals you wish to fulfill in each area of your life. Be as specific as you can. Reviewing the Functional Status Worksheet you used earlier in this chapter will help you recall specific weaknesses and strengths. If you are satisfied with your current efforts and functional status in a given dimension, simply indicate that in the appropriate column.

Once you have completed this worksheet, you have, in effect, listed your *long-term goals* for becoming the "you" you want to be. Chances are your list of goals to be accomplished may seem rather overwhelming. To turn "overwhelming" into "achievable," prioritize the goals in each dimension in terms of their importance to your

FORM

13.3 Long-Term Goal Worksheet: How I Would Like to Be.

Directions: First review your completed Functional Status Worksheet. Then, for each dimension of life, indicate how you would like to be as compared to what your Functional Status Worksheet indicates. Use the worksheet to help you be specific. If you are satisfied with your current status in any dimension, place a checkmark in the designated column. Finally, rank the goals in each dimension in terms of their importance to your overall health and well-being. Use #1 for the most important goal; #2 for next most important, and so on.

GOALS

Dimension of Life	I would like to be:	Importance ranking	I am how I want to be
Physical	_____	_____	_____
	_____	_____	
	_____	_____	
	_____	_____	
	_____	_____	
Emotional	_____	_____	_____
	_____	_____	
	_____	_____	
	_____	_____	
	_____	_____	
Social	_____	_____	_____
	_____	_____	
	_____	_____	
	_____	_____	
	_____	_____	
Mental	_____	_____	_____
	_____	_____	
	_____	_____	
	_____	_____	
Spiritual	_____	_____	_____
	_____	_____	
	_____	_____	
	_____	_____	
	_____	_____	

overall health and well-being. Your #1 long-term goal in each dimension then will be your focus in planning how to *start* becoming the person you want to be.

FORMULATING SHORT-TERM GOALS

Having identified your most important goal in each dimension, the next step is to break down that goal into smaller, short-term goals or actions you believe you can actually achieve. The Short-Term Goal Worksheet (Form 13.4) is designed to help you do this.

Focusing only on your #1 goal in each dimension, make a list of possible actions you could take to start becoming more like your goal describes you. Each action on your list must be stated as specifically as possible in measurable or observable behaviors. For example, "I will walk 30 minutes, three times per week" can be observed and

---

FORM

13.4   Short-Term Goal Worksheet: The Small Steps to Success.

Directions: For each dimension, first list your #1 long-term goal (from Long-Term Goal Worksheet), and then list *specific actions* you think you could do now to start achieving your #1 goal. State your short-term goals in a way that allows you to measure or record your progress. Finally, rank your goals according to their importance to your health and well-being and indicate your readiness to start doing the specified action *now* by circling "yes" or "no."

PHYSICAL DIMENSION

#1 Long-Term Goal _____

_____

Short-Term Goals	*Importance ranking*	*Readiness*	
1. _____	_____	yes	no
_____			
2. _____	_____	yes	no
_____			
3. _____	_____	yes	no
_____			
4. _____	_____	yes	no
_____			

EMOTIONAL DIMENSION

#1 Long-Term Goal _____

_____

Short-Term Goals	*Importance ranking*	*Readiness*	
1. _____	_____	yes	no
_____			
2. _____	_____	yes	no
_____			
3. _____	_____	yes	no
_____			
4. _____	_____	yes	no
_____			

(continued)

FORM
13.4 Continued.

SOCIAL DIMENSION

#1 Long-Term Goal _____

_____

Short-Term Goals	Importance ranking	Readiness	
1. _____	_____	yes	no
2. _____	_____	yes	no
3. _____	_____	yes	no
4. _____	_____	yes	no

MENTAL DIMENSION

#1 Long-Term Goal _____

_____

Short-Term Goals	Importance ranking	Readiness	
1. _____	_____	yes	no
2. _____	_____	yes	no
3. _____	_____	yes	no
4. _____	_____	yes	no

SPIRITUAL DIMENSION

#1 Long-Term Goal _____

_____

Short-Term Goals	Importance ranking	Readiness	
1. _____	_____	yes	no
2. _____	_____	yes	no
3. _____	_____	yes	no
4. _____	_____	yes	no

recorded precisely. "I'll start doing some exercise" is too vague; you haven't said how much "some exercise" is or even what "exercise" means. Similarly, "I can eat a piece of fruit instead of my usual afternoon candy bar" is sufficiently specific to be measurable, but "I want to eat better" is not.

Use what you've learned in this book to help you formulate your list of short-term goals. The preceding chapters offer many recommendations regarding what you can do to improve your health and well-being and how you can do it safely and effectively. These suggestions range from simply gathering more information (through behavior diaries or talking with others who have made changes in their lives, for example) to actually attempting a behavior change (such as substituting 10 minutes of deep breathing at times when you usually snack, hungry or not). More than likely, your short-term goals will include a similar range of possible actions because considering and attempting are the first two steps in the behavior change process (see the illustrations in the book's Introduction). If you already have achieved your ideal functional status in any one dimension, your list of short-term goals will consist of the actions you need to take to *maintain* your capacities.

When you have finished the action list for each of your priority long-term goals, you will have created an array of possible steps you might undertake in the process of becoming how you want to be. The next step is to prioritize these short-term goals according to their importance to your health and well-being *and* your readiness to do them. The instructions for doing this are given on the Short-Term Goal Worksheet (Form 13.4).

If many of the goals you are most ready to attempt are also ranked as most important to you, you are at a somewhat advanced stage of the "consideration process" of behavior change. Probably you have been thinking about trying a different behavior for some time; perhaps you have even attempted it once or twice. If, on the other hand, the actions you are most ready to attempt are not the goals you rated as most important, you may simply be at an earlier point in the "consideration process," or perhaps some of your short-term goals need to be stated in smaller steps to become "accomplishable." You also may find that the action for which you *do* feel ready is actually a step *toward* your important goals, even if it is not the most direct step. Whatever the case, make your top priority the action you are most ready to take at this point in time. It is the step with which you are most likely to succeed, and accomplishing one change may give you the confidence and incentive to try another, perhaps your most important one.

TAKING ACTION: MAKING A CONTRACT WITH YOURSELF

At this point you have identified at least one long-term goal and one short-term goal you feel ready to pursue in each dimension of your life. Though you could succeed at making all of these changes at the same time, successful change is more likely if you use the *one-step-at-a-time* approach. Thus, to give yourself the best chance to succeed, select just one dimension of your life to work on for the moment. Use the same criteria to prioritize the dimensions as you used for prioritizing and selecting goals within each dimension—that is, prioritize according to the importance of that aspect to your health and well-being and according to your readiness to try the action specified.

Once you have identified that dimension of your life most important to you right now, it is time to take action. As suggested in Chapter 2, making a contract with yourself is one of the best ways to do this because it helps you plan for all the things that seem to increase your chances for success. A good contract form asks you to specify exactly what you will do and when, how you will avoid potential pitfalls, who will be your support person or group, how you will reward yourself, and when you will evaluate and revise your action plan. An example of a completed contract form such as the one just described was shown and discussed in detail in Chapter 2, Figure 2.4.

Your contract form is provided on the following page. Filling it out can be your key to action—action that leads to becoming and being all you can be. Before you close this book and lay it aside, choose to do that for yourself.

Choosing to grow is valuing and honoring your life. It is quality living. It is your choice, your life. Give it your best.

> *Each of us experiences life in our own context, but for all of us there is a struggle to balance the reality of life with our needs and our dreams. Perhaps the most difficult thing of all is to value our life and who we are, and to direct our life in a manner that honors it . . .*
>
> Laurie Harper, *A Taste for Life*

A CONTRACT WITH MYSELF

I, _____, hereby declare that I am ready and willing to commit myself to the following goals and activities. I realize that to achieve my long-term goals, I must be willing to work for small gains, I must seek support, and I must be adequately prepared. Therefore, for the next week I resolve to myself to do the following:

1. Long-term goal(s): _____
   _____

2. Specific goal: During the next week, I plan to: _____
   _____
   _____

3. I will ask my helper to assist me by: _____
   _____
   _____

4. I realize I can easily avoid fulfilling my action plan by: _____
   _____
   _____

5. So I plan to avoid doing this by: _____
   _____
   _____

6. My reward to myself when I fulfill the terms of my action plan each day will be:_____
   _____
   _____

TODAY'S DATE: _____   SIGNATURE: _____

REVIEW DATE: _____   HELPER:_____

7. Action plan evaluation/revision
   a. After working on my action plan for one week, I found that:_____
      _____
      _____
      _____
      _____
      _____

   b. To continue working toward my goal in small steps during the next week, I plan to:
      _____   Follow the same action plan because: _____
                       _____
                       _____
                       _____

      _____   Expand my action plan to include: _____
                       _____
                       _____

      _____   Cut back on my original plan for now because:_____
                       _____
                       _____
                       _____

Source: Adapted from *The American Way of Life Need Not Be Hazardous to Your Health* by James Farquhar. Copyright © 1978 by Stanford Alumni Association.

Exercises to Build a Healthy Back and Neck

The following photographs illustrate flexibility and strengthening exercises that are used to build a healthy back and neck. If done correctly, these exercises are safe for anyone of any age and starting level.

a. Neck Stretch

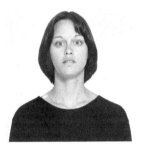 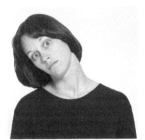 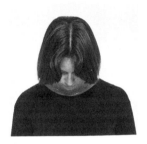 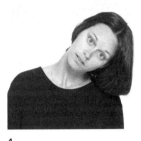

1

Position one: Head erect, eyes looking forward.

2

Position two: Roll head to one side, then return to position one.

3

Position three: Roll head forward, then return to position one.

4

Position four: Roll head to the other side, then return to position one.

b. Lateral Flexion of Neck

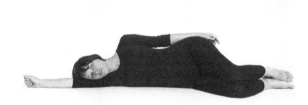 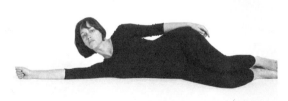

1

Position one: Lying on side, legs comfortably bent, head supported by outstretched bottom arm, top arm resting on hip.

2

Position two: Raise ear to shoulder, hold for two seconds, and return to position one. Repeat on opposite side.

c. Neck Rotation

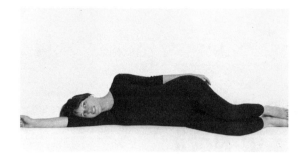

1

Position one: Same position as in exercise b, eyes looking straight ahead.

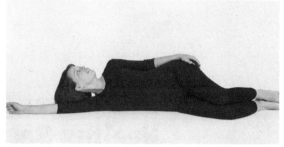

2

Position two: Rotate chin so eyes look up. Repeat on opposite side.

d. Hamstring Stretch

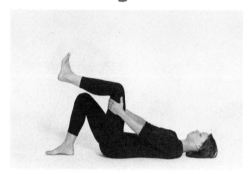

1

Position one: Lying on back, one leg bent with foot on floor, other leg bent at 90° with hips at 90°, support bent leg at thigh with hands.

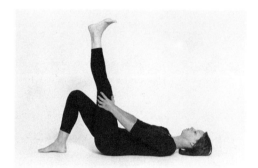

2

Position two: Straighten leg slowly. Return extended leg to starting position. Repeat with other leg.

e. Pelvic Tilt

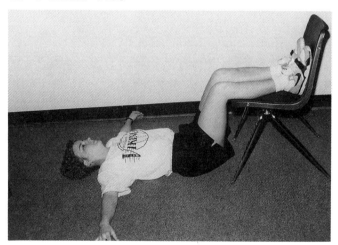

Lying on back with arms stretched to side and legs elevated to chair, flatten small of back onto floor.

f. Knees to Chest

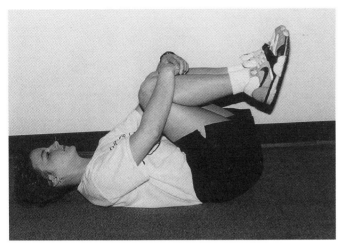

Lying on back, raise both knees toward chest as far as possible and hold knees with arms.

g. Body Curl Extension

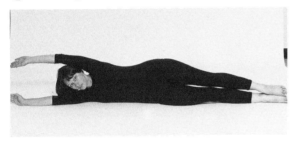

1

Position one: Lying on side, both arms overhead, head neutral.

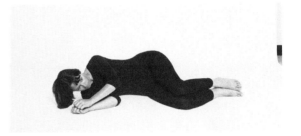

2

Position two: Head, torso, and hips bending toward mid-tuck position.

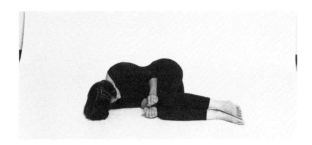

3

Position three: Full-tuck position, then return to position one.

h. Upper Back Stretch

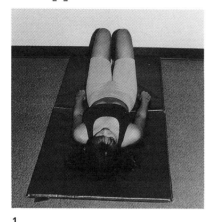

1

Position one: Lying on back, legs bent at knees, arms by side.

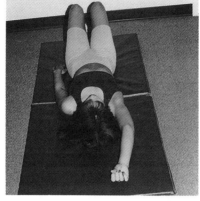

2

Position two: Sweep right arm up right side to above-head position.

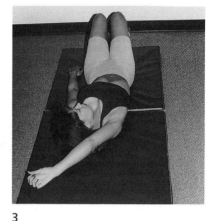

3

Position three: Continue right arm sweep with left lateral bending of trunk to left. Repeat with left arm and lateral bending of trunk to right.

i. Cat Curl

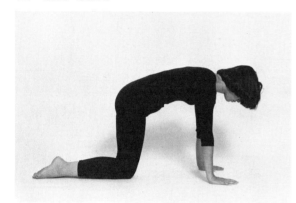

1

Position one: Begin on all fours, knees together, arms extended shoulder-width apart, back and neck rounded, head forward, eyes looking between hands.

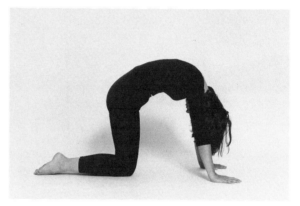

2

Position two: Tighten stomach muscles and arch back, dropping head between elbows.

j. Partial Curl-Up

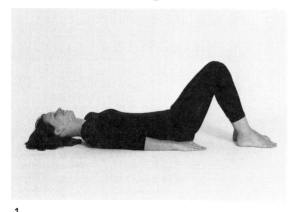

1

Position one: Lying on back, legs bent at knees, feet slightly apart, arms at sides, head on floor.

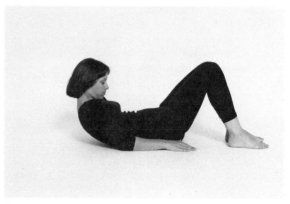

2

Position two: Curl head and trunk forward and upward. Do not raise pelvis off floor.

k. Back Raise

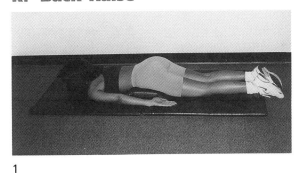

1

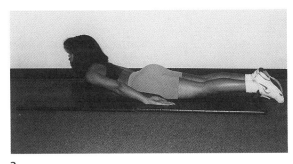

2

Position one: Lying face down, pillow support under pelvis, legs straight and together, arms by sides, palms up, head neutral, chin resting on floor.

Position two: Raise up head and upper back, feet down, hold for 10 seconds.

l. Double Leg Raise

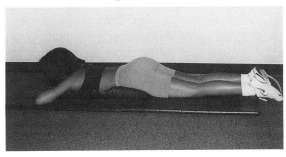

1

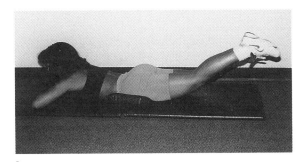

2

Position one: Lying face down, arms folded under chin supporting head, legs relaxed and straight.

Position two: Raise both legs upward and hold for 10 seconds.

Exercises to Avoid

The exercises in Appendix 2 have been associated with chronic pain and the likelihood of developing exercise-related injuries. Although many books and exercise leaders still advocate some or all of these exercises, it would seem prudent to avoid them and substitute the safer flexibility exercises presented in Appendix 3.

a. The *yoga plow* and related exercises (such as vertical bicycling) are particularly dangerous because they can overstretch the cervical region of the spine, possibly resulting in disc injuries. These exercises also can restrict the carotid artery, which supplies blood to the brain.

b. The *hurdler's stretch* and related exercises can lead to overstretching the muscles and ligaments in the groin region, making them more susceptible to a groin pull. In addition, these exercises overstretch the medial collateral ligament, which stabilizes the inner side of the knee. This can lead to instability of the knee. The sciatic nerve also may be stretched, producing back pain.

c. The *deep knee bend* and *duck walk* put great pressure on the lateral meniscus of the knee. (The meniscus is the cartilage within the knee joint on the outer side; it acts as a cushion between upper and lower leg bones.) This can damage the meniscus, resulting in permanent disability or the need for surgery.

d. *Toe-touching* puts excessive stress on one of the main supporting ligaments in the spine and also can put undue stress on the spinal discs, possibly causing them to rupture. These exercises also stretch the sciatic nerve, often leading to back pain. Note also that doing the *Sit-and-Reach* exercise, though safe enough to do as a test occasionally, stretches the posterior longitudinal ligament and elongates the sciatic nerve, which can lead to back pain.

e. For the person untrained in ballet, *ballet stretches* place excessive demands on the hips, knees, ankles, and feet. They overstretch the sciatic nerve and are a common cause of back and leg pain.

f. *Stiff-leg raises* and *double-leg raises*, especially if they are done with added weights on the feet, put excessive stress on the hip flexor muscles. Also, most people cannot do them without arching the lower back. Because this arching strains the structures in the lower back, it should be avoided.

g. *Knee stretches* can cause the range of motion of the knee to be exceeded; they can overstretch the patellar and collateral ligaments of the knee, reducing stability in this region. As the knee is one of the most easily injured joints, these exercises should be avoided as they serve no useful purpose.

h. The *straight-legged* and *hands-behind-the-head* sit-ups are generally recognized to put undue strain on the lower back because of arching. Bending the legs (knees up) into the "hook-lying position" lessens the strain on the sciatic nerve, making the exercise safer. When doing the hands-behind-the-head sit-up, particularly when doing the exercise rapidly, the head and neck are pulled into hyperflexion, stretching the posterior ligaments. A safer form of abdominal exercise is described in Appendix 1, photo (j).

i. *Back-arching exercises*: Activities that cause hyperextension of the lower back are not recommended, as they can stretch or compress the nerves and other support structures in that region, leading to low-back pain.

j. *Neck circling* generally is not recommended because hyperextension of the neck can pinch nerves in that region. The alternate neck stretches shown in Appendix 1, (a), done slowly to the left and right, are safer.

EXERCISES TO AVOID

a. Yoga "Plow" and Variations

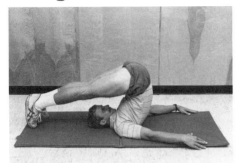 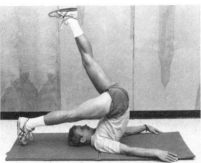 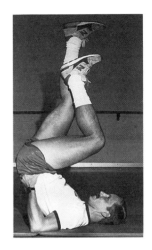

b. Hurdler's Stretch and Related Exercises

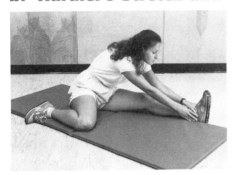 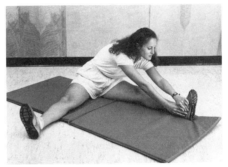 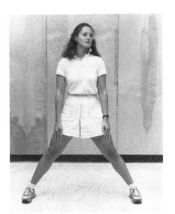

c. Deep Knee Bend and Duck Walk

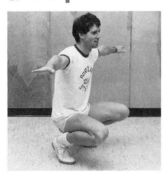 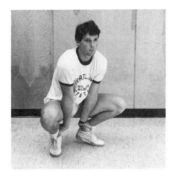

d. Toe-Touching

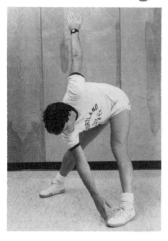
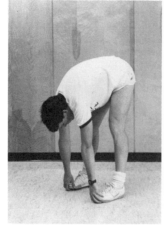
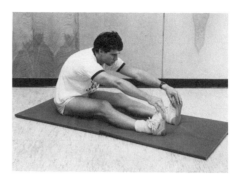

e. Ballet Stretches

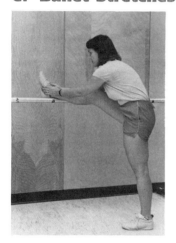

EXERCISES TO AVOID

f. Leg Raises: Stiff   Leg Raises: Double

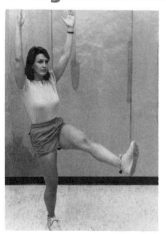
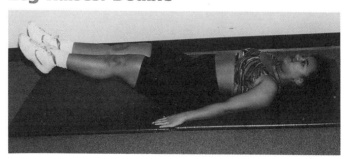

g. Knee stretches

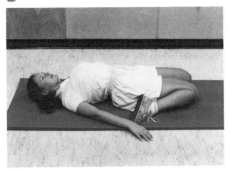
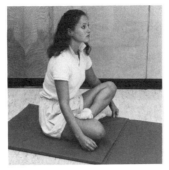
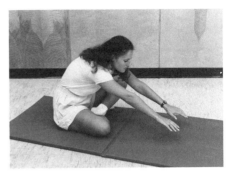

EXERCISES TO AVOID

h. Straight leg sit-ups/sit and reach

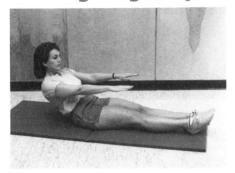

Hands-behind-the-head curl-up

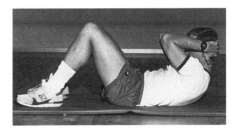

i. Back-arching exercises

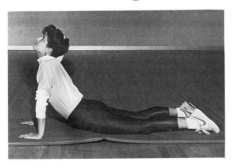
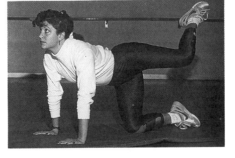

j. Neck circling exercise

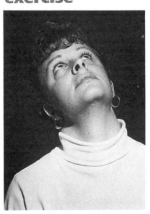

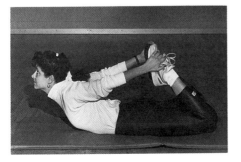
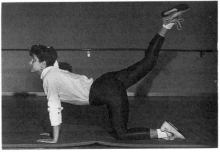

Exercises for Building Strength, Muscle Endurance, and Flexibility

These exercises, used to build strength, muscle endurance, and flexibility, are safe for anyone of any age and starting fitness level.

MILD RESISTIVE EXERCISES

a. Incline Press

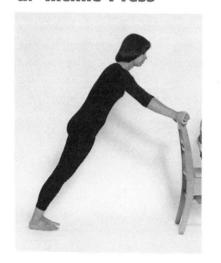 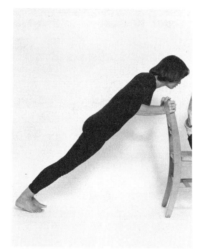

1

Position one: Support the inclined body with the arms, body inclined at a 45° angle.

2

Position two: Keep body straight while bending arms to touch chin to support surface, then return to position one.

b. Shoulder Extension

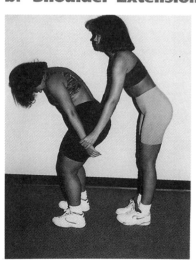 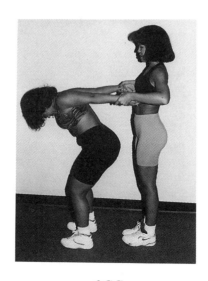

1

Position one: Standing position with legs bent, hips bent, back rounded, arms hanging down. Partner supports wrists from the rear.

2

Position two: Maintaining body position, pull arms slowly to the rear as partner offers partial resistance to the motion.

c. Toe Raise—One Leg

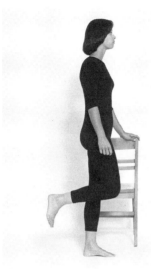

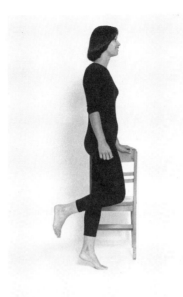

1

Position one: Standing position, weight balanced on one foot, other foot in bent leg position, one hand providing support.

2

Position two: Raise on toes, then return to position one. Repeat with opposite leg.

d. Ski Squat

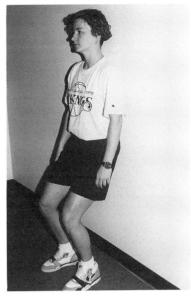

Stand in a partial squat position with hips against support, hips flexed at 45°, feet apart, arms parallel to floor. Hold this position for 30 seconds.

e. Hip Extension

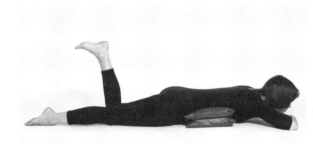

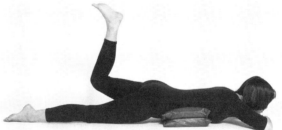

1

Position one: Lying face down, pillow support under stomach, one leg bent at knee at 90° angle, arms folded under chin, body relaxed.

2

Position two: Raise bent leg toward ceiling. Lower and repeat opposite leg.

f. Hip Abduction

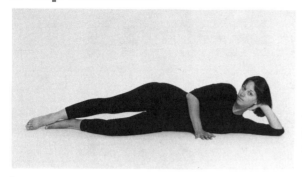

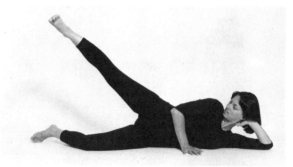

1

Position one: Lying on your side, bottom leg bent for balance, top leg straight, bottom arm supporting head, top arm supporting body.

2

Position two: Elevate top leg to approximately a 45° angle while keeping pelvis forward; ankle position is neutral.

MILD FLEXIBILITY EXERCISES

a. Side Arm Raise

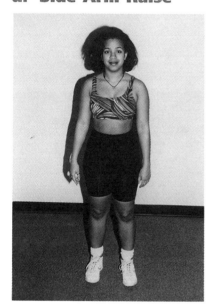

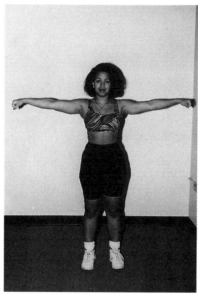

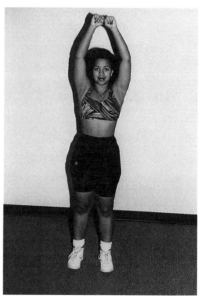

1

Position one: Standing, fists clenched slightly, thumbs forward, body relaxed.

2

Position two: Raise arms to the sides to shoulder level.

3

Position three: Continue to raise arms to the side and up until hands touch. Return to position one.

b. Forward Arm Raise

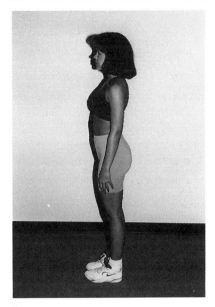 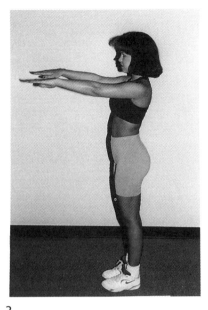 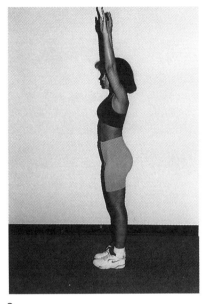

1

Position one: Standing, fists clenched slightly, thumbs forward, body relaxed.

2

Position two: Raise arms forward slowly, level with shoulders.

3

Position three: Continue to raise arms forward and upward to a point above head. Return arms to position one.

c. Back Arm Raise

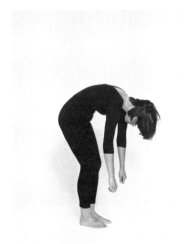 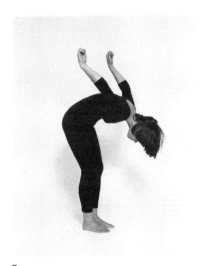

1

Position one: Body bent forward, arms hanging down from shoulders, fists lightly clenched, palms facing backward, bending at hips and knees, back rounded.

2

Position two: Pull arms back.

d. Heel Cord Stretch

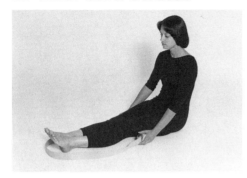

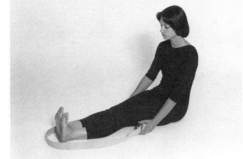

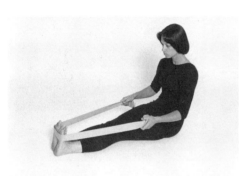

1

Position one: Long-sit position, feet relaxed, strap unattached.

2

Position two: Pull toes back toward shins as far as possible.

3

Position three: Hold previous position, attach strap to balls of feet, and apply additional stretch.

e. Seated Stretch

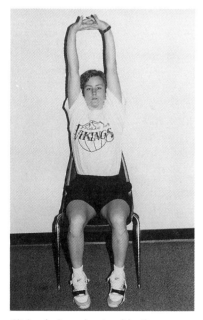

Sit in chair and extend both arms over head fingers grasped lightly.

f. Standing Knee Stretch

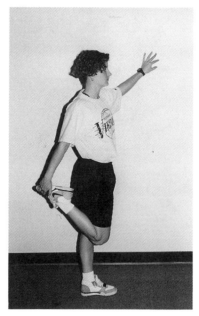

Standing on one leg next to wall, use one arm to aid balance. Bend other leg at knee and grasp with downstretched hand. Use hand pressure to accentuate stretch.

g. Lower Back Stretch

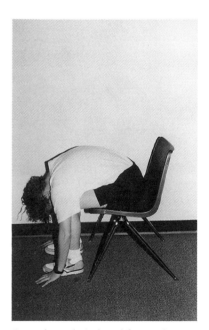

Seated on chair, bend forward at hip and place hands on floor.

h. Back-Lying Hip Stretch

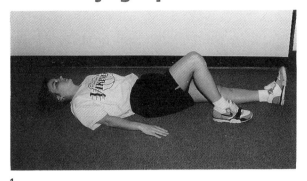 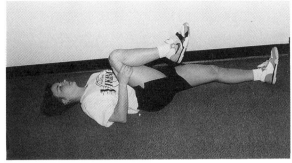

1

Position one: Lying on back with knee bent.

2

Position two: Raise one knee to chest. Repeat with other leg.

DYNAMIC EXERCISES

These exercises should be considered as more rigorous. They are designed for individuals who have the initial fitness to permit doing them without injury. Resistance machines available in many gyms can be used in place of barbells.

a. Dead Lift and Vertical Press

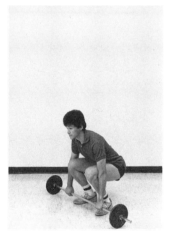 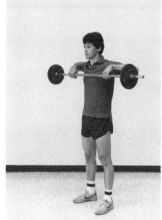 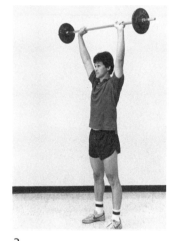

1

Position one: To do this exercise correctly, keep your back straight and hold the bar with an overhand grip.

2

Position two: Lift the barbell to chest level and drop your elbows.

3

Position three: Lift the barbell vertically. Reverse motions to return the barbell to the floor.

This exercise can be used effectively with light weights as a warm-up exercise because it involves many of the major muscle groups of the body.

b. Elbow Curl

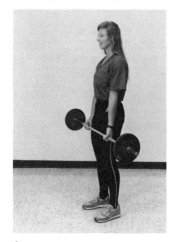

1

Position one: Keep your back straight when doing this exercise. Hold the bar with an underhand grip.

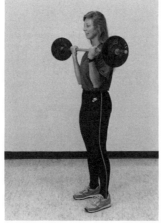

2

Position two: Lift the barbell upward by flexing the elbows, and return to position one.

c. Seated Vertical Press

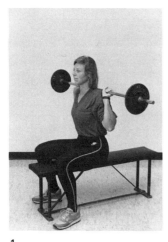

1

Position one: Do this exercise with the barbell placed behind the head as pictured, or in front of the head.

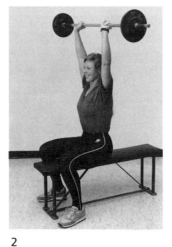

2

Position two: Lift vertically, keeping the back straight, and return. Do not arch the back.

d. Bench Press

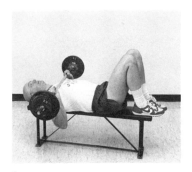

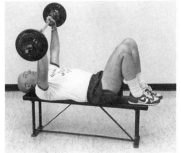

1

Position one: To keep the lower back flat, do this exercise with the knees bent as pictured.

2

Position two: Lift the barbell vertically overhead, and return.

e. Bent-Over Row

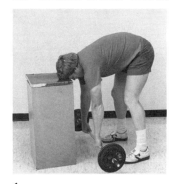

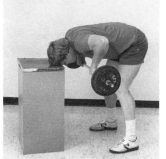

1

Position one: In this exercise support the head as pictured.

2

Position two: Raise barbell to the chest and then lower it.

f. Half Squat

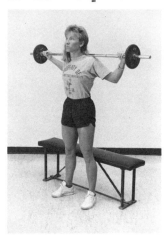

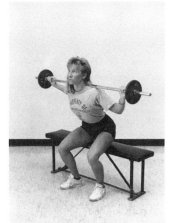

1

Position one: Support barbell on your shoulders.

2

Position two: Squat to a bench and return. Keep your back as straight as possible, and do not bend your knees more than 90°.

g. Heel Raises

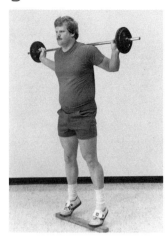

With the barbell supported on your shoulder and your toes placed on a board as pictured, raise your heels as high as you can, and return.

h. Back Extensions

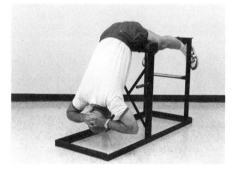

1

Position one: With your feet supported, place your hands behind your head, and bend your trunk at the waist.

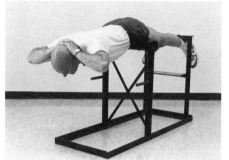

2

Position two: Lift upward until your spine is horizontal, and return. Do not lift above the horizontal plane. Use extra weights behind the head, if desired.

i. Bench Dip

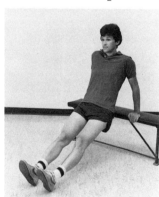

1

Position one: Place your hands on a bench and extend your feet in front of you.

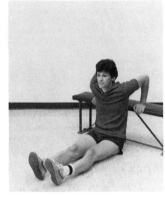

2

Position two: Lower yourself to the floor, and return.

j. Pull-Up

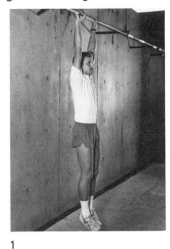 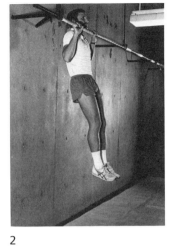

1

Position one: With your
hands placed in the
forward grip, hang
from a bar.

2

Position two: Raise yourself
upward until your chin is
above the bar, and return.
If you are unable to do this
exercise, an assistant can
help you partially by lifting
up on your legs.

k. Reverse Curl

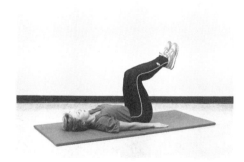 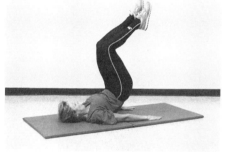

1

Position one: Lie on your back with
arms placed at your sides and with your
legs elevated.

2

Position two: Lift your lower spine
upward as far as you can, and return.

Caloric Expenditure for Selected Physical Activities

The caloric values listed below are estimates of caloric expenditure per minute per pound (or kilogram) for selected activities. The values were formulated based on performing the activity under steady-state conditions. In many instances, however, the estimates are based upon the results of only one individual's activity. This is significant because for some activities (running, for example) research has indicated that (a) caloric expenditure differs from individual to individual and (b) the intensity of the exercise greatly influences the rate of energy expenditure. This is true for virtually every activity (gardening, tennis, sweeping, and so on), although research has demonstrated it for only a few selected activities. Other factors such as fitness, skill, and body composition, to name a few, also influence the rate of energy expenditure profoundly. With these factors in mind, individuals using the following table should recognize that the figures are approximations at best.

In cases where the table presents a range of caloric values for one activity, choose the value that best describes your circumstances. Chapter 7 is devoted to the overall topic of caloric expenditure and its relation to weight management.

Example: for 20 minutes of driving a car to work for a person who weighs 110 lbs (50 kg), the tabled value is .020 cal/min/lb, or

$$[.020][20 \text{ min}][110 \text{ lbs}] = 44 \text{ calories}$$

	CAL/MIN/LB	CAL/MIN/KG
Daily Activities		
Classwork, lecture	.011	.024
Conversing	.012	.026
Driving car	.020	.044
Driving motorcycle	.024	.053
Kneeling	.008	.018
Lying at ease	.008–.010	.018–.022
Making bed	.026	.057
Personal necessities	.013–.023	.029–.051
Resting in bed	.008	.018
Showering	.021	.046
Sitting, eating	.009	.020
Sitting, light activity	.012	.026
Sitting, playing cards	.010	.022
Sitting, reading	.008	.018
Sitting, writing	.012	.026
Sleeping	.008	.018
Squatting	.013	.028
Standing at ease	.009–.013	.020–.029
Standing, light activity	.016	.035
Washing and dressing	.017–.021	.037–.046
Washing and shaving	.019	.042
Domestic Activities		
Bed making/stripping	.031	.068
Carpentry	.026	.057
Chopping wood	.050	.110
Cleaning floor (kneeling and bending)	.032	.070
Cleaning windows	.028	.062
Farming chores	.026	.057
Farming, planting, hoeing, raking	.031	.068

	CAL/MIN/LB	CAL/MIN/KG
Gardening:		
weeding	.035	.077
digging	.062	.136
Hand sewing	.011	.024
House painting	.023	.051
Ironing clothes	.029	.064
Kneading dough	.023	.051
Knitting	.011	.024
Machine sewing	.017	.037
Metal working	.023	.051
Mopping floors	.030	.066
Pick-and-shovel work	.045	.099
Scrubbing (kneeling)	.026	.057
Stirring	.016	.036
Sweeping floors	.024	.053
Truck and automobile repair	.028	.062
Musical Instrument Playing (Standing)		
Bass	.016	.035
Conducting	.018	.040
Trumpet	.014	.031
Musical Instrument Playing (Seated)		
Accordion	.015	.033
Cello	.019	.042
Drums	.030	.066
Flute	.016	.035
Horn	.013	.028
Organ	.024	.053
Piano	.018	.040
Violin	.020	.044
Woodwind	.015	.033

	CAL/MIN/LB	CAL/MIN/KG		CAL/MIN/LB	CAL/MIN/KG
Exercises/Recreational Activities/Sports			Running (treadmill):		
Archery	.034	.075	5.0 mph (12:00 min/mi)	.056	.123
Baseball (except pitcher)	.031	.069	7.0 mph (8:34/mi)	.078–.093	.172–.205
Basketball	.047	.103	8.7 mph (6:54/mi)	.103	.227
Bowling	.044	.098	9.0 mph (6:40/mi)	.111	.244
Calisthenics:			11.60 mph (5:10/mi)	.131	.288
abdominal	.020	.044	cross-country running		
arm swinging, hopping	.043	.095	(speed not specified)	.074	.163
balancing exercises	.016	.035	running on grade (treadmill):		
trunk bending	.023	.051	8.70 mph on 2.5% grade (6:54/mi)	.121	.266
Canoeing:			8.70 mph on 3.8% grade (6:54/mi)	.127	.279
2.5 mph (24:00/mi)	.020	.044	sprinting	.155	.342
4.0 mph (15:00/mi)	.047	.103	Sculling:		
Circuit weight-training:			51 m/min	.028	.062
females	.045	.100	68 m/min	.048	.106
males	.053	.117	87 m/min	.052	.114
Cross-country skiing:			97 m/min	.077	.169
level, hard snow, moderate speed	.054–.127	.119–.279	Snow-shoeing:		
uphill, hard snow, max speed	.125	.274	soft snow, 4 km/hr	.076	.166
Cycling:			Squash	.069	.152
5.5 mph (10:54/mi)	.029	.064	Stairmaster:		
9.4 mph (6:23/mi)	.045	.099	machine workrate:		
13.1 mph (4:35/mi)	.084	.185	level 5	.055	.122
own pace	.045–.068	.099–.150	level 7	.068	.149
Dancing:			level 9	.081	.178
aerobic (low-impact)	.060	.12–.130	level 11	.093	.204
fox trot	.029	.064	Swimming:		
petronella	.031	.068	back crawl (speed unknown)	.077	.169
rumba	.046	.101	backstroke: 25 yd/min	.025	.055
square	.045	.099	30 yd/min	.035	.077
waltz	.034	.075	35 yd/min	.045	.099
Football (American)	.054	.118	40 yd/min	.055	.121
Football (soccer)	.060	.131	breaststroke: 20 yd/min	.032	.070
Golfing	.036	.079	30 yd/min	.048	.106
Gymnastic routines (male):			40 yd/min	.064	.141
free exercise	1.477	3.249	breaststroke (speed unknown)	.074	.163
horizontal bars	2.493	5.485	crawl: 45 yd/min	.058	.128
parallel bars	2.196	4.831	55 yd/min	.071	.156
pommel horse	2.584	5.685	side stroke: 40 yd/min	.055	.121
still rings	1.825	4.015	Tennis	.046	.101
vault	9.480	20.856	Volleyball (recreational)	.023	.051
Hill climbing:			Walking on different surfaces:		
(17.5% grade)			asphalt (1.15 mph)	.037	.081
11 lb load	.059	.130	grass track (1.16 mph)	.041	.090
22 lb load	.064	.141	potato furrows (1.12 mph)	.045	.100
44 lb load	.067	.147	stubble field (1.08 mph)	.045	.099
(21% grade)			plowed field (1.10 mph)	.050	.110
11 lb load	.066	.145	Walking downstairs	.020	.044
22 lb load	.069	.152	Walking on level (treadmill):		
44 lb load	.072	.158	2 mph (30:00/mi)	.021	.046
Horseback riding:			2.27 mph (26:26/mi)	.023	.051
gallop	.062	.136	2.5 mph (24:00/mi)	.025	.055
trot	.050	.110	3.0 mph (20:00/mi)	.018–.029	.040–.064
walking	.019	.042	3.20 mph (18:45/mi)	.031	.068
Horseshoes	.024	.052	3.50 mph (17:08/mi)	.033	.073
Mountain climbing	.067	.147	4.47 mph (13:25/mi)	.044	.097
Ping-pong	.026	.057	4.60 mph (13:02/mi)	.055	.121
Pool	.014	.030	5.18 mph (11:35/mi)	.063	.139
Rowing for pleasure	.033	.073	5.80 mph (10:20/mi)	.076	.167
			Walking upstairs	.052	.115

BIBLIOGRAPHY

Butts, N. K., Dodge, C., and McAlpine, M. 1995. "Effect of Stepping Rate on Energy Costs During Stairmaster Exercise," *Medicine and Science in Sports* 25(3): 378–382.

Carroll, M. W., Otto, R. M., and Wygand, J. 1991. "The Metabolic Cost of Two Ranges of Arm Position Height With and Without Hand Weights." *Research Quarterly for Exercise and Sport* 62(4): 420–423.

Consolazio, C. F., Johnson, R. E., and Pecora, L. J. 1963. *Physiological Measurements of Metabolic Functions in Man.* New York: McGraw Hill.

Fellingham, G. W., Roundy, E. S., Fisher, A. G., and Bryce, G. R. 1978. "Caloric Cost of Walking and Running." *Medicine and Science in Sports* 10(2): 132–136.

Hoeger, W., and Fisher, A. G. 1981. "Energy Costs for Men's Gymnastic Routines." *International Gymnast Technical Supplement* (No 5) 11(1): 1–3.

Howley, E. T., and Glover, M. E. 1974. "The Caloric Costs of Running and Walking One Mile for Men and Women." *Medicine and Science in Sports* 6(4): 235–237.

Passmore, R., and Durnin, J. V. G. A. 1955. "Human Energy Expenditure." *Physiological Reviews* 35: 801–840.

Wilmore, J. H., Parr, R. B., Ward, P., Vodak, P. A., Barstow, T. J., Pipes, T. V., Grimditch, G., and Leslie, P. 1978. "Energy Cost of Circuit Weight Training." *Medicine and Science in Sports* 10(2): 75–78.

Table of Weights and Measures

1 ounce	=	28.3 grams			
1 pound	=	16 ounces	=	454 grams	= .454 kilograms
1 kilogram	=	1,000 grams	=	2.2 pounds	
1 gram	=	1,000 milligrams			

1 tablespoon	=	3 teaspoons			
1 teaspoon	=	5 milliliters			
1 cup	=	16 tablespoons	=	8 fluid ounces	
1 quart	=	2 pints	=	4 cups	= .95 liters
1 liter	=	1000 milliliters			
1 milliliter	=	.0338 ounces			

1 meter	=	100 centimeters	=	1,000 millimeters	= 39.37 inches
1 inch	=	2.54 centimeters			
1 yard	=	36 inches	=	.914 meters	
1 mile	=	1,609 meters	=	1,760 yards	

1 lb	=	.455 kg
1 kg	=	2.2 lbs
1 kg·m	$\cong$	1.8 ml O_2
1,000 ml O_2	$\cong$	5 cal

Recommended Dietary Allowances (RDA) Tables*

TABLE
A6.1 Median heights and weights and recommended energy intake.

CATEGORY	AGE (YEARS) OR CONDITION	WEIGHT		HEIGHT		REE[a] (kcal/day)	AVERAGE ENERGY ALLOWANCE (kcal)[b]		
		(kg)	(lb)	(cm)	(in)		MULTIPLES of REE	Per kg	Per day[c]
Infants	0.0–0.5	6	13	60	24	320		108	650
	0.5–1.0	9	20	71	28	500		98	850
Children	1–3	13	29	90	35	740		102	1,300
	4–6	20	44	112	44	950		90	1,800
	7–10	28	62	132	52	1,130		70	2,000
Males	11–14	45	99	157	62	1,440	1.70	55	2,500
	15–18	66	145	176	69	1,760	1.67	45	3,000
	19–24	72	160	177	70	1,780	1.67	40	2,900
	25–50	79	174	176	70	1,800	1.60	37	2,900
	51+	77	170	173	68	1,530	1.50	30	2,300
Females	11–14	46	101	157	62	1,310	1.67	47	2,200
	15–18	55	120	163	64	1,370	1.60	40	2,200
	19–24	58	128	164	65	1,350	1.60	38	2,200
	25–50	63	138	163	64	1,380	1.55	36	2,200
	51+	65	143	160	63	1,280	1.50	30	1,900
Pregnant	1st trimester								+0
	2nd trimester								+300
	3rd trimester								+300
Lactating	1st 6 months								+500
	2nd 6 months								+500

[a] REE = Resting Energy Expenditure
[b] In the range of light to moderate activity, the coefficient of variation is ±20%.
[c] Figure is rounded.

*Reprinted by permission from *Recommended Dietary Allowances*, 10th edition, by the National Academy of Sciences, published by National Academy Press, 1989.

TABLE A6.2 Food and Nutrition Board, National Academy of Sciences—National Research Council Recommended Dietary Allowances, revised 1989.

							FAT-SOLUBLE VITAMINS				WATER-SOLUBLE VITAMINS							MINERALS						
CATEGORY	AGE (YEARS) OR CONDITION	WEIGHT[b] (kg)	WEIGHT[b] (lb)	HEIGHT[b] (cm)	HEIGHT[b] (in)	PROTEIN (g)	VITAMIN A μg RE[c]	VITAMIN D (μg[d])	VITAMIN E (mg α-TE[e])	VITAMIN K (μg)	VITAMIN C (mg)	THIAMIN (mg)	RIBOFLAVIN (mg)	NIACIN (mg NE[f])	VITAMIN B$_6$ (mg)	FOLATE (μg)	VITAMIN B$_{12}$ (μg)	CALCIUM (mg)	PHOSPHORUS (mg)	MAGNESIUM (mg)	IRON (mg)	ZINC (mg)	IODINE (μg)	SELENIUM (μg)
Infants	0.0–0.5	6	13	60	24	13	375	7.5	3	5	30	0.3	0.4	5	0.3	25	0.3	400	300	40	6	5	40	10
	0.5–1.0	9	20	71	28	14	375	10	4	10	35	0.4	0.5	6	0.6	35	0.5	600	500	60	10	5	50	15
Children	1–3	13	29	90	35	16	400	10	6	15	40	0.7	0.8	9	1.0	50	0.7	800	800	80	10	10	70	20
	4–6	20	44	112	44	24	500	10	7	20	45	0.9	1.1	12	1.1	75	1.0	800	800	120	10	10	90	20
	7–10	28	62	132	52	28	700	10	7	30	45	1.0	1.2	13	1.4	100	1.4	800	800	170	10	10	120	30
Males	11–14	45	99	157	62	45	1,000	10	10	45	50	1.3	1.5	17	1.7	150	2.0	1,200	1,200	270	12	15	150	40
	15–18	66	145	176	69	59	1,000	10	10	65	60	1.5	1.8	20	2.0	200	2.0	1,200	1,200	400	12	15	150	50
	19–24	72	160	177	70	58	1,000	10	10	70	60	1.5	1.7	19	2.0	200	2.0	1,200	1,200	350	10	15	150	70
	25–50	79	174	176	70	63	1,000	5	10	80	60	1.5	1.7	19	2.0	200	2.0	800	800	350	10	15	150	70
	51+	77	170	173	68	63	1,000	5	10	80	60	1.2	1.4	15	2.0	200	2.0	800	800	350	10	15	150	70
Females	11–14	46	101	157	62	46	800	10	8	45	50	1.1	1.3	15	1.4	150	2.0	1,200	1,200	280	15	12	150	45
	15–18	55	120	163	64	44	800	10	8	55	60	1.1	1.3	15	1.5	180	2.0	1,200	1,200	300	15	12	150	50
	19–24	58	128	164	65	46	800	10	8	60	60	1.1	1.3	15	1.6	180	2.0	1,200	1,200	280	15	12	150	55
	25–50	63	138	163	64	50	800	5	8	65	60	1.1	1.3	15	1.6	180	2.0	800	800	280	15	12	150	55
	51+	65	143	160	63	50	800	5	8	65	60	1.0	1.2	13	1.6	180	2.0	800	800	280	10	12	150	55
Pregnant						60	800	10	10	65	70	1.5	1.6	17	2.2	400	2.2	1,200	1,200	320	30	15	175	65
Lactating	1st 6 months					65	1,300	10	12	65	95	1.6	1.8	20	2.1	280	2.6	1,200	1,200	355	15	19	200	75
	2nd 6 months					62	1,200	10	11	65	90	1.6	1.7	20	2.1	260	2.6	1,200	1,200	340	15	16	200	75

[a] The allowances, expressed as average daily intakes over time, are intended to provide for individual variations among most normal persons as they live in the United States under usual environmental stresses. Diets should be based on a variety of common foods in order to provide other nutrients for which human requirements have been less well defined.

[b] Weights and heights of Reference Adults are actual medians for the U.S. population of the designated age, as reported by NHANES II. The use of these figures does not imply that the height-to-weight ratios are ideal.

[c] Retinol equivalents. 1 retinol equivalent = 1 μg retinol or 6 μg β-carotene.

[d] As cholecalciferol. 10 μg cholecalciferol = 400 IU of vitamin D.

[e] α-Tocopherol equivalents. 1 mg d-α tocopherol = 1 α-TE.

[f] NE (niacin equivalent) is equal to 1 mg of niacin or 60 mg of dietary tryptophan.

**TABLE
A6.3** Estimated sodium, chloride, and potassium—minimum requirements of healthy persons.*

AGE	WEIGHT (kg)[a]	SODIUM (mg)[a,b]	CHLORIDE (mg)[a,b]	POTASSIUM (mg)[c]
Months				
0–5	4.5	120	180	500
6–11	8.9	200	300	700
Years				
1	11.0	225	350	1,000
2–5	16.0	300	500	1,400
6–9	25.0	400	600	1,600
10–18	50.0	500	750	2,000
>18[d]	70.0	500	750	2,000

[a] No allowance has been included for large, prolonged losses from the skin through sweat.
[b] There is no evidence that higher intakes confer any health benefit.
[c] Desirable intakes of potassium may considerably exceed these values (~3,500 mg for adults).
[d] No allowance included for growth. Values for those below 18 years assume a growth rate at the 50th percentile reported by the National Center for Health Statistics and averaged for males and females.

**TABLE
A6.4** Estimated safe and adequate daily dietary intakes of selected vitamins and minerals.*

CATEGORY	AGE (years)	VITAMINS	
		BIOTIN (mg)	PANTOTHENIC ACID (mg)
Infants	0–0.5	10	2
	0.5–1	15	3
Children and	1–3	20	3
adolescents	46	25	3–4
	7–10	30	4–5
	11+	30–100	4–7
Adults		30–100	4–7

CATEGORY	AGE (years)	TRACE ELEMENTS[b]				
		COPPER (mg)	MANGANESE (mg)	FLUORIDE (mg)	CHROMIUM (µg)	MOLYBDENUM (µg)
Infants	0–0.5	0.4–0.6	0.3–0.6	0.1–0.5	10–40	15–30
	0.5–1	0.6–0.7	0.6–1.0	0.2–1.0	20–60	20–40
Children and	1–3	0.7–1.0	1.0–1.5	.05–1.5	20–80	25–50
adolescents	4–6	1.0–1.5	1.5–2.0	1.0–2.5	30–120	30–75
	7–10	1.0–2.0	2.0–3.0	1.5–2.5	50–200	50–150
	11+	1.5–2.5	2.0–5.0	1.5–2.5	50–200	75–250
Adults		1.5–3.0	2.0–5.0	1.5–4.0	50–200	75–250

[a] Because there is less information on which to base allowances, these figures are not given in the main table of RDA and are provided here in the form of ranges of recommended intakes.
[b] Since the toxic levels for many trace elements may be only several times usual intakes, the upper levels for the trace elements given in this table should not be habitually exceeded.

"Eating Smart" Shopping Guide

Eat less fat, eat more fiber, eat less salt and sugar. Many consumers are learning that following this advice can reduce their risk of heart disease, stroke, colon and breast cancer, obesity, and other health problems. But supermarkets don't have aisles labeled "fat" or "salt," and few cooks prepare "fiber" for dinner!

You can't follow vital dietary advice unless someone translates it into food. That's why we've compiled this "Eating Smart Shopping Guide."

These excerpts from *Nutrition Action Healthletter* go right to the heart of the matter. They focus on the basic foods that you eat:

➥ **Fruits** ➥ **Vegetables** ➥ **Beans** ➥ **Grains** ➥ **Poultry and Meats** ➥ **Cereals**

There are no vague generalities. These articles tell you which breakfast cereals are best, which vegetables are healthiest, which meats contain the least fat, and which fruits will give you the most vitamins.

The "Eating Smart Shopping Guide" makes shopping easy — and healthy eating a pleasure.

The Fruit Stand

We came up with a "score" for each fruit by adding up its percent of the U.S. Recommended Daily Allowance (USRDA) for nine nutrients plus fiber. (We only printed five, because the others were usually low.) There is no USRDA for fiber, so we made up our own of 25 grams. Ditto for potassium (we used 3,500 mg).

For example, a quarter of a cantaloupe has 86 percent of the USRDA for vitamin A (86 points), 94 percent for vitamin C (94 points), 12 percent for potassium (12 points), 6 percent for folate (6 points), 4 percent each for fiber and niacin (8 points), 3 percent for thiamin (3 points), 2 percent each for iron and riboflavin (4 points), and 1 percent for calcium (1 point). After rounding, that works out to a score of 213. Numbers for canned fruit are for two halves or slices, including the juice.

If no number was available for a nutrient (folate for blackberries, for example), we assigned it a value of 0. That could make the scores for some fruits lower than they should be. Fruits are ranked from highest to lowest score.

Fruit	Score	Calories	Vit. A	Vit. C	Folate	Potassium	Fiber
Grapefruit, white (½)	84	39	*	✓		*	✓
Honeydew melon (⅒)	81	46		✓	na	✓	✓
Peaches (2)	77	74	✓	✓	na	*	✓
Pineapple (1 cup)	77	77		✓		*	*
Star fruit (1)	73	42	✓	✓	na	*	na
Blueberries (1 cup)	68	82		✓			✓
Cherries, sweet (1 cup)	64	104	*	✓		✓	✓
Nectarines (1)	64	67	✓	✓	*	*	*
Pomegranates (1)	61	104	na	✓	na	✓	✓
Bananas (1)	60	105		✓	*	*	*
Plums (2)	60	72	*	✓			✓
Prunes, dried (5)	59	101	✓			✓	✓
Apples, w/skin (1)	58	124		✓		*	✓
Boysenberries (1 cup)	57	66		*		*	na
Pears (1)	48	98		✓			✓
Grapes, green (60)	46	90		✓		*	
Peaches, canned in juice	43	68	✓	*	na	*	*
Apples, no skin (1)	42	111		✓		*	✓
Pineapple, canned in juice	40	70		✓	na		✓
Figs, dried (2)	39	95					
Currants, dried (¼ cup)	36	102				✓	
Rhubarb, cooked (½ cup)	36	139		✓	*	*	na
Raisins (¼ cup packed)	35	124				*	*
Dates (5)	30	114				*	*
Pears, canned in juice	16	76			na		na

Fruit	Score	Calories	Vit. A	Vit. C	Folate	Potassium	Fiber
Papaya (½)	252	59	✓	✓	na	✓	✓
Cantaloupe (¼)	213	47	✓	✓	*	✓	✓
Strawberries (1 cup)	186	45		✓	*	*	✓
Oranges (1)	169	62	*	✓	*	*	✓
Tangerines (2)	168	74	✓	✓	*	*	✓
Kiwis (1)	154	46		✓	na	*	✓
Mango (½)	153	68	✓	✓	na	✓	*
Apricots (4)	143	68	✓	✓		✓	✓
Persimmons (1)	134	118	✓	✓		*	✓
Watermelon (2 cups)	122	100	✓	✓		✓	*
Raspberries (1 cup)	117	61		✓	na	*	✓
Grapefruit, red or pink (½)	103	37	*	✓			
Blackberries (1 cup)	101	74		✓	na	*	✓
Apricots, dried (10)	97	83	✓			✓	✓

✓ = contains at least 10 percent of the USRDA   na = not available
* = contains between 5 and 9 percent of the USRDA

Sources: USDA and Plant Fiber in Foods by James W. Anderson.

The Healthiest Vegetables? Beets Us

We came up with a "Score" for each vegetable by adding up its percent of the U.S. Recommended Daily Allowance (USRDA) for six nutrients plus fiber.

There is no USRDA for fiber, so we made up our own of 25 grams.

For example, one medium raw carrot has 405 percent of the USRDA for vitamin A (405 points), 11 percent for vitamin C (11 points), 9 percent for fiber (9 points), 3 percent for folate (3 points), and 2 percent each for calcium, iron, and copper (6 points). That gives it a score of 434 points.

If no number was available for a nutrient (folate or copper for leaf lettuce, for example), we assigned it a value of 0. That could make the scores of some vegetables lower than they should be. Vegetables are ranked from highest to lowest score.

Vegetable (1/2 cup fresh, cooked, unless noted)

Vegetable	Score	Vit. A	Vit. C	Folate	Iron	Copper	Calcium	Fiber
Sweet potato, no skin (1 whole)	582	✓	✓	*		✓		✓
Carrot, raw (1 whole)	434	✓	✓					*
Carrots	408	✓	✓	✓	✓	*		*
Spinach	241	✓	✓	✓	✓	*	✓	*
Collard greens, frozen	181	✓	✓	✓	*		✓	na
Red pepper, raw (1/2 pepper)	166	✓	✓					
Kale	161	✓	✓	na	*	*	✓	✓
Dandelion greens	156	✓	✓	✓	*	na	*	*
Spinach, raw (1 cup)	152	✓	✓	✓	✓		✓	✓
Broccoli	145	✓	✓	✓	*	*	*	*
Brussels sprouts	128	✓	✓	✓	*			✓
Broccoli, frozen	127	✓	✓	✓	*	*	*	*
Potato, baked, w/skin (1 whole)	114	na	✓	*	✓	✓		✓
Mixed vegetables, frozen	111	✓	*					✓
Winter squash	110	✓	✓	*	*	*	*	*
Swiss chard	105	✓	✓	na	✓	na	*	*
Broccoli, raw	100	✓	✓	*	*		*	*
Snow peas	90	✓	✓	na	*			*
Mustard greens	85	✓	✓	na		na	*	*
Kohlrabi	82		✓	na		na		
Romaine lettuce (1 cup)	78	✓	✓	✓	*	na		*
Cauliflower	77		✓	*				
Cauliflower, raw	77	✓	✓	*		*		*
Asparagus	75	✓	✓	✓	*	*		*

Vegetable (1/2 cup fresh, cooked, unless noted)

Vegetable	Score	Vit. A	Vit. C	Folate	Iron	Copper	Calcium	Fiber
Green peppers, raw (1/2 pepper)	67	*	✓					*
Potato, baked, no skin (1 whole)	67	na	✓	✓	*	✓		✓
Parsley, raw (1/4 cup)	66	✓	✓	*	*			*
Green peas, frozen	64	✓	✓	✓	*	*		✓
Avocado, California (1/2 avocado)	63	✓	✓	✓	*	✓		*
Okra	61	*	✓	✓	*		*	✓
Collard greens	57	✓	✓					*
Endive, raw (1 cup)	56	✓	*	✓		✓		✓
Parsnips	53		✓	✓		✓		✓
Rutabaga	48		✓	✓				*
Cabbage	47		✓					*
Artichoke (1/2 artichoke)	46		✓	*		*		✓
Mushrooms	43		*			✓		*
Cabbage, raw	39		✓	*				*
Corn	39	*	*	✓	*			✓
Boston lettuce, raw (1 cup)	38	✓	*	✓	*		*	*
Green beans	37	*	*	*				*
Tomato, raw (1/2 tomato)	37	*	✓					*
Beets	32			✓				*
Summer squash	31	*	✓			*		*
Onions	27		*					*
Green beans, canned	26	*	*					*
Turnips	26		✓			na		*
Lettuce, leaf (1 cup)	25	✓	*	na		na		*
Corn, frozen	23			*				*
Lettuce, Iceberg (1 cup)	22		✓	*				✓
Radishes, raw (1/4 cup)	17		✓					*
Celery, raw (1 stalk)	14							*
Onions, raw (1/4 cup)	14						*	*
Eggplant	12							✓
Alfalfa sprouts (1/2 cup)	11							*
Cucumber, raw	11					na		*
Mushrooms, raw	10							*
Garlic, raw (1 clove)	3					na		*

✓ = contains at least ten percent of the USRDA

* = contains between five and nine percent of the USRDA

na = not available

Source: *USDA Handbook 8*

The Bean Bag

All beans are nutritional powerhouses, but some are a bit more "powerhousey" than others.

We came up with a score for each bean by adding its percent of the U.S. Recommended Daily Allowance (USRDA) for seven nutrients plus fiber and potassium. There are no USRDAs for fiber or potassium, so for fiber we used the new Daily Value (DV) of 25 grams, which will soon appear on food labels. For potassium we used our "Nutrition Action RDA" (NARDA) of 3,500 milligrams.

For example: A cup of cooked lentils has 57 percent of the DV for fiber (57 points) and 19 percent of the NARDA for potassium (19 points). It also has 81 percent of the USRDA for folic acid (81 points), 16 percent for magnesium (16 points), 33 percent for iron (33 points), 23 percent for copper (23 points), 15 percent for zinc (15 points), 25 percent for protein (25 points), and 16 percent for vitamin B-6 (16 points). That adds up to a score of 285.

Small differences in score (25 points or less) are meaningless. Potassium and vitamin B-6 values are included in each score but don't appear on the chart. Numbers are for canned or cooked dried beans. Beans are ranked from highest to lowest score.

Bean (1 cup, cooked)	Score	Fiber	Folic Acid	Magnesium	Iron	Copper	Zinc	Protein
Black beans (turtle beans)	265	●	●	◐	○	○	○	◐
Small white beans *	263	●	●	◐	◐	○	○	◐
White beans	253	◐	◐	◐	◐	◐	○	◐
Lima beans, baby	252	●	●	○	◐	○	○	○
Kidney beans, all types	243	◐	●	○	◐	○	○	○
Adzuki beans *	238	◐	◐	○	○	◐	○	○
Great northern beans	228	●	◐	○	○	○	○	○
Mung beans *	226	●	●	○	○	○	○	○
Lima beans, large	224	●	◐	○	○	○	○	○
Broadbeans (fava beans) *	197	◐	◐	○	○	○	○	○
Peas, split (green)	192	●	◐	○	○	○	○	○
Tofu, raw, (4 oz.) ‡	144	—	—	◐	●	○	○	◐

Bean (1 cup, cooked)	Score	Fiber	Folic Acid	Magnesium	Iron	Copper	Zinc	Protein
Soybeans ‡	300	◐	○	◐	●	◐	○	◐
Pinto beans	287	●	●	◐	●	○	○	○
Chickpeas (garbanzos, ceci)	286	●	●	○	◐	◐	○	◐
Lentils	285	●	●	○	◐	◐	○	●
Cranberry beans *	278	●	●	○	○	◐	○	◐
Black-eyed peas (cowpeas)	273	◐	●	○	○	◐	○	○
Pink beans *	269	◐	●	○	◐	○	○	◐
Navy beans *	266	●	●	◐	◐	◐	○	○

● = contains at least 50 percent of the USRDA
◐ = contains between 25 and 49 percent of the USRDA
○ = contains between 10 and 24 percent of the USRDA
— = contains less than 10 percent of the USRDA

* Values for one or more nutrients are estimates.
‡ Soybeans are the only fatty bean. A cup has 15 grams of fat. A four-ounce serving of tofu, which is made from soybeans, can have anywhere from 2 to 7 grams of fat.

Source: USDA Handbook 8

Grains & Losses

We calculated a "score" for each grain by adding up its percent of the U.S. Recommended Daily Allowance (USRDA) for five nutrients plus fiber. There is no USRDA for fiber, so we used the new Daily Value (DV)—25 grams—that will soon appear on food labels.

For example, a five-ounce serving of quinoa has 9 percent of the DV for fiber (9 points), and 20 percent of the USRDA for magnesium (20 points), 4 percent for vitamin B-6 (4 points), 8 percent for zinc (8 points), 14 percent for copper (14 points), and 18 percent for iron (18 points). That adds up to a score of 73.

We included potatoes and pastas for comparison. (Yes, pastas are made from grains, and they're quite healthy.) The ten grains with the highest scores are our "Best Bites." Grains are ranked from highest to lowest score.

Grain (5 ounces, cooked)

Grain	Score	Fiber	Magnesium	B-6	Zinc	Copper	Iron
✓ Brown rice	51	+	+	+	*	*	-
✓ Triticale [1]	47	+	+	-	*	*	-
Spaghetti	42	+	*	+	*	*	+
✓ Wheat berries [1]	41	+	*	-	*	*	*
Macaroni	39	*	*	-	*	*	+
Kamut [1]	37	na	+	-	*	*	*
Oats, rolled	33	+	*	-	*	*	*
Spelt [1]	33	+	+	na	na	*	*
White rice, converted	26	-	-	-	-	*	*
Couscous	23	*	-	-	-	-	-
White rice, instant	18	-	-	-	-	*	*
Soba noodles	12	na	-	-	-	-	-
Corn grits	10	-	-	-	-	-	*

Grain (5 ounces, cooked)

Grain	Score	Fiber	Magnesium	B-6	Zinc	Copper	Iron
Potato, with skin	81	+	*	+	-	+	+
✓ Quinoa [1]	73	*	+	-	*	+	+
Macaroni or Spaghetti, whole wheat	69	+	+	*	*	+	*
✓ Amaranth [1]	66	+	+	-	*	+	+
✓ Buckwheat groats [2]	64	+	+	*	*	+	*
Spaghetti, spinach	61	na	+	*	+	*	*
✓ Bulgur	60	+	+	*	*	*	*
✓ Barley, pearled [2]	59	+	*	*	*	*	+
✓ Wild rice [2]	58	+	+	+	+	*	*
✓ Millet	53	*	+	*	*	+	*

✓ = "Best Bite"
+ = contains at least 10 percent of the USRDA
* = contains between 5 and 9 percent of the USRDA
- = contains less than 5 percent of the USRDA
na = not available.

[1] score is based on USDA estimates of all nutrients.
[2] fiber value is a USDA estimate.

Source: *USDA Handbook 8*

The Meat Market

The numbers in the chart are for four ounces of the meat from cooked, skinless poultry or (scrupulously) trimmed meat, unless otherwise noted. Four ounces is about how much meat is on a typical chicken breast. A typical chicken thigh contains 1.8 oz. of meat, a typical drumstick 1.6 oz., and a typical wing 0.7 oz. Products are ranked from lowest saturated fat to highest. Ideally, most people should eat no more than 15 grams of saturated fat in a day. To help non-red-meat eaters, we've marked (with a ◆) the poultry & fish products.

Food (four ounces, cooked)	Calories	Saturated Fat (g)	Total Fat (g)
Less than 1 gram of saturated fat			
Turkey breast† ◆	153	0.3	0.8
Shady Brook Farms Ground Breast of Turkey* ◆	170	1.0	3.0
1 to 2 grams of saturated fat			
Healthy Choice Extra Lean Ground Beef	120	1.1	3.2
Chicken breast ◆	187	1.1	4.0
Turkey wing† ◆	185	1.2	3.9
Veal leg, top round steak	170	1.4	3.8
Beef top round (Select)	192	1.4	4.2
Turkey leg† ◆	180	1.4	4.3
Beef eye of round (Select)	181	1.6	4.5
Chicken drumstick ◆	195	1.7	6.4
Pork tenderloin	186	1.9	5.5
2 to 3 grams of saturated fat			
Beef top round (Choice)	214	2.3	6.7
Beef bottom round (Select)	203	2.4	7.0
Turkey breast, with skin ◆	214	2.4	8.4
Beef tip round (Select)	204	2.5	7.3
Chicken breast, with skin ◆	223	2.5	8.8
Shady Brook Farms Ground Turkey, with skin* ◆	259	2.5	14.7
Veal shoulder, arm steak	186	2.6	6.6
Chicken wing ◆	230	2.6	9.2
Beef top sirloin (Select) ◆	211	2.7	7.0
Veal sirloin	191	2.7	7.1
Lamb shank	204	2.7	7.6
Veal shoulder, blade steak	194	2.9	7.8
Veal loin	198	2.9	7.9
3 to 4 grams of saturated fat			
Pork top loin	230	3.1	8.8
Pork center loin	229	3.3	9.2
Ham, leg, rump half	234	3.3	9.2
Chicken thigh ◆	237	3.4	12.3
Beef top sirloin (Choice) ◆	229	3.5	9.1
Turkey leg, with skin ◆	236	3.5	11.1
Chicken drumstick, with skin ◆	248	3.5	12.6
Lamb sirloin	231	3.7	10.4
Beef chuck arm pot roast (Choice)	255	3.8	10.5
Turkey wing, with skin ◆	260	3.8	14.1
Veal shoulder, blade steak, untrimmed	211	3.9	9.8
Lamb loin	245	3.9	11.0
Pork loin, center rib	248	3.9	11.0
4 to 5 grams of saturated fat			
Pork loin or sirloin, whole	240	4.1	11.3
Beef top loin (Choice)	243	4.4	11.5
Beef top round, untrimmed (Choice)	254	4.5	12.0
Lamb shoulder, blade	239	4.6	12.8
Duck ◆	228	4.7	12.7
Beef tenderloin (Choice)	252	4.8	12.7
Pork shoulder, arm, picnic	259	4.9	14.3
Chicken thigh, with skin ◆	280	4.9	17.6
5 to 10 grams of saturated fat			
Veal sirloin, untrimmed	229	5.1	11.9
Pork center loin, untrimmed	272	5.4	14.8
Perdue Ground Chicken, with skin ◆	270	5.5	16.5
Chicken wing, with skin ◆	329	6.2	22.1
Beef chuck blade roast (Choice)	298	6.3	16.3
Pork loin, center rib, untrimmed	298	6.5	17.6
Pork sirloin, untrimmed	294	6.7	18.2
Ground beef, extra lean (83% lean)	290	7.3	18.5
Ground beef, lean (80% lean)	308	8.2	20.9
Ground beef, regular (73% lean)	328	9.2	23.5
Beef top loin, untrimmed (Choice)	336	9.4	23.8
More than 10 grams of saturated fat			
Porterhouse steak, untrimmed (Choice)	346	10.1	25.1
Duck, with skin ◆	382	11.0	32.1
Lamb loin, untrimmed	358	11.1	26.2
Beef chuck blade roast, untrimmed (Choice)	412	12.6	31.5
Pork spareribs, untrimmed	450	12.6	34.4
Beef short ribs, untrimmed (Choice)	534	20.2	47.6
For comparison			
Flounder ◆	133	0.4	1.7
Pink Salmon ◆	169	0.8	5.0

* Estimate from raw values.
◆ Poultry & fish products.
† Fryers and roasters. On average, other types are twice as fatty.
Sources: USDA and manufacturers.

Source: "Copyright 1994, CSPI. Reprinted from *Nutrition Action Healthletter* (1875 Connecticut Avenue, N.W., #300, Washington, DC 20009-5728." $24.00 for 10 issues).

Cereal Square-off

Our chart lists nutrition numbers for one ounce of cereal. Yet surveys show that most people eat 3/4 oz. (about a cup) of light cereals—like Rice Krispies or Corn Flakes—and two or three ounces (1/2 to 2/3 cup) of dense cereals—like Grape-Nuts or granola. We have added, in parentheses following each name, how many cups of cereals equal one ounce. That way, you can figure out how much is in a serving of your cereal. For example, 1/3 cup of Kellogg's Bran Buds weighs an ounce. So if you typically eat about two-thirds of a cup, multiply the numbers in the chart by 2. "Best Bite" criteria: (1) predominantly whole grain, (2) at least 2.5 grams of fiber, (3) no more than two grams of fat, five grams of sugar, or 250 mg of sodium, and (4) free of BHA, BHT, and aspartame. Within each category, products are ranked from highest to lowest fiber.

Product	Fat (g)	Fiber (g)	Sugar (g)
Whole Grain Cereal (50 to 120 calories)			
Kellogg's All-Bran w/Extra Fiber (1/2) a, b	0	14	0
General Mills Fiber One (1/2) a	1	13	0
Kellogg's Bran Buds (1/3) b	1	11	8
Kellogg's All-Bran (1/3)	1	9	5
Health Valley Raisin Bran Flakes (1/2)	0	6	na
✓ Kellogg's Bran Flakes (2/3)	0	5	5
Kellogg's Fiberwise (2/3) b	1	5	5
Erewhon Right Start (1/3) *	0	5	na
Köln Oat Bran Crunch (1/3)	1	5	na
Barbara's 100% Oat Bran (1/4) *	4	5	na
Nabisco Shredded Wheat 'n Bran (2/3) b	1	4	0
Kellogg's Nutri-Grain Raisin Bran (3/4)	1	4	6
Kellogg's Cracklin' Oat Bran (1/2)	3	4	7
Post Fruit & Fibre Dates and Raisins (1/2) b	2	4	8
Kellogg's Fruitful Bran (1/2)	0	4	9
Kellogg's Raisin Bran (1/2)	1	4	9
Post Natural Raisin Bran (1/2)	1	4	9
Health Valley Oat Bran Flakes or O's (1/2)	0	4	na
✓ Puffed Kashi (1 1/3)	0	3	0
Nabisco Shredded Wheat (1 biscuit) b	1	3	0
✓ Kellogg's Nutri-Grain Wheat (2/3)	0	3	2
✓ Weetabix (1 3/4 biscuits)	1	3	2
✓ Post Grape-Nuts (1/4)	0	3	3

Product	Fat (g)	Fiber (g)	Sugar (g)
General Mills Total or Wheaties (1) b	1	3	3
Ralston Whole Grain Wheat Chex (2/3) b	1	3	3
Nabisco Fruit Wheats (1/2) b	0	3	5
Quaker Life (2/3) b	2	3	5
Kellogg's Frosted Mini Wheats (4 biscuits) b	0	3	6
General Mills Raisin Nut Bran (1/2) b	3	3	8
Health Valley Real Oat Bran Raisin (1/4)	1	3	na
Grainfield's Oat Bran Flakes (3/4)	2	3	na
General Mills Cheerios (1 1/4)	2	2	1
General Mills Honey Nut Cheerios (3/4)	2	2	10
New Morning Oatios (1 1/4) *	2	2	na
Kellogg's Kenmei Rice Bran (3/4) b	1	1	4
General Mills Oatmeal Raisin Crisp (1/3) b	2	1	8
General Mills Wheaties Honey Gold (3/4) b	0	1	10
Granola and Muesli (90 to 130 calories)			
Arrowhead Mills Maple Nut Granola (1/4)	5	6	na
Familia 25% Bran (1/3)	2	5	6
Health Valley Healthy Crunch (1/4) *	1	4	na
✓ Alpen (no salt/no sugar) (1/4)	2	3	5
Familia (1/3)	1	3	6
Kellogg's Müeslix Golden Crunch (1/3) b	2	3	6
Breadshop Fat Free Granola (1/3)	0	3	na
Health Valley Fat-Free Granola (1/4) *	0	3	na
Health Valley Real Oat Bran Crunch (1/4)	1	3	na
Rainforest Granola (1/3)	5	3	na
Quaker 100% Natural (1/4) *	5	2	7
Kellogg's Low-Fat Granola (1/3) b	2	2	8
Ralston Muesli (1/3) *, b	2	2	8
Nature Valley 100% Natural (1/3) *	5	1	6
Refined Cereal (90 to 110 calories)			
Ralston Multi-Bran Chex (2/3) b	0	4	6
General Mills Basic 4 (1/2) b	2	2	6
Post Honey Bunches of Oats (2/3) b	2	2	6
Kellogg's Corn Flakes (1) b	0	1	2
Kellogg's Product 19 or Special K (1) b	0	1	3
Kellogg's Frosted Flakes (3/4) b	0	1	11
Kellogg's Rice Krispies (1) b	0	0	3
Kellogg's Nut & Honey Crunch (2/3) b	1	0	9

✓ = Best Bite   * = average for the entire line   na = not available
a = sweetened with aspartame   b = contains BHA or BHT

All information obtained from manufacturers.

Nutritional Information for Selected Fast-Food Outlets

	serving size (in grams unless otherwise noted)	calories	protein (g)	carbo (g)	total fat (g)	sat. fat (g)	cholesterol (mg)	% calories from fat	sodium (mg)
BURGER KING									
Whopper® Sandwich	270	630	27	45	39	11	90	56	850
Hamburger	103	260	14	28	10	4	30	35	500
Cheeseburger	115	300	17	28	14	6	45	43	710
BK Big Fish Sandwich	255	720	25	59	43	8	60	54	1090
BK Broiler® Chicken Sandwich	248	540	30	41	29	6	48	480	
Chicken Tenders® (6 pieces)	88	250	16	14	12	3	35	44	530
French Fries (medium, salted)	116	400	5	43	20	5	0	45	240
Chocolate Shake (medium)	284	310	9	54	7	4	20	19	230
Croissan'wich® w/ bacon, egg, & cheese	118	350	15	18	24	8	225	63	790
Croissan'wich® w/ sausage, egg, & cheese	159	530	20	21	41	14	225	70	1000
MCDONALD'S									
Hamburger	102	255	12	30	9	3	37	32	490
Cheeseburger	116	305	15	30	13	5	50	38	725
McLean Deluxe™	206	320	22	35	10	4	60	28	670
Big Mac®	215	500	25	42	26	9	100	47	890
Filet-O-Fish®	141	370	14	38	18	4	50	44	730
McChicken®	187	415	19	39	20	4	50	43	830
Medium French Fries	97	320	4	36	17	3.5	0	48	150
Egg McMuffin®	135	280	18	28	11	4	235	35	710
Sausage Biscuit	118	420	12	32	28	8	44	60	1040
Vanilla Lowfat Frozen Yogurt Cone	3 oz.	105	4	22	1	0.5	3	8	80

continued

	serving size (in grams unless otherwise noted)	calories	protein (g)	carbo (g)	total fat (g)	sat. fat (g)	cholesterol (mg)	% calories from fat	sodium (mg)
TACO BELL									
Soft Taco	—	223	12	19	11	5	32	45	539
Taco	—	180	10	10	11	5	32	56	276
Chicken Soft Taco	—	223	14	19	10	4	58	40	553
Tostada	—	242	9	27	11	4	14	41	593
7-Layer Burrito	—	485	15	59	21	8	28	39	1115
Bean Burrito	—	391	13	58	12	4	5	28	1138
Burrito Supreme™	—	443	18	50	19	9	47	38	
Taco Salad	—	838	31	55	55	16	79	58	1132
KFC									
Original Recipe® breast	137	360	33	12	20	5	115	50	870
Original Recipe® thigh	92	260	19	9	17	5	110	58	570
Original Recipe® drumstick	51	130	13	4	7	2	70	46	210
Extra Tasty Crispy™ breast	168	470	31	25	28	7	80	53	930
Extra Tasty Crispy™ thigh	118	370	19	18	25	6	70	59	540
Extra Tasty Crispy™ drumstick	67	190	13	8	11	3	60	53	260
Mashed Potatoes w/ Gravy	120	109	1	16	5	<1	<1	41	368
Cole Slaw	90	114	1	13	6	1	<5	47	177
Potato Salad	125	180	3	18	11	2	11	55	423
PIZZA HUT									
Pepperoni— Thin 'N Crispy crust*	84	215	11	21	10	4	25	42	627
Pepperoni—Pan crust	104	265	11	28	12	4	24	41	569
Veggie Lover's— Thin 'N Crispy crust	112	186	9	22	7	3	17	33	545
Veggie Lover's—Pan crust	133	243	10	29	10	3	17	36	512
Supreme— Thin 'N Crispy crust	116	257	14	21	13	5	31	45	795
Supreme—Pan crust	136	311	15	28	15	6	30	45	764

*all pizza figures are per slice

	serving size	calories	protein (g)	carbo (g)	total fat (g)	sat. fat (g)	cholesterol (mg)	% calories from fat	sodium (mg)
BASKIN-ROBBINS									
Ice Cream—chocolate	½ cup	150	3	19	8	5	25	47	65
Sherbet—rainbow	½ cup	120	1	25	1.5	1	5	1.5	25
Light Ice Cream— praline dream	½ cup	120	3	18	4	1.5	10	33	65
Fat Free Ice Cream— jamoca swirl	½ cup	110	4	24	0	0	2	0	70
Frozen Yogurt— chocolate	½ cup	120	5	23	1.5	1	5	12.5	75
"TCBY"®									
Regular Frozen Yogurt	½ cup	130	4	23	3	2	10	23	50
Nonfat Frozen Yogurt	½ cup	110	4	23	0	0	<5	0	45
Sorbet	½ cup	100	0	25	0	0	0	0	5
No Sugar Added Nonfat Yogurt	½ cup	80	4	19	0	0	<5	0	35

Laboratory Activities

LAB 3

A Biographical Sketch, 2025+

Assume that 25–30 years from now, around 2025, you have become so successful that a biographer wants to write about your life.

For each dimension of your life (as described in Chapter 2) what would you hope this biographer would use to describe the person you have become?

_____

_____

_____

_____

_____

_____

_____

_____

_____

_____

_____

_____

_____

_____

_____

_____

_____

_____

_____

_____

_____

_____

_____

_____

_____

_____

_____

_____

Using a red marker, underline the adjectives that describe you now. Then circle those that do not describe you now. If you have any circles on your page, you have some things you want to change about yourself.

LAB 5

The Pathway to Change

We all have the power to change ourselves, but many of us never find a way to do it. This worksheet provides a step-by-step process that can help you design a personal behavior change plan that will work for you. Although the example that follows focuses on exercise (a physical aspect of your life), you may wish to focus on a nutritional or a stress-management or a social interaction aspect, or any other aspect of your life for which you would like to implement changes.

Following the example below is a blank worksheet. You may wish to photocopy it so you can formulate new "pathways to change" as you progress through this course. Also, we have included a more formal "Contract with Myself." If your instructor agrees, use this contract to focus on the one area of change that is most important to you.

SAMPLE WORKSHEET

Step 1:

State what you want to work on or change as a *behavior* you do or do not do, and not *as an issue or object*. For example:

"Not exercising enough." ("Out of shape" would not be an appropriate response, as it is not a behavior that can be changed. Focus on a behavior.)

Step 2:

List your immediate and long-term reasons for wanting to change your current behavior. For example:

Short-term reasons:

I'm gaining weight.
I don't have much energy.
I get winded quickly.
I feel sluggish.

Long-term reasons:

I'm probably going to get fat.
I won't have as much vigor and vitality as I get older.
I'll be a good candidate for heart disease and maybe diabetes.

Step 3:

List any reasons you have for not wanting to change the behavior you listed in #1. For example:

I'm too busy already to add something else.
I don't have a lot of money to spend for exercise equipment or clubs or classes.
It's dark before I go to work and after I come home; I don't want to be out in the dark.
I don't have anybody to exercise with.

Step 4:

List alternative behaviors you would consider trying in place of your current behavior. For example:

The types of exercise I might like to do:

walking, aerobics, weight-training, tennis, downhill skiing

continued

L15

L A B O R A T O R Y

Step 5:

Compare #3, your list of reasons for not wanting to change, with your #4 list of possible behavior alternatives. Note which alternative behaviors will allow you to avoid most of the reasons you listed for not wanting to change. For example:

Walking:

+ −   no cost except for shoes
+   no equipment/facilities needed
+   maybe could walk at lunch to avoid dark and to fit it in my schedule
   −   no companion

Downhill skiing:

−   need equipment and transportation
−   need money for ticket
−   need lots of time

Aerobics:

+ −   small cost for each class
+ −   need shoes
+   can find a class that fits my schedule
+   avoids the darkness problem
+   lots of people there

Although our sample comparisons will end here, you should analyze each alternative on your list however many you have.

Step 6:

Decide which behavior alternative(s) to try, and specify long-term (one or more months away) and specific short-term (one week) goals. State your goals in measurable, observable terms so you can determine readily if you've accomplished them. *Note:* If no alternative behavior you listed in #4 seemed to be workable after you did your analysis in #5, you may want to discuss it with your instructor or someone who has accomplished the behavior change you are interested in making, to get some additional ideas.

For example:

I will increase my exercise by attending aerobics classes.

Long-term goal:

By the end of three months, I will be attending at least three aerobics classes per week.

Short-term goal:

By Friday of this next week, I will have located at least two facilities near my home or school offering aerobics classes and will have visited them to get their schedules and to see if I like either of them.

I will also repeat to myself the affirmative statements to be developed in Step #7 at least two to three times each day.

At the end of this week, I will review my success in completing this goal and establish what I must do next to keep progressing toward my long-term goal.

continued

LAB 6

What's Your Risk of Heart Attack?

How To Find Out

*Every year about 1.5 million Americans suffer a heart attack. And almost 500,000 of them die. The fact is, **heart attack claims more lives than any other single cause**. Are you at risk? Take the following quiz to find out! If your score is high, don't despair. You can lower your risk by following the steps listed on the back page.*

Instructions: In each category, circle the number next to the statement that's most true for you.

Cigarette Smoking

I never smoked or stopped smoking three or more years ago.	**1**
I don't smoke but live and/or work with smokers.	**2**
I stopped smoking within the last three years.	**3**
I smoke regularly.	**4**
I smoke regularly and live and/or work with other smokers.	**5**

Total Blood Cholesterol

Use the number from your most recent blood cholesterol measurement.

Less than 160	**1**
160–199	**2**
Don't know	**3**
200–239	**4**
240 or higher	**5**

HDL ("Good") Cholesterol

Use the number from your most recent HDL cholesterol measurement.

Over 60	**1**
56–60	**2**
Don't know	**3**
35–55	**4**
Less than 35	**5**

Systolic Blood Pressure

Use the first (highest) number from your most recent blood pressure measurement.

Less than 120	**1**
120–139	**2**
Don't know	**3**
140–159	**4**
160 or higher	**5**

Excess Body Weight

I am within 10 pounds of my desirable weight.	**1**
I am 10–20 pounds above my desirable weight.	**2**
I am 21–30 pounds above my desirable weight.	**3**
I am 31–50 pounds above my desirable weight.	**4**
I am more than 50 pounds above my desirable weight.	**5**

continued

L
A
B
O
R
A
T
O
R
Y

Physical Activity

Choose the column (A, B or C) that best describes your usual level of physical activity.

A Highly Active	B Moderately Active	C Inactive
My job requires very hard physical labor (such as digging or loading heavy objects) at least four hours a day **OR** I do vigorous activities (jogging, cycling, swimming, etc.) at least three times per week for 30–60 minutes or more **OR** I do at least one hour of moderate activity such as brisk walking at least four days a week	My job requires that I walk, lift, carry or do other moderately hard work for several hours per day (day care worker, stock clerk or busboy/waitress) **OR** I spend much of my leisure time doing moderate activities (dancing, gardening, walking or housework)	My job requires that I sit at a desk most of the day **AND** Much of my leisure time is spent in sedentary activities (watching TV, reading, etc.) **AND** I seldom work up a sweat and I cannot walk fast without having to stop to catch my breath

Rating your activity level:

If your physical activity is more like:	*Circle*
Column A	**1**
Between Column A and B	**2**
Column B	**3**
Between Column B and C	**4**
Column C	**5**

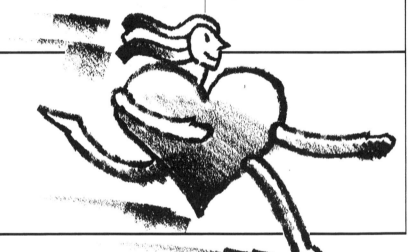

Scoring

Add your answers for each question to get your total score.

If your total score is:	*Your heart attack risk is:*
6–13	Low
14–22	Moderate
23–30	*High*

Your score is simply an estimate of your possible risk. A high score does not mean you will surely have a heart attack, and a low score doesn't mean you're safe from heart disease. Check your individual category scores to see which factors are increasing your risk of heart attack the most. Then go to the back page to learn how to lower your risk.

LAB 7

Cancer: Assessing Your Risk

▪ INTRODUCTION ▪

You can reduce your risk of getting some types of cancer, such as lung cancer, by changing your life-style behaviors. For other types of cancer, such as breast and colorectal cancers, your chance for cure is greatly increased if the cancer is found at an early stage through periodic screening examinations.

This questionnaire has been designed by the American Cancer Society to help you learn about (1) your risk factors for certain types of cancer and (2) the chances that cancer would be found at an early stage when a cure is possible.

▪ TEST SCORE CARD DIRECTIONS ▪

Read each question concerning each site and its specific risk factors. Be honest in your responses. Place the number in parenthesis in the correct space on your score panel to the right.

For example, Question #2 on lung cancer, above right: if you are 53 years old (age 50-59) then enter 5 as your score.

▪ FOR WOMEN ▪

Complete the score panel for lung, colon/rectum and breast cancer on this page, then continue to the next page. The major cancer sites for women are included with space to enter the score totals.

▪ ABOUT YOUR ANSWERS ▪

You may check your own risks with the answers contained in this folder.

You are advised to discuss this folder with your physician if you are at higher risk.

IMPORTANT:
▪ REACT TO EACH STATEMENT ▪

Individual numbers for specific questions are not to be interpreted as a precise measure of relative risk, but the totals for a given site should give a general indication of your risk.

---

continued

L A B O R A T O R Y

LUNG CANCER

1. **SEX:**   a. Male (2)   b. Female (1)

2. **AGE:**   a. 39 or less (1)   b. 40-49 (2)   c. 50-59 (5)   d. 60+ (7)

3. **EXPOSURE TO ANY OF THESE:**
   a. Mining (3)   b. Asbestos (7)   c. Uranium & radioactive products (5)   d. None (0)

4. **HABITS:**   a. Smoker (10)*   b. Nonsmoker (0)*

5. **TYPE OF SMOKING:**
   a. Cigarettes or little cigars (10)   b. Pipe and/or cigar, but not cigarettes (3)   c. Nonsmoker (0)

6. **NUMBER OF CIGARETTES SMOKED PER DAY:**
   a. 0 (1)   b. Less than ½ pack per day (5)   c. ½-1 pack (9)   d. 1-2 packs (15)   e. 2+ packs (20)

7. **TYPE OF CIGARETTE:**
   a. High tar/nicotine (10)**   b. Medium tar/nicotine (9)**   c. Low tar/nicotine (7)**   d. Nonsmoker (1)

8. **LENGTH OF TIME SMOKING:**
   a. Nonsmoker (1)   b. Up to 15 years (5)   c. 15-25 years (10)   d. 25+ years (20)

SUBTOTAL _____

REDUCING YOUR RISK — * If you stopped smoking more than 10 years ago, count yourself as a nonsmoker. If you have stopped smoking in the past 10 years, you are an **ex-smoker**. Ex-smokers should answer questions 5 through 8 according to how they previously smoked. Then ex-smokers may **reduce** their point total on questions 5 through 8 by 10% for each year they have not smoked. Current smokers also answer questions 5 through 8.

I am stopping smoking today. (Subtract 2 points.)   TOTAL _____

** High Tar/Nicotine: 20 mg. or more tar / 1.3 mg. or more nicotine   Medium Tar/Nicotine: 16-19 mg. tar / 1.1-1.2 mg. nicotine   Low Tar/Nicotine: 15 mg. or less tar / 1.0 mg. or less nicotine

COLON RECTUM CANCER

RISK FACTORS

1. **AGE:**   a. 40 or less (2)   b. 40-49 (7)   c. 50 and over (12)

2. **HAS ANYONE IN YOUR FAMILY EVER HAD:**
   a. Colon cancer (18)   b. Colon polyps (18)   c. Neither (1)

3. **HAVE YOU EVER HAD:**
   a. Colon cancer (25)   b. Colon polyps (25)   c. Ulcerative colitis for more than seven years (18)
   d. Cancer of the breast, ovary, uterus, or stomach (13)   e. None of the above (1)

TOTAL _____

SYMPTOMS

1. Do you have bleeding from the rectum?   Yes _____ No _____

2. Have you had a change in bowel habits (such as altered frequency, size, consistency, or color of stool)?   Yes _____ No _____

REDUCING YOUR RISKS AND DETECTING CANCER EARLY

1. I have altered my diet to include less fat and more fruits, fiber, and cruciferous vegetables, (broccoli, cabbage, cauliflower, Brussels sprouts).   Yes _____ No _____

2. I have had a negative test for blood in my stool within the past year.   Yes _____ No _____

3. I have had a negative examination for colon cancer and polyps within the past year (proctosigmoidoscopy, colonscopy, barium enema x-rays).   Yes _____ No _____

BREAST CANCER

1. **AGE GROUP:**   a. Under 35 (10)   b. 35-39 (20)   c. 40-49 (50)   d. 50 and over (90)

2. **RACE:**   a. Oriental (10)   b. Hispanic (10)   c. Black (20)   d. White (25)

3. **FAMILY HISTORY:**   a. None (10)   b. Mother, sister, daughter with breast cancer (30)

4. **YOUR HISTORY:**
   a. No breast disease (10)   b. Previous lumps or cysts (15)   c. Previous breast cancer (100)

5. **MATERNITY:**
   a. 1st pregnancy before 30 (10)   b. 1st pregnancy at 30 or older (15)   c. No pregnancies (20)

SUBTOTAL _____

REDUCING YOUR RISK

6. I practice breast self-examination monthly. (Subtract 10 points.)

7. I have had a negative mammogram and examination by a physician within the past year. (Subtract 25 points.)

TOTAL _____

continued

SKIN CANCER

1. Live in the southern part of the U.S.:   Yes   No
2. Frequent work or play in the sun: Yes   No
3. Fair complexion or freckles; (natural hair color of blonde, red, or light brown, or eye color of grey, green, blue, or hazel):   Yes   No
4. Work in mines, around coal tars or radioactivity: Yes   No
5. Experienced a severe, blistering sunburn before the age of 18:   Yes   No
6. Have any family members with skin cancer or history of melanoma: Yes   No
7. Had skin cancer or melanoma in the past: Yes   No
8. Use or have used tanning beds or sun lamps: Yes   No
9. Have large, many, or changing moles: Yes   No

REDUCING YOUR RISK

10. I cover up with a wide-brimmed hat and wear long-sleeved shirts and pants.   Yes   No
11. I use sun screens with an SPF rating of 15 or higher when going out in the sun.   Yes   No
12. I examine my skin once a month for changes in warts or moles.   Yes   No

CERVICAL CANCER

(Lower Portion of Uterus) — These questions do not apply to a woman who has had a total hysterectomy.

1. **AGE GROUP:**
   a. Less than 25 (10)   b. 25-39 (20)   c. 40-54 (30)   d. 55 and over (30)
2. **RACE:**   a. Oriental or white (10)   b. Black (20)   c. Hispanic (20)
3. **NUMBER OF PREGNANCIES:**   a. 0 (10)   b. 1 to 3 (20)   c. 4 and over (30)
4. **VIRAL INFECTIONS:**
   a. Viral infections of the vagina such as Venereal warts, herpes or ulcer formations (10)
   b. Never (1)
5. **AGE AT FIRST INTERCOURSE:**
   a. Before 15 (40)   b. 15-19 (30)   c. 20-24 (20)
   d. 25 and over (10)   e. Never had intercourse (5)
6. **BLEEDING BETWEEN PERIODS OR AFTER INTERCOURSE:**
   a. Yes (40)   b. No (1)
7. **SMOKER:**   Non-smoker (2)   b. Smoker (3)

SUBTOTAL _____

REDUCING YOUR RISK

8. I have had a negative Pap smear and pelvic examination within the past year. (Subtract 50 points.)

TOTAL _____

ENDOMETRIAL CANCER

(Body of Uterus) — These questions do not apply to a woman who has had a total hysterectomy.

1. **AGE GROUP:**   a. 39 or less (5)   b. 40-49 (20)   c. 50 and over (60)
2. **RACE:**   a. Oriental (10)   b. Black (10)   c. Hispanic (10)   d. White (20)
3. **BIRTHS:**   a. None (15)   b. 1 to 4 (7)   c. 5 or more (5)
4. **WEIGHT:**
   a. 50 or more pounds overweight (50)   b. 20-49 pounds overweight (15)
   c. Normal or underweight for height (10)
5. **DIABETES (elevated blood sugar):**   a. Yes (3)   b. No (1)
6. **ESTROGEN HORMONE INTAKE*:**
   a. Yes, regularly (15)   b. Yes, occasionally (12)   c. None (10)
7. **ABNORMAL UTERINE BLEEDING:**   a. Yes (40)   b. No (1)
8. **HYPERTENSION (high blood pressure):**   a. Yes (3)   b. No (1)

SUBTOTAL _____

REDUCING YOUR RISK

9. I have had a negative pelvic examination and Pap smear or endometrial tissue sampling (endometrial biopsy) performed within the past year. (Subtract 50 points.)

TOTAL _____

*NOTE: This excludes birth control pills.

continued

L U N G   A n s w e r s

1. Men have a higher risk of lung cancer than women. Since more women may also be smoking more, their incidence of lung and upper respiratory tract (mouth, tongue and voice box) cancer is increasing.
2. The occurrence of lung and upper respiratory tract cancer increases with age.
3. Cigarette smokers may have 20 times or even greater risk than nonsmokers. However, **the rates of ex-smokers who have not smoked for ten years approach those of nonsmokers.**
4. Pipe and cigar smokers are at a higher risk for lung cancer than nonsmokers. Cigarette smokers are also at a much higher risk for lung cancer than nonsmokers or than pipe and cigar smokers. All forms of tobacco, including chewing or dipping, markedly increase the user's risk of developing cancer of the mouth.
5. Male smokers of less than ½ pack per day have a five times higher lung cancer rate than nonsmokers. Male smokers of 1-2 packs per day have a 15 times higher lung cancer rate than nonsmokers. Smokers of more than 2 packs per day are 20 times more likely to develop lung cancer than nonsmokers.
6. Smokers of low tar/nicotine cigarettes have slightly lower lung cancer rates. Please note however that smokers of low tar/nicotine cigarettes may unconsciously smoke in a manner that **increases** their exposure to these chemicals.
7. The frequency of lung and upper respiratory tract cancer increases with the duration of smoking.
8. Exposures to materials used in these and other industries have been shown to be associated with lung cancer, especially in smokers.

If your total is:

24 or less...... You have a low risk for lung cancer.

25-49...... You may be a light smoker and would have a good chance of kicking the habit.

50-74...... As a moderate smoker, your risks of lung and upper respiratory tract cancer are increased. The time to stop is now!

75-over...... As a heavy cigarette smoker, your chances of getting lung cancer and cancer of the upper respiratory or digestive tract are greatly increased.

REDUCING YOUR RISK — Make a decision to quit today. Join a smoking cessation program. If you are a heavy drinker of alcohol, your risks for cancer of the head and neck and esophagus are further increased. Use of "smokeless" tobacco increases your risks of cancer of the mouth. Your best bet is not to use tobacco in any form. See your doctor if you have a nagging cough, hoarseness, persistent pain or sore in the mouth or throat or lumps in the neck.

C O L O N   R E C T U M   A n s w e r s

1. Colon cancer occurs more often after the age of 50.
2. Colon cancer is more common in families with a previous history of this disease.
3. Polyps and bowel diseases are associated with colon cancer. Cancer of the breast, ovaries or stomach may also be associated with an increased risk of colon cancer.
4. Rectal bleeding may be a sign of colon/rectum cancer.

I. **RISK FACTORS* — If your total is:**

5 or less...... You are currently at low risk for colon and rectum cancer. Eat a diet high in fiber and low in fat and follow cancer checkup guidelines.

6-15...... You are currently at moderate risk for colon and rectum cancer. Follow the American Cancer Society guidelines for early detection of colorectal cancer. These are: (1) a digital rectal exam** every year after 40 and (2) a stool blood test every year and a sigmoidoscopic exam every 3 - 5 years after age 50.

16 or greater...... You are in the high risk group for colon and rectum cancer. This rating requires a life-time, on-going screening program that includes periodic evaluation of your entire colon. See your doctor for more information.

* If your answers to any of these questions change, you should REASSESS YOUR RISK.

II. **SYMPTOMS** — The presence of rectal bleeding or a change in bowel habits may indicate colon/rectum cancer. See your physician right away if you have either of these symptoms.

III. ### REDUCING YOUR RISKS AND DETECTING CANCER EARLY — Regular tests for hidden blood in the stool and appropriate examinations of the colon will increase the likelihood that colon polyps are discovered and removed early and that cancers are found in an early, curable state. Modifying your diet to include more fiber, cruciferous vegetables, and foods rich in Vitamin A; and less fat and salt-cured foods may result in a reduction of cancer risk.

** This test has an additional advantage in that it is also an early detection method for cancer of the prostate in men.

B R E A S T   A n s w e r s

If your total is:

Under 100...... Low risk women (and all others). You should practice monthly Breast Self-Examination, have your breasts examined by a doctor as part of a regular cancer-related checkup, and have mammography in accordance with ACS guidelines.

100-199...... Moderate risk women. You should practice monthly BSE and have your breasts examined by a doctor as part of a cancer-related checkup, and have periodic mammography in accordance with American Cancer Society guidelines, or more frequently as your physician advises.

200 or higher...... High risk. You should practice monthly BSE and have your breasts examined by a doctor, and have mammography more often. See your doctor for the recommended frequency of breast physical examinations and mammography.

REDUCING YOUR RISK — One in 10 American women will get breast cancer in her lifetime. Being a woman is a risk factor! Most women (75%) who get breast cancer don't have other risk factors. BSE and mammography may diagnose a breast cancer in its earliest stage with a greatly increased chance of cure. When detected at this stage, cure is more likely and breast-saving surgery may be an option.

continued

SKIN   Answers

1. The sun's rays are more intense the closer one lives to the equator.
2. Excessive ultraviolet light from the sun causes cancer of the skin.
3. These materials can cause cancer of the skin.
4. Persons with light complexions are at greater risk for skin cancer.
5. A severe sunburn while growing up may increase one's risk for melanoma.
6. A tendency to have pre-cancerous moles or melanomas may occur in certain families.
7. Persons with a previous skin cancer or melanoma are at increased risk for developing a skin cancer or melanoma.
8. Tanning beds use a type of ultraviolet ray which adds to the skin damage caused by the sun, contributing to skin cancer formation.
9. Any change in a mole may be a sign of melanoma.

The key is if you answered "yes" to any of the first nine questions, you need to use protective clothing and use a sun screen with an SPF rating of 15 or greater whenever you are out in the sun and check yourself monthly for any changes in warts or moles. An answer of "yes" to questions 10, 11, and 12 can help reduce your risk of skin cancer.

REDUCING YOUR RISK — Numerical risks for skin cancer are difficult to state. For instance, a person with dark complexion can work longer in the sun and be less likely to develop cancer than a person with a light complexion. Furthermore, a person wearing a long-sleeved shirt and wide-brimmed hat may work in the sun and be at less risk than a person who wears a bathing suit for only a short time. The risk for skin cancer goes up greatly with age.
Melanoma, the most serious type of skin cancer, can be cured when it is detected and treated at a very early stage. Changes in warts or moles are important and should be checked by your doctor. For more information, ask for the American Cancer Society pamphlet, "Melanoma/Skin Cancer, You Can Recognize the Signs."

CERVICAL   Answers

1. The numbers represent the relative risks for invasive cancer in different age groups. The highest incidence of invasive cancer is among women over 40 years of age. However, abnormal changes and early noninvasive cancers occur more commonly in the 20's and 30's age groups. These early changes can be found with the Pap test.
2. Puerto Ricans, Blacks, and Mexican Americans have higher rates of cervical cancer.
3. Women who have delivered more children have a higher occurrence.
4. Viral infections of the cervix and vagina are associated with cervical cancer.
5. Women with earlier age at first intercourse and with more sexual partners are at a higher risk.
6. Irregular bleeding may be a sign of uterine cancer.

   If your total is:
   40-69...... This is a low risk group. Ask your doctor for a Pap test and advice about frequency of subsequent testing.
   70-99...... In this moderate risk group, more frequent Pap tests may be required.
   100 or more...... You are in a high risk group and should have a Pap test (and pelvic exam) as advised by your doctor.

REDUCING YOUR RISK — Early detection of this cancer by the Pap test has markedly improved the chance of cure. When this cancer is found at an early stage, the cure rate is extremely high and uterus-saving surgery and child-bearing potential may be preserved.

ENDOMETRIAL   Answers

1. Endometrial cancer is seen among women in older age groups. Numbers in parentheses by the age groups represent approximate relative rates of endometrial cancer at different ages.
2. Caucasians have a higher occurrence.
3. The fewer children one has delivered the greater the risk of endometrial cancer.
4. Women who are overweight are at greater risk.
5. Cancer of the endometrium is associated with diabetes.
6. Cancer of the endometrium may be associated with prolonged continuous estrogen hormone intake which occurs in only a small number of women. You should consult your physician before starting or stopping any estrogen medication. The medical use of estrogen in combination with progesterone does not appear to increase risk and may have other health benefits in this case.
7. Women who do not have cyclic regular menstrual periods are at greater risk. Any bleeding after menopause may be a sign of this cancer.
8. Cancer of the endometrium is associated with high blood pressure.

   If your total is:
   45-59...... You are at very low risk for developing endometrial cancer.
   60-99...... Your risks are slightly higher. Report any abnormal bleeding immediately to your doctor. Tissue sampling at menopause is recommended.
   100 and over...... Your risks are much greater. See your doctor for tests as appropriate.

REDUCING YOUR RISK — Once again, early detection is a key to your chance of a cure for this cancer. Regular pelvic examinations may find other female cancers such as cancer of the ovary.

continued

LABORATORY

YOUR TEST SCORES

Check your own risks with the answers contained in this folder. Individual numbers for specific questions are not to be interpreted as a precise measure of relative risk, but the totals for a given site should give you a general indication of your risk.

Additional educational information is available from your American Cancer Society.

1-800-ACS-2345

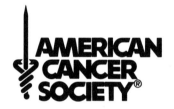

You are advised to discuss this folder with your physician if you are at high risk.

LAB 8

Are You at Risk for Diabetes?

Write in the points next to each statement that is *true* for you. If a statement is *not true* for you, put a zero. Then add up your total score.

1. I have been experiencing one or more of the following symptoms on a regular basis:
   - excessive thirst   Yes 3 _____
   - frequent urination   Yes 3 _____
   - extreme fatigue   Yes 1 _____
   - unexplained weight loss   Yes 3 _____
   - blurry vision from time to time Yes 2 _____

2. I am over 30 years old.   Yes 1 _____

3. My weight is equal to or above that listed in the chart. Yes 2 _____

4. I am a woman who has had more than one baby weighing over 9 lbs. at birth. Yes 2 _____

5. I am of American Indian descent. Yes 1 _____

6. I am of Hispanic or Black American descent. Yes 1 _____

7. I have a parent with diabetes.   Yes 1 _____

8. I have a brother or sister with diabetes. Yes 2 _____

Total _____

Weight Chart
(shows 20% over maximum weight)

Height (without shoes)		Weight in Pounds (without clothing)	
Feet	Inches	Women	Men
4	9	127	
4	10	131	
4	11	134	
5	0	138	
5	1	142	146
5	2	146	151
5	3	151	155
5	4	157	158
5	5	162	163
5	6	167	168
5	7	172	174
5	8	176	179
5	9	181	184
5	10	186	190
5	11		196
6	0		202
6	1		208
6	2		214
6	3		220

These charts show weights that are 20% heavier than the maximum recommended for both men and women with a medium frame. If your weight is at or above the amount listed for your height, you may be at risk for developing diabetes.

Scoring 3–5 points:
If you scored 3–5 points, you probably are at low risk for diabetes. But don't just forget about it. Especially if you're over 30, overweight, or of Black American, Hispanic, or american Indian descent.

What to do about it:
Be sure you know the symptoms of diabetes. If you experience any of them, contact your doctor for further testing.

Scoring over 5 points:
If you scored over 5 points, you may be at high risk for diabetes. You even may already have diabetes.

What to do about it:
See your doctor promptly. Find out if you have diabetes. Even if you don't have diabetes, know the symptoms. If you experience any of them in the future, you should see your doctor immediately.

The American Diabetes Association urges all pregnant women to be tested for diabetes between the 24th–28th weeks of pregnancy.

This test is meant to educate and make you aware of the serious risks of diabetes. Only a medical doctor can determine if you do have diabetes.

Check with your local American Diabetes Association chapter or affiliate for more information about diabetes, healthy eating, and exercise. (Numbers are listed in the White pages of the phone book.)

LAB 9

Exercise, Health Risks, and Aging Changes

A 16-year study of 16,936 Harvard alumni aged 35–74 revealed that those who spent between 1500 and 2000 calories per week doing something active were significantly healthier, had fewer heart attacks, and lived longer than those who were more sedentary. There was some additional reduction in death rates among those who spent up to 3500 calories per week, but beyond that, death rates actually increased slightly. Even among those who spent only 500–1500 calories per week, there was some reduction in death rate compared to those who spent less than 500 calories per week.*

A listing of activities a 150-lb person could do to accrue 1800 calories in one week is shown below. As you can see, marathon efforts are not necessary on any day to accumulate 1800 calories, and in fact household chores such as gardening, washing the car, mowing the lawn, and even house cleaning (done as if company were coming in an hour) contribute to the total.

Your task is to keep a record for one week of all the active things you do, and how long you do them. At the end of the week, consult a calorie expenditure table for the number of calories you expended per activity. Add these together to get your "active expenditure" per day and then per week. Calorie expenditure tables can be found in many nutrition and exercise-related texts (and in Appendix 4 of this textbook).

If your caloric expenditure is below what seems desirable to you given the information in the opening paragraph of this worksheet, you simply need to add to your life some new, active things you enjoy doing. As a guide to the type of activities you might want to consider, see Lab 10, "What Am I Using/What Am I Losing?"

If you were pleased with your weekly expenditure total, Lab 10 should help you determine if the kinds of activities you are doing are providing all the benefits you want for yourself now and in the future.

THE EASY ROAD TO FITNESS

DAY	ACTIVITY	CALORIES
Monday	Brisk walking, to and from work, 30 minutes Stair climbing, 5 minutes	160 35
Tuesday	Cycling, stationary, 15 minutes (10 mph)	105
Wednesday	Brisk walking, to and from work, 30 minutes	160
Thursday	30 minutes at gym: Stair climbing, fast, 10 minutes Rowing, on machine, 10 minutes Running, treadmill, 10 minutes	85 65 95
Friday	Swimming, 20 minutes Cycling, 20 minutes	180 135
Saturday	Brisk walking, 30 minutes Gardening, 20 minutes Housecleaning, 20 minutes	160 110 80
Sunday	Brisk walking, 15 minutes Mowing lawn, 20 minutes Raking grass and yard work, 20 minutes Washing car, 20 minutes	80 150 135 65
GRAND TOTAL (150-lb person)		1800 (in about 5 hours)

Excerpted from the University of California, Berkeley *Wellness Letter*, Health Letter Associates, 1992. Used by permission.

*R. Paffenbarger, et al. 1986. "Physical Activity, All-Cause Mortality, and Longevity of College Alumni." *New England Journal of Medicine* 314: 605–613.

LAB 9 Continued.

LABORATORY

DAY	ACTIVITY	CALORIES
Monday		
Tuesday		
Wednesday		
Thursday		
Friday		
Saturday		
Sunday		
GRAND TOTAL		

LAB 10

What Am I Using/What Am I Losing?

There is absolutely no question about it: The human body thrives on use and deteriorates with disuse. No pill or anti-aging therapy currently known has the power of exercise to maintain vigor and vitality with age. So as each day goes by, the issue truly is: What are we using, and what are we losing? This worksheet will help you determine if you are using everything today that you would like to be using in the future.

Directions: Indicate any **deliberate** attempt to exercise the muscles or muscle groups listed below by recording in the appropriate box the type of activity/exercise and how long you did it.

BODY PART	MON	TUES	WED	THURS	FRI	SAT	SUN
Arms							
Legs							
Abdominals							
Back							
Heart							
Most strenuous activity today (List activity and give heart rate)							

LAB 12

Calculating Target Heart Rate Zone

PURPOSE:

Knowing your target heart rate zone will enable you to monitor your aerobic exercise intensity safely and effectively. Working within your zone has been found to result in optimal improvement in cardiovascular fitness.

DIRECTIONS:

1. Determine your predicted maximum heart rate:

   220 – age = _____ b/min
   (predicted max HR)

2. Determine your resting heart rate under truly resting conditions:

   resting heart rate = _____ b/min

3. Estimate your heart rate reserve as follows:

   maximum heart rate – resting heart rate = _____ beats
   (HR reserve)

4. Calculate:

   .5 (HR Reserve) = _____ beats

   .85 (HR Reserve) = _____ beats

5. Calculate your minimum target heart rate:

   .5 (HR Reserve) + resting HR = _____ b/min
   (minimum target HR)

6. Calculate your maximum target heart rate:

   .85 (HR Reserve) + resting HR = _____ b/min
   (maximum target HR)

(See Figure 5.6 on page 91 for an example.)

Source: American College of Sports Medicine. 1990. "Position Stand: The Recommended Quantity and Quality of Exercise for Developing and Maintaining Cardiorespiratory and Muscular Fitness in Healthy Adults." *Medicine & Science in Sports and Exercise* 22(3): 265–274.

LAB 13

Warm-Up/Cool-Down Routine

WARM-UP

As a general rule, any exercise program should begin with a warm-up lasting 5–10 minutes. You should begin to move slowly and gently at first, the goal being to raise your core temperature and the temperature of your muscles and joints. Toward the latter part of the warm-up, you can elect to increase the intensity of exercise. Several examples are given below to illustrate how to personalize your warm-up:

Warm-up for a running program:

1. Begin by walking slowly for 5 minutes.
2. Increase the pace to a fast walk that moves gradually into a slow jog for the next 5 minutes.

Note: A similar procedure can be used to warm up for swimming, cycling, skiing, rowing, and like activities.

Warm-up for a weight-lifting program:

1. Begin by walking slowly for 5 minutes.
2. For each muscle group you plan to use, begin lifting very low weights for several repetitions before attempting heavier weights.

Warm-up for general fitness program:

1. Begin by performing the target activity gently for 5 minutes.
2. Follow by performing gentle exercises for the next 5–10 minutes.

COOL-DOWN

In general, cool-down activities should be performed for 5–10 minutes following vigorous exercise. Engaging in cool-down activities hastens recovery, prevents blood pooling in the lower extremities (which can lead to lightheadedness), and puts less strain on the heart during recovery.

The most common procedure is to continue doing the activity at a very slow pace. For example, runners walk around, cyclers pedal easily, swimmers stroke easily, before heading for the shower or other activities. Do not stand still.

Following cool-down is a good time to engage in stretching exercises to enhance flexibility, because muscle and connective tissue are more receptive to stretching when warm.

LAB 15

Rockport Walk Test

PURPOSE:

This test will enable you to determine your cardiovascular endurance in a simple submaximal field test that you can repeat at intervals to document your progress. Also, you will be able to predict your maximum oxygen consumption (VO_2 max) and compare it to gender- and age-specific norms.

DIRECTIONS:

1. After an adequate warm-up of 5–10 minutes, complete a 1-mile walk on a measured track as fast as you can, and record the elapsed time.
2. Within 5 seconds of completing the walk, take a 10-second pulse count, and multiply by 6 to determine your pulse rate in beats/minute.
3. Calculate your VO_2 max in ml/kg/min, using the formula below:
$$VO_2 \text{ max} = 132.853 - 0.0769(BW) - 0.3877(age) + 6.3150(sex) - 3.2649(T) - 0.1565(HR)$$
where: BW = body weight in pounds
     age = age in years
     sex = 0 for females, 1 for males
     T = time for 1-mile track walk in minutes and hundredths
    HR = heart rate in beats/min at the end of the walk

(*Note:* The error associated with the prediction of VO_2 max is 5 ml/kg/min, which means that approximately 68% of persons actually will have their true VO_2 max within ±5 ml/kg/min of their predicted value on this test.)

4. Use the table provided to determine how fit you are with regard to maximal oxygen consumption.
5. Use the Summary at the end of this lab to keep track of changes in your cardiovascular endurance.

RESULTS:

1. Walk time: minutes: seconds _____   minutes: hundredths _____

2. Immediate postexercise heart rate:

   _____ beats/10 sec × 6 = _____ beats/minute

3. VO_2 max =   132.853 =   132.853

            − 0.0769 (   ) = − _____

            − 0.3877 (   ) = − _____

            + 6.3150 (   ) = + _____

            − 3.2649 (   ) = − _____

            − 0.1565 (   ) = − _____

                          = _____ ml/kg/min.

   (*Note:* use time in minutes, and hundredths only.)

4. Fitness Category: _____ (Refer to the table for age- and gender-specific norms.)

continued

TABLE 1 Aerobic capacity norms based on age and gender.

			MAXIMAL OXYGEN CONSUMPTION (ml/kg/min)				
	Excellent	*Very good*	*Good*	*Average*	*Fair*	*Poor*	*Very poor*
Women							
20	53	47–52	43–51	37–42	33–36	27–32	26
30	47	44–46	38–43	34–37	30–33	25–29	24
40	42	38–41	34–37	30–33	26–29	22–25	21
50	37	34–36	30–33	26–29	23–25	19–22	18
60	31	28–30	25–27	22–24	19–21	16–18	15
70	26	24–25	21–23	18–20	15–17	13–14	12
Men							
20	64	56–63	51–55	45–50	38–44	32–37	31
30	57	52–56	46–51	41–45	35–40	29–34	28
40	53	47–51	42–45	37–41	32–36	27–31	26
50	47	42–46	37–41	33–36	28–32	24–27	23
60	42	37–42	34–36	28–33	25–27	21–24	20
70	36	32–35	28–31	25–27	22–24	18–21	17

Adapted from "Aerobic Fitness Norms for Males and Females Aged 6 to 75 Years: A Review," by E. Shrantz and R. C. Reibold, 1990, *Aviation, Space and Environmental Medicine* 61: 3–11.

SUMMARY:

Date	$\dot{V}O_2$ max	Percentile
_____	_____	_____
_____	_____	_____
_____	_____	_____

LAB 16

Cooper 12-Minute Run

PURPOSE:

This lab provides you with an opportunity to determine your current level of cardiovascular fitness using an endurance run. As little technical equipment is required, you can repeat this test on any track at intervals of your own choosing to see what improvements you achieve as you continue your exercise program.

Note: Because of its difficulty, this test should not be completed unless you have moderate aerobic fitness or better or if you have been training aerobically for 1–2 months or more.

DIRECTIONS:

1. Begin with an adequate warm-up for 5–10 minutes.
2. Count the number of full laps plus fractions of lap completed in 12 minutes. If you are unable to complete the test by running continuously for the full 12 minutes, you may run/walk. Refer to Figure 1 and Table 1 to change the number of laps; both full and partial, into the distance covered.

   a. Type of track (check one): ¼ mile _____ ⅛ mile _____

   b. Number of full laps: _____ Equivalent distance _____

   c. Partial lap (letter circled on track diagram): _____ Equivalent distance _____

   d. Total distance completed (add b + c) _____

3. Based on your distance completed and the norms in Tables 2 and 3, determine your fitness category:
   _____ *(see Tables 2 (men) or 3 (women))*

DISTANCE CALCULATIONS

FIGURE 1   Track diagram.

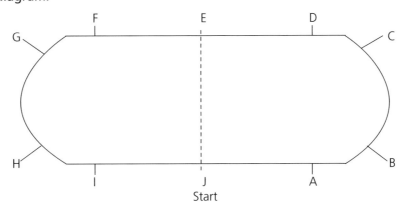

Note: Each letter represents ¹/₁₀ of a lap.

continued

TABLE 1   Conversion of laps to distance.

NUMBER OF FULL LAPS	DISTANCE (MILES) 1/8 MI. TRACK	DISTANCE (MILES) 1/4 MI. TRACK	PARTIAL LAPS	DISTANCE (MILES) 1/8 MI. TRACK	DISTANCE (MILES) 1/4 MI. TRACK
1	.125	.25			
2	.25	.5	A	.0125	.025
3	.375	.75			
4	.5	1.0	B	.025	.05
5	.625	1.25			
6	.75	1.5	C	.0375	.075
7	.875	1.75			
8	1.0	2.0	D	.05	.10
9	1.125	2.25			
10	1.25	2.5	E	.0625	.125
11	1.375				
12	1.5		F	.075	.150
13	1.625				
14	1.75		G	.0875	.175
15	1.875				
16	2.0		H	.10	.20
17	2.125				
18	2.25		I	.1125	.225

TABLE 2   12-Minute Test for Men (distance in miles covered in 12 minutes).

FITNESS CATEGORY	AGE 13–19	20–29	30–39	40–49	50–59	60 +
Very Poor	<1.30	<1.22	<1.18	<1.14	<1.03	<0.87
Poor	1.30–1.37	1.22–1.31	1.18–1.30	1.14–1.24	1.03–1.16	0.87–1.02
Fair	1.30–1.56	1.32–1.49	1.31–1.49	1.25–1.39	1.17–1.30	1.03–1.20
Good	1.57–1.72	1.50–1.64	1.46–1.56	1.40–1.53	1.31–1.44	1.21–1.32
Excellent	1.73–1.86	1.65–1.76	1.57–1.69	1.54–1.65	1.45–1.58	1.33–1.55
Superior	>1.87	>1.77	>1.70	>1.66	>1.59	>1.56

Note: < means "less than," > means "more than"

TABLE 3   12-Minute Test for Women (distance in miles covered in 12 minutes).

FITNESS CATEGORY	AGE 13–19	20–29	30–39	40–49	50–59	60 +
Very Poor	<1.00	<0.96	<0.94	<0.88	<0.84	<0.78
Poor	1.00–1.18	0.96–1.11	0.95–1.05	0.88–0.98	0.84–0.93	0.78–0.86
Fair	1.19–1.29	1.12–1.22	1.06–1.18	0.99–1.11	0.94–1.05	0.87–0.98
Good	1.30–1.43	1.23–1.34	1.19–1.29	1.12–1.24	1.06–1.18	0.99–1.09
Excellent	1.44–1.57	1.35–1.45	1.30–1.39	1.25–1.34	1.19–1.30	1.10–1.18
Superior	>1.58[a]	>1.46	>1.40	>1.35	>1.31	>1.19

Note: < means "less than," > means "more than"

Source: Tables 2 and 3 are from *The Aerobics Program for Total Well-Being.* Kenneth H. Cooper, M.D., M.P.H. Copyright © 1982 by Kenneth H. Cooper. Used by permission of Bantam Books, a division of Bantam Doubleday Dell Publishing Group, Inc.

LAB 18

Strength Tests

STATIC STRENGTH: THE GRIP TEST

DIRECTIONS:

1. Using a grip dynamometer (pictured below), adjust the grip size to fit your hand comfortably. Squeeze as hard as you can for 1–2 seconds. Your strength score will be registered on the device.
2. Repeat after a 1–2 minute rest, and then follow the same procedure for your other hand.
3. Compute an average for each hand and then the sum of the averages.
4. Use Table 1 to determine your percentile ranking based on your gender and age.

	Trial 1	Trial 2	Trial 3	Average
Date: _____				
Left hand	_____	_____	_____	_____
Right hand	_____	_____	_____	_____
Sum of averages				_____
Percentile				_____

continued

LAB 18   Continued.

TABLE 1   Norms and percentiles by age groups and sex for combined righthand and lefthand grip strength (kg)

AGE	15–19		20–29		30–39		40–49		50–59		60–69	
SEX	M	F	M	F	M	F	M	F	M	F	M	F
Excellent	⩾ 113	⩾ 71	⩾ 124	⩾ 71	⩾ 123	⩾ 73	⩾ 119	⩾ 73	⩾ 110	⩾ 65	⩾ 102	⩾ 60
Above Average	130–112	64–70	113–123	65–70	113–122	66–72	110–118	65–72	102–109	59–64	93–191	54–59
Average	95–102	59–63	106–112	61–64	105–112	61–65	109–109	59–64	96–101	55–58	86–92	51–53
Below Average	84–94	54–58	97–105	55–60	97–104	56–60	94–101	55–58	87–95	51–54	79–85	48–50
Weak	⩽ 83	⩽ 53	⩽ 96	⩽ 54	⩽ 96	⩽ 55	⩽ 93	⩽ 54	⩽ 86	⩽ 50	⩽ 78	⩽ 47

AGE (YRS.)	15–19		20–29		30–39		40–49		50–59		60–69	
SEX	M	F	M	F	M	F	M	F	M	F	M	F
Percentiles												
95	125	78	136	78	135	80	128	80	119	72	111	67
90	119	74	127	74	127	76	123	76	114	69	106	62
85	113	71	124	71	123	73	119	73	110	65	102	60
80	110	69	120	70	120	71	117	71	108	63	99	58
75	108	67	118	68	117	69	115	69	105	62	96	56
70	105	65	115	67	115	68	112	67	103	60	94	55
65	103	64	113	65	113	66	110	65	102	59	93	54
60	101	63	111	64	111	65	108	64	100	58	91	53
55	99	61	109	63	109	63	106	62	99	57	89	52
50	97	60	107	62	107	62	104	61	97	56	88	52
45	95	59	106	61	105	61	102	59	96	55	86	51
40	93	58	104	59	104	60	100	58	94	54	84	50
35	90	57	102	58	101	59	98	57	92	53	82	49
30	87	56	100	56	99	58	96	56	90	53	81	49
25	84	54	97	55	97	56	94	55	87	51	79	48
20	81	53	95	53	94	55	91	53	85	50	76	47
15	77	51	91	52	91	53	89	51	83	48	73	45
10	73	49	87	50	87	51	84	49	80	46	69	43
5	67	45	81	47	81	48	76	46	74	42	62	39

Source: Canada Fitness Survey 1981, from *Standardized Tests of Fitness,* 2d edition, Fitness and Amateur Sport, Quebec, Canada, 1981.

continued

DYNAMIC STRENGTH: ONE REPETITION MAXIMUM TEST

DIRECTIONS:

1. After a sufficient warm-up—including warming up the specific muscle group you are about to measure using easy repetitions with a light weight—guess a weight you think is close to your maximum. If you find you can lift it easily, then after a rest period of a few minutes, adjust the next trial upward accordingly and try again. Making adjustments upward or downward as necessary, you should be able to determine your 1 RM in five trials or fewer, as reliability decreases after too many trials.

    You may use free weights or weight machines for this measurement. Weight machines are of many different types; no one brand is necessarily better than another, and the technique for measuring strength is the same with all of them.

2. Record your maximum weight for one repetition in the appropriate space below.

SUMMARY

	Result (lbs)			
Date	Bench Press	Standing Press	Curl	Leg Press
_____	_____	_____	_____	_____
_____	_____	_____	_____	_____
_____	_____	_____	_____	_____
_____	_____	_____	_____	_____

3. The norms given in Tables 2 through 5* are broken into age categories for adults of both sexes. They are applicable only to 1 RM tests for the *bench press exercise* and the *leg press exercise* on a Universal Gym machine. To standardize the norms for body weight, divide your strength score in pounds by your body weight, and then compare it to the appropriate table and age category.

*Norms are used with permission from the Institute for Aerobics Research, 12330 Preston Rd., Dallas, TX 75230.

continued

TABLE 2   Absolute strength: 1 repetition maximum bench press: Female.*

BENCH PRESS-WEIGHT RATIO $\dfrac{\text{WEIGHT PUSHED IN LBS.}}{\text{BODY WEIGHT IN LBS.}}$

%	< 20	20–29	30–39	40–49	50–59	60 +	
			AGE				
99	> .88	> 1.01	> .82	> .77	> .68	> .72	S
95	.88	1.01	.82	.77	.68	.72	
90	.83	.90	.76	.71	.61	.64	
85	.81	.83	.72	.66	.57	.59	E
80	.77	.80	.70	.62	.55	.54	
75	.76	.77	.65	.60	.53	.53	
70	.74	.74	.63	.57	.52	.51	G
65	.70	.72	.62	.55	.50	.48	
60	.65	.70	.60	.54	.48	.46	
55	.64	.68	.58	.53	.47	.46	
50	.63	.65	.57	.52	.46	.45	F
45	.60	.63	.55	.51	.45	.44	
40	.57	.59	.53	.50	.44	.43	
35	.56	.58	.52	.48	.43	.41	
30	.56	.56	.51	.47	.42	.40	P
25	.55	.53	.49	.45	.41	.39	
20	.53	.51	.47	.43	.39	.39	
15	.52	.50	.45	.42	.38	.36	
10	.50	.480	.42	.38	.37	.33	VP
5	.41	.436	.39	.35	.305	.26	
1	< .41	< .436	< .39	< .35	< .305	< .26	
N	20	191	379	333	189	42	TOTAL 1154

TABLE 3   Absolute strength: 1 repetition maximum bench press: Male.*

BENCH PRESS-WEIGHT RATIO $\dfrac{\text{WEIGHT PUSHED IN LBS.}}{\text{BODY WEIGHT IN LBS.}}$

%	< 20	20–29	30–39	40–49	50–59	60 +	
			AGE				
99	> 1.76	> 1.63	> 1.35	> 1.20	> 1.05	> .94	S
95	1.76	1.63	1.35	1.20	1.05	.94	
90	1.46	1.48	1.24	1.10	.97	.89	
85	1.38	1.37	1.17	1.04	.93	.84	E
80	1.34	1.32	1.12	1.00	.90	.82	
75	1.29	1.26	1.08	.96	.87	.79	
70	1.24	1.22	1.04	.93	.84	.77	G
65	1.23	1.18	1.01	.90	.81	.74	
60	1.19	1.14	.98	.88	.79	.72	
55	1.16	1.10	.96	.86	.77	.70	
50	1.13	1.06	.93	.84	.75	.68	F
45	1.10	1.03	.90	.82	.73	.67	
40	1.06	.99	.88	.80	.71	.65	
35	1.01	.96	.86	.78	.70	.65	
30	.96	.93	.83	.76	.68	.63	P
25	.93	.90	.81	.74	.66	.60	
20	.89	.88	.78	.72	.63	.57	
15	.86	.84	.75	.69	.60	.56	
10	.81	.80	.71	.650	.57	.53	VP
5	.76	.72	.65	.590	.53	.49	
1	< .76	< .72	< .65	< .590	< .53	< .49	
N	60	425	1909	2090	1279	343	TOTAL 6106

*When using the Universal DVR machine, use the number on the *right* side of the weight plate to determine maximum lift.

continued

TABLE 4   Absolute strength: 1 repetition maximum leg press: Female.*

LEG PRESS-WEIGHT RATIO <u>WEIGHT PUSHED IN LBS.</u>
BODY WEIGHT IN LBS.

%	< 20	20–29	30–39	40–49	50–59	60 +	
99	> 1.88	> 1.98	> 1.68	> 1.57	> 1.43	> 1.43	S
95	1.88	1.98	1.68	1.57	1.43	1.43	
90	1.85	1.82	1.61	1.48	1.37	1.32	
85	1.81	1.76	1.52	1.40	1.31	1.25	E
80	1.71	1.68	1.47	1.37	1.25	1.18	
75	1.69	1.65	1.42	1.33	1.20	1.16	
70	1.65	1.58	1.39	1.29	1.17	1.13	G
65	1.62	1.53	1.36	1.27	1.12	1.08	
60	1.59	1.50	1.33	1.23	1.10	1.04	
55	1.51	1.47	1.31	1.20	1.08	.99	
50	1.45	1.44	1.27	1.18	1.05	.99	F
45	1.42	1.40	1.24	1.15	1.02	.97	
40	1.38	1.37	1.21	1.13	.99	.93	
35	1.33	1.32	1.18	1.11	.97	.90	
30	1.29	1.27	1.15	1.08	.95	.90	P
25	1.25	1.26	1.12	1.06	.92	.86	
20	1.22	1.22	1.09	1.02	.88	.85	
15	1.19	1.18	1.05	.97	.84	.80	
10	1.09	1.14	1.0	.94	.78	.72	VP
5	1.06	.99	.96	.85	.72	.63	
1	< 1.06	< .99	< .96	< .85	< .72	< .63	
							TOTAL
N	20	192	381	337	192	44	1166

TABLE 5   Absolute strength: 1 repetition maximum leg press: Male.*

LEG PRESS-WEIGHT RATIO <u>WEIGHT PUSHED IN LBS.</u>
BODY WEIGHT IN LBS.

%	< 20	20–29	30–39	40–49	50–59	60 +	
99	> 2.82	> 2.40	> 2.20	> 2.02	> 1.90	> 1.80	S
95	2.82	2.40	2.20	2.02	1.90	1.80	
90	2.53	2.27	2.07	1.92	1.80	1.73	
85	2.40	2.18	1.99	1.86	1.75	1.68	E
80	2.28	2.13	1.93	1.82	1.71	1.62	
75	2.18	2.09	1.89	1.78	1.68	1.58	
70	2.15	2.05	1.85	1.74	1.64	1.56	G
65	2.10	2.01	1.81	1.71	1.61	1.52	
60	2.04	1.97	1.77	1.68	1.58	1.49	
55	2.01	1.94	1.74	1.65	1.55	1.46	
50	1.95	1.91	1.71	1.62	1.52	1.43	F
45	1.93	1.87	1.68	1.59	1.50	1.40	
40	1.90	1.83	1.65	1.57	1.46	1.38	
35	1.89	1.78	1.62	1.54	1.42	1.34	
30	1.82	1.74	1.59	1.51	1.39	1.30	P
25	1.80	1.68	1.56	1.48	1.36	1.27	
20	1.70	1.63	1.52	1.44	1.32	1.25	
15	1.61	1.58	1.48	1.40	1.28	1.21	
10	1.57	1.51	1.43	1.35	1.22	1.16	VP
5	1.46	1.42	1.34	1.27	1.15	1.08	
1	< 1.46	< 1.42	< 1.34	< 1.27	< 1.15	< 1.08	
							TOTAL
N	60	424	1909	2089	1286	347	6115

*When using the Universal DVR machine, use the number on the *right* side of the weight plate to determine maximum lift.

L53

LAB 20

Body Mass Index and Waist-to-Hip Ratio

PURPOSE:

Body mass index (BMI) often is used to determine relative risk from excess weight. It is not a measure of body composition but it is correlated highly to risk of death associated with excess fat. The ratio of your waist circumference to your hip circumference also is linked to greater risk for a number of diseases.

DIRECTIONS:

1. BMI = $\dfrac{wt_{kg}}{ht^2_m}$

   A simple method of calculating BMI is shown in Figure 1. Locate your height in the lefthand column and your weight at the bottom. Draw perpendicular lines from these points. At the point where the lines intersect, move upward along the nearest curved line to find body mass index.

RESULTS: Date: _____

My BMI: _____
   • Normal BMI is between 20 and 25.
   • Adults with a BMI in excess of 26 have an increase in health risk associated with obesity.

2. Waist/hip ratio

   Waist circumference: This is obtained with a tape measure placed around the natural waist (narrowest part of the torso as seen from the front).

   Hip circumference: This is obtained by placing the tape measure around the maximum extension of the buttocks as seen from the side.

   Note: To minimize error, both circumferences should be taken without clothing or over tight-fitting clothing.

RESULTS: Date: _____

My waist circumference: _____

My hip circumference:_____

My waist/hip ratio:_____

   A waist-to-hip ratio greater than .8 in women and .9 in men is associated with increased risk, independent of total weight.

SUMMARY:

Date	BMI	Waist/hip ratio
_____	_____	_____
_____	_____	_____
_____	_____	_____

continued

L
A
B
O
R
A
T
O
R
Y

FIGURE 1   Body mass index for specified heights and weights.

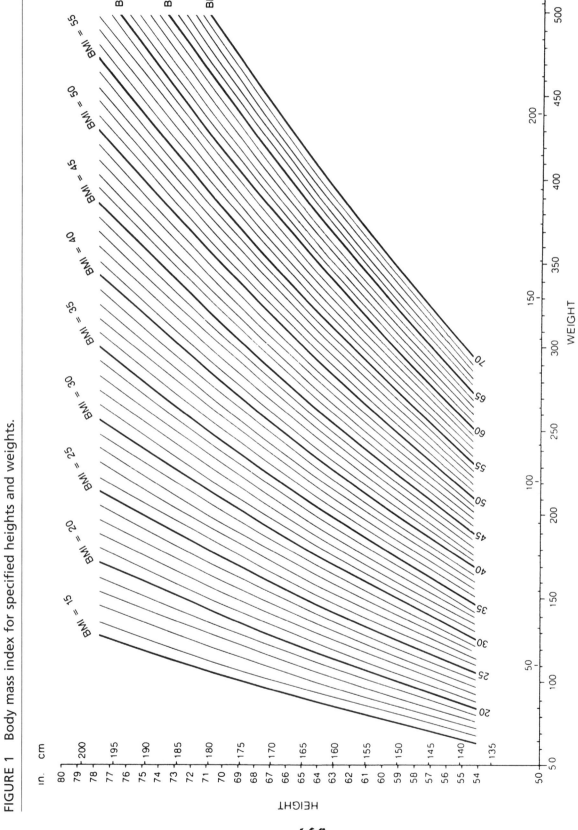

Source: Used by permission of H.M. Frankel, Portland Health Institute, Portland, OR.

LAB 21

Estimating Body Composition via Skinfold Fat

PURPOSE:

This technique involves measuring skinfold fat thickness at specific sites on the body and substituting the scores into an appropriate regression equation for predicting body density. The equations are different for each sex, and age is one of the variables. Once density is determined, another regression equation can be used to predict percent body fat.

Research has shown that skinfold thickness can be used to make predictions in the average individual, assuming that the measurements are taken by someone who is skilled in this technique. Even with a skillful technician, error is estimated to range between 4% and 5.5% fat because of assumptions not holding true for all individuals. Without a skillful technician, errors can be considerably larger. Therefore, if you elect to use this procedure, inquire about the background of the person measuring you. Note also that the limits of accuracy described above are most applicable for people who fall nearer the middle ranges of skinfold thickness. This means that for those who have extremely small or extremely large skinfold thicknesses, the errors can be larger than reported above.

DIRECTIONS:

1. Determine which three sites to use from the instructions given below. Photos a–e illustrate each of the sites and give a close-up view of the technique for measuring skinfold thickness:
   Male sites: (a) chest, (b) abdomen, (c) thigh
   Female sites: (d) triceps, (e) suprailiac, (c) thigh

2. Sum the three measurements. Tables 1 and 2 have been developed to simplify your calculations and require only the sum of your three measurements and your age to the nearest year. Your answer will be an estimate of your percent fat. The formulas used to develop these tables are as follows:

   Males: Density* = 1.0994921 − (0.0009929) (sum)
   + (0.0000023) (sum)^2 − 0.0001392 (age)

   Females: Density* = 1.1093800 − (0.0008267) (sum)
   + (0.0000016) (sum)^2 − 0.0002574 (age)

   where: sum = sum of your three skinfolds
   age = age in years

3. Once density is known, the Siri formula** is used to predict percent fat from density:

   percent fat = [(4.95/density) − 4.5][100]

Example: Assume Geoff, age 27 years and body weight 167 lbs., had his skinfold fat measured as follows:

   chest = 17 mm   abdomen = 18 mm   thigh = 22 mm

   percent fat = 16.5   (from Table 2)

   Fat weight = (% fat) x (body weight)
   ⎯⎯⎯⎯⎯⎯⎯⎯⎯
   100

---

*"Generalized Equations for Predicting Body Density of Men." 1978. A. S. Jackson and M. L. Pollock, *British Journal of Nutrition* 40: 497–504; and "Generalized Equations for Predicting Body Density of Women." 1980. A. S. Jackson, M. L. Pollock, and A. Ward, Medicine and Science Sports Exercise 12: 175–182.

**W. E. Siri. 1956. "Gross Composition of the Body." In *Advances in Biological and Medical Physics*, vol. 4, J. M. Lawrence and C. A. Tobias, (Eds.) New York: Academic Press.

continued

**L
A
B
O
R
A
T
O
R
Y**

$$= \frac{16.5}{100} \times (167 \text{ lbs}) = .165 \times (167) = 27.56 \text{ lbs}$$

Fat-free weight = (body weight) − (fat weight)

$$= 167 − 27.56 = 139.44 \text{ lbs}$$

Minimal weight $= \dfrac{\text{fat-free weight}}{1.0 − \dfrac{\text{(essential \% fat)*}}{100}}$

$$= \frac{139.44 \text{ lbs}}{1.0 − \dfrac{3}{100}} = \frac{139.44}{1.0 −.03} = \frac{139.44}{.97} = 143.75 \text{ lbs}$$

Storage fat = (body weight) − (minimal weight)

$$= 167 − 143.75 = 23.25 \text{ lbs}$$

Desired weight $= \dfrac{\text{fat-free weight}}{1.0 − \dfrac{\text{(desired \% fat)}}{100}}$

(at 15% fat) $= \dfrac{139.44 \text{ lbs}}{1.0 − \dfrac{15}{100}} = \dfrac{139.44}{1.0 − .15} = \dfrac{139.44}{.85} = 164.05 \text{ lbs}$

(at 10% fat) $= \dfrac{139.44 \text{ lbs}}{1.0 − \dfrac{10}{100}} = \dfrac{139.44}{1.0 −.10} = \dfrac{139.44}{.90} = 154.93 \text{ lbs}$

Therefore, assuming Geoff were to lose only fat weight from his 23.25 lbs of total storage fat, his weight loss would be:

(at 15% fat) 167 − 164.05 = 2.95 lbs

(at 10% fat) 167 − 154.93 = 12.07 lbs

*Essential fat is estimated to be 3%–5% for adult males and 8%–12% for adult females.

continued

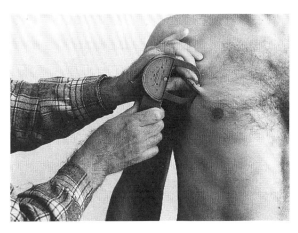

a

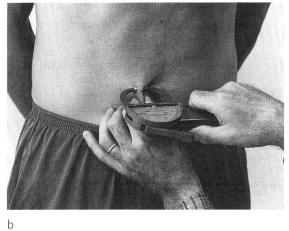

b

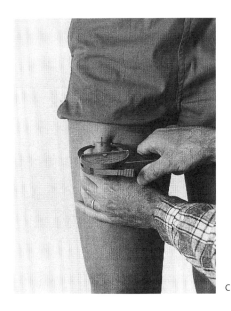

c

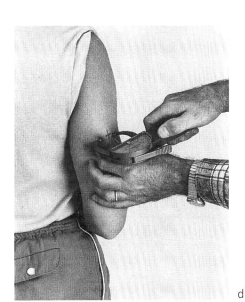

d

e

continued

L A B O R A T O R Y

TABLE 1 Percentage of body fat estimation from age and the sum of triceps, suprailium, and thigh skinfolds: Women.

SUM OF SKINFOLDS (MM)	AGE TO THE LAST YEAR								
	UNDER 22	23–27	28–32	33–37	38–42	43–47	48–52	53–57	OVER 58
23–25	9.7	9.9	10.2	10.4	10.7	10.9	11.2	11.4	11.7
26–28	11.0	11.2	11.5	11.7	12.0	12.3	12.5	12.7	13.0
29–31	12.3	12.5	12.8	13.0	13.3	13.5	13.8	14.0	14.3
32–34	13.6	13.8	14.0	14.3	14.5	14.8	15.0	15.3	15.5
35–37	14.8	15.0	15.3	15.5	15.8	16.0	16.3	16.5	16.8
38–40	16.0	16.3	16.5	16.7	17.0	17.2	17.5	17.7	18.0
41–43	17.2	17.4	17.7	17.9	18.2	18.4	18.7	18.9	19.2
44–46	18.3	18.6	18.8	19.1	19.3	19.6	19.8	20.1	20.3
47–49	19.5	19.7	20.0	20.2	20.5	20.7	21.0	21.2	21.5
50–52	20.6	20.8	21.1	21.3	21.6	21.8	22.1	22.3	22.6
53–55	21.7	21.9	22.1	22.4	22.6	22.9	23.1	23.4	23.6
56–58	22.7	23.0	23.2	23.4	23.7	23.9	24.2	24.4	24.7
59–61	23.7	24.0	24.2	24.5	24.7	25.0	25.2	25.5	25.7
62–64	24.7	25.0	25.2	25.5	25.7	26.0	26.7	26.4	26.7
65–67	25.7	25.9	26.2	26.4	26.7	26.9	27.2	27.4	27.7
68–70	26.6	26.9	27.1	27.4	27.6	27.9	28.1	28.4	28.6
71–73	27.5	27.8	28.0	28.3	28.5	28.8	28.0	29.3	29.5
74–76	28.4	28.7	28.9	29.2	29.4	29.7	29.9	30.2	30.4
77–79	29.3	29.5	29.8	30.0	30.3	30.5	30.8	31.0	31.3
80–82	30.1	30.4	30.6	30.9	31.1	31.4	31.6	31.9	32.1
83–85	30.9	31.2	31.4	31.7	31.9	32.2	32.4	32.7	32.9
86–88	31.7	32.0	32.2	32.5	32.7	32.9	33.2	33.4	33.7
89–91	32.5	32.7	33.0	33.2	33.5	33.7	33.9	34.2	34.4
92–94	33.2	33.4	33.7	33.9	34.2	34.4	34.7	34.9	35.2
85–97	33.9	34.1	34.4	34.6	34.9	35.1	35.4	35.6	35.9
98–100	34.6	34.8	35.1	35.3	35.5	35.8	36.0	36.3	36.5
101–103	35.3	35.4	35.7	35.9	36.2	36.4	36.7	36.9	37.2
104–106	35.8	36.1	36.3	36.6	36.8	37.1	37.3	37.5	37.8
107–109	36.4	36.7	36.9	37.1	37.4	37.6	37.9	38.1	38.4
110–112	37.0	37.2	37.5	37.7	38.0	38.2	38.5	38.7	38.9
113–115	37.5	37.8	38.0	38.2	38.5	38.7	39.0	39.2	39.5
116–118	38.0	38.3	38.5	38.8	39.0	39.3	39.5	39.7	40.0
119–121	38.5	38.7	39.0	39.2	39.5	39.7	40.0	40.2	40.5
122–124	39.0	39.2	39.4	39.7	39.9	40.2	40.4	40.7	40.9
125–127	39.4	39.6	39.9	40.1	40.4	40.6	40.9	41.1	41.4
128–130	39.8	40.0	40.3	40.5	40.8	41.0	41.3	41.5	41.8

Percentage of fat calculated by the formula of Siri. Percentage of fat = $[(4.95/Db) - 4.5] \times 100$, where Db = body density.

Source: "Measurement of Cardiorespiratory Fitness and Body Composition in the Clinical Setting." 1980. M. L. Pollock, D. H. Schmidt, and A. S. Jackson. *Comprehensive Therapy* 6(9):12–27. Used by permission of the Laux Company, Ayer, MA.

continued

TABLE 2   Percentage of body fat estimation from age and the sum of chest, abdominal, and thigh skinfolds: Men.

SUM OF SKINFOLDS (MM)	AGE TO THE LAST YEAR								
	UNDER 22	23–27	28–32	33–37	38–42	43–47	48–52	53–57	OVER 58
8–10	1.3	1.8	2.3	2.9	3.4	3.9	4.5	5.0	5.5
11–13	2.2	2.8	3.3	3.9	4.4	4.9	5.5	6.0	6.5
14–16	3.2	3.8	4.3	4.8	5.4	5.9	6.4	7.0	7.5
17–19	4.2	4.7	5.3	5.8	6.3	6.9	7.4	8.0	8.5
20–22	5.1	5.7	6.2	6.8	7.3	7.9	8.4	8.9	9.5
23–25	6.1	6.6	7.2	7.7	8.3	8.8	9.4	9.9	10.5
26–28	7.0	7.6	8.1	8.7	9.2	9.8	10.3	10.9	11.4
29–31	8.0	8.5	9.1	9.6	10.2	10.7	11.3	11.8	12.4
32–34	8.9	9.4	10.0	10.5	11.1	11.6	12.2	12.8	13.3
35–37	9.8	10.4	10.9	11.5	12.0	12.6	13.1	13.7	14.3
38–40	10.7	11.3	11.8	12.4	12.9	13.5	14.1	14.6	15.2
41–43	11.6	12.2	12.7	13.3	13.8	14.4	15.0	15.5	16.1
44–46	12.5	13.1	13.6	14.2	14.7	15.3	15.9	16.4	17.0
47–49	13.4	13.9	14.5	15.1	15.6	16.2	16.8	17.3	17.9
50–52	14.3	14.8	15.4	15.9	16.5	17.1	17.6	18.2	18.8
53–55	15.1	15.7	16.2	16.8	17.4	17.9	18.5	19.1	19.7
56–58	16.0	16.5	17.1	17.7	18.2	18.8	19.4	20.0	20.5
59–61	16.9	17.4	17.9	18.5	19.1	19.7	20.2	20.8	21.4
62–64	17.6	18.2	18.8	19.4	19.9	20.5	21.1	21.7	22.2
65–67	18.5	19.0	19.6	20.2	20.8	21.3	21.9	22.5	23.1
68–70	19.3	19.9	20.4	21.0	21.6	22.2	22.7	23.3	23.9
71–73	20.1	20.7	21.2	21.8	22.4	23.0	23.6	24.1	24.7
74–76	20.9	21.5	22.0	22.6	23.2	23.8	24.4	25.0	25.5
77–79	21.7	22.2	22.8	23.4	24.0	24.6	25.2	25.8	26.3
80–82	22.4	23.0	23.6	24.2	24.8	25.4	25.9	26.5	27.1
83–85	23.2	23.8	24.4	25.0	25.5	26.1	26.7	27.3	27.9
86–88	24.0	24.5	25.1	25.7	26.3	26.9	27.5	28.1	28.7
89–91	24.7	25.3	25.9	25.5	27.1	27.6	28.2	28.8	29.4
92–94	25.4	26.0	26.6	27.2	27.8	28.4	29.0	29.6	30.2
95–97	26.1	26.7	27.3	27.9	28.5	29.1	29.7	30.3	30.9
98–100	26.9	27.4	28.0	28.6	29.2	29.8	30.4	31.0	31.6
101–103	27.5	28.1	28.7	29.3	29.9	30.5	31.1	31.7	32.3
104–106	28.2	28.8	29.4	30.0	30.6	31.2	31.8	32.4	33.0
107–109	28.9	29.5	30.1	30.7	31.3	31.9	32.5	33.1	33.7
110–112	29.6	30.2	30.8	31.4	32.0	32.6	33.2	33.8	34.4
113–115	30.2	30.8	31.4	32.0	32.6	33.2	33.8	34.5	35.1
116–118	30.9	31.5	32.1	32.7	33.3	33.9	34.5	35.1	35.7
119–121	31.5	32.1	32.7	33.3	33.9	34.5	35.1	35.7	36.4
122–124	32.1	32.7	33.3	33.9	34.5	35.1	35.8	36.4	37.0
125–127	32.7	33.3	33.9	34.5	35.1	35.8	36.4	37.0	37.6

Percentage of fat calculated by the formula of Siri. Percentage of fat = $[(4.95/Db) - 4.5] \times 100$, where Db = body density.

Source: "Measurement of Cardiorespiratory Fitness and Body Composition in the Clinical Setting." 1980. M. L. Pollock, D. H. Schmidt, and A. S. Jackson. *Comprehensive Therapy* 6(9): 12–27. Used by permission of the Laux Company, Ayer, MA.

continued

NAME _____   SECTION _____   DATE _____

DATA SHEET

Age (years) _____   Body Weight (lbs)_____

Skinfold fat scores:

	TRIAL			
	1	2	3	Average
Female Measure 1: triceps	_____	_____	_____	_____
Measure 2: suprailiac	_____	_____	_____	_____
Measure 3: thigh	_____	_____	_____	_____
Sum of 3:				_____
Male Measure 1: chest	_____	_____	_____	_____
Measure 2: abdomen	_____	_____	_____	_____
Measure 3: thigh	_____	_____	_____	_____
Sum of 3:				_____

Percent fat _____ (from Table 1 or 2)

Fat weight (lbs) = $\dfrac{(\%fat)}{100}$ (body weight) = _____

Fat-free weight = (body weight) − (fat weight) = _____

Minimal weight (lbs): = $\dfrac{\text{fat-free weight}}{1.0 - \dfrac{\text{(essential fat)}}{100}}$ Desired weight = $\dfrac{\text{fat-free weight}}{1.0 - \dfrac{\text{(desired \%fat)}}{100}}$

$= \dfrac{\rule{2cm}{0.4pt}}{1.0 - \dfrac{(\_\_\_)}{100}} = \rule{2cm}{0.4pt}$ $= \dfrac{\rule{2cm}{0.4pt}}{1.0 - \dfrac{(\_\_\_)}{100}}$

$= \rule{2cm}{0.4pt}$

Note: essential fat for females = 8%–12% fat
males = 3%–5% fat

Storage fat = (body weight) − (minimal weight)

= _____ − _____ = _____

SUMMARY:

Date	Body Weight	% fat	Fat-free weight
_____	_____	_____	_____
_____	_____	_____	_____
_____	_____	_____	_____
_____	_____	_____	_____

LAB 22

Personalized Exercise Prescription

PURPOSE:

The following forms are designed to assist you in developing your personalized plan for exercise. Experience has shown that it is often helpful for people to identify their goals and plans in writing. The questions on this form will assist you in that process. To be successful, your plan of action must be something that you choose to engage in voluntarily, not something dictated to you from elsewhere.

MY LONG-TERM GOALS:

Where do I wish to be in 6 months with regard to regular exercise/fitness?

_____

_____

_____

_____

I plan to develop/maintain myself in the following areas of fitness (check those that apply):

_____ Cardiorespiratory
_____ Strength/Muscle Endurance
_____ Flexibility
_____ Body Composition

For each area that you intend to focus on, list briefly:

	CR Fitness Endurance	Strength/Muscular Endurance	Flexibility	Body Composition
Type of activity	_____ _____	_____ _____	_____ _____	_____ _____
Days/week (specify)	_____	_____	_____	_____
Location	_____ _____	_____ _____	_____ _____	_____ _____
Time of day	_____	_____	_____	_____

continued

**L
A
B
O
R
A
T
O
R
Y**

EXERCISE PRESCRIPTION SPECIFIC PROGRAM PLANS

For each area of fitness I plan to work on (describe specifically):

My warm-up activities: _____

_____

_____

   Duration:_____

My workout activity (describe): _____

_____

_____

_____

_____

_____

_____

_____

I plan to exercise the following number of times per week: _____

_____

My plans to set exercise intensity are (describe): _____

_____

_____

_____

Each session, I plan to exercise for: _____

_____

_____

_____

My cool-down activities will be:_____

_____

_____

   Duration:_____

Other plans: _____

_____

_____

_____

_____

_____

_____

continued

EVALUATING MY PROGRESS

Date: _____

Comments: _____

_____

_____

_____

_____

_____

_____

_____

Date: _____

Comments: _____

_____

_____

_____

_____

_____

_____

_____

Date: _____

Comments: _____

_____

_____

_____

_____

_____

_____

_____

L
A
B
O
R
A
T
O
R
Y

LAB 23

Exercise Log

This sample exercise log can be used to keep track of all your activities.

CHARTING MY EXERCISE BEHAVIOR

Date	Activity done	Duration	Personal notes

LABORATORY

Date	Activity done	Duration	Personal notes

LAB 25

Nutritional Assessment: Analyzing Your Diet

One of the more accurate techniques for analyzing your diet is the food diary. You simply record everything you eat, and the amounts, for a 24-hour period. If your dietary intake varies a lot from day to day, do this for a minimum of 3 days and preferably for an entire week. Once you have recorded your food intake for at least a day, you will need to determine the nutrient content of what you've eaten. You can do this by consulting the *Nutritive Value of Foods,* available in most libraries and from the Government Printing Office in Washington, D.C. You then can compare the nutrient quality of the foods you have eaten with the Recommended Dietary Allowances (RDAs) and the Dietary Goals for Americans. These comparisons will provide at least an indicator of how well you are eating to optimize body functioning and to minimize risk of chronic disease.

You also can compare the total calories you consume in a day with your caloric expenditure. This should help in analyzing present weight control and in preventing future weight problems. Instructions for calculating your daily caloric expenditure are given in Chapter 7. It would be best, of course, to calculate your expenditure for the same day or days you recorded your food intake. If done carefully, this should provide the most accurate estimate of your caloric expenditure. You can, however, estimate your expenditure using the formula shown in Table 1.

Inaccuracy in recording the amounts of food you eat greatly diminishes the value of the food diary. Before beginning your food diary, you may need some practice in estimating amounts of food. It is fairly easy to say how many slices of bread or how many bananas you have eaten, although even with these, sizes vary. An extra-thick slice of bread, for example, should be listed in your food diary as 1½ or 2 slices to indicate the quantity of bread accurately. Thus, you will have to pay close attention to the size of the item you consume. Estimating the amount of roast beef you eat in ounces, the amount of milk your favorite mug holds, or the amount of rice on your plate requires more than just close attention. You will have to have some idea what standard serving sizes look like on your plate or in your glass.

When you feel reasonably confident about estimating portions of food, you are ready to begin your food diary. You should eat just as you normally would on the day or days you record your intake. People have a tendency to eat less when they know they have to record the information; in fact, this is one of the techniques used to help people lose weight. For the purpose of analyzing your diet, however, avoid this tendency.

On Forms 1 and 2 you can record your food intake and energy expenditure. Forms 3 through 7 are provided to assist you in comparing the nutrient value of your diet with the RDAs and Dietary Goals for Americans. You will note that Form 4, for recording the nutrient content of the foods you have eaten, provides space only for specific vitamins and minerals; the reason is that diets providing adequate amounts of these key nutrients *usually* also contain the other essential nutrients you need.

TABLE 1   **Estimated daily caloric need.**

ACTIVITY LEVEL	CALORIES PER POUND EXPENDED
1. Very sedentary: no activity; confined to house	13
2. Sedentary: typical American with office job/light work	14
3. Moderate: #2 plus weekend recreation	15
4. Very active: complies with American College of Sports Medicine standards of vigorous exercise 3 times per week	16
5. Competitive athlete: vigorous activity	17+

Formula: Weight in pounds × Activity level expenditure
Example: 120 lb. female × Sedentary activity level
         120 lb. × 14 = 1680 calories
         Estimated daily caloric need = 1680 calories

Source: American Heart Association, Dallas, TX, 1986.

continued

L
A
B
O
R
A
T
O
R
Y

Using Form 3, you can determine if your calorie intake is in balance with your expenditure and, if not, what the impact of this imbalance would be on your weight over time if you were to eat and exert yourself similarly every day. You also can calculate the number of pounds you might gain or lose in a year if you choose to modify your intake or expenditure patterns.

If there is a large difference between your intake and expenditure and you are not gaining or losing weight, you probably have erred in recording or calculating your data. Or maybe you did not eat or exercise as you normally do during the time you recorded your data. Either way, you might want to recheck your initial calculations or even repeat your data collection before proceeding further with the analysis, so you know you are working with accurate information.

When you have completed Form 4, you will have gathered all the nutrient data you need to analyze how well you are eating. The next step in analyzing your diet is to determine if you are eating the proportions of protein, fat, and carbohydrate suggested in the Dietary Goals for Americans as important for minimizing the incidence of major chronic disease. Use Form 5 to calculate the percent of your total calories each of these major nutrients comprises and to compare these proportions to the Dietary Goals for Americans. By determining your cholesterol–saturated fat index (CSI) on Form 6, you can check to see if the kind of fat you are eating minimizes or increases your risk of heart disease.

The last step is to determine if your diet provides the RDAs for eight key nutrients that, as explained previously, are general indicators of the overall quality of your diet in terms of essential nutrients. Use Form 7 to compare the amounts of the key nutrients you consumed with the RDAs for your sex and age groups (Appendix 6). You also might want to identify the best source of each key nutrient in your diet, as well as some additional foods you could eat that would contribute these nutrients. Space to do this is provided on the form. Making sure you get some of these foods every day can help maintain or improve the quality of your diet.

continued

FORM 1   CALORIC INTAKE RECORD

Directions: Keep a 24-hour diary of all foods and beverages consumed. Be specific as to type, method of preparation, and quantity. For mixed dishes, estimate amount of each ingredient. Check package labels or *Nutritive Value of Foods* (available in libraries) to assess calorie content. Include all butter, dressings, mayonnaise, etc.

FOOD ITEM	QUANTITY (tsp, cup, oz)	CALORIES	TOTALS

Breakfast

Breakfast Total: _____

Snack

Snack Total: _____

Lunch

Lunch Total: _____

Snack

Snack Total: _____

Dinner

Dinner Total: _____

Snack

Snack Total: _____

DAILY TOTAL:_____

continued

LABORATORY

L
A
B
O
R
A
T
O
R
Y

FORM 2   CALORIC EXPENDITURE RECORD

Directions: Keep a 24-hour diary of your activities. Be sure to include sleeping and sitting so that your records show the full 24 hours. Find calories expended per activity (Appendix 4). Add calorie column to find daily totals.

ACTIVITY	LENGTH OF TIME	CALORIES EXPENDED

Morning

Afternoon

Evening

Night

TOTAL HRS = 24   Daily Calorie Total _____

continued

FORM 3   CALORIC BALANCE COMPUTATION SHEET

Directions: Refer to caloric intake record and caloric expenditure record for determining energy balance and body weight change.

A. Total calories consumed in 24-hour period: _____ cal

B. Total calories expended in 24-hour period: _____ cal

C. Caloric balance (difference between A and B): _____ cal

D. Indicate whether negative (expenditure greater than intake) or positive (intake greater than expenditure) caloric balance.

   Circle one: Negative   Positive

E. Weight change should take place at a rate of 1 pound for every 3500 calories in excess or deficit. A negative balance produces weight loss, and a positive balance yields weight gain. If this 24-hour calorie pattern would continue unchanged, the following body weight changes could be expected:

   1. Weekly weight change: $\dfrac{\text{(Caloric Balance)} \times 7}{3500}$ = _____ lbs

   2. Monthly weight change: $\dfrac{\text{(Caloric Balance)} \times 30}{3500}$ = _____ lbs

   3. Annual weight change: $\dfrac{\text{(Caloric Balance)} \times 365}{3500}$ = _____ lbs

F. List two modifications you could make in your eating and activity patterns, and project the effect of each on your weight for a period of one year.

$$\text{lbs/year} = \frac{\text{(cal/wk} \times 52)}{3500}$$

   1. Eating modifications:

Food	Calories	Servings/wk	Cal/wk		
_____	_____	_____	_____	=	_____ lbs/yr
_____	_____	_____	_____	=	_____ lbs/yr

   2. Activity modifications:

Activity	Time	Calories	Periods/wk	Cal/wk		
_____	_____	_____	_____	_____	=	_____ lbs/yr
_____	_____	_____	_____	_____	=	_____ lbs/yr

continued

L87

L A B O R A T O R Y

FORM 4 NUTRIENT COMPONENTS OF FOODS

Directions: Make a nutritional evaluation of foods consumed during a 24-hour period. List food, precise amount, and quantity of each component listed below. Use *Nutritive Value of Foods* (available in libraries) for nutrient quantities. Add columns to find daily totals.

(A) Food	(B) Approx. Measure or Weight	(D) Food Energy (Calories)	(E) Protein (gm)	(F) Fat (gm)	(J) Carbo-hydrate (gm)	(K) Calcium (mg)	(M) Iron (mg)	(O) Vitamin A (I.U.)	(P) Thiamin (mg)	(Q) Ribo-flavin (mg)	(R) Niacin (mg)	(S) Ascorbic Acid (Vit. C) (mg)
TOTALS												

continued

FORM 5   PERCENT OF CALORIES FROM PROTEIN, FAT, AND CARBOHYDRATE

The contribution that protein, fat, and carbohydrates make toward total caloric intake is an important health consideration. Typical American diets are quite high in fat (40%–45% of total calories). Recommendations from the National Research Council Report, *Diet and Health,* are 12% protein, less than 30% fat, and 55+% carbohydrates.

Directions: Use the following formula and example to assist you in computing your own percentages:

$$\text{PERCENT OF TOTAL CALORIES} = \frac{\text{calories from energy nutrient}}{\text{TOTAL CALORIES}} \times 100$$

Example: A diet of 100 grams protein (4 cal/gm), 145 grams fat (9 cal/gm), and 300 grams carbohydrates (4 cal/gm) is evaluated as follows:

calories from protein	$= 100 \times 4 =$	400 calories
calories from fat	$= 145 \times 9 =$	1305 calories
calories from carbohydrates	$= 300 \times 4 =$	1200 calories
	TOTAL CALORIES $=$	2905

$$\text{percent from protein} = \frac{400}{2905} \times 100 = 13.77\%$$

$$\text{percent from fat} = \frac{1305}{2905} \times 100 = 44.92\%$$

$$\text{percent from carbohydrates} = \frac{1200}{2905} \times 100 = 41.31\%$$

Make computations using your data from the previous pages.

Grams of protein _____, Grams of fat _____, Grams of carbohydrates _____

calories from protein	= _____
calories from fat	= _____
calories from carbohydrates	= _____
percent from protein	= _____
percent from fat	= _____
percent from carbohydrates	= _____

How do your percentages compare to recommendations of the National Research Council Report, *Diet and Health?* Rate your diet as "equal," "over," or "below" for each nutrient.

	PROTEIN	FAT	CARBOHYDRATE
U.S. Dietary Goals	12%	<30%	55+%
Your Diet	%	%	%
Your Rating			

continued

L A B O R A T O R Y

FORM 6   CHOLESTEROL–SATURATED FAT INDEX (CSI)

A new way to estimate the cholesterol-raising effect of food is to calculate the Cholesterol–Saturated Fat Index (CSI). Because this formula considers *both* of the dietary fats known to increase blood cholesterol, it offers a more precise evaluation of your diet as a risk for cardiovascular disease. You will need to look up the grams of saturated fat and the milligrams of cholesterol in the food(s) you are examining; use the *Nutritive Values of Food* table described on p. 178 and found in any nutrition text.

To compute the CSI, you simply multiply the grams of saturated fat in food by 1.01 and the milligrams of cholesterol by .05 and add the two products together. The larger the result, the more risky the food!

For Example:

A. 3 oz regular hamburger has 6.9 g saturated fat and 76 mg cholesterol
CSI = 6.9g (1.01) + 76 mg (.05) = **10.77**

B. 3 oz water-packed tuna has 0.3 g saturated fat and 48 mg cholesterol
CSI = .3g (1.01) + 48 mg (.05) = **2.7**

The CSI of an average American's daily diet ranges from 51–60 for women and children and 69–82 for men and teenagers. A more healthy diet for your heart would yield a CSI of 16–19 for most women and children and 23–26 for men and teenagers.

Calculate the CSI for two of your favorite foods.

1. CSI for _____ = _____ g (1.01) + _____ mg (.05) = _____

2. CSI for _____ = _____ g (1.01) + _____ mg (.05) = _____

continued

FORM 7   COMPARISONS OF NUTRIENT INTAKE TO RDA

Compare your daily intake of nutrients to the recommended dietary allowances listed for your sex and age (Appendix 6). Note foods that were consumed and could be consumed that provide high levels of each nutrient.

	Calories	Protein (gm)	Calcium (mg)	Iron (mg)	Vitamin A (I.U.)	Thiamin (Vit. B$_1$) (mg)	Riboflavin (Vit. B$_2$) (mg)	Niacin (mg)	Ascorbic Acid (Vit. C) (mg)
Daily total of nutrients in your 24-hour period									
Recommended daily allowance									
Evaluation of your totals ("Below" "Equal" or "Above" the RDA)									
Food in your diet that is highest in each nutrient									
List another food in each column that would add significantly to that nutrient.									

167

LAB 26

STDs: Reducing Your Risk

1. List any behaviors that, in a pressure situation, you might take part in that could place you at risk of contracting a sexually transmitted disease.

_____

_____

_____

_____

2. For each circumstance you listed, create a "screen play," complete with dialogue and action directions, in which you avoid or extricate yourself safely from the tempting/risky situation.

_____

_____

_____

_____

_____

_____

_____

_____

_____

_____

_____

_____

_____

_____

_____

_____

_____

_____

_____

_____

_____

_____

_____

_____

_____

L A B O R A T O R Y

**L
A
B
O
R
A
T
O
R
Y**

LAB 27

HIV Risk Checklist

Evidence shows that HIV, the virus that causes AIDS, has been in the United States at least since 1978. The following are known risk factors for contracting HIV. If you answer *yes* to any of these questions, you definitely should seek counseling and testing. You may be at increased risk of infection if any of the following apply to you since 1978.

_____ Have you shared needles or syringes to inject drugs or steroids?

_____ If you are a male, have you had sex with other males?

_____ Have you had sex with someone you know or suspect was infected with HIV?

_____ Have you had a sexually transmitted disease (STD)?

_____ Have you received blood transfusions or blood products between 1978 and 1985?

_____ Have you had sex with someone who would answer yes to any of the above questions?

If you have had sex with someone and you didn't know his or her risk behavior, or you have had many sexual partners in the last 10 years, you have increased the chances that you might be HIV-infected.

If you are a woman in any of the above risk categories and plan to become pregnant, counseling and testing are important. HIV-infected women have about a one-in-four chance of infecting their baby during pregnancy or delivery.

Source: *America Responds to AIDS,* Centers for Disease Control and Prevention, U. S. Public Health Service.

LAB 28

Alcohol Quiz

Although alcohol is the most commonly used psychoactive drug in the world, many misconceptions surround its use and abuse. Test your knowledge about alcohol. After scoring the quiz, pay particular attention to areas in which you had misconceptions (T = True F = False).

T   F   1. Alcohol is correctly classified as a drug.

T   F   2. After a drink, a person is pepped up because alcohol in small amounts is a stimulant.

T   F   3. Excessive ingestion of alcohol can cause death by overstimulating the nerve cells to the point of exhaustion.

T   F   4. Alcohol is absorbed into the system and digested in the same way as food.

T   F   5. Alcohol has no nutritional value.

T   F   6. Alcohol has caloric value and can be used to produce energy.

T   F   7. An alcohol hangover can be eliminated by eating high levels of carbohydrates before or during drinking.

T   F   8. Drinking black coffee accelerates the sobering-up process.

T   F   9. Between 50% and 75% of all alcoholics eventually develop cirrhosis of the liver.

T   F   10. Alcohol cannot cross the placenta; thus, even excessive drinking cannot affect the fetus significantly.

T   F   11. For the average 150-pound individual, it would take the accumulation of five drinks to significantly affect driving skills.

T   F   12. Social drinking is the primary cause of alcoholism.

T   F   13. The development of alcoholism usually proceeds through predictable stages.

T   F   14. Only individuals with seriously maladjusted personalities become alcoholics.

T   F   15. Women become alcoholics primarily because they try to keep up with the drinking behavior of significant men in their lives.

T   F   16. Alcoholism has no effective treatment.

T   F   17. Among teenagers 12 to 17 years old, alcohol is second only to marijuana as the most widely used drug.

T   F   18. Alcoholics Anonymous has been replaced by more modern treatments and now is used seldom as a treatment modality.

T   F   19. Because alcoholism is rare among employed individuals, few companies have developed employee alcohol programs.

T   F   20. Accentuating guilt feelings is the most effective way to help a friend who is a problem drinker.

Answer Key: **1. T**   **2. F**   **3. F**   **4. F**   **5. T**   **6. T**   **7. F**   **8. F**   **9. F**   **10. F**   **11. F**
12. F   **13. T**   **14. F**   **15. F**   **16. F**   **17. F**   **18. F**   **19. F**   **20. F**

LAB 29

Why Do You Smoke?

Here are some statements made by people to describe what they get out of smoking cigarettes. How often do you feel this way when smoking? Circle one number for each statement. *Answer every question.*

	Always	Frequently	Occasionally	Seldom	Never
A. I smoke cigarettes to keep myself from slowing down.	5	4	3	2	1
B. Handling a cigarette is part of the enjoyment of smoking it.	5	4	3	2	1
C. Smoking cigarettes is pleasant and relaxing.	5	4	3	2	1
D. I light up a cigarette when I feel angry about something.	5	4	3	2	1
E. When I have run out of cigarettes, I find it almost unbearable until I can get more.	5	4	3	2	1
F. I smoke cigarettes automatically without even being aware of it.	5	4	3	2	1
G. I smoke cigarettes to stimulate myself, to perk myself up.	5	4	3	2	1
H. Part of the enjoyment of smoking a cigarette comes from the steps I take to light up.	5	4	3	2	1
I. I find cigarettes pleasurable.	5	4	3	2	1
J. When I feel uncomfortable or upset about something, I light up a cigarette.	5	4	3	2	1
K. I am very much aware of the fact when I am not smoking a cigarette.	5	4	3	2	1
L. I light up a cigarette without realizing I still have one burning in the ashtray.	5	4	3	2	1
M. I smoke cigarettes to give myself a lift.	5	4	3	2	1
N. When I smoke a cigarette, part of the enjoyment is watching the smoke as I exhale it.	5	4	3	2	1
O. I want a cigarette most when I am comfortable and relaxed.	5	4	3	2	1

Test written by Daniel H. Horn, National Clearinghouse for Smoking and Health, U. S. Department of Health and Human Services.

continued

L
A
B
O
R
A
T
O
R
Y

	Always	Frequently	Occasionally	Seldom	Never
P. When I feel blue or want to take my mind off my cares and worries, I smoke cigarettes.	5	4	3	2	1
Q. I get a real gnawing hunger for a cigarette when I haven't smoked for a while.	5	4	3	2	1
R. I've found a cigarette in my mouth and didn't remember putting it there.	5	4	3	2	1

SCORING

1. Enter the number you have circled for each question in the spaces below, putting the number you have circled to Question A over line A, to Question B over line B, etc.

2. Add the three scores on each line to get your totals. For example, the sum of your scores over lines A, G, and M gives you your score on Stimulation, lines B, H, and N give the score on Handling, etc.

TOTALS

+		+	=	
A	G	M		STIMULATION
+		+	=	
B	H	N		HANDLING
+		+	=	
C	I	O		PLEASURABLE RELAXATION
+		+	=	
D	J	P		CRUTCH: TENSION REDUCTION
+		+	=	
E	K	Q		CRAVING: PSYCHOLOGICAL ADDICTION
+		+	=	
F	L	R		HABIT

Scores can vary from 3 to 15. A score of 11 and above is high; a score of 7 and below is low.

LAB 30

Drugs: Motivations and Alternatives

List 10 effects of drugs that motivate people to take them.

1. _____

2. _____

3. _____

4. _____

5. _____

6. _____

7. _____

8. _____

9. _____

10. _____

For each effect, write down three alternative non-drug behaviors that would fulfill each of the 10 motivations listed above.

1. a._____   6. a._____

   b._____   b._____

   c._____   c._____

2. a._____   7. a._____

   b._____   b._____

   c._____   c._____

3. a._____   8. a._____

   b._____   b._____

   c._____   c._____

4. a._____   9. a._____

   b._____   b._____

   c._____   c._____

5. a._____   10. a._____

   b._____   b._____

   c._____   c._____

LAB 31

Check Out Your House or Apartment

Think about the safety of each item below that is in or around your home. Give each item a safety rating from 1 to 5, with 5 being the highest mark (safe) and 1 being the lowest mark (unsafe). For items scored lower than 5, think of ideas to make the item safer. (Some of the items below may apply only to houses or only to apartments.)

SCORE   **IDEAS**

_____ Windows (access) _____

_____ Door locks (spring latch, deadbolt, 2 locks/door) _____

_____ Type of doors (hollow core, solid wood, metal) _____

_____ Peephole _____

_____ Security system _____

_____ Lighting _____

_____ Shrubs/trees _____

_____ Fenced yard _____

_____ Elevators/stairs _____

_____ Laundry area (away from central location) _____

_____ Recreation room (away from central location) _____

_____ Storage areas _____

_____ Parking _____

_____ Neighborhood watch program _____

LABORATORY

Potentially Threatening Situations: What Could You Do?

Think about the hypothetical situations below that are potentially dangerous. What might you do to prevent a dangerous situation from developing?

1. Walking down the street, you see a group of five tough-looking men who appear to have been drinking, one block ahead in the direction you need to go.

   _____

   _____

   _____

   _____

2. Upon arriving home, you see your front door is open and things look disturbed.

   _____

   _____

   _____

   _____

3. You pull into your parking spot at work/school, and you think you see someone duck behind a nearby car.

   _____

   _____

   _____

   _____

4. There are two parking spots at the shopping mall in which you can park. The first one is next to a van and the second is between two unoccupied cars. Which one should you choose?

   _____

   _____

   _____

   _____

5. You pull into a shopping mall and park. But as you are getting ready to get out you look around and see two people sitting in a parked car next to you. They don't seem out of place but your "sixth sense" is alerting you. What do you do?

   _____

   _____

   _____

   _____

continued

LABORATORY

6. You are at a public place with a new date. He makes several derogatory remarks about other women around you.

_____

_____

_____

_____

7. You are at a shopping mall buying gifts for Christmas. You have purchased most of your gifts. You want to take these to your car and then return to finish your shopping. How might you do this to avoid inviting a break-in?

_____

_____

_____

_____

8. While you are driving home late at night you think you are being followed.

_____

_____

_____

_____

9. You are walking down the street and a street person asks you for money.

_____

_____

_____

_____

NAME _____ SECTION _____ DATE _____

LAB 39

A Contract with Myself

I, _____, hereby declare that I am ready and willing to commit myself to the following goals and activities. I realize that to achieve my long-term goals, I must be willing to work for small gains, I must seek support, and I must be adequately prepared. Therefore, for the next week I resolve to myself to do the following:

1. Long-term goal(s):_____
   _____

2. Specific goal: During the next week, I plan to: _____
   _____
   _____

3. I will ask my helper to assist me by: _____
   _____
   _____

4. I realize I can easily avoid fulfilling my action plan by: _____
   _____
   _____

5. So I plan to avoid doing this by: _____
   _____
   _____

6. My reward to myself when I fulfill the terms of my action plan each day will be: _____
   _____
   _____

TODAY'S DATE:_____   SIGNATURE:_____
REVIEW DATE:_____   HELPER: _____

- -

7. Action plan evaluation/revision
   a. After working on my action plan for one week, I found that:_____
      _____
      _____
      _____
      _____

   b. To continue working toward my goal in small steps during the next week, I plan to:
      _____ Follow the same action plan because: _____
      _____
      _____
      _____

      _____ Expand my action plan to include: _____
      _____
      _____
      _____

      _____ Cut back on my original plan for now because: _____
      _____
      _____
      _____

Source: Adapted from *The American Way of Life Need Not Be Hazardous to Your Health*. James Farquhar. Copyright © 1978 by Stanford Alumni Association.

L117

Glossary

Absolute muscle endurance — the number of correctly completed repetitions one can do with a standard weight before being unable to continue.

Adaptation — the tendency of the body to fight to restore homeostasis in the face of forces that upset the natural bodily balance.

Adaptive stress — the stress imposed on the body during attempts to cope with or adapt to stressful situations.

Aerobic — the production of energy within exercising muscles with the use of oxygen.

Aerobic capacity — see *maximum oxygen intake*.

Aerobic fitness — see *cardiorespiratory fitness*.

Affirmation (constructive) — positive self-talk in the form of behavior-specific, present-tense "I" statements written/spoken to affirm and remind ourselves of what we want to become.

Aggressive communication — a demanding, bossy, patronizing, or demeaning style that insists that someone obey your wishes.

Agility — the ability to move the body rapidly in different and often changing directions.

Aging/aging process — changes attributed to the passage of time, usually applied only to the post-maturational period of adulthood.

AIDS (acquired immune deficiency syndrome) — a viral (human immunodeficiency virus) disease that incapacitates the immune system and usually causes death by opportunistic infections; intimate sexual contact and shared needles among IV drug users are the dominant modes of transmission, with blood transfusions currently a minor mode.

Altered state — the state of consciousness, often called the meditative state, that is opposite the normal "take care of business" state of consciousness.

Amino acids — the building blocks of protein linked together in chains to form protein; 9 of the 22 known amino acids are *essential* (must be obtained from food).

Anabolic steroids — synthetically produced drugs that have growth-promoting properties similar to those of the male sex hormone testosterone. Ingesting anabolic steroids, particularly in large quantities, can be dangerous to one's health in a number of ways.

Anaerobic — the production of energy within exercising muscles without the use of oxygen.

Anaerobic threshold — the level of exercise intensity that just avoids a rapid rise of lactic acid in the blood.

Aneurysm — an extremely dangerous condition in which a section of blood vessel has bulged or ballooned outward, making the vessel weak and susceptible to rupture.

Angina pectoris — pain in the chest area resulting from insufficient blood (oxygen) flow in some part of the heart.

Anorexia nervosa — self-induced starvation arising out of an intense fear of becoming obese.

Antigravity muscle — muscle responsible for helping the body maintain an erect posture.

Anxiety — acute or chronic arousal, usually fear, but often undirected.

Anxious-reactivity — the body reacting to feelings of anxiety with more anxiety and more arousal, making resolution difficult.

Arteriosclerosis — the hardening and narrowing of artery walls.

Arthritis — inflammation of joint tissue, often causing pain and swelling and ultimately permanent joint damage.

Assertiveness — saying what is liked or disliked about someone or something without using degradation; getting what is wanted, but not at the expense of someone else.

Atherosclerosis — the gradual accumulation of fat on blood vessel walls; the most common form of arteriosclerosis.

Autogenics — self-generating; the body responding to self talk or visual imagery.

Average life expectancy — expected length of life for the average person, given current mortality rates from diseases and accidents.

Ballistic stretching — a common procedure encountered when doing certain calisthenics, in which one moves through a full range of motion explosively. Ballistic stretching should be avoided because of the danger of overstressing and injuring tissues.

Beta-carotene — plant precursor of vitamin A; destroys harmful free radicals.

Biofeedback — a change technique that uses electrical instrumentation to magnify the subtle signals from the body so they become more noticeable and thus more controllable. Electrical impulses from muscles, brain waves, and/or skin temperature are most commonly used.

Biological rhythms — naturally recurring cycles of biological activity governed by the nervous and hormonal systems.

BMI — see *body mass index*.

Body composition — the relative proportion of fat and non-fat tissue in the body.

Body mass index (BMI) — body weight in kg, divided by height in meters, squared. BMI is used to estimate health risk from obesity.

Bulimia — a condition characterized by binge eating, preoccupation with body weight, repeated efforts to lose weight, and sometimes also by purging.

Calisthenics — exercises in which your body weight serves as the resistance.

Caloric balance equation — the relationship between the amount of energy consumed and the amount of energy expended by an individual.

Caloric expenditure — the number of calories one uses in a 24-hour day.

Caloric intake — the number of calories one consumes in a 24-hour day.

Calorie — the amount of heat required to raise one kilogram of water one degree centigrade in temperature. In common usage, a "calorie" is the same as a "kilocalorie" in scientific literature.

Cancer — a large number of diseases characterized by development, uncontrolled growth, and spread (metastasis) of abnormal cells.

Carbohydrate — a nutrient compound consisting of molecules of sugar linked together in large complexes (called complex carbohydrate or starch) or in pairs or existing as single molecules (called simple carbohydrate or sugars).

Carcinogens — Cancer-producing substances.

Cardiorespiratory fitness — the combined abilities of the respiratory and circulatory systems to provide adequate oxygen to large and small muscle groups while they engage in continuous, rhythmic exercise for extended periods of time.

Cardiovascular disease (CVD) — diseases of the heart and blood vessels including heart attack, stroke, and hypertension.

Cerebral thrombosis — formation of a blood clot in an artery of the brain.

Cerebrovascular disease — a blood vessel disorder that results in insufficient blood being available to the brain; commonly termed *stroke*.

Cholesterol — a form of fat found in every animal cell and a major constituent of human bile and sex hormones; the liver makes all the body needs; high levels in the blood are associated with increased risk of cardiovascular disease.

Cholesterol–Saturated Fat Index (CSI) — a calculation that uses the amounts of saturated fat and cholesterol consumed or in a certain food to estimate the likelihood of one's diet or a certain food to increase blood cholesterol levels and, thus, risk of cardiovascular disease.

Chronic conditions — diseases and conditions that tend to take a long time to develop and usually require continuing treatment.

Circuit training — a form of overall training in which stations of strength or muscle endurance exercises, with or without weights, are arranged and completed in a series, with short rests of 15–30 seconds between stations; rest periods allow moving to the next station.

Competent coping — meeting demands while managing stress levels.

Complementary proteins — incomplete proteins from various foods which complement each other when eaten together with other incomplete or complete proteins; that is, in combination they provide all 9 essential amino acids (e.g., black beans and rice, cereal with milk, peanut butter on bread).

Complete protein — any protein containing all 9 essential amino acids in sufficient amounts for the body to use to build the proteins it needs. Proteins from animals and animal products are complete.

Constructive affirmation — see *affirmation (constructive)*.

Cool-down — a period of continued activity (e.g., walking, stretching) following vigorous exercise, done to avoid blood pooling, dizziness, and promote recovery.

Coronary thrombosis — a clot that blocks an artery in the heart.

CVD — see *Cardiovascular disease*.

Deprivational stress — the psychophysiological stress response caused by states of boredom or loneliness.

Diabetes — a metabolic disease that diminishes the body's ability to metabolize glucose, either because of inadequate production of insulin (Type I diabetes, usually occurring in children and young adults) or inability to utilize available insulin (Type II diabetes, usually occurring in adults aged 40 and older).

Diaphragmatic breathing — deep, but not exaggerated, breathing in which air is taken to the bottom lobes of the lungs, during which you can feel the diaphragm move up and down with each breath.

Diastolic pressure — the lowest blood pressure level that occurs when the heart is resting between beats.

Distress — debilitating or harmful stress with which the individual is not coping well; also referred to as negative stress.

Duration of exercise — how long one engages in exercise.

Dynamic strength — the heaviest weight a person can lift at one time.

Dysrhythmias — one of a variety of irregular patterns of electrical activity in the heart which can be, but not always is, health-threatening.

Electrocardiogram (ECG) — a medical examination in which the electrical activity of the heart is recorded and compared to standard values; often an ECG test is taken while undergoing a stress test.

Embolism — a clot floating through the vascular system until lodging in (blocking) a vessel too small to allow its passage.

Emotional health — the ability to control emotions and express them appropriately and comfortably.

Enabling factors — the personal skills, resources, and facilities needed to successfully try one behavior versus another.

Energy balance — a state in which the caloric intake equals the caloric expenditure over time.

Environmental stress — stimuli arising out of the environment that produce a stress response in most individuals.

Enzymes — special proteins that facilitate the chemical reaction in cells that keep the body functioning.

Epinephrine — one of two hormones (the other is norepinephrine) secreted by the body under conditions of stress including vigorous exercise; also termed *adrenalin*.

Essential fat — the minimum amount of fat needed for optimal health (3%–5% in males and 8%–12% in females).

Essential nutrient — a substance that the body needs for proper function but that it cannot make; the nutrient must be obtained through food or water.

Eustress — positive, action-enhancing stress.

Eutrophication — bacteria breaking down dead plant material and using up the oxygen in the water, which kills active life in lakes.

Exercise — regular physical activity engaged in for health and fitness. Moderate exercise is exercise that is well within your current capacity and that can be sustained for at least 60 minutes. Vigorous exercise is an intensity of exercise that an untrained person could not sustain for more than 15–20 minutes continuously. Moderate exercise programs are relatively safe for persons of all ages. Vigorous exercise programs should not be started without a medical exam above the age of 40 years for men and 50 years for women.

Fat-free weight — the weight of all bodily tissues except fat.

Fat weight — the weight of all the deposits of fat in the body.

Fiber — compounds in plant foods that human digestive enzymes cannot digest (e.g., pectins, gums, hemicelluloses); formerly called crude fiber.

Flexibility — the ability of body segments to move through a range of motion.

Fluid-replacement beverage — a drink taken during the heat, particularly during prolonged exercise in the heat, to replace lost fluids and minerals.

Frequency of exercise — how often one engages in exercise.

Frustration — excessive stress that occurs when we are blocked from doing what we want to do.

Fuel — foodstuffs (fat, carbohydrate, protein) used by the muscles during various types of exercise.

General Adaptation Syndrome (GAS) — the theory of stress arousal developed by Hans Selye, involving three stages: (1) the alarm reaction, (2) the stage of resistance, and (3) the stage of exhaustion.

Geriatrics — a medical specialty that focuses on the diseases and physical problems of old age.

Gerontology — study of the aging process, spanning all adulthood.

Hatha yoga — a form of yoga that uses body positions and exercises to promote physical and mental harmony.

HDLs (high density lipoproteins) — compounds that are composed of about equal amounts of protein and fat that seem to carry excess cholesterol from the cells back to the liver for reformulation or disposal; called "good cholesterol" because high levels in the blood are associated with decreased risk of cardiovascular disease.

Health — conceptual term referring to overall level of functioning at any particular point in time, including the physical, emotional, social, mental, and spiritual dimensions of life. See also *physical health*, *emotional health*, *social health*, *mental health*, *spiritual health*.

Health Belief Model — a conceptual schema consisting of a series of five sequential beliefs that lead to successful behavior change.

Health-related fitness — those components of fitness that are related to health and well-being. They include cardiorespiratory fitness, body composition, strength and muscle endurance, flexibility of the lower back and hip region.

Heart rate reserve — the difference between the maximum heart rate and the resting heart rate.

HIV (Human Immunodeficiency Virus) — the virus that causes AIDS.

Homeostasis — the state of the body in which exists stable equilibrium of internal functions.

Hydrogenation — a chemical process manufacturers use to artificially saturate (i.e., add hydrogens and reduce the number of double bonds in mono- or polyunsaturated fats); makes unsaturated fat solid at room temperature.

Hydrostatic weighing — a common laboratory method for estimating body composition that involves weighing one's body weight on land and under water to determine density; also commonly referred to as "underwater weighing."

Hypertension (high blood pressure) — blood pressure levels chronically higher than 140 systolic and 90 diastolic.

Hypertrophy — the growth in muscle size that occurs after extensive weight-training.

Hypokinetic degeneration — a degenerative process that occurs because of too little movement. Typical outcomes include loss of muscle and flexibility, osteoporosis, and cardiovascular, respiratory, bladder, and bowel malfunction.

Incomplete protein — protein containing insufficient amounts of or completely lacking one or more essential amino acids; proteins from vegetables and grains are usually incomplete, although those from legumes closely resemble animal proteins.

Intensity of exercise — how hard one engages in exercise.

Internal environment — the "world" within the body; as discussed in stress management the term usually refers to the nervous system. Quieting the internal environment is a goal of relaxation activities.

Interval training — a procedure involving periods of work (e.g., jogging/sprinting) interspersed with periods of rest or light exercise (e.g., walking).

Involuntary muscle system — muscles not under direct mental control; deals primarily with the gastrointestinal system and the cardiovascular system.

Ischemia — inadequate blood flow to a certain body area, leaving that tissue without sufficient oxygen.

Isokinetic strength — the peak force (or "torque") that a person is able to exert while pushing against an isokinetic machine. Isokinetic exercise is a method of training to improve muscle function (e.g., strength/endurance) by using an isokinetic machine, which allows only constant speed movement regardless of the force exerted against the machine.

Lactic acid — a byproduct of incomplete carbohydrate metabolism, associated with muscle fatigue.

LDLs (low density lipoproteins) — compounds composed of a small amount of protein and large amount of fat, with cholesterol as the major component, formed by the liver and conversion of VLDLs for distribution of fat to cells; called "bad cholesterol" because high levels of LDLs in the blood are associated with the build-up of fatty deposits on blood vessel walls.

Life span — length of time the average person would live if there were no diseases or accidents.

Lifestyle — how one lives in the sociocultural environment, the events of one's life as well as daily work and play activities; often mentioned as the most important determinant of stress.

Lipoprotein — a compound of fat and protein found in the blood, the purpose of which is to transport fat; three types best known for their association with cardiovascular disease are VLDLs, LDLs, and HDLs.

Maximum cardiac output — the maximum amount of blood the heart can pump per minute.

Maximum heart rate — the highest heart rate value one can attain; usually measured during heavy exercise.

Maximum oxygen intake ($\dot{V}O_2$ max) — the highest amount of oxygen an individual can consume while engaging in heavy exercise; $\dot{V}O_2$ max is considered an important measure of an individual's cardiorespiratory fitness.

Meditation — exercises, postures, and other rituals developed in an attempt to slow body activities to a point at which the mind would also be allowed to become quiet.

Mental health — the ability to learn and to use intellectual capabilities.

Mineral — inorganic substance naturally present on earth; 21 minerals are known to be essential for proper body functioning.

Mitochondria — subcellular sites where aerobic energy is produced in tissues.

Mode of exercise — the type of exercise activity that is chosen.

Moderate exercise — see *exercise*.

Monounsaturated fatty acids — compounds of varying numbers of carbons and enough hydrogens to fill all but two receptor sites on the carbons, creating a double bond between the two carbons missing the hydrogens.

Muscle endurance — the ability of a muscle group to engage in repetitive exercise for long periods of time with little fatigue.

Muscle soreness — muscular pain that arises one or two days after some form of strenuous exercise.

Muscle strain — a tear to muscle fiber surrounding tissue.

Muscle viscosity — see *viscosity*.

Myocardial infarction — death of heart muscle tissue from prolonged lack of oxygen.

Negative stress — see *distress*.

Neuromuscular relaxation training — systematic exercises that train not only the muscles but also the nervous system components that control muscle activity. The objective is to reduce the tension in the muscles.

Norepinephrine — see *epinephrine*.

Obesity — excess body fat above a level that most experts consider as healthy.

1 RM — see *repetition maximum*.

Optimal stress — a point between eustress and distress that promotes a maximal level of performance.

Osteoarthritis — gradual wearing away of the cartilage pads protecting the ends of the bones forming the joint, often resulting in thickening of bone ends, growth of bone spurs, and pain.

Osteoporosis — loss of calcium from bone, making it porous and easily fractured; classified as senile (Type I) osteoporosis, resulting from aging process, or post-menopausal (Type II) osteoporosis, caused by loss of estrogen.

Overload (stress) — a state in which the demands of life exceed one's capacity to meet them.

Overload principle — the training maxim that describes the body's adaptive response to physical stress applied regularly.

Overtraining — excessive training that leads to poorer performance, sleep disturbance, injury, or illness.

Overweight — excess weight relative to the average person of the same sex and stature. Persons who are overweight often, but not always, have excess body fat.

Passive behavior — nonassertive action, lacking skill to ask for what is wanted; mode of operation is to manipulate.

Performance-related fitness — those components of fitness that enhance performance but are not necessarily related to health, including flexibility (except the lower back and hips), power, speed, and agility.

Personality — may be thought of as the summation of personal characteristics, attitudes, and values, and behavior patterns that individuals manifest in interactions with the environment. The dynamics of an individual's self-perception and characteristic attitudes and behaviors that may somehow contribute to excessive stress are called personality stressors.

Physical fitness — the capacity to meet the demands of modern-day life with relatively little strain.

Physical health — the ability to carry out daily tasks with energy remaining for unforeseen circumstances; biological integrity.

Physical stress — strain, pressure, or force on a person.

Phytochemicals — the chemicals in plants that appear to inhibit cancer.

Plyometric training — a form of resistance training in which the muscle must decelerate a mass prior to contracting explosively. An example is rebound jumping where an individual jumps off and onto a 2-foot box.

PNF — see *proprioceptive neuromuscular facilitation*.

Polyunsaturated fatty acids (PUFA) — compounds of varying numbers of carbons and attached hydrogens lacking a minimum of four hydrogens to saturate carbon receptor sites and having a minimum of two double bonds between carbons.

Positive stress — see *eustress*.

Power — ability to exert force explosively; the application of force per unit of time. Great power comes from maximizing force and speed simultaneously.

Predisposing factors — the basis for our motivation or predisposition to act one way versus another, including our knowledge, beliefs, attitudes, and values.

Progressive exercise — the training principle describing incremental application of overload stress over time.

Proprioceptive neuromuscular facilitation (PNF) — a technique for improving flexibility in which one stretches a muscle, then contracts the same muscle while a partner resists any movement, and then stretches the muscle once more immediately afterward without resistance.

Protein — basic structural substance of the human body, composed of carbon, hydrogen, oxygen, and nitrogen arranged into amino acid strands.

Psychosocial stressors — a function of the complex interaction between social behavior and the way our senses and our minds interpret those behaviors.

Psychosomatic disease — any condition thought to be the result of excess emotional arousal, maladaptive coping, and chronic distress.

Rate of perceived exertion (RPE) — the relative value assigned by an individual when asked to grade the level of physical exertion during exercise, on a scale ranging from 6 to 20.

Recommended Dietary Allowance (RDA) — recommendations of the Food and Nutrition Board of the National Academy of Sciences National Research Council for the daily intake of essential nutrients adequate to meet the needs of practically all healthy people.

REE — see *resting metabolic rate*.

Reinforcing factors — persons or events who/that support or encourage certain behaviors.

Relative muscular endurance — the number of correctly executed repetitions one can do with a weight that is a specified fraction of one's 1 RM (e.g., 70% 1 RM) or a specified fraction of one's body weight.

Repetition maximum (RM) — the maximum amount of weight an individual can successfully lift a specified number of times, as in a 1 RM or a 10 RM. 1 RM is a common way of measuring dynamic strength.

Resting heart rate — the heart rate under resting conditions.

Resting metabolic rate (RMR) — the number of calories one expends at rest under standardized testing conditions but without fasting. RMR is also referred to as resting energy expenditure (REE).

RMR — see *resting metabolic rate*.

RPE — see *rate of perceived exertion*.

Saturated fat — triglyceride that carries almost all saturated fatty acids; solid at room temperature.

Saturated fatty acids — compounds of varying numbers of carbons and sufficient hydrogen to saturate, or completely fill all receptor sites on the carbons.

Sciatica — pain commonly attributable to pressure on the sciatic nerve, which runs through the spinal column and into the leg.

Self-actualization — the process of being and becoming the most one can be; developing one's fullest potential.

Self-contract — a motivational device in the form of a written promise to yourself to try a specific plan of action for a designated time period.

Sexually transmitted diseases (STDs) — diseases that are transmitted primarily by sexual contact, direct person-to-person contact, and exposure to bodily fluids.

Skinfold fat — the layer of fat just beneath the skin, which can be measured for thickness using skinfold fat calipers.

Social health — the ability to interact well with people and the environment; having satisfying interpersonal relationships.

Specificity principle — the training principle that describes training outcomes as uniquely determined by the type, speed, and angle of training and occurring only within the muscle groups involved in the training.

Speed — the ability to move the body rapidly, usually in a straight line, as in sprinting.

Sphygmomanometer — an air pressure cuff used to measure blood pressure in units of millimeters of mercury (mmHg).

Spiritual health — the belief in some unifying force such as nature, scientific laws, or a godlike entity.

Spot-reducing — the mistaken notion that by exercising a specific body part, localized fat stores will be lost from that site.

Static strength — measurement of strength in a fixed position, usually with the use of a tool such as a grip dynamometer for grip strength. In static exercise, the person executes a maximal contraction against an immovable object while in a fixed position.

Static stretching — a common procedure employed to improve flexibility, in which one moves to a position of stretch and holds that position for a short time.

Strength — the capacity of a muscle group to exert force under maximal conditions.

Stress — the body's reaction to outside pressures manifested by mental and physical arousal, increased blood pressure, and muscle tension, which can fatigue body systems to the point of malfunction and disease.

Stress management — a pattern of behavior that involves understanding the stress response, recognizing stressors, developing stress reduction skills, and regularly incorporating these into one's lifestyle.

Stressor — any condition or event that causes a stress response; may be physical, social, or psychological, including imaginary.

Stress test — a test on a motor-driven treadmill, designed to determine the fitness of an individual during exercise; stress tests usually involve electrocardiographic evaluation of the heart.

Submaximal — less than one's limit; in exercise, a test that doesn't require maximum effort.

Super circuit weight-training — circuit training in which periods of aerobic activity are regularly interspersed between stations focusing on strength/muscle endurance. Super circuit training serves as a more aerobic stimulus than does strict circuit training, while also providing benefits to the muscular system.

Sympathomimetic agents — chemical substances that mimic the sympathetic stress response.

Systolic pressure — the highest blood pressure level that occurs when the heart is contracting, or beating.

Target heart rate — a heart-rate value during exercise which falls within your training-sensitive zone. (See *training-sensitive zone.*)

Tendinitis — inflammation of connective tissue (tendons) that attaches muscle to bone.

Thought-stopping — a technique whereby the stressed person intentionally breaks the anxious cycle by abruptly leaving the obsessional thoughts.

Thrombus — a clot forming in a blood vessel and causing partial or complete obstruction of blood flow; often precipitated by fatty deposits on blood vessel walls.

Time-urgency personality trait — extensively studied as part of the famous cardiovascular Type A–prone personality construct describing individuals who tend to be impatient, driven by an excessive time and task orientation, and are more often prone to excessive feelings of anger and hostility.

Training — a process of regular activity directed toward building up or maintaining the components of fitness.

Training-sensitive zone — the region of exercise-induced heart rate values that falls between 50% and 85% of the heart rate reserve. Exercise done within the training sensitive zone is thought to provide optimal stimulus for improving one's cardiorespiratory fitness.

Trans-fatty acid — a fatty acid created during the partial hydrogenation process.

Triglyceride — comprises 95% of the fats we consume; composed of a glycerol stem with three (tri) fatty acids attached; if the attached fatty acids are almost all saturated, the fat tends to be solid, or if mostly unsaturated, the fat will be a liquid oil.

Unsaturated fat — triglycerides that carry almost all mono- or polyunsaturated fatty acids; liquid at room temperature unless partially hydrogenated to solidify it.

U.S. Dietary Goals — recommendations of the nation's foremost nutrition and health experts for reducing the incidence of disability and death, especially from cardio-vascular disease, cancer, and diabetes; first issued in 1977 and revised in 1989.

U.S. Dietary Guidelines — practical suggestions/practices for achieving the U.S. Dietary Goals; issued by the U.S. Department of Agriculture in 1985 and revised in 1990.

U.S. Recommended Daily Allowances (USRDAs) — Food and Drug Administration (FDA) standards that manufacturers must use if they list the nutrient content of their product on the label; the adult standard actually is the RDA for an adult man, although for the nutrient iron the RDA for adult women is used.

Valsalva maneuver — holding one's breath while lifting a heavy weight or otherwise exerting oneself maximally; doing so raises blood pressure, can lead to lightheadedness, and should be avoided.

Vigorous exercise — see *exercise.*

Viscosity — resistance to movement, as in muscle viscosity or blood viscosity.

Visual imagery — a relaxation technique involving self-directed mental images of relaxed states.

Vitamin — an organic compound that is necessary for growth and for proper body functioning, but provides no calories for energy.

VLDLs (very low density lipoproteins) — triglyceride compounds composed of a very large amount of fat and a very small amount of protein, formed by the liver and released into the blood stream for distribution of fat to cells; converts to LDLs (low density lipoproteins).

$\dot{V}O_2$ **max** — see *maximum oxygen intake.*

Voluntary muscular systems — muscles that allow us to move our limbs.

Waist-to-hip ratio — a measure of body composition in which the waist and hip measurements are compared; should not exceed 0.9 in men and 0.8 in women.

Warm-up — a process of gradually preparing the body for more vigorous exercise by beginning with gentle activities that emphasize range of motion at slow to moderate speeds.

Weight control — refers to maintaining a stable body weight.

Weight loss — loss of weight, as when dieting or exercising. Most people wish weight loss to be the same as fat loss but this is not always the case as it can occur from water loss and/or loss of fat-free tissue.

Wellness — a state of well-being in each dimension of life—the physical, emotional, social, mental, and spiritual.

Index